Tumors of the Intestines

AFIP Atlas
of
Tumor Pathology

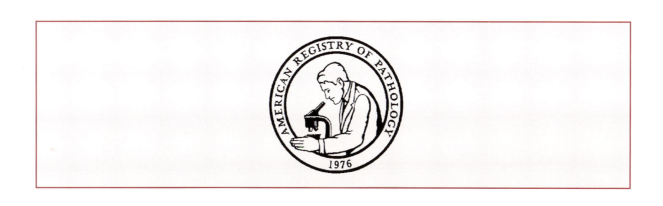

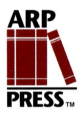

ARP PRESS

Washington, DC

Editorial Director: Mirlinda Q. Caton
Production Editor: Dian S. Thomas
Publications Subscriptions Manager: Magdalena C. Silva
Editorial Assistant: Alana N. Black
Copyeditor: Audrey Kahn

Available from the American Registry of Pathology
Washington, DC 20006
www.arppress.org
ISBN 1-933477-39-3
978-1-933477-39-8

Printed in South Korea

AFIP ATLAS OF TUMOR PATHOLOGY

Fourth Series
Fascicle 26

TUMORS OF
THE INTESTINES

by

Elizabeth A. Montgomery, MD
Professor of Pathology, Oncology, and Orthopedic Surgery
The Johns Hopkins Medical Institutions
Baltimore, Maryland

Rhonda K. Yantiss, MD
Professor of Pathology and Laboratory Medicine
Department of Pathology and Laboratory Medicine
Weill Cornell Medicine and New York Presbyterian Hospital
New York, New York

Dale C. Snover, MD
Pathologist, Fairview Southdale Hospital and
Adjunct Professor of Laboratory Medicine and Pathology
The University of Minnesota Medical School
Minneapolis, Minnesota

Laura H. Tang, MD, PhD
Attending Pathologist
Memorial Sloan-Kettering Cancer Center
New York, New York

Published by the
American Registry of Pathology
Washington, DC
2017

AFIP ATLAS OF TUMOR PATHOLOGY

EDITOR
Steven G. Silverberg, MD
Department of Pathology
University of Maryland School of Medicine
Baltimore, Maryland

ASSOCIATE EDITOR
Ronald A. DeLellis, MD
Warren Alpert Medical School
of Brown University
Providence, Rhode Island

ASSOCIATE EDITOR
Leslie H. Sobin, MD
Armed Forces Institute of Pathology
Washington, DC

EDITORIAL ADVISORY BOARD

Manuscript reviewed by:
Ronald A. DeLellis, MD
Lysandra Voltaggio, MD
Jason Hornick, MD, PhD

EDITORS' NOTE

The Atlas of Tumor Pathology has a long and distinguished history. It was first conceived at a cancer research meeting held in St. Louis in September 1947, as an attempt to standardize the nomenclature of neoplastic diseases. The first series was sponsored by the National Academy of Sciences-National Research Council. The organization of this formidable effort was entrusted to the Subcommittee on Oncology of the Committee on Pathology, and Dr. Arthur Purdy Stout was the first editor-in-chief. Many of the illustrations were provided by the Medical Illustration Service of the Armed Forces Institute of Pathology (AFIP), the type was set by the Government Printing Office, and the final printing was done at the Armed Forces Institute of Pathology. The American Registry of Pathology (ARP) purchased the Fascicles from the Government Printing Office and sold them virtually at cost. Over a period of 20 years, approximately 15,000 copies each of nearly 40 Fascicles were produced. The worldwide impact of these publications over the years has largely surpassed the original goal. They quickly became among the most influential publications on tumor pathology, primarily because of their overall high quality, but also because their low cost made them easily accessible the world over to pathologists and other students of oncology.

Upon completion of the first series, the National Academy of Sciences-National Research Council handed further pursuit of the project over to the newly created Universities Associated for Research and Education in Pathology (UAREP). A second series was started, generously supported by grants from the AFIP, the National Cancer Institute, and the American Cancer Society. Dr. Harlan I. Firminger became the editor-in-chief and was succeeded by Dr. William H. Hartmann. The second series' Fascicles were produced as bound volumes instead of loose leaflets. They featured a more comprehensive coverage of the subjects, to the extent that the Fascicles could no longer be regarded as "atlases" but rather as monographs describing and illustrating in detail the tumors and tumor-like conditions of the various organs and systems.

Once the second series was completed, with a success that matched that of the first, ARP, UAREP, and AFIP decided to embark on a third series. Dr. Juan Rosai was appointed as editor-in-chief, and Dr. Leslie Sobin became associate editor. A distinguished Editorial Advisory Board was also convened, and these outstanding pathologists and educators played a major role in the success of this series, the first publication of which appeared in 1991 and the last (number 32) in 2003.

The same organizational framework applies to the current fourth series, but with UAREP and AFIP no longer functioning, ARP is now the responsible organization. New features include a hardbound cover and illustrations almost exclusively in color. There is also an increased emphasis on the cytopathologic (intraoperative, exfoliative, or fine needle aspiration) and molecular features that are important in diagnosis and prognosis. What does not change from the three previous series, however, is the goal of providing the practicing pathologist with thorough, concise, and up-to-date information on the nomenclature and classification; epidemiologic, clinical, and pathogenetic features; and, most importantly, guidance in the diagnosis of the tumors and tumorlike lesions of all major organ systems and body sites.

As in the third series, a continuous attempt is made to correlate, whenever possible, the nomenclature used in the Fascicles with that proposed by the World Health Organization's Classification of Tumors, as well as to ensure a consistency of style. Close cooperation between the various authors and their respective liaisons from the Editorial Board will continue to be emphasized in order to minimize unnecessary repetition and discrepancies in the text and illustrations.

Particular thanks are due to the members of the Editorial Advisory Board, the reviewers, the editorial and production staff, and the individual Fascicle authors for their ongoing efforts to ensure that this series is a worthy successor to the previous three.

Steven G. Silverberg, MD
Ronald A. DeLellis, MD
Leslie H. Sobin, MD

PREFACE AND ACKNOWLEDGMENTS

There have been many advances in the pathology of intestinal tumors since the publication of the Third Series Intestines Fascicle in 2003, but many of the foundations of intestinal tumor diagnosis remain tried and true. Tubular adenomas are still tubular adenomas, but better understanding of serrated polyps has been a key advance in the years since the publication of the Third Series volume. Additionally, developments in molecular biology of colorectal carcinoma have allowed for targeted therapy and refinements to our evaluation of Lynch syndrome, which was termed hereditary nonpolyposis colorectal carcinoma (HNPCC) in the past. Our understanding of other polyposis syndromes has similarly blossomed in the past 15 years. Neuroendocrine tumors have been reclassified in the 2010 World Health Organization classification of gastrointestinal tumors. The molecular basis of gastrointestinal stromal tumors of the intestines has been a subject of great interest as well. In producing this update, this group of authors has enjoyed working together in gathering images and information to update this edition of the Intestines atlas. In doing so, we stand on the shoulders of giants before us, namely Drs. Robert H. Riddell, Robert E. Petras, Geraint T. Williams, and Leslie H. Sobin.

While many areas of intestinal tumor pathology are without controversy, the classification and nomenclature for appendiceal tumors remain a subject of debate, including among ourselves. We have attempted to offer information on the various divergent viewpoints where they exist for this topic and others. Our efforts have been synergistic, and we hope that readers will enjoy the many interesting illustrations that we were able to amass.

Lastly, we would like to thank those who have helped see this volume to production. These colleagues include the American Registry of Pathology Press team, consisting of Magdalena Silva, Dian Thomas, Alana Black, and Audrey Kahn, all under the able leadership of Mirlinda Caton. We also thank Drs. Lysandra Voltaggio, Jason Hornick, and Ronald DeLellis for their critical review of the manuscript. Lastly, we thank Dr. Steven G. Silverberg for his tireless support of the Fourth Series of these wonderful guides to tumor pathology.

Elizabeth A. Montgomery, MD
Rhonda K. Yantiss, MD
Dale C. Snover, MD
Laura H. Tang, MD, PhD

Dedications

*To our colleagues and trainees who share
our love of gastrointestinal pathology.*
Drs. Montgomery, Snover, Tang, and Yantiss

To Zachary and Madeleine, the best part of me.
Rhonda K. Yantiss

CONTENTS

1 NORMAL ANATOMY AND HISTOLOGY

SMALL INTESTINE

Anatomy

The length of the adult small intestine is 300 to 900 cm. The small intestine is divided into the duodenum, the jejunum, and the ileum.

The duodenum, the most proximal portion, is approximately 25 cm in length and, except for its first portion, is retroperitoneal. It is divided in four parts: the first portion includes the duodenal bulb and extends from the gastric outlet to the second (descending) portion; the second portion includes the ampulla of Vater and extends to the level of the fourth lumbar vertebra on the right side of the spine; the third portion again crosses the spine to complete a C shape, which surrounds the head and body of the pancreas; the fourth part rises slightly and terminates at the duodenojejunal junction, which is moored by the ligament of Treitz.

The pancreatic and bile ducts usually empty into the common bile duct, which opens at the ampulla of Vater on the medial wall of the descending duodenum. The opening of the accessory pancreatic duct of Santorini is found 2 to 3 cm proximal to the ampulla of Vater in up to 70 percent of normal individuals.

The remaining small intestine is mobile and situated on a narrow mesentery; the proximal 40 percent is arbitrarily designated as the jejunum while the distal 60 percent is the ileum. The jejunum is located in the left upper quadrant, the jejunoileal transition point is in the mid-abdomen, and the terminal ileum is in the right lower quadrant. The root of the small bowel mesentery passes obliquely downward and to the right across the abdomen. The diameter of the proximal jejunum is about 3.5 cm, and the ileum is approximately 2.5 cm.

The luminal surface of the small bowel is arranged in mucosal folds that vary from 3 to 10 mm in height and run transversely around the bowel. These circumferential folds are known as valvulae conniventes (a misnomer: they are neither valves nor do they stopper the lumen), plicae circularis, or the folds of Kerckring (fig. 1-1). These gradually become less conspicuous through the distal jejunum and may be absent in the distal ileum.

Lymphoid follicles form tiny nodules (0.1 to 0.3 cm) that become more numerous distally, coalescing to form Peyer patches in the

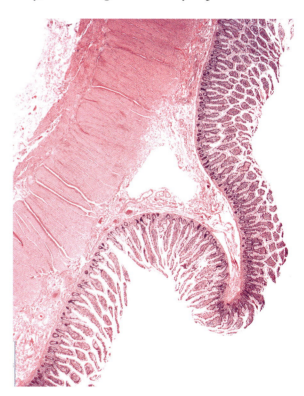

Figure 1-1

NORMAL SMALL INTESTINE

The mucosa (consisting of epithelium, lamina propria, and muscularis mucosae) is at the top (lumen side) and the submucosa is below. The muscularis propria consists of a double layer of smooth muscle. In the center of the field is a fold of tissue projecting into the lumen known as a fold of Kerckring (valvula connivente).

terminal ileum; these measure up to 1.5 cm in width and can extend longitudinally for up to 12 cm. Lymphoid follicles are prominent in young individuals but begin to atrophy in adulthood, so that they may be inapparent in older individuals. They may enlarge as the result of inflammation or neoplasia.

Like the rest of the gastrointestinal tract, the small bowel is composed of mucosa, muscularis mucosae, muscularis propria, and serosa. The muscularis propria consists of inner circular and outer longitudinal layers. In most of the small intestine, the muscularis propria is separated from the peritoneal surface by a layer of connective tissue and a variable amount of fat.

The ileocecal valve creates a large papilla-like structure, the orifice of which folds down to produce a stellate appearance. It behaves like a physiologic sphincter when closed and prevents coloileal reflux. Prominent lymphoid aggregates at the orifice may result in a thickened appearance, particularly among pediatric patients. Accumulation of fat in the submucosa of the ileocecal valve region is common and is termed lipohyperplasia/lipomatous hypertrophy. Fat accumulation in this area may radiographically mimic a neoplasm.

The duodenal blood supply is derived from celiac and superior mesenteric arteries. The proximal duodenum is supplied by the superior pancreaticoduodenal branch of the gastroduodenal artery, which originates from the celiac axis; the distal duodenum is supplied by the inferior pancreaticoduodenal branch of the superior mesenteric artery. The jejunum and ileum are supplied by the superior mesenteric artery, which gives rise to overlapping arterial arcades within the mesentery. Vasa recta emanating from the arcade vessels penetrate the bowel wall. The ileocolic branch of the superior mesenteric artery supplies the terminal ileum, along with the proximal colon. Arteries in the bowel wall give rise to vessels that supply the muscularis propria directly or penetrate the muscularis propria, supplying the submucosa and mucosa.

The venous drainage of the small bowel includes a submucosal venous plexus, penetrating intramural veins that leave the bowel wall as serosal veins. These merge to form mesenteric veins that drain into the portal system. Arteries and veins travel together at all levels within the bowel wall; histologic sections should always demonstrate paired vessels.

The lymphatic drainage of the duodenum is to the pancreaticoileal and pyloric groups of lymph nodes. The jejunal and ileal lymphatics drain into the superior mesenteric lymph nodes, and the terminal ileum drains into the ileocolic lymph nodes. There are approximately 200 lymph nodes in the small bowel mesentery. Lymph draining from these nodes enters the cisterna chyli, and ultimately reaches the thoracic duct. The presence of chylomicrons imparts a milky appearance to the lymphatic fluid draining the small bowel.

Histology

The small intestinal mucosa consists of epithelium and lamina propria organized in finger-like villi that project into the lumen (fig. 1-2), and crypts of Lieberkühn that extend toward the muscularis mucosae. Villi vary from 0.3 to 1.0 mm in length, depending on anatomic location, and span approximately 0.1 mm in width. Villi are shorter in the duodenal bulb and the descending duodenum where Brunner glands are abundant. They are tallest in the distal duodenum and proximal jejunum, and then become progressively shorter from the jejunum to the terminal ileum. Villi overlying the randomly scattered mucosal lymphoid follicles and Peyer patches are commonly distorted. Villous cores consist of lamina propria; each villus contains an arteriole, venule, capillary network, central lymphatic (lacteal) vessel, and some nerve fibers. Delicate longitudinal strands of smooth muscle are also found in the cores of the villi, allowing them to move and maximize absorption of nutrients.

The crypts of Lieberkühn are about 170 μm in length and contain the epithelial stem cells in a zone close to their bases (1). The daughters of these stem cells undergo differentiation as they extend toward the lumen, ultimately differentiating into the goblet cells and absorptive cells that surface the villi. Multiple crypts merge luminally into a zone from which villi arise (2). The process of epithelial cell migration from crypt base to villus tip occurs over 4 to 6 days. The proliferative compartment, as seen by MIB-1 (Ki-67) immunolabeling, is found toward the base of the crypts (fig. 1-3).

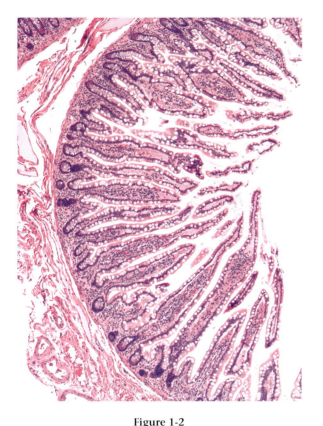

Figure 1-2

**NORMAL SMALL INTESTINAL
MUCOSA AND SUBMUCOSA**

The villi are long and slender and goblet cells outnumber absorptive cells, suggesting a distal location in the jejunum (the villi are stubby in the ileum).

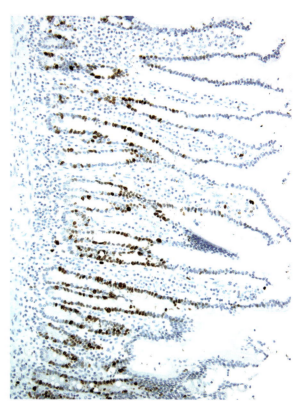

Figure 1-3

**NORMAL SMALL INTESTINAL MUCOSA:
MIB-1 IMMUNOHISTOCHEMICAL STAIN**

This pattern conforms to the proliferative compartment of the small bowel. The bases of the crypts and the villi lack labeling but labeling is present in the crypts.

Four epithelial types are found in the small intestine: enterocytes, goblet cells, Paneth cells, and endocrine cells. Enterocytes are tall, columnar absorptive cells that mostly cover the villi and occupy the upper portions of the crypts. They are arranged in a monolayer attached to the basement membrane and are interspersed with goblet cells, which are present in variable numbers (fig. 1-4). Enterocytes contain uniform basal nuclei, eosinophilic cytoplasm, and a microvillous brush border that can be accentuated by a periodic acid–Schiff (PAS)–alcian blue stain (fig. 1-5). The microvillous brush border can be highlighted with CD10, EPCAM, and villin immunohistochemical stains (fig. 1-6) (4,5). The microvilli contain a core of actin filaments that are cross-linked by fimbrin and villin, and tethered to the plasma membrane by myosin 1 and calmodulin. The microvilli contain enzymes, including alkaline phosphatase, aminopeptidases, and disaccharidases. On the outer surface of the microvilli is the glycocalyx, a glycoprotein coat produced by the enterocytes.

Enterocytes are closely associated with the mucosa-associated lymphoid tissue (MALT) of the small bowel. The epithelium normally contains scattered T lymphocytes that express CD3, CD5, and CD8. Intraepithelial lymphocytes number up to 20 per 100 enterocytes in the proximal small bowel, but are less numerous distally. Intraepithelial lymphocytes are normally present overlying lymphoid aggregates. Enterocytes produce a secretory component, which facilitates epithelial translocation of immunoglobulin (Ig) A. The epithelium that overlies the B-cell–rich zones of lymphoid follicles and Peyer patches consists of specialized M cells that govern the presentation of luminal antigens to the mucosal

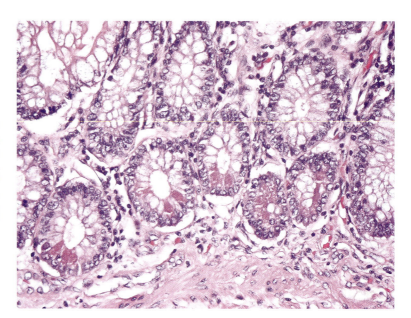

Figure 1-4

NORMAL SMALL INTESTINAL MUCOSA

There are many Paneth cells in each crypt. These are at the base of the crypts and contain prominent magenta granules. At the upper left, both goblet cells and absorptive cells can be seen, but overall, goblet cells, containing clear droplets, predominate in keeping with distal small bowel.

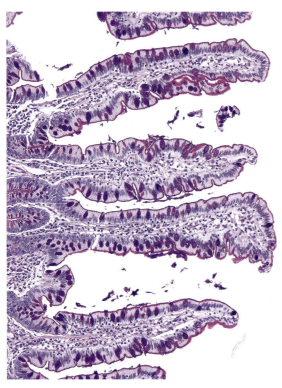

Figure 1-5

NORMAL SMALL INTESTINAL MUCOSA: PERIODIC ACID–SCHIFF (PAS), ALCIAN BLUE (AB) STAINS

The goblet cells stain with a combination of PAS and AB, imparting a purple color to their cytoplasm. The intervening absorptive cells lack cytoplasmic mucin with the PAS stain highlighting the slender brush border. Since absorptive enterocytes predominate, it can be assumed that this sample is from the proximal small intestine.

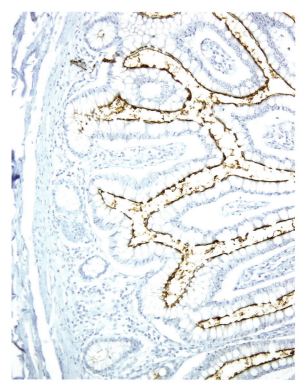

Figure 1-6

NORMAL SMALL INTESTINAL MUCOSA: CD10 IMMUNOHISTOCHEMICAL STAIN

The CD10 stain highlights the brush border. Goblet cells are numerous, suggesting a distal origin. This sample is from the ileum.

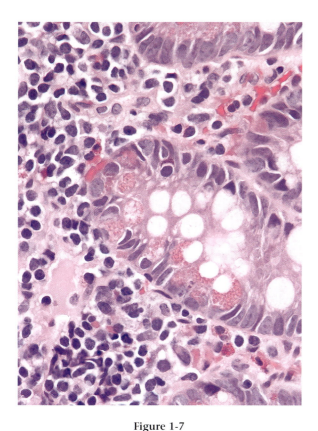

Figure 1-7

NORMAL SMALL INTESTINAL MUCOSA

Paneth cell granules are highlighted. Also seen are lamina propria lymphoid cells and plasma cells.

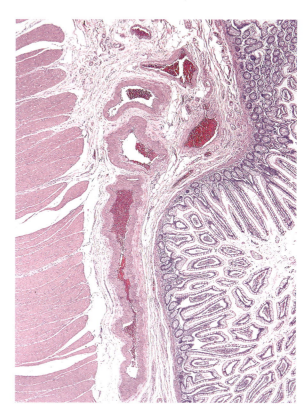

Figure 1-8

NORMAL SMALL INTESTINE

Prominent submucosal blood vessels are seen in the center of the field.

immune system. M cells have a luminal membrane that is arranged in microfolds rather than regular microvilli (3). M cells are distinguished from adjacent enterocytes by their coexpression of CK18 and vimentin (3).

Goblet cells are present throughout the small intestine. They are abundant in the crypts and progressively decrease in density toward the tips of villi. They are cylindrical cells containing a well-marginated collection of mucin in the luminal aspect of the cytoplasm (the "goblet"). Their proportion in relation to enterocytes is highest in the ileum and lowest in the distal duodenum and jejunum (figs. 1-4, 1-7). They extrude mucus that consists of sialylated (but not sulfated or O-acetylated) glycoproteins that are alcian blue and PAS positive, and they express mucin core protein 2 (MUC2).

The deep crypts of the small bowel contain Paneth cells and endocrine cells (fig. 1-7). Paneth cells are columnar in shape with basal nuclei, and they contain large eosinophilic granules rich in growth factors and antimicrobial proteins. Endocrine cells also contain eosinophilic granular cytoplasm, although the granules are much finer and contain a variety of peptides and bioactive compounds. Endocrine cells have a pyramidal shape with apically oriented nuclei and basal cytoplasm.

The mucosal lamina propria consists of loosely arranged collagen and elastin fibers containing small blood vessels, nerve fibrils, lymphatic vessels, and mucosal lymphoid follicles. Mucosal arteries arise from the submucosal arterial plexuses, giving rise to two networks of capillaries: one is loose, ramifying, and surrounds the crypts, and the other is richer and denser within the cores of the villi. Villous capillaries drain into a single venule, which, in turn, drains into the submucosal venous plexus (fig. 1-8), and finally into the portal vein. Mucosal lymphatics begin as central villous lacteals that feed into a submucosal

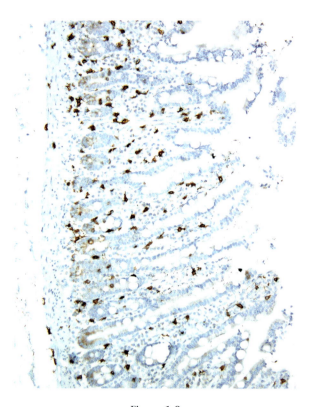

Figure 1-9

**NORMAL SMALL INTESTINAL MUCOSA:
CD117 IMMUNOHISTOCHEMICAL STAIN**

This preparation highlights scattered mast cells in the lamina propria.

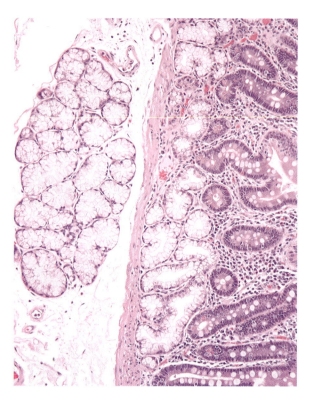

Figure 1-10

NORMAL DUODENAL MUCOSA

Submucosal Brunner glands are seen at the left of the field. These plump glands produce abundant neutral mucin. Although it is not strictly normal for them to be in the lamina propria (note the slim band of muscularis mucosae separating the submucosa from the lamina propria, which contains inflammatory cells), most individuals have scattered mucosal Brunner glands.

lymphatic plexus and then to the cisterna chyli. The central villous lacteal is inconspicuous unless it is pathologically enlarged; the lacteals are close to the basement membranes of the enterocytes of the villi to allow the transfer of chylomicrons and fat droplets.

The small intestinal lamina propria houses much of the gut-associated lymphoid tissue. It contains numerous plasma cells, lymphocytes, and macrophages, as well as scattered mast cells (fig. 1-9) (6). The plasma cells mostly produce IgA and are concentrated in the intercryptal region. Other cell types are more sparsely distributed throughout the lamina propria. Mature lymphocytes are mostly T cells with a CD4-positive helper cell phenotype, but some have a CD8-positive suppressor-cytotoxic phenotype. Occasional eosinophils are normally present, but neutrophils are rare.

As in other parts of the gastrointestinal tract, the small bowel muscularis mucosae consists of a slender zone of smooth muscle with inner circular and outer longitudinal layers. The bases of the crypts end on the muscularis mucosae. The submucosa is situated beneath the mucosa and consists of loose connective tissue that supports large caliber vessels and the Meissner nerve plexus of parasympathetic ganglion cells and sympathetic neurons. The duodenal submucosa also contains Brunner glands filled with neutral mucin that is alcian blue negative and PAS positive (figs. 1-1, 1-10–1-12). When these glands are crushed, they can be mistaken for mesenchymal tumors or even for Whipple disease (fig. 1-12).

The submucosa is also rich in lymphoid aggregates, often with germinal centers (figs. 1-13–1-15). These lymphoid aggregates are linear in most of the small bowel, but are

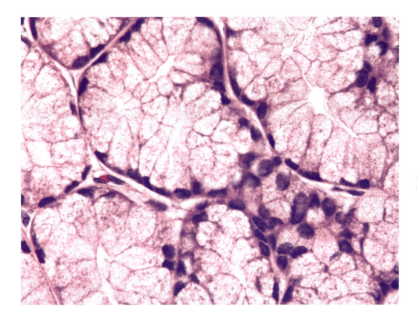

Figure 1-11

BRUNNER GLANDS

The cytoplasm has a granular appearance. These glands are only found in the duodenum.

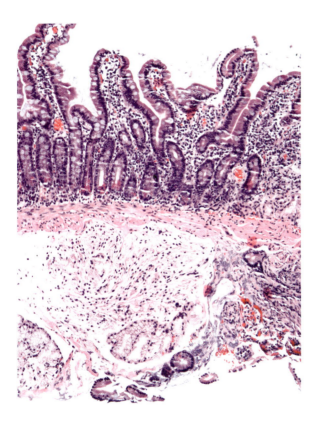

Figure 1-12

BRUNNER GLANDS

The glands are crushed, imparting an appearance reminiscent of a myxoid mesenchymal neoplasm.

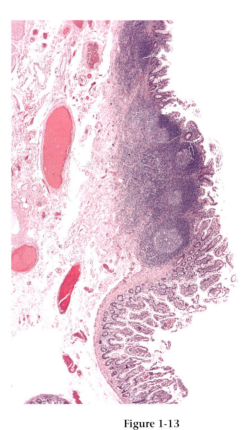

Figure 1-13

**ILEAL MUCOSA AND
SUBMUCOSA WITH PEYER PATCHES**

The villi at the bottom are regularly spaced without the slight disarray of those associated with the lymphoid aggregates (Peyer patches). Four pale germinal centers are seen in the center. There is rich submucosal vascularity.

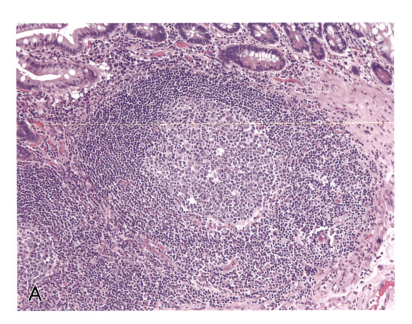

Figure 1-14

ILEAL MUCOSA AND SUBMUCOSA WITH LYMPHOID FOLLICLE

A: The mucosa at the top of the field features prominent Paneth cells. There is a germinal center at the middle of the image.

B: A CD20 immunohistochemical stain shows numerous B cells.

C: The CD3-expressing T cells cuff the germinal center.

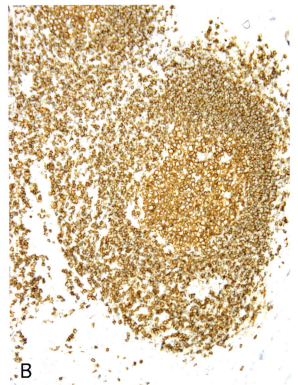

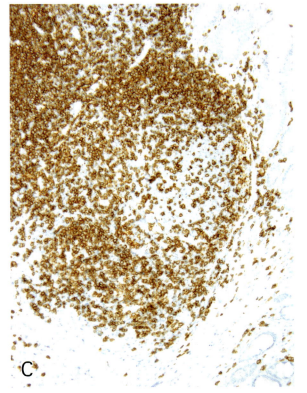

circumferential in the ileum, such that intussus-ception in the ileum with lymphoid hyperplasia as the lead point can be encountered, often in children with viral infections (7). The lymphoid aggregates often extend into or even originate in the lamina propria. It is important to re-member that finding numerous lymphocytes in the epithelium overlying the Peyer patches is normal and scattered T cells are normally found in the small intestinal epithelium (fig. 1-16). Although not a normal finding, the ileal lymphoid tissue often contains macrophages containing titanium derived from toothpaste and some foods (fig. 1-17).

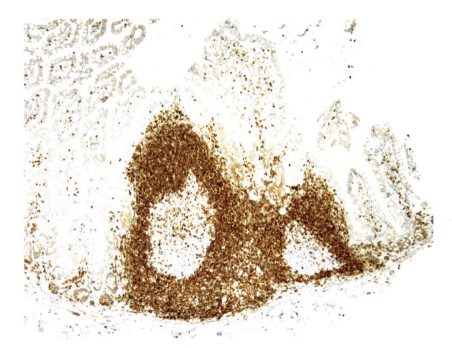

Figure 1-15

ILEAL MUCOSA AND SUBMUCOSA WITH LYMPHOID FOLLICLES: BCL2 IMMUNOHISTOCHEMICAL STAIN

The normal germinal centers contain only scattered labeled cells.

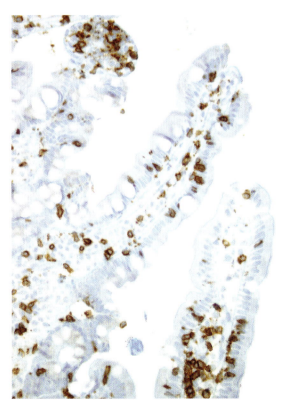

Figure 1-16

NORMAL SMALL INTESTINAL SURFACE EPITHELIUM: CD3 IMMUNOHISTOCHEMICAL STAIN

Scattered T cells are a normal component of the epithelium. There are also a few T cells in the lamina propria.

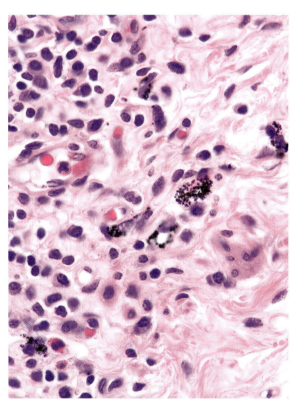

Figure 1-17

ILEAL SUBMUCOSA

Most people have black pigment that has been engulfed by macrophages in their terminal ileum; this corresponds to the titanium found in toothpaste and packaged foods.

9

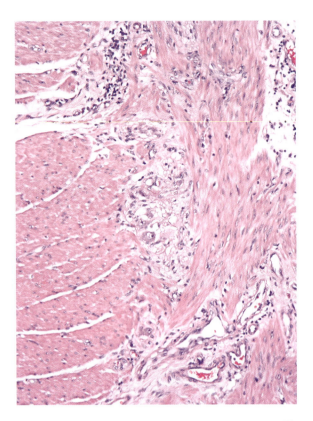 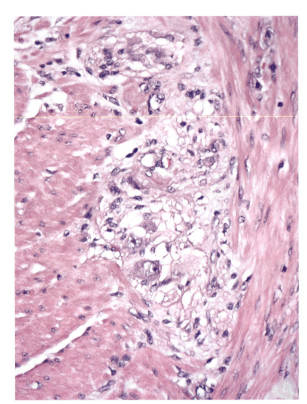

Figure 1-18

MUSCULARIS PROPRIA, SMALL INTESTINE

Left: Ganglion cells in Auerbach plexus are present between the inner and outer layers of muscularis propria.
Right: The plexus of ganglion cells with spindled Schwann cells is seen.

The muscularis propria is the thick double-layered muscle beneath the submucosa and provides most of the contractile function of the bowel wall (figs. 1-1, 1-18, 1-19). It consists of inner circular and outer longitudinal layers; the Auerbach nerve plexus containing parasympathetic ganglion cells is between the layers.

The intraperitoneal portions of the small bowel (jejunum, ileum, and proximal duodenum) have a serosa consisting of loose connective tissue with a mesothelial lining. The retroperitoneal portion of the duodenum is surfaced by mesothelium anteriorly; the posterior surface consists of the loose connective tissue of the adventitia.

COLON

Anatomy

The colon (large intestine) begins at the ileocecal valve. Its diameter is about twice that of the small intestine proximally, but diminishes distally to the rectal ampulla. The function of the colon is to absorb electrolytes and other components that result from bacterial degradation. About 1 L of fluid enters the colon from the ileocecal valve daily, which is reduced to approximately 100 mL in feces. The colorectum is 120 to 150 cm in length; it consists of the right, transverse, and left colon, and terminates in the rectum.

The right colon is defined as the cecum and ascending colon. The cecum is usually completely surrounded by peritoneum and contains the appendiceal orifice on its medial wall, approximately 2 cm below the ileocecal valve. The ascending colon measures 15 to 20 cm and extends to the hepatic flexure. It lacks a mesentery except anteriorly and laterally along the right paracolic gutter. The colon acquires a mesentery at the hepatic flexure and becomes the transverse colon, which is 30 to 60 cm long. At the splenic flexure, the posterior part of the colon again becomes retroperitoneal and fixed.

Figure 1-19

**MUSCULARIS PROPRIA, SMALL INTESTINE:
CD117/KIT IMMUNOHISTOCHEMICAL STAIN**

There are fewer Cajal cells in the small bowel muscularis propria than in that of the colon and appendix. The long slender cells are the so-called gastrointestinal pacemaker cells of Cajal, whereas the two plump cells at the left of the field are mast cells.

The left colon consists of the descending and sigmoid colons. The descending colon lies on the posterior abdominal wall and extends for 20 to 25 cm until it crosses the pelvic brim, reacquires a mesentery, and becomes the sigmoid colon. The sigmoid colon measures between 20 and 85 cm, with an average length of about 40 cm. The rectosigmoid junction is opposite the level of the sacral promontory.

The rectum is 10 to 15 cm, ending at the dentate (or pectinate) line, which traditionally marks the anatomic anorectal junction. Its upper third is peritonealized both anteriorly and laterally, losing serosa more distally, first laterally and then anteriorly, as the peritoneum drapes over the posterior aspect of the bladder in the male or the uterus in the female.

The posterior (retroperitoneal) rectum is enveloped by mesorectum that contains fat and all of the regional lymph nodes of the rectum. It is surfaced by an embryologic plane of cleavage (mesorectal fascia). This whole mesorectal compartment is resected during a total mesorectal excision for rectal carcinoma; the pathologist is required to examine its entire circumferential margin after marking it with ink to address the completeness of excision. A similar approach is necessary to assess the nonperitoneal resection margins of right and left hemicolectomy specimens for cancer (8).

The large bowel is characterized by the presence of three slim external bands of longitudinal smooth muscle: the teniae coli, which are condensations of the longitudinal muscle layer of the muscularis propria. One is close to the mesentery (mesocolic tenia), and the other two are almost equidistant from each other and the mesenteric tenia on the antimesenteric aspect of the colon. The teniae unite at the base of the appendix, completely investing it. In the proximal rectum, all three flare out, forming an external muscle coat, similar to that of the small intestine. The inner circular layer of the muscularis propria and the teniae are thin in the proximal colon and become thicker toward the rectosigmoid junction.

The external colon also has appendices epiploicae, which represent protuberances of subserosal fat, the abundance of which correlates with overall adiposity. Two rows of epiploicae are present in the ascending and descending colon, but only a single row is found on the undersurface of the transverse colon. The greater omentum is a large peritoneal fold that contains abundant fat. It hangs from the greater curvature of the stomach into the abdominal cavity, where it folds over and returns to attach to the transverse colon; the lesser omentum extends superiorly between the stomach and the liver. The large intestine contains a series of haustra, which are saccules between the teniae that impart a segmented appearance to the outer aspect of the colon and produce the appearance of semilunar folds (plicae semilunaris) when viewed from the mucosal surface, analogous to the folds of Kerckring in the small bowel.

The vascular supply for the cecum and proximal colon to the splenic flexure consists of the

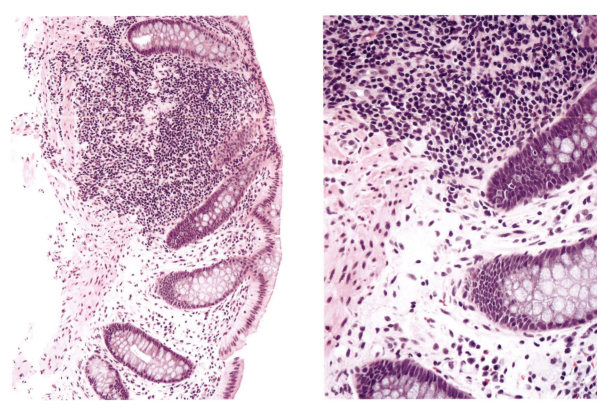

Figure 1-20

NORMAL COLON MUCOSA

Left: Normal rectal mucosa with lymphoid aggregate. The overlying epithelium contains more numerous lymphocytes than the adjacent epithelium. Muciphages are present in the lamina propria adjacent to the lymphoid aggregate.

Right: Muciphages are highlighted in this higher power image.

ileocolic, right colic, and middle colic branches of the superior mesenteric artery. The rest is supplied by the inferior mesenteric artery (left colic and sigmoid branches). There are numerous anastomosing arcades that link the superior and inferior mesenteric arteries, and these are joined by the marginal artery of Drummond, which courses close and parallel to the mesenteric surface of the colon. This vessel can be attenuated in the region of the splenic flexure, such that the blood supply to this part of the colon is readily compromised. The rectum is vascularized by the superior rectal branch of the inferior mesenteric artery, the middle rectal arteries from the internal iliac vessels, and the inferior rectal arteries from the internal pudendal vessels. The vessels of the large bowel become increasingly tortuous over time. The veins that pair with the arteries are similarly named. All drain into the portal system, with the exception of those from

the distal rectum, which drain into the systemic circulation. Portal-systemic anastomoses occur by communication of the superior rectal with the middle and inferior rectal veins.

Lymph nodes draining the large bowel consist of those that are immediately adjacent to the bowel wall (paracolic and pararectal nodes), and those that follow the vascular channels. The lymphatic drainage of the lower rectum consists of lymph nodes along the superior rectal artery and nodes along the middle rectal vessels; these ultimately drain to the internal iliac nodes, and occasionally, to the inguinal nodes, presumably via presacral lymphatic channels.

Histology

The layers of the colon include the mucosa, muscularis mucosae, submucosa, muscularis propria, and serosa or adventitia, depending on whether the segment is surfaced by peritoneum.

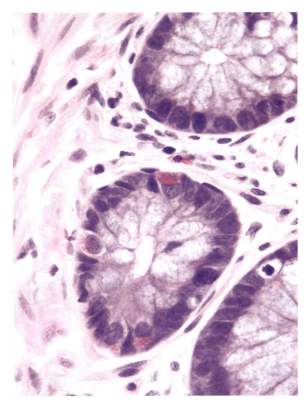

Figure 1-21

COLONIC MUCOSA

Endocrine cells are in the center of the field. In contrast to the Paneth cells, best seen in figures 1-4 and 1-7, the granules of the endocrine cells are smaller, red, and oriented away from the lumen whereas the granules of Paneth cells empty into the lumen.

A key function of the colon is to absorb water and electrolytes, and thus, its mucosa has a different architecture from that of the small bowel (figs. 1-20–1-22). The colonic mucosa is flat, unlike the small bowel mucosa, although it may display smooth undulations (anthemic folds). There are no villi; the epithelium of the colon consists of straight, regularly spaced invaginations, the architecture of which has been likened to "test tubes in a rack." The crypts are lined predominantly by goblet cells, punctuated by scattered absorptive cells.

Intraepithelial lymphocytes are a normal finding throughout the colon. Endocrine cells, Paneth cells, and progenitor cells are found at the crypt bases. The Paneth and endocrine cells have the same morphology as those in the small intestine. Colonic Paneth cells are normal con-

stituents of the ascending and transverse colons, but they are absent in the normal descending and sigmoid colons.

Although the rectal mucosa has the same components as the rest of the colon, this mucosa also shows some characteristic features. The crypts in the rectum are often shorter, with less regular and wider spacing that those more proximally situated. They may be reduced in number and show mild dilation or irregular shapes. The rectal lamina propria is sometimes more cellular than that of the descending and sigmoid colons, with lymphocytes, plasma cells, neutrophils, and muciphages; the latter are found in about 40 percent of evaluated samples (fig. 1-20) (9). Mild fibrosis of the lamina propria may be noted in the rectum.

Beneath the surface epithelium, the colonic lamina propria contains lymphocytes, plasma cells, and eosinophils. These cells are more abundant in the lamina propria of the right colon than the left colon so that correlation with biopsy location is necessary to accurately assess inflammatory findings. Importantly, the lamina propria of the colon lacks significant lymphatic vessels (they are present but not a prominent feature), a critical point when staging neoplasms that invade the lamina propria, as discussed in chapter 4.

Beneath the lamina propria is the thin muscularis mucosae. It has inner circular and outer longitudinal smooth muscle layers. The crypt bases extend to the top of the muscularis mucosae. The submucosa is composed of loose connective tissue, large caliber vessels, and the Meissner nerve plexus containing parasympathetic ganglion cells and sympathetic neurons.

The colonic muscularis propria provides the key contractile force for the colon. It consists of inner circular and outer longitudinal smooth muscle components. The Auerbach nerve plexus lies between these smooth muscle layers and contains parasympathetic ganglion cells. The colonic inner circular smooth muscle is continuous throughout its length and circumference, while the outer longitudinal layer is discontinuous and contains three bundles of longitudinal smooth muscle distributed evenly around the circumference of the colon (the tinea coli).

Beneath the muscularis propria is the final layer of the colon, the serosa. This layer

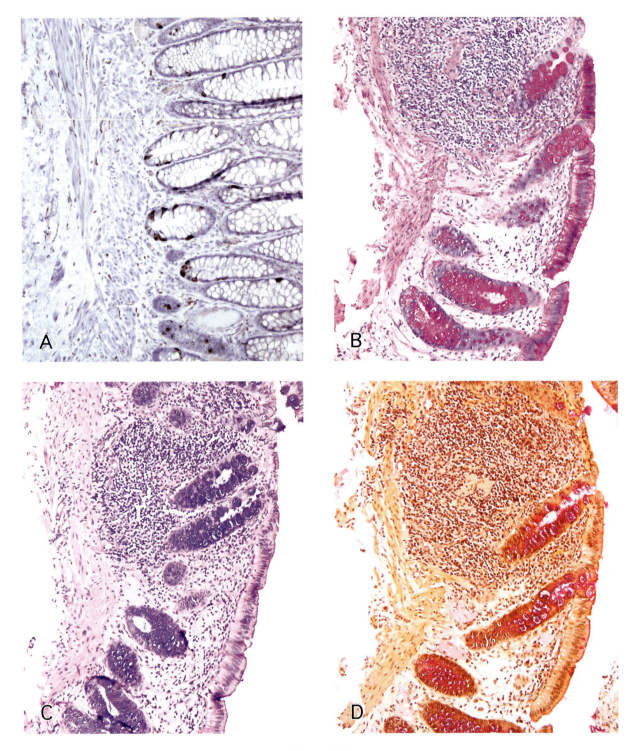

Figure 1-22

COLONIC MUCOSA

A: With the chromogranin immunostain, scattered labeled endocrine cells toward the bases of the crypts are seen.
B: With the PAS stain, goblet cells are seen.
C: With the PAS/AB stain, the goblet cells are dark blue to purple.
D: With the mucicarmine stain, the goblet cells are stained well while the muciphages are only faintly stained.

includes loose connective tissue as well as the mesothelium that lines the peritonealized portions of the colon.

The proximal portion of the rectum lies in the abdominal cavity and is covered anteriorly by peritoneum, but the distal portion is embedded in the soft tissue of the pelvis and lacks a peritoneal covering. This point is important when evaluating rectal specimens, as the external surface of the distal portion is a true surgical margin, as discussed in chapter 4.

APPENDIX

Anatomy

The appendix has no known function. It arises from the medial cecal wall and measures 6 to 7 cm in adults, with a diameter of approximately 0.7 cm. It may be as small as 2 cm in length in pediatric patients, particularly infants. The teniae coli of the large bowel coalesce at the base of the appendix, investing it completely.

The appendiceal orifice is approximately 2.5 cm below the ileocecal valve in adults, but the location of the appendix in the abdomen is variable. It usually lies posterior to the cecum or ascending colon; the next most frequent site is overhanging the pelvic brim where it may directly impinge on the bladder. It may also follow the cecum, either in front of or behind the terminal ileum, or it may sit on the psoas muscle. Rarely, it is subhepatic (with incomplete rotation of the bowel resulting in failed descent of the cecum). In patients with situs inversus, the appendix is in the left iliac fossa.

The mesoappendix consists of adipose tissue containing the appendiceal vasculature and occasional small lymph nodes. The appendix is supplied by the posterior cecal branch of the ileocolic artery, a distal branch of the superior mesenteric artery. The venous drainage is into the superior mesenteric vein and the portal vein. Occasional lymph nodes may be present in the mesoappendix, which then drain to the pericolic and superior mesenteric nodes.

Histology

The mucosa of the appendix is like that in the colon (figs. 1-23–1-25), although it has more prominent lymphoid tissue, often with lymphoid follicles that fill the lumen and result in distorted crypt architecture (fig. 1-23). The appendiceal submucosa lacks fat in the neonate; submucosal "fibrosis" uniting the muscularis mucosae and propria is normal in children. The submucosal nerve plexus is frequently inconspicuous and, although ganglion cells and nerves are normally present between the circular and longitudinal layers of the muscularis propria, ganglion cells are also normally present, scattered throughout the muscularis propria.

ANUS

Anatomy

The anal canal is an anteroposterior opening located between the rectum and perianal skin. It usually spans 3 to 4 cm and is separated from the coccyx by fibromuscular tissue (the anococcygeal ligament) posteriorly. The perineal body lies between the anus and the membranous part of the urethra and the bulb of the penis in the male, or the lower end of the vagina in the female. On each side lies an ischiorectal fossa.

Descriptions of anal anatomy and histology can be confusing because of terminology. From proximal to distal, the anal region is divided into the anal transition zone, the dentate line, the pecten, and the perianal skin (10). The anal transition zone is the area between colorectal-type mucosa and squamous mucosa. It is most commonly covered by noncolumnar, transitional-type epithelium and ranges from 0.5 to 2.0 cm in length, although it may be shorter or even absent.

The dentate line (pectinate line) is the single, wavy line that circumnavigates the anal mucosa. It is easily visible in resected specimens and at endoscopy. Six to 10 anal columns (of Morgagni) merge with the rectal mucosa above the dentate line. These vertical columns are joined at their bases by semilunar valves that form papillae at the dentate line. Immediately behind them, anal sinuses (or crypts) are found. These correspond to the anal ducts that open onto the surface. The dentate line may be difficult to identify when valves and papillae are obscured, or in older patients in whom the anal columns are less prominent; it is defined in these cases by the opening of the lowest visible sinus. The dentate line and the columns of Morgagni usually have thin transitional-type mucosa that

Figure 1-23

NORMAL APPENDIX

A: This sample was from an opportunistic appendectomy performed at the time of a gynecologic procedure. There are prominent lymphoid aggregates that distort the mucosa.

B: This section was taken to highlight the tip but shows the lymphoid aggregates to advantage.

C: The muscularis propria can be seen to have two layers. Crypt distortion is expected in this site.

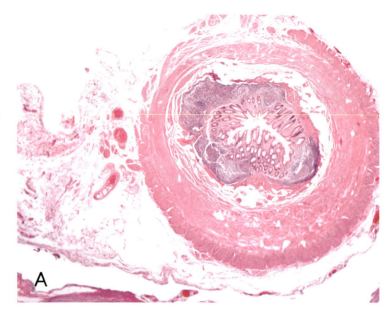

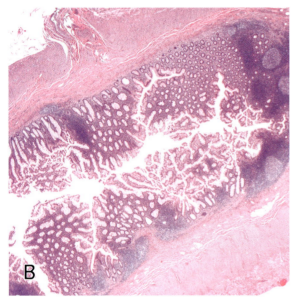

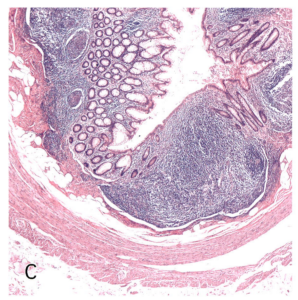

may extend downward for a few millimeters beyond the dentate line.

The pecten is the zone that extends between the dentate line and the hair-bearing perianal skin. It lacks hair and is covered by nonkeratinizing squamous epithelium. Smooth and glistening in situ, it appears wrinkled in resected specimens. The term "histologic anal canal" is sometimes used to describe the anal transition zone and pecten together. This part of the anal region is covered by transitional and squamous epithelium, lacks hair or sweat glands, and is enclosed by the external sphincter muscle. The connective tissue of the transition zone is loose, but in the pecten, denser fibroelastic tissue attaches the epithelium firmly to the internal sphincter. This creates a submucosal barrier at the dentate line that is important in containing the spread of cancer in this region. The pecten merges imperceptibly with the perianal skin, sometimes called the anal verge or anal margin, which is hair bearing. Tumors arising in the transitional zone and the pecten are regarded as tumors of the anal canal. Those arising in the hair-bearing perianal skin are called tumors of the anal margin.

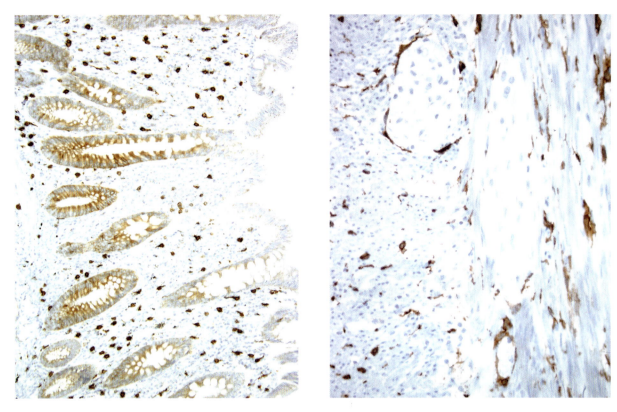

Figure 1-24

NORMAL APPENDIX: CD117/KIT IMMUNOHISTOCHEMICAL STAIN

Left: Scattered mast cells are entirely normal. The mucosa in this field is indistinguishable from colorectal mucosa.

Right: The muscularis propria contains abundant Cajal cells, similar to the colon. In this field, they are in intimate association with Auerbach plexus.

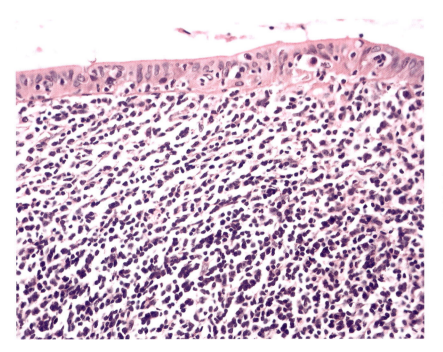

Figure 1-25

NORMAL APPENDIX

This epithelium over a lymphoid aggregate contains numerous lymphocytes actively communicating with the M cells to interface with the gut immune system.

The anal musculature consists an internal anal sphincter, an external anal sphincter, and the levator ani. The internal sphincter is composed of smooth muscle that is a continuation and modification of the circular muscle of the rectum. The external anal sphincter surrounds the internal sphincter and is composed of skeletal muscle with subcutaneous, superficial, and deep portions. The subcutaneous portion is immediately related to the perianal skin and the most external parts of the anal canal; the superficial portion extends around to reinforce the internal sphincter on all sides; and the deep part runs into the levator ani muscles, which form the pelvic floor and are attached to the lateral pelvic walls. Part of levator ani is a sling of muscle called the puborectalis, which contracts to cause forward angulation of the rectum, helping to maintain continence. This muscle is tethered posteriorly by the anococcygeal ligament and anteriorly ends on the perineal body.

The innervation of the internal sphincter consists of autonomic sympathetic nerves arising from the upper two or three spinal nerves that synapse in the inferior mesenteric ganglion, and parasympathetic fibers from the sacral spinal cord that synapse in the myenteric plexus above the dentate line. The parasympathetic fibers create the emptying reflex. The external sphincter is somatically innervated by the inferior hemorrhoidal nerve, branches of the fourth sacral nerve, and the pudendal nerves. The mucosa of the pecten is supplied by somatic sensory nerves and is highly sensitive to touch and pain.

The blood supply of the upper part of the anal canal derives from the inferior mesenteric artery via the superior rectal artery, which bifurcates on the posterior surface of the rectum, each branch passing laterally (the lateral rectal arteries), piercing the muscle at several sites to enter the submucosa down to the level of the columns of Morgagni. The middle sacral artery arises from the posterior wall of the aorta immediately above its bifurcation and supplies a branch to the posterior rectal wall. The distal anal vasculature is from the internal pudendal arteries, which divide into the inferior rectal artery and several other branches that supply the sphincter muscles and then the mucosa. These anastomose with branches from the lateral rectal, gluteal, and perineal arteries.

There are two major venous plexi, the internal and external, which communicate with each other across the dentate line. The internal plexus is immediately above the dentate line. Both internal and external venous plexi are submucosal. They can become engorged and give rise to hemorrhoids.

The greatest concentration of veins is immediately above the dentate line in the columns of Morgagni, where they are modified into three specialized vascular anal cushions that bulge into the anal canal; these may enlarge and prolapse to give rise to hemorrhoids. The external hemorrhoidal plexus is submucosal and drains through the inferior and middle hemorrhoidal veins back into the internal pudendal veins, and then into the internal iliac veins and vena cava. Tumors of the anal canal are thus more prone to systemic metastases than their rectal counterparts. In addition, communication between the internal and external hemorrhoidal plexuses form an anastomosis between the portal and systemic venous systems, so that hemorrhoidal bleeding may be a reflection of portal hypertension.

The lymphatic drainage from the pecten is primarily to the inguinal lymph nodes and then to the iliac nodes. Above the dentate line, lymphatic vessels go both to the internal iliac nodes and the inferior mesenteric nodes, the latter via the lateral (perirectal) and superior rectal artery groups of nodes. Tumors of the anal canal, therefore, always require careful observation of these nodes. Fortunately, the inguinal nodes are superficial and therefore accessible to fine needle aspiration or excision biopsy should they be considered to be pathologically enlarged.

Histology

The mucosa of the anus is roughly divided into three regions based on the type of epithelium; there is striking variation, however, in the proportion and locations of these epithelial types. Proximally, the anal epithelium is similar to the columnar epithelium of the rectum, with crypts lined mostly by goblet cells. Most distally, the anal epithelium consists of nonkeratinizing stratified squamous epithelium, which becomes keratinized skin with adnexal structures distal to the anal verge. The transition from columnar and squamous epithelia, usually located in the region

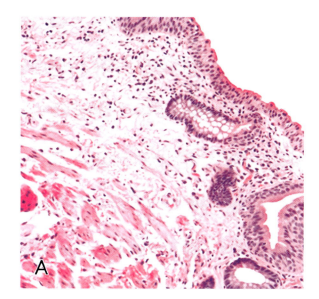

Figure 1-26

ANAL TRANSITIONAL MUCOSA

A: There are pockets with goblet cells of colorectal-type mucosa adjoining epithelium reminiscent of urothelial epithelium.

B: The epithelium has features of both squamous and columnar epithelium.

C: At high magnification, the similarity to urothelial epithelium is striking.

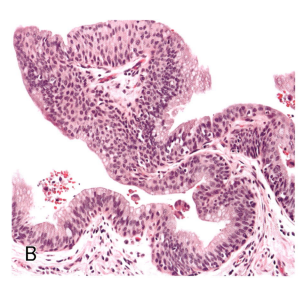

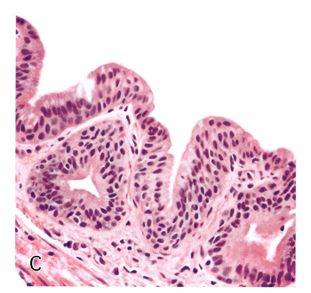

of the dentate line, is highly variable between individuals. In some persons, the columnar rectal epithelium is located directly adjacent to stratified squamous epithelium, with little if any intervening transitional epithelium. In other cases, the columnar and squamous epithelia are separated by a transitional epithelium (fig. 1-26) consisting of four to nine layers of stratified cuboidal cells that are neither squamous nor columnar (with a similar morphology to the epithelium of the urinary bladder).

The nonkeratinizing squamous epithelium of the pectin has short, thick dermal papillae without skin appendages. Langerhans cells,

Merkel cells, and melanocytes can be found, particularly more distally. The perianal skin is keratinizing, with a granular layer, and has abundant hair follicles/skin appendages. The anal glands (fig. 1-27) are often within the internal sphincter muscle at the level of the dentate line. If immunolabeling is performed, they express CK7 but not CK20. They are tubular mucous glands that empty behind the cusps of the anal valves through anal ducts lined by epithelium, identical to that of the anal transition zone, although scattered goblet cells can be found. These glands are typically surrounded by lymphocytes and plasma cells.

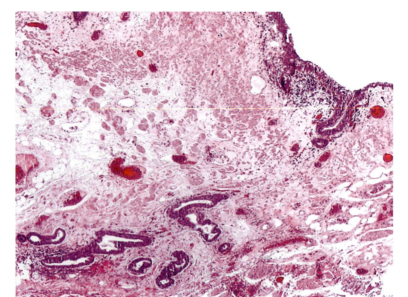

Figure 1-27

ANAL GLANDS AND DUCTS

These glands are seen within muscle (left), opening onto the lumen at the right of the field.

REFERENCES

1. King SL, Dekaney CM. Small intestinal stem cells. Curr Opin Gastroenterol 2013;29:140-145.

2. Cocco AE, Dohrmann MJ, Hendrix TR. Reconstruction of normal jejunal biopsies: three-dimensional histology. Gastroenterology 1966;51:24-31.

3. Gebert A, Rothkotter HJ, Pabst R. M cells in Peyer's patches of the intestine. Int Rev Cytol 1996;167:91-159.

4. Groisman GM, Amar M, Livne E. CD10: a valuable tool for the light microscopic diagnosis of microvillous inclusion disease (familial microvillous atrophy). Am J Surg Pathol 2002;26:902-907.

5. Ranganathan S, Schmitt LA, Sindhi R. Tufting enteropathy revisited: the utility of MOC31 (EpCAM) immunohistochemistry in diagnosis. Am J Surg Pathol 2014;38:265-272.

6. Doyle LA, Sepehr GJ, Hamilton MJ, Akin C, Castells MC, Hornick JL. A clinicopathologic study of 24 cases of systemic mastocytosis involving the gastrointestinal tract and assessment of mucosal mast cell density in irritable bowel syndrome and asymptomatic patients. Am J Surg Pathol 2014;38:832-843.

7. Montgomery EA, Popek EJ. Intussusception, adenovirus, and children: a brief reaffirmation. Hum Pathol 1994;25:169-174.

8. Amin M, Edge S, Greene F, et al. AJCC Cancer Staging Manual, 8th ed. Switzerland: Springer International Publishing; 2017.

9. Bejarano PA, Aranda-Michel J, Fenoglio-Preiser C. Histochemical and immunohistochemical characterization of foamy histiocytes (muciphages and xanthelasma) of the rectum. Am J Surg Pathol 2000;24:1009-1015.

10. Fenger C. The anal transitional zone. Acta Pathol Microbiol Immunol Scand Suppl 1987;289:1-42.

2 HAMARTOMATOUS POLYPS, HETEROTOPIAS, UNCLASSIFIED POLYPS, AND TUMOR-LIKE LESIONS

BRUNNER GLAND POLYPS

Definition. A *Brunner gland polyp* is a mass-producing lesion consisting of glands that differentiate along the lines of duodenal submucosal glands. Such lesions are most commonly hyperplastic or hamartomatous (1), but some are neoplastic (adenomas and carcinomas). Since it may be difficult to determine whether the process is hyperplastic, hamartomatous, or neoplastic, the noncommittal term Brunner gland polyp is used. Some authors have also used the term *Brunner gland proliferating lesions* (1) for these polyps. Most are benign and, in some cases, the proliferation of Brunner glands is simply a reparative phenomenon that coexists with gastric mucin cell metaplasia and is part of so-called nodular duodenitis.

General Features. Since the Brunner glands are located in the duodenum, Brunner gland polyps arise in the duodenum. They are native to the submucosa but often extend into the mucosa, presumably due to cycles of damage and repair. Sometimes the polyps coalesce into sessile or nodular lesions, which account for 5 to 10 percent of duodenal masses (2).

Clinical Features. Most patients are asymptomatic and the polyps are detected during upper endoscopy performed for another indication. Occasionally, however, these tumors become large and may present clinically as pancreatic carcinoma because they result in obstruction and a mass lesion detected on imaging studies. In one series (1), the median age of patients with Brunner gland lesions was about 50 years, but a few young adults were included. Most lesions were found in the duodenal bulb. The majority of patients had no symptoms; melena, abdominal pain, nausea, and dyspepsia were noted in a minority. In this study, lesions regarded as Brunner gland hamartomas were more common in women in contrast to a male predominance for Brunner gland hyperplasia, but the histo-logic overlap in the described lesions casts some doubt on whether there was a clear separation between the two types.

The occasional Brunner gland lesions that are believed to be truly neoplastic (adenomas and adenocarcinomas) tend to be reported as single case reports rather than large series. The age range of patients with Brunner gland adenocarcinoma culled from the literature (3–12) was 54 to 85 years, with a median of 70 years, far older than the median age of 50 for apparently non-neoplastic lesions. Assessment of adenomas is difficult because some lesions reported as Brunner gland adenomas are non-neoplastic or pyloric gland adenomas (13–15), and Brunner gland adenomas are difficult to distinguish, so reported cases may be heterogeneous.

Gross Findings. Brunner gland lesions are unremarkable macroscopically (fig. 2-1). They are often recognized as submucosal-based tumors. The polyp is a firm, whitish, fairly well-marginated tumor on cut surface.

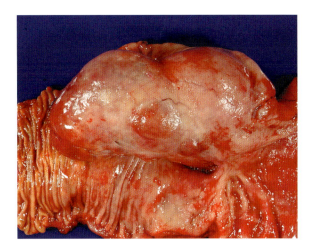

Figure 2-1

BRUNNER GLAND POLYP

The overlying duodenal mucosa is eroded but largely intact. This example resulted in obstruction that required resection.

21

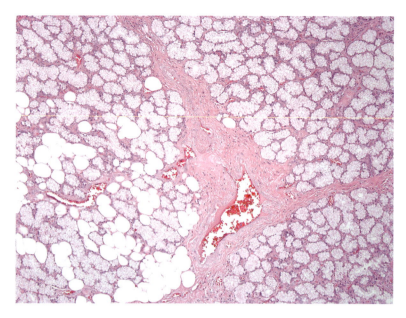

Figure 2-2

BRUNNER GLAND HAMARTOMA

The criteria used to separate hamartoma, hyperplasia, and adenoma are not entirely clear, but the presence of adipose tissue in this lesion and the thick bands of smooth muscle would lead some to regard it as a hamartoma.

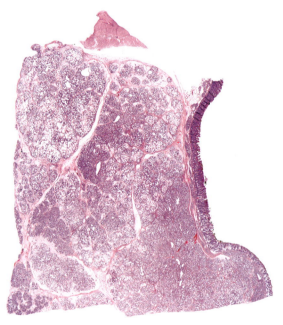

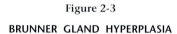

Figure 2-3

BRUNNER GLAND HYPERPLASIA

This lobulated lesion lacks adipose tissue and the thick bands of smooth muscle noted in figure 2-2. The overlying small bowel mucosa appears reactive and the lobules of the overlying Brunner glands are far smaller.

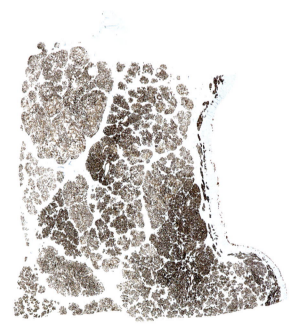

Figure 2-4

BRUNNER GLAND HYPERPLASIA

Both the markedly hyperplastic glands as well as the normal ones express MUC6.

Microscopic Findings. Lesions regarded as hamartomas show Brunner glands, large ducts, thick smooth muscle bundles, and admixed adipose tissue (fig. 2-2). Hyperplasias are believed to have predominantly Brunner glands with negligible amounts of the other components (figs. 2-3, 2-4) (1). Either type of lesion can display overlying gastric mucin cell metaplasia.

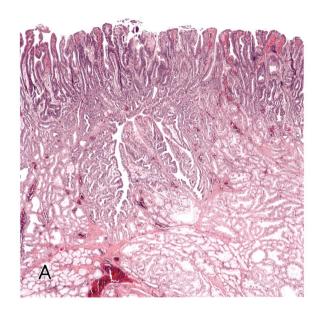

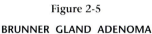

Figure 2-5

BRUNNER GLAND ADENOMA

A: The glands at the bottom left of the field appear hyperplastic but those in the center and to the right appear to be composed of cells with larger nuclei.

B: High magnification shows the glands to the right of the field have enlarged nuclei and a cribriform appearance. The nuclei are round and have lost their polarity, features of high-grade dysplasia.

C: A Ki-67 stain shows a zone of intensified proliferation.

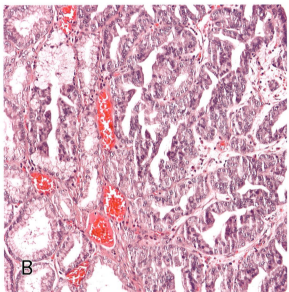

Tumors classified as adenomas (figs. 2-5, 2-6) have larger nuclei than those associated with hyperplasias and hamartomas, but, it may be impossible to be certain whether a lesion is a hamartoma, a hyperplastic lesion, or an adenoma. Lesions reported as carcinomas and adenomas adjoining Brunner glands (8,16–18) have features that overlap morphologically, immunohistochemically, and genetically with pyloric gland adenomas (14,15).

Immunohistochemical Findings. Brunner glands express MUC6, so it is not surprising that lesions showing Brunner gland differentia-

tion also express MUC6 (figs. 2-4, 2-6C). MUC5 is seen in areas of gastric foveolar metaplasia overlying Brunner gland lesions but can also be found in the Brunner gland lesions themselves, regardless of the apparent biologic potential. Lesions believed to be malignant sometimes show aberrant p53 expression.

Molecular Genetic Findings. The molecular profile of Brunner gland lesions is not well understood. Loss of *Lrig* has been reported to trigger the production of duodenal adenomas that show gastric-type differentiation (18). Activating *GNAS* and *KRAS* mutations have been

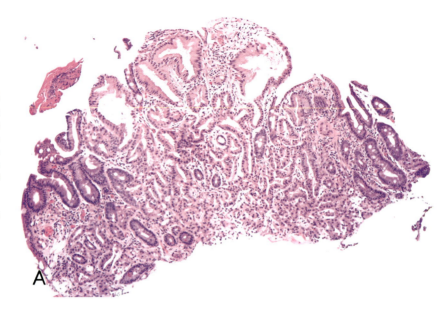

Figure 2-6

BRUNNER GLAND CARCINOMA

A: The glands have a complex architecture. The lack of surface involvement supports an interpretation of Brunner gland carcinoma over a lesion arising in a pyloric gland adenoma, but the distinction is not always clear.

B: High magnification image.

C: The lesion is stained with MUC6.

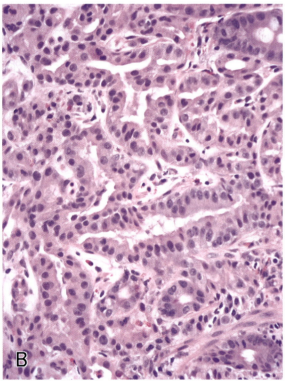

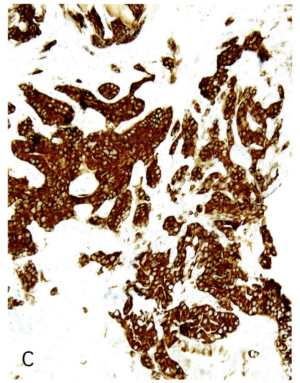

reported in gastric foveolar metaplasia, gastric heterotopia, and adenocarcinoma in the duodenum (16), but the malignant lesions reported were not illustrated in the study. The presence of *GNAS* mutations in such duodenal lesions is of interest, since *GNAS* mutations are characteristic of pyloric gland adenomas. As such,

at least some Brunner gland adenocarcinomas reported in the literature may be the same as neoplasms regarded as duodenal pyloric gland adenomas (15).

Differential Diagnosis. The entities in the clinical differential diagnosis of Brunner gland lesions include intestinal-type tubular adenomas,

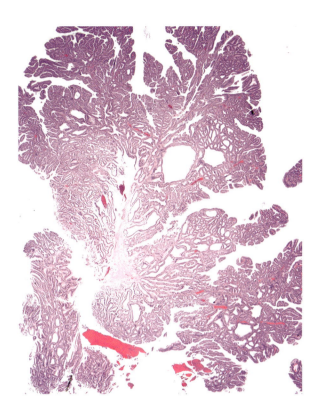
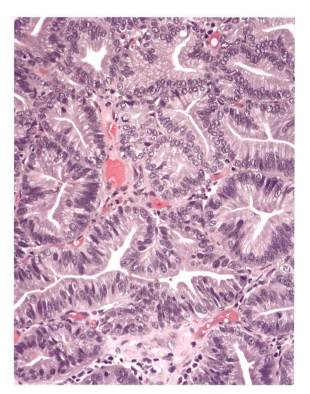

Figure 2-7

PYLORIC GLAND ADENOMA

Left: The tumor appears similar to Brunner gland lesions but is composed of closely packed tubules with metachromatic ground-glass cytoplasm and the lesion involves the surface.

Right: The cytoplasm has a ground glass appearance and the rounded nuclei are arranged in a monolayer along the base of the cells.

gastrointestinal stromal tumors of the duodenum, and ampullary carcinomas. The pathologic differential diagnosis includes hamartomas, hyperplasias, and adenomas. In cases that are clearly neoplastic, pancreatobiliary lesions need to be differentiated from primary duodenal ones. Brunner gland neoplasms are submucosal and extend into the lamina propria and muscularis propria, whereas pancreatobiliary carcinomas appear more "bottom heavy."

As suggested above, the distinction between Brunner gland neoplasms and pyloric gland neoplasms is unclear. The latter consist of tightly packed, round tubules featuring cells with round, basally oriented nuclei and ground-glass cytoplasm; they co-label with MUC6 and MUC5 (fig. 2-7). Standard intestinal-type adenomas contain goblet cells and involve the surface epithelium.

Treatment and Prognosis. Most cases are managed by endoscopic polypectomy/resec-tion, but some large lesions can result in obstruction and require surgery. Those that appear malignant on biopsies should be resected.

Most Brunner gland polyps are benign. The rare reported carcinomas have generally been associated with a favorable outcome following resection.

CRONKHITE-CANADA POLYPOSIS

Definition. *Cronkhite-Canada syndrome* (CCS) is a rare protein-losing gastroenterocolopathy typically characterized by diffuse gastrointestinal polyposis and characteristic ectodermal changes, such as hair loss, skin pigmentation, and nail dystrophy (onycholysis) (19). The latter changes stem from persistent protein loss.

General Features. A detailed review of the literature concerning this lesion has been published by Slavik (20). Although most recent studies favor an autoimmune etiology, the precise cause of CCS remains unknown (20). Patients

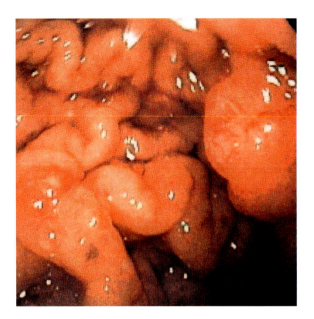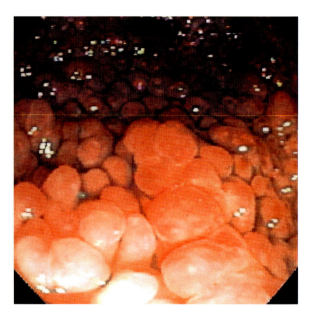

Figure 2-8

CRONKHITE-CANADA SYNDROME

Left: These polyps carpet the small bowel.
Right: An endoscopic image of the right colon.

acquire mucus-producing polyps throughout their tubular gastrointestinal tract (except the esophagus), which result in a syndrome of severe protein loss.

Clinical Features. More than 80 percent of patients are diagnosed at age 50 years or older; in other words, the disease is acquired rather than congenital. As above, it is believed to be an immunologic condition but the antigenic trigger remains undiscovered. Typically, the polyposis in CCS is diffuse throughout the entire gastrointestinal tract, sparing only the esophagus.

The most common presenting symptoms are diarrhea, weight loss, nausea, vomiting, hypogeusia, and anorexia. Paraesthesias, seizures, and tetany, apparently related to electrolyte abnormalities, have also been reported. Mucoid diarrhea results in the depletion of the patient's protein reserves such that the patient loses his (usually) hair and nails. Nail dystrophy, with thinning, splitting, and separation from the nailbeds, is typical. Both scalp and body hair alopecia may be present. Diffuse hyperpigmentation of the skin, manifested by light to dark brown macular lesions, is seen most frequently on the extremities, face, palms, soles, and neck. Microscopic examination of biopsied skin reveals abnormally increased melanin deposition, with or without increased melanocyte proliferation.

Gross Findings. The polyps are broad based and sessile, and are a few millimeters to 1.5 cm in size. There is either diffuse mucosal thickening or polyposis (fig. 2-8). In gastric disease, the presence of diffuse disease can suggest malignancy (lymphoma or linitis plastica) or gastric infection rather than CCS polyposis (21).

Microscopic Findings. Microscopically, the polyps of CCS show marked epithelial hyperplasia with cystically dilated glands, abundant stromal edema, and a predominantly mononuclear inflammatory infiltrate (fig. 2-9). Eosinophils may be prominent.

Differential Diagnosis. The differential diagnosis is primarily with hamartomatous polyposis syndromes as described below. Especially in the stomach, CCS polyps may be difficult to discriminate from hyperplastic, juvenile or Peutz-Jeghers polyps, and those in the small bowel and colon also resemble juvenile polyps (22). Of key diagnostic importance for this differential diagnosis is the fact that the intervening mucosa between polyps in CCS is also affected and shows marked lamina propria edema, an inflammatory infiltrate, and gland distortion, which distinguish

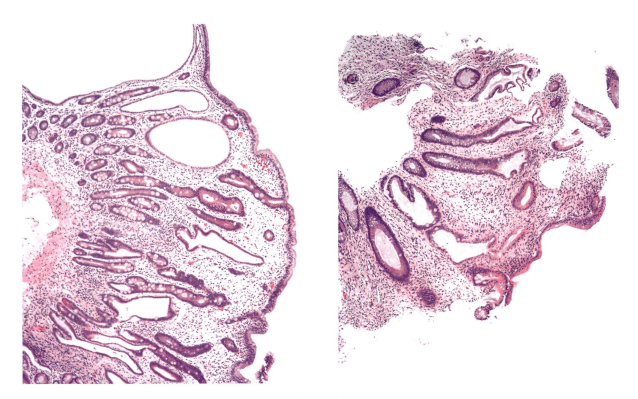

Figure 2-9

CRONKHITE-CANADA SYNDROME

Left: The appearance of this small bowel polyp is nonspecific and overlaps with that of a juvenile polyp. Diagnosing the syndrome requires correlation with the clinical features and endoscopic appearance.

Right: The colon biopsy shows nonspecific features as well.

the polyps from those in Peutz-Jeghers syndrome and juvenile polyposis in which the mucosa is normal (20,22). In addition, correlation with clinical manifestations, in particular the typical ectodermal changes in CCS, is key to a correct diagnosis (22). For example, patients with juvenile polyposis or Peutz-Jeghers syndrome are generally not clinically ill with diarrhea and protein loss. They also tend to present at a younger age than those with CCS since CCS is acquired. Gastric CCS has overlap with Ménétrier disease, but the latter affects the gastric body and not the entire gastrointestinal tract.

Treatment and Prognosis. There is no standard therapy but limited success has been reported with antibiotics, steroids, and partial gastrectomy. The prognosis is poor. Less than 5 percent of patients have complete remission and the 5-year mortality rate of 55 percent is due primarily to gastrointestinal bleeding, sepsis, and congestive heart failure. Electrolyte abnormalities, dehydration, protein-losing

enteropathy, and other nutritional deficiencies due to malabsorption complicate the course of the disease. CCS patients are prone to recurrent infections, but it is not known whether this is related to malnutrition or is a primary immunologic deficiency.

The polyps in CCS are non-neoplastic but coexisting adenomas and adenocarcinomas have been reported. Patients may be at increased risk of colorectal cancer, possibly secondary to chronic mucosal inflammation. Assessment of the gastrointestinal cancer risk is limited by the rarity of this syndrome and it remains inconclusive whether CCS patients are truly at increased risk of gastrointestinal malignancy (20).

ENDOMETRIOSIS INVOLVING THE INTESTINES

Definition. *Endometriosis* is an estrogen-dependent gynecologic condition in which patients have ectopic endometrial tissue. This tissue is often associated with inflammation and results in

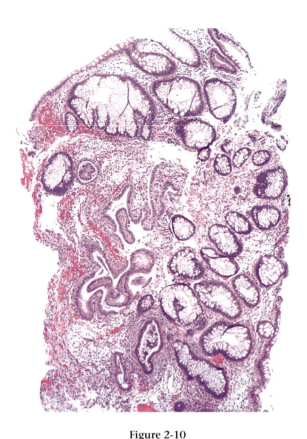

Figure 2-10

ENDOMETRIOSIS

This lesion presented as a rectal polyp. Endometrial glands and stroma are present in the center of the image.

was made at the time of a bowel biopsy or resection. These women presented with bowel obstruction or abdominal pain and 7 percent had fecal blood. The clinical diagnoses include diverticulitis, appendicitis, Crohn disease, tubo-ovarian abscess, irritable bowel syndrome, carcinoma, and lymphoma (27). Most cases of intestinal endometriosis affect the sigmoid colon or rectum, followed by the ileocecum. The incidence of appendiceal involvement is not clear from available reports.

Gross Findings. Most examples of intestinal endometriosis show bowel wall thickening, strictures, or ulceration. Only occasionally are cysts containing degenerating blood (so-called chocolate cysts) identified macroscopically.

Microscopic Findings. Endometriosis involving the intestines has the same appearance as that elsewhere in the body, but the diagnosis of lesions in the gastrointestinal tract requires awareness of the possibility of encountering it. Intestinal endometriosis consists of endometrial glands and endometrial-type stroma in varying proportions (figs. 2-10–2-12). Nevertheless, it is a challenge to diagnose in the intestines because only about two thirds of cases show involvement of the lamina propria or submucosa, so that mucosal biopsies may not be diagnostic.

Since mucosal disease is accompanied by features of chronic injury (architectural distortion, dense lymphoplasmacytic infiltrates, pyloric metaplasia of the ileum) and fissures, endometriosis can mimic inflammatory bowel disease histologically (27). Additionally, mucosal prolapse, ischemic changes, and ulceration may be present. Changes to the muscularis propria include marked concentric smooth muscle hyperplasia and hypertrophy, neuronal hypertrophy and hyperplasia, and fibrosis of the muscularis propria with serositis (27). In pregnant patients, decidualization of the lesion can be present (fig. 2-13).

An important pitfall is the occasional presence of intestinal metaplasia in endometriosis itself (figs. 2-14, 2-15), a phenomenon that has been described in appendiceal and cecal endometriosis (28). In this form of endometriosis, the epithelium of the intestinalized glands shows goblet cells and loses the expression of hormone receptors (estrogen receptor and progesterone receptor). The importance of this

severe and chronic pain as well as infertility (23). The term *bowel endometriosis* is used to describe endometriosis in the intestinal subserosa to the mucosa; *peritoneal endometriosis* is endometriosis restricted to the bowel serosa.

General Features. Endometriosis is believed to affect about 5.5 million women in the United States (23). Patients are usually diagnosed during a laparoscopic procedure. The diagnosis requires the presence of endometrial glands and stroma on biopsies. The condition was believed to result from "retrograde menstruation" but it is now apparent that mutations in several genes can be detected (24). Between 15 and 37 percent of patients with endometriosis are estimated to have intestinal involvement (25,26).

Clinical Features. In a consecutive series of 100 patients with intestinal endometriosis (25), most (73 percent) had a prior clinical history of endometriosis; for the rest, the diagnosis

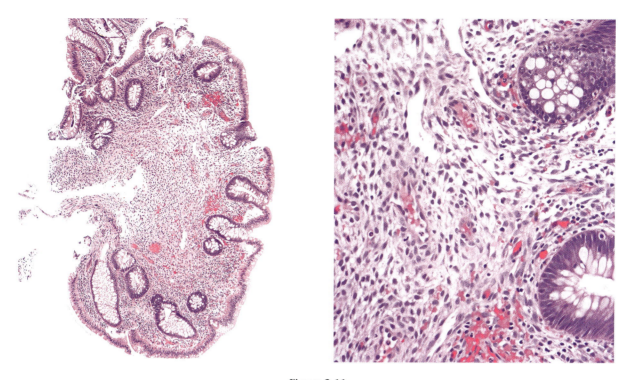

Figure 2-11

ENDOMETRIOSIS

Left: The lack of glands in this case suggests a sarcoma.
Right: At high magnification, reactive changes are seen in the overlying colonic mucosa.

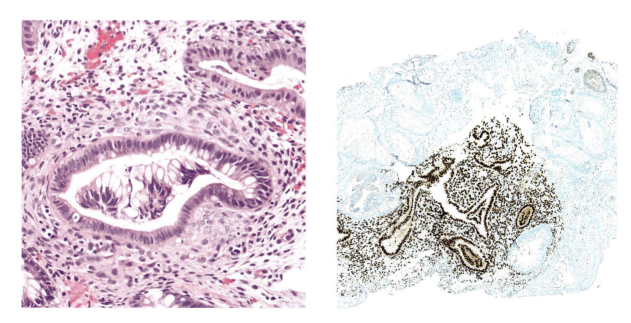

Figure 2-12

ENDOMETRIOSIS

Left: Both endometrial glands and stroma are seen. Some rectal epithelium has been artifactually pressed into the lumen of the endometrial gland in the center of the field.
Right: This is an estrogen receptor immunostain from the polyp shown in figure 2-10.

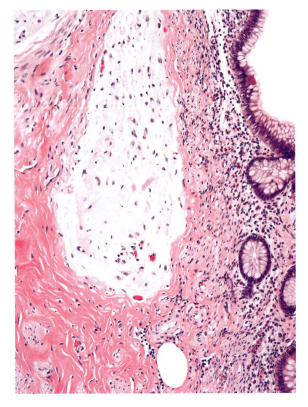

Figure 2-13

ENDOMETRIOSIS

This example has become decidualized in a pregnant patient. There are no visible glands in this field.

phenomenon is that it can mimic appendiceal mucinous neoplasms.

Immunohistochemical Findings. As in endometriosis in general, intestinal endometriosis expresses hormone receptors (estrogen and progesterone receptors) and the stroma shows CD10 immunolabeling.

Differential Diagnosis. Endometriosis can easily mimic neoplasms when it is encountered in the intestines, especially on biopsies, since they are often taken based on the presence of a mass. If the stroma is not readily identified and the endometrial glands are closely packed, the appearance overlaps with that of colorectal adenoma. Detecting the stroma is key. If the stroma is present without the endometrial-type glands, however, the appearance is readily mistaken for sarcoma. Recutting sections to search for glands and immunolabeling for hormone receptors help resolve this issue.

If intestinal metaplasia is encountered in appendiceal examples, it is easily confused with low-grade appendiceal mucinous neoplasms, a concern resolved by searching for the stroma, which can be subtle. Often, typical endometriosis is found in the same appendectomy specimen, a further clue to the correct diagnosis.

Treatment and Prognosis. The treatment for intestinal endometriosis mirrors that for endometriosis in general, namely, medical and surgical. The medical therapies include gonadotropin-releasing hormone analogues, progestins, combined oral contraceptive pills, synthetic androgens (danazol), and aromatase inhibitors. Surgical treatment includes nodulectomies for lesions involving the muscularis propria or surgical resections. Which of these is best is unclear but most surgical colleagues do not advise removal of small lesions restricted to the serosa. Nevertheless, patients with bowel endometriosis tend to have improvement of symptoms following surgery (27,29).

GASTRIC HETEROTOPIA, PANCREATIC HETEROTOPIA, AND MECKEL DIVERTICULA

With the exception of *Meckel diverticula*, these developmental lesions are generally incidental findings encountered as nodules during endoscopy for other reasons; sometimes, however, they produce clinically significant lesions. *Pancreatic heterotopia,* especially in the gastric antrum in children, can result in gastric outlet obstruction (30), and there are rare examples of pancreatic-type carcinomas that arise in association with pancreatic heterotopia (31–33). *Gastric heterotopia* may present as incidental colorectal polyps detected during screening colonoscopy, an incidental finding that we have termed "outlet patch" (in jest) to underscore the distinction from the so-called inlet patch of the esophagus, which consists of residual gastric tissue that has remained during the development of the esophagus. Some examples of gastric heterotopia in both the small and large bowel are symptomatic, depending on the size and location (34–37).

Grossly, pancreatic heterotopia tends to produce a submucosal mass whereas gastric heterotopia produces an eroded mucosal mass or polyp (figs. 2-16, 2-17). Microscopically these heterotopias have the same appearance as

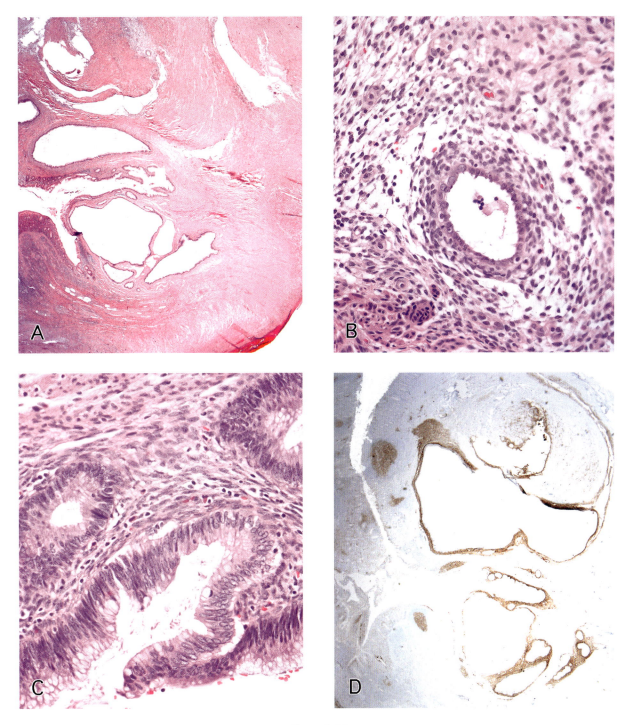

Figure 2-14

**APPENDICEAL ENDOMETRIOSIS WITH INTESTINAL METAPLASIA
MIMICKING LOW-GRADE APPENDICEAL MUCINOUS NEOPLASM**

A: At low magnification, typical endometriosis is seen on the top. The intestinalized component below it appears similar to an appendiceal mucinous neoplasm.

B: The typical endometriosis component.

C: The part with intestinal metaplasia. The diagnostic clue is the presence of endometrial stroma.

D: A CD10 stain highlights the endometrial stroma that forms a cuff around the endometriotic glands.

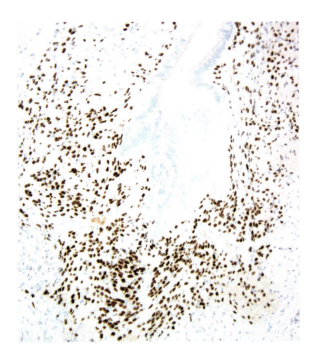

Figure 2-15

APPENDICEAL ENDOMETRIOSIS WITH INTESTINAL METAPLASIA MIMICKING LOW-GRADE APPENDICEAL MUCINOUS NEOPLASM

An estrogen receptor stain labels the endometrial stroma but not the glands that have undergone intestinal metaplasia.

pancreatic or gastric tissue (fig. 2-18), with the full complement of pancreatic acini and islets in the case of pancreatic heterotopia and fully developed oxyntic or antral-type mucosa in the case of gastric heterotopia. Oxyntic mucosa may become eroded since it produces acid, or result in erosions in the adjoining intestinal tissue.

Meckel Diverticula

Meckel diverticula are likely to come to clinical attention (38,39). They are believed to be the most common congenital anomaly of the gastrointestinal tract (39,40), although it is impossible to know the incidence of small foci of gastric and pancreatic heterotopia since most examples are microscopic findings of no clinical relevance. Meckel diverticula are true diverticula that encompass all the layers of the bowel wall, distinct from the pseudodiverticula that arise in the sigmoid colon and generally lack muscularis propria.

Most Meckel diverticula are asymptomatic; the lifetime risk for complications is about 5 percent. The so-called rules of 2 for these lesions state that the incidence of these lesions is about 2 percent, the diverticula themselves measure about 2 inches, they are usually found within 2 feet proximal to the ileocecal junction in the

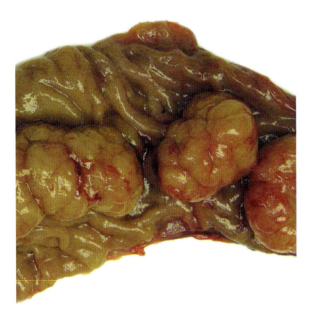

Figure 2-16

PANCREATIC HETEROTOPIA

This example involves the small bowel and is coated by normal intestinal mucosa.

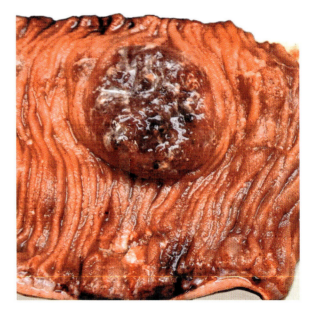

Figure 2-17

GASTRIC HETEROTOPIA

This lesion presented as a hemorrhagic rectal polyp. A resection was performed to address local hemorrhage.

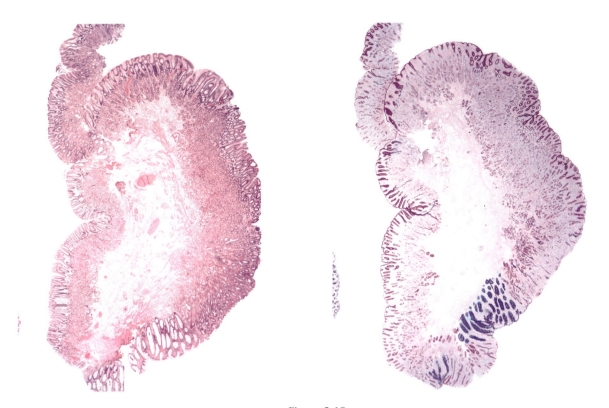

Figure 2-18

GASTRIC HETEROTOPIA

Left: This rectal lesion was treated by polypectomy. The colorectal type mucosa is on the bottom.

Right: With a periodic acid–Schiff (PAS)/alcian blue stain, the blue colorectal mucosa on the bottom contrasts with the pink gastric-type mucosa.

small intestine, and they tend to manifest in patients under 2 years of age (39,41).

Meckel diverticula are remnants of the omphalomesenteric (vitteline) duct which connects the yolk sac with the developing gut. During the process of embryonic development, the midgut returns to the abdominal cavity around the 10th to 12th week of gestation, at which time the omphalomesenteric duct involutes into a slender fibrous band. Failure of complete involution results in the formation of a Meckel diverticulum. In more dramatic failures, an ileo-umbilic fistula can result, and manifest clinically as discharge of feces from the umbilicus.

Meckel diverticula are often asymptomatic and detected during operations for another condition. Some studies report a male predominance in symptomatic cases but there is probably no gender predominance in asymptomatic examples (38,39). Most symptomatic cases present in children under 10 years of age. Presenta-

tions include bleeding per rectum, abdominal pain, obstructive symptoms, and fever.

Plain films are of little value in diagnosing these lesions, but they can be detected on barium studies, ultrasonography, computerized tomography (CT) imaging, or scintigraphy (if there is gastric mucosa). The latter (so-called Meckel scan) revolves around the uptake of ^{99m}Tc-pertechnetate by the mucus-secreting cells of the gastric mucosa, which is often present in Meckel diverticula (42). The sensitivity of this method is 80 to 90 percent in children but lower (closer to 60 percent) in adults.

Macroscopically, specimens consist of outpouched intestine (fig. 2-19), with or without inflammation or neoplasm. The diverticula are generally lined by small intestinal-type mucosa, but about 20 percent are lined, at least in part, by gastric mucosa, about 2 percent by pancreatic tissue, and about 5 percent by both pancreatic and gastric tissue (38). Any type of neoplasm that

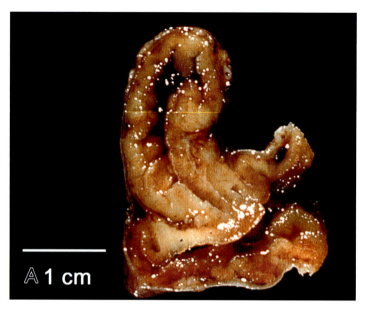

Figure 2-19

MECKEL DIVERTICULUM

A: Luminal hemorrhage is seen.
B: The diverticulum is lined by gastric-type mucosa.
C: Foci of pancreatic-type components are seen.

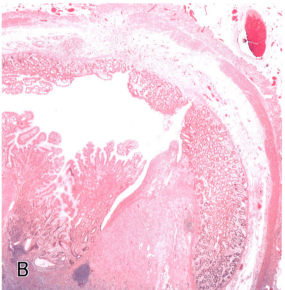

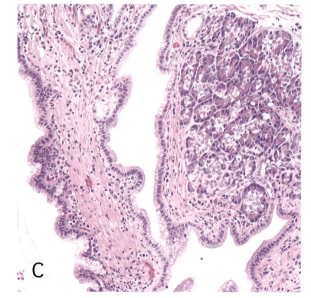

can be encountered in small bowel, pancreas, or stomach, or the muscularis propria thereof, has been reported in association with Meckel diverticula, including carcinomas, endocrine tumors, and gastrointestinal stromal tumors. An example of a gastric-type adenocarcinoma arising in a Meckel diverticulum is shown in figure 2-20.

Complications of Meckel diverticula, in descending order of likelihood, include hemorrhage, intussusception, intestinal obstruction, perforation, strangulation secondary to a diverticular band, diverticulitis, volvulus, hernia, neoplasm, enterolith, and chronic intermittent pain (39). Symptomatic Meckel diverticula are managed by excision.

HAMARTOMATOUS POLYPS

Hamartomatous polyps contain non-neoplastic epithelial and stromal elements. They occur as solitary lesions in otherwise healthy patients, or herald the presence of a heritable polyposis disorder. Although hamartomatous polyps are not considered to represent neoplasms, individuals who have hamartomatous polyposis syndromes are at increased cancer risk compared to the general population.

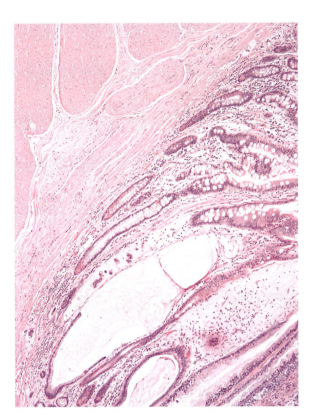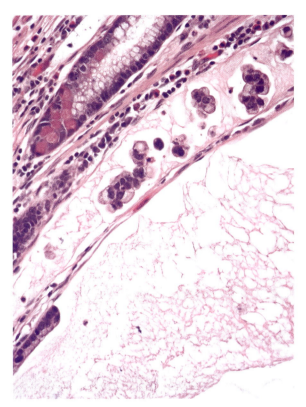

Figure 2-20

MECKEL DIVERTICULUM

Left: A gastric-type adenocarcinoma is arising in a gastric component. Clusters of signet cells are in the center left of the field. There is small intestinal-type mucosa to the left.

Right: High magnification of a signet ring cell gastric-type adenocarcinoma arising in gastric heterotopia within the diverticulum.

Clinical symptoms in adolescence and early adulthood are generally related to the benign complications of the disease, such as bleeding or intussusception; older patients usually have symptoms related to malignancy. In addition to gastrointestinal polyposis, patients with hamartomatous syndromes may have a history of similarly affected family members, extraintestinal disease manifestations, and characteristic germline DNA alterations.

The clinical, pathologic, and molecular criteria are not entirely sensitive or specific. Many patients without a polyposis disorder have solitary polyps that are indistinguishable from those of heritable syndromes, whereas others clearly have a hamartomatous syndrome, but lack a family history of polyposis. Moreover, many patients lack detectable germline mutations. Thus, accurate classification often requires care-

ful correlation between clinical manifestations, pathologic findings, and molecular data.

Juvenile Polyps and Juvenile Polyposis Syndrome

Definition. *Juvenile polyps* develop sporadically or in association with *juvenile polyposis syndrome*. Juvenile polyposis syndrome is a phenotypically heterogeneous, autosomal dominant heritable disorder affecting 1/100,000-160,000 persons in the United States. The diagnostic criteria include: 1) three or more colorectal juvenile polyps, 2) any number of extracolonic juvenile polyps, or 3) any number of juvenile polyps in a patients with a family history of the syndrome (43).

Clinical Features. Sporadic juvenile polyps affect 1 to 2 percent of children and adolescents, but can, rarely, affect adults; detection of one or two colorectal lesions does not necessarily imply the presence of a heritable disorder. Sporadic lesions only develop in the colorectum and more than 50 percent are confined to the rectum (44,45). Pedunculated polyps readily auto-amputate and may be passed in the stool. Most signs and symptoms are related to gastrointestinal bleeding (e.g., occult blood loss, hematochezia, anemia), although occasional patients present with symptoms related to mucosal prolapse.

Infantile juvenile polyposis is the least common form of juvenile polyposis and typically occurs in patients without a family history. Patients present in infancy or early childhood with life-threatening gastrointestinal bleeding, diarrhea, malnutrition, and protein-losing enteropathy (46). Most patients (98 percent) have multiple polyps of the colorectum, whereas hamartomas of the stomach, jejunum and ileum, and duodenum are less common, occurring in 14, 7, and 7 percent of patients, respectively (47).

Congenital abnormalities are seen in 15 to 20 percent of patients with juvenile polyposis. These include cardiac abnormalities, cleft lip and cleft palate, polydactyly, intestinal malrotation, and pulmonary arteriovenous malformations (48,49). Some patients have hereditary hemorrhagic telangiectasia with vascular malformations affecting multiple organs; this combination has been described as *juvenile polyposis syndrome-hereditary hemorrhagic telangiectasia* (50).

Gross Findings. Juvenile polyps are pedunculated or sessile, mucosa-based lesions with a smooth, friable surface. Sporadic colorectal polyps often display an erythematous, ulcerated surface with adherent fibrin, which appears as a white exudate (fig. 2-21). They have a sponge-like cut surface with numerous cysts, reflecting the presence of markedly dilated crypts. Juvenile polyps that occur in patients with juvenile polyposis syndrome may show these classic features or have a multinodular, mulberry-like appearance (fig. 2-22). The latter are termed atypical, or epithelial, juvenile polyps, as described below. Gastric polyposis can be severe, resulting in the marked expansion of rugal folds by confluent, sessile polyps (fig. 2-23).

Microscopic Findings. Sporadic juvenile polyps classically contain dilated crypts enmeshed in edematous and inflamed lamina propria (fig. 2-24). They are frequently ulcerated and display

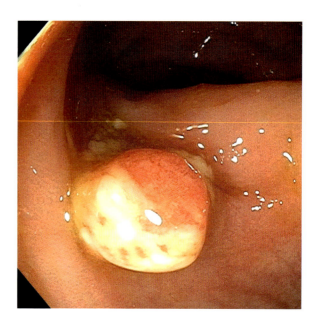

Figure 2-21

SPORADIC JUVENILE POLYP

This sessile polyp has a smooth, round surface, with white exudate and hemorrhage reflecting an erosion.

numerous delicate capillaries intimately associated with an eosinophil-rich, mixed inflammatory cell infiltrate (fig. 2-25). Occasional polyps contain ganglion cells that are arranged singly or in small clusters; they are unassociated with a spindle cell component.

Syndromic juvenile polyps may be histologically indistinguishable from sporadic juvenile polyps, although the former tend to show a lesser degree of crypt dilatation and lamina propria edema (fig. 2-26). Early syndromic polyps may be difficult to recognize because they show only mild crypt dilation, with increased cellularity in the lamina propria. Epithelial, or atypical, juvenile polyps of the colorectum contain less stroma, with crowded, irregularly shaped crypts, and may show low- or high-grade dysplasia; they tend to be more common among patients with *SMAD4* mutations (fig. 2-27).

Adenocarcinomas that develop in juvenile polyposis syndrome can arise from dysplastic foci in hamartomatous polyps or from adenomatous polyps of tubular or villous type (51,52). Gastric polyps are indistinguishable from sporadic hyperplastic/regenerative polyps; they display striking foveolar hyperplasia with

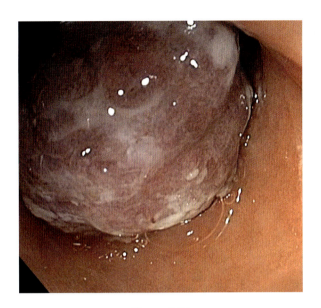

Figure 2-22

SYNDROMIC JUVENILE POLYP

A large polyp has a nodular surface with an inflammatory exudate.

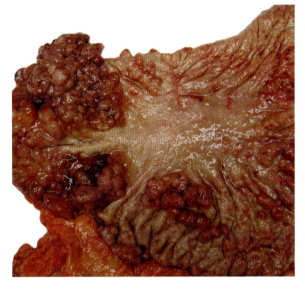

Figure 2-23

JUVENILE POLYPOSIS SYNDROME OF THE STOMACH

Innumerable, erythematous polyps form confluent plaques that stud the mucosal surfaces of the body and antrum.

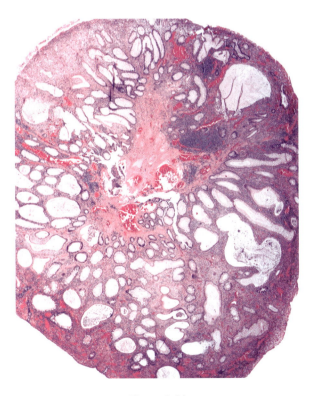

Figure 2-24

SPORADIC JUVENILE POLYP OF THE RECTUM

The polyp has a smooth, round surface and contains cystically dilated crypts. The surface epithelium is eroded and the lamina propria is expanded by granulation tissue.

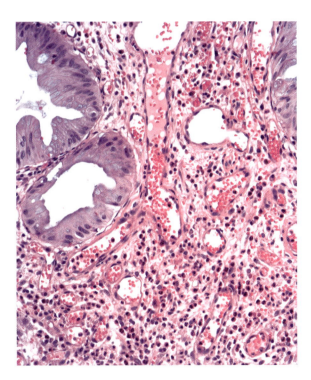

Figure 2-25

SPORADIC JUVENILE POLYP OF THE RECTUM

Numerous thin-walled capillaries are associated with eosinophil-rich inflammation. A few hyperplastic crypts are slightly serrated.

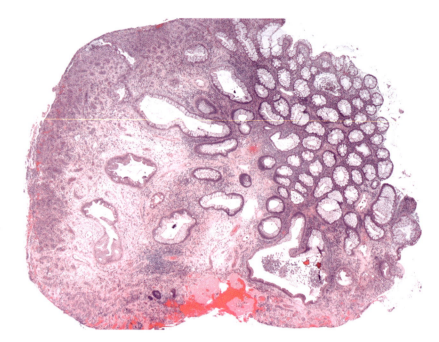

Figure 2-26

SYNDROMIC JUVENILE POLYP OF THE COLON

The polyp contains hyperplastic, slightly dilated crypts associated with inflammation and granulation tissue.

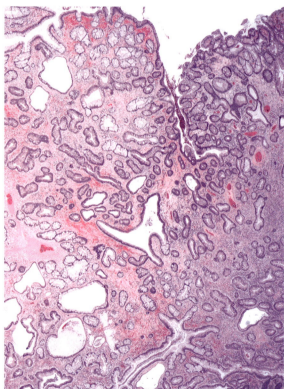
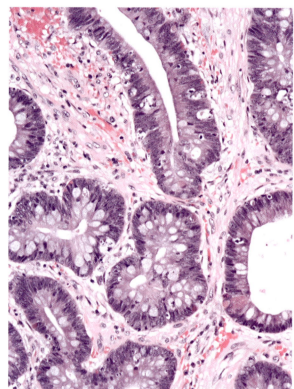

Figure 2-27

EPITHELIAL JUVENILE POLYP OF JUVENILE POLYPOSIS SYNDROME

Left: Scattered dilated crypts are lined by non-neoplastic epithelium and associated with increased numbers of epithelial elements. Some irregularly branching and dilated crypts are lined by low-grade dysplastic epithelium.

Right: At high magnification, enlarged, crowded, hyperchromatic nuclei and scattered apoptotic debris are seen in the neoplastic epithelium.

tortuous or cystic gastric pits, edematous lamina propria, and frequent erosions (fig. 2-28).

Molecular Genetic Findings. Approximately 60 percent of patients with clinically defined juvenile polyposis syndrome have germline abnormalities in the signal transduction pathway initiated by transforming growth factor-β. These are equally represented by alterations in *SMAD4,* located on chromosome 18q21.1, and *BMPR1A* (bone morphogenic protein receptor 1A), located on chromosome 10q22.3 (53–55). Approximately 25 percent of patients develop de novo germline mutations and the remaining patients have a family history.

Specific molecular alterations are associated with variable phenotypic manifestations: *SMAD4* mutations are more common among patients with severe gastric polyposis, gastrointestinal carcinoma, and hereditary hemorrhagic telangiectasia, whereas *BMPR1A* mutations are associated with cardiac defects (56). Infantile juvenile polyposis can result from large deletions affecting two contiguous tumor suppressor genes, *BMPR1A* and *PTEN* (phosphatase and tensin homolog [mutated in multiple advanced cancers 1]), or *ENG* mutations (54,57). Germline *SMAD9* mutations have been described in some patients with juvenile polyposis syndrome, ganglioneuromatous polyps, and wild-type *BMPR1A* and *PTEN*; these mutations result in decreased PTEN expression (58).

Differential Diagnosis. The polyps of juvenile polyposis syndrome mimic those of other hamartomatous syndromes and inflammatory conditions. Juvenile polyps tend to contain edematous and inflamed lamina propria, rather than the prominent smooth muscle component of Peutz-Jeghers polyps, although traumatized juvenile polyps can show fibromuscularization of the lamina propria that simulates the arborizing aggregates of smooth muscle cells characteristic of Peutz-Jeghers polyps. Colorectal juvenile polyps are often indistinguishable from the inflammatory polyps that develop in association with inflammatory bowel disease, inflammatory "cap" polyposis, and CCS, whereas diffuse gastric polyposis simulates hypertrophic gastropathies, such as Ménétrier disease. The differential diagnosis is usually resolved with adequate sampling of the intervening, nonpolypoid mucosa; inflammation-related polyps are

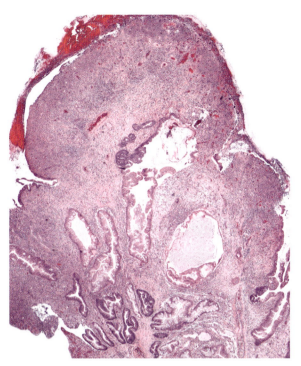

Figure 2-28

JUVENILE POLYPOSIS SYNDROME OF THE STOMACH

Striking foveolar hyperplasia is associated with lamina propria edema, ulcers, and granulation tissue.

associated with similar changes in the nonpolypoid mucosa, whereas the intervening mucosa is normal in patients with juvenile polyposis syndrome. Ménétrier disease generally spares the antrum and is associated with some degree of oxyntic gland atrophy, whereas juvenile polyposis may affect any part of the stomach and is accompanied by normal oxyntic glands.

Treatment and Prognosis. Approximately one third of patients with juvenile polyposis syndrome develop dysplasia in their colorectal polyps, presumably due to the local effects of cytokine elaboration by inflammatory cells. The cumulative colorectal cancer risk is estimated to be 68 percent by 60 years of age, although patients are also at increased risk for carcinomas of the stomach, pancreas, and proximal small intestine (59). For these reasons, patients with juvenile polyposis syndrome undergo complete endoscopic examination in late adolescence, or with the onset of symptoms, followed by endoscopic surveillance of the upper and lower gastrointestinal tract at 3-year intervals.

PTEN Hamartoma Tumor Syndrome

Definition. The *PTEN hamartoma tumor syndrome* affects approximately 1/200,000 persons/year. It includes *Cowden syndrome* and related disorders that result from germline *PTEN* abnormalities (60,61).

The International Cowden Consortium (62) compiled diagnostic criteria for the PTEN hamartoma tumor syndrome. These are classified as pathognomonic criteria (mucocutaneous lesions, facial trichilemmomas, acral keratosis, papillomatous lesions, and papules), major criteria (breast cancer, thyroid cancer, macrocephaly, and Lhermitte-Duclos disease), and minor criteria (thyroid nodules or goiter, intellectual disability, and gastrointestinal hamartomas). A combination of these findings in a patient or in a family member of a patient with the disorder, is used to diagnose PTEN hamartoma tumor syndrome.

Clinical Features. Virtually all patients with PTEN hamartoma tumor syndrome develop mucocutaneous lesions in early adulthood, but only 35 to 40 percent have hamartomatous polyps of the gastrointestinal tract. Other common manifestations include thyroid abnormalities, fibrocystic breast disease and mammary carcinoma, and uterine leiomyomata (63). Lhermitte-Duclos disease is characterized by dysplastic gangliocytoma of the cerebellum in addition to the abovementioned features of PTEN hamartoma tumor syndrome. Patients with Bannayan-Ruvalcaba-Riley syndrome have a variety of fatty and/or vascular tumors of the skin and viscera, as well as down-slanting palpebral fissures, ocular hypertelorism, pseudopapilledema and prominent corneal nerves, café au lait spots, acanthosis nigricans, and wart-like lesions of the face (64–66). More than 50 percent of affected males with Bannayan-Ruvalcaba-Riley syndrome have pigmented penile macules. Variably severe hypotonia is common and results from abnormal lipid accumulation in proximal muscles. Joint hyperextensibility, scoliosis, and pectus excavatum, as well as other skeletal abnormalities, have been described (55,67,68). Some autism spectrum disorders associated with microcephaly are also included under the umbrella of PTEN hamartoma tumor syndrome (69).

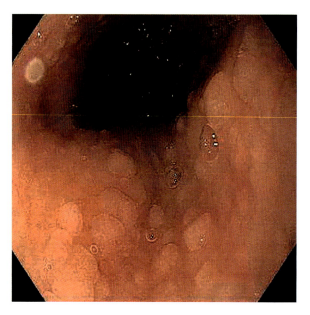

Figure 2-29

GLYCOGENIC ACANTHOSIS OF PTEN HAMARTOMA TUMOR SYNDROME

Innumerable, slightly raised white plaques are present throughout the esophagus.

Gross Findings. Endoscopic abnormalities are common in patients with PTEN hamartoma tumor syndrome. Approximately 80 percent of patients who undergo endoscopy have diffuse glycogenic acanthosis of the esophagus, and most have gastrointestinal polyps (69). In fact, the combination of diffuse esophageal glycogenic acanthosis and gastrointestinal polyposis is virtually pathognomonic of PTEN hamartoma tumor syndrome (figs. 2-29–2-31). Hamartomatous polyps of the stomach, small intestine, and colon appear as raised, slightly erythematous nodules or sessile polyps. They tend to be less numerous and often smaller than polyps associated with other hamartomatous polyposis disorders.

Microscopic Findings. Diffuse glycogenic acanthosis appears as innumerable white esophageal plaques; these reflect increased numbers of hypertrophic squamous cells filled with glycogen (fig. 2-32). Hamartomatous polyps occur throughout the gastrointestinal tract, particularly the stomach and colorectum. Gastric polyps contain tortuous, occasionally cystic, regenerative pits supported by slightly inflamed lamina propria, often with increased numbers of myofibroblastic spindle cells that

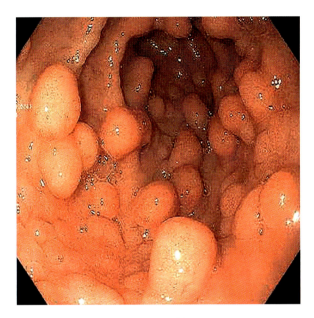

Figure 2-30

**GASTRIC POLYPS OF
PTEN HAMARTOMA TUMOR SYNDROME**

The gastric body is studded by numerous sessile polyps. These lesions have a normal or slightly erythematous appearance.

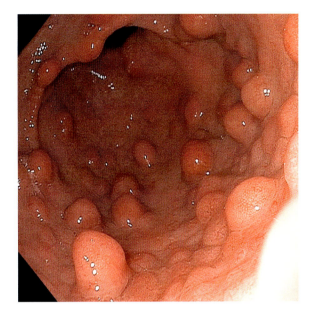

Figure 2-31

**COLONIC POLYPS OF
PTEN HAMARTOMA TUMOR SYNDROME**

Smooth, sessile polyps are present throughout the colon. Most are small, spanning only a few millimeters.

impart pink discoloration to the lamina propria (fig. 2-33). Intestinal lesions may resemble juvenile polyps when they contain cystic crypts and inflamed lamina propria, but they tend to show additional scattered or clustered ganglion cells and mesenchymal elements, including my-ofibroblasts, smooth muscle cells, nerve fibers, and fat (fig. 2-34). Other colonic polyps include lipomas, ganglioneuromas, lymphoid nodules, and adenomas.

Molecular Genetic Findings. More than 80 percent of patients with PTEN hamartoma tumor syndrome have germline mutations affecting *PTEN*, which encodes a 403 amino acid phosphatase (62,68,70). This important protein functions as a lipid phosphatase integral to the cell cycle, apoptosis, cell migration, and genomic stability. It also cleaves phosphatidylinositol-3,4,5-triphosphate (PIP3), a component of the PI3 kinase pathway that mediates cell survival via AKT/PKB (71). Some patients who meet the clinical criteria for PTEN hamartoma tumor syndrome lack *PTEN* mutations, but have germline mutations affecting succinate dehydrogenase complex subunit B (*SDHB*) or D (*SDHD*) located on 1p35-36 and 11q23, respectively (72).

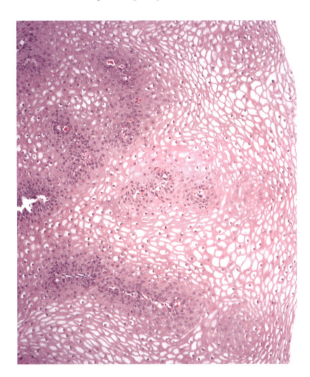

Figure 2-32

GLYCOGENIC ACANTHOSIS

The squamous mucosa is expanded by squamous cells with clear cytoplasm, reflecting glycogen accumulation.

Figure 2-33

GASTRIC POLYP OF PTEN HAMARTOMA TUMOR SYNDROME

Hamartomatous polyps show subtle abnormalities including foveolar hyperplasia with mucin depletion or dilated pits. This polyp appears pink owing to the myofibroblasts proliferating in the mucosa in association with the fibrosis.

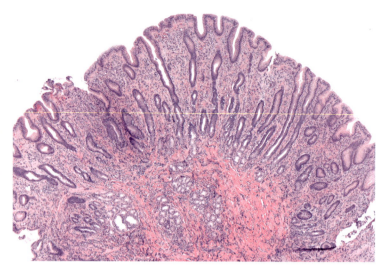

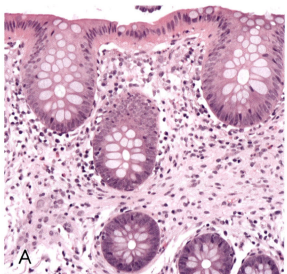

Figure 2-34

COLONIC GANGLIONEUROMA OF PTEN HAMARTOMA TUMOR SYNDROME

A: The lamina propria contains short fascicles of spindle cells and a cluster of ganglion cells (left).

B: The findings in this polyp are subtle: the colonic crypts are mildly dilated and the lamina propria is expanded by a spindle cell proliferation around the crypts.

C: This polyp contains mildly dilated, disorganized crypts and a lymphoid aggregate; a very nonspecific appearance.

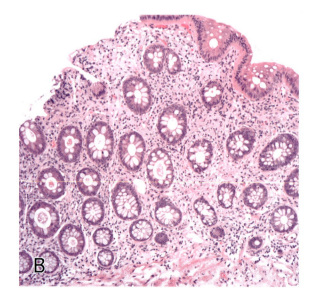

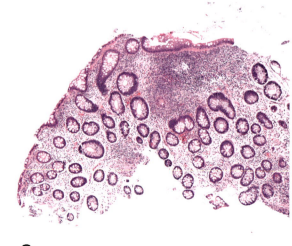

Differential Diagnosis. The endoscopic features of diffuse esophageal glycogenic acanthosis simulate eosinophilic esophagitis or *Candida* infection, but both entities are readily excluded following mucosal biopsy analysis. Because the PTEN hamartoma tumor syndrome is associated with a variety of different polyp types, the differential diagnosis is broad and includes a number of unrelated conditions. All of the polyps that occur in association with the syndrome may also be incidentally discovered in otherwise healthy patients. Isolated ganglioneuromas are common and do not signify an underlying heritable disorder, but multiple lesions should raise suspicion for PTEN hamartoma tumor syndrome. A diagnosis of PTEN hamartoma tumor syndrome should be considered in patients with multiple "hyperplastic" polyps, lymphoid aggregates, lipomas, and adenomas.

All of the hamartomatous polyposis syndromes can produce polyps that are similar to the polyps of PTEN hamartoma tumor syndrome, and it can be difficult to distinguish these entities based on polyp morphology. Indeed, there is considerable overlap between juvenile polyposis syndrome and PTEN hamartoma tumor syndrome with respect to gastrointestinal manifestations; the final classification often requires consideration of clinical and molecular features. Features of PTEN hamartoma tumor syndrome-related lesions include a prominent spindle cell component, ganglion cells, neuromatous elements, and fat within a polyp that shows reparative/regenerative changes, such as hyperplastic, serrated, or dilated glands and lamina propria inflammation. Hamartomatous polyps with a prominent spindle cell component may be misinterpreted to represent mucosal prolapse polyps, although the mesenchymal elements of the former tend to be more cellular than aggregates of smooth muscle cells emanating from the muscularis mucosae in mucosal prolapse.

Treatment and Prognosis. Women with PTEN hamartoma tumor syndrome have an increased risk for cancer of the breast: the estimated lifetime risk is 25 to 50 percent for breast cancer compared to only 10 percent among women in the general population. Affected men and women are at risk for carcinomas of the thyroid gland, ovary, endometrium, uterine cervix, urinary bladder, and colorectum. The lifetime risk for thyroid cancer may be as high as 10 percent; follicular carcinomas are more common than papillary neoplasms (73–75). Surveillance includes complete endoscopic examination of the gastrointestinal tract beginning at age 15 years, with subsequent studies depending on findings and annual thyroid examinations beginning in adolescence. Female patients are encouraged to undergo annual breast examinations starting at 25 years of age as well as annual mammography beginning at age 30.

Peutz-Jeghers Syndrome

Definition. *Peutz-Jeghers syndrome* is an autosomal dominant polyposis disorder that affects 1/200,000 persons in the United States. Affected patients have gastrointestinal hamartomatous polyps, melanotic mucocutaneous pigmentation, and an increased cancer risk affecting multiple organs (76). The diagnostic criteria include: 1) three or more Peutz-Jeghers polyps, 2) any number of Peutz-Jeghers polyps in a patient with affected family members, 3) mucocutaneous pigmentation in a patient with affected family members, or 4) any number of Peutz-Jeghers polyps occurring in a patient with mucocutaneous pigmentation (44).

Clinical Features. Patients with Peutz-Jeghers syndrome generally present with symptoms related to gastrointestinal polyposis: polyps of the small intestine cause recurrent abdominal pain secondary to intermittent intussusception, whereas large polyps may infarct or ulcerate and produce signs and symptoms related to gastrointestinal bleeding. Polyps begin to develop in the first decade of life, but do not produce symptoms until adolescence or young adulthood (77,78). Pigmentation of the lips and perioral mucosa are common: at least 95 percent of affected patients show some degree of mucocutaneous melanin deposition. Perioral freckling may occur in patients unaffected by the syndrome, but macules that cross the vermillion border are rare in the sporadic setting and raise the possibility of Peutz-Jeghers syndrome. Macules tend to be clustered and more deeply pigmented than common freckles. Pigmentation of fingers, soles of feet, palms, anus, periorbital skin, buccal mucosa, and conjunctiva may be observed. Cutaneous pigmentation may fade

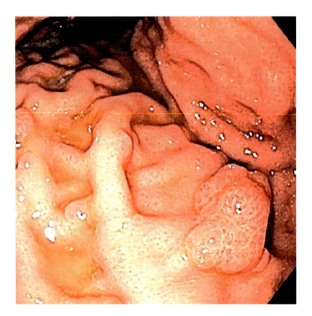

Figure 2-35

GASTRIC PEUTZ-JEGHERS POLYPS

Two sessile hamartomatous polyps are present on the crests of rugal folds.

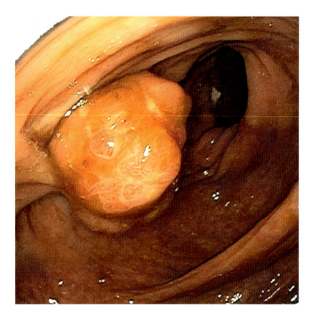

Figure 2-36

COLONIC PEUTZ-JEGHERS POLYPS

A large, multinodular polyp is present on a thick, broad stalk.

after puberty, but macules on the buccal mucosa and conjunctiva tend to persist into mid-adulthood and may be evident even when perioral lesions are lacking.

Gross Findings. Virtually all affected patients (88 to 100 percent) have gastrointestinal polyps. Most patients with hamartomas of the colon, stomach, or appendix have polyps in the small bowel as well (figs. 2-35, 2-36). Polyps may be sessile or pedunculated, and the latter may have abnormally long stalks. The stalk of a Peutz-Jeghers polyp is often thick, reflecting an abundance of smooth muscle cells emanating from the muscularis propria. The polyps may be round with smooth surfaces or erosions, but often have a multinodular appearance.

Microscopic Findings. Isolated hamartomatous polyps resembling Peutz-Jeghers polyps have been described in the older literature. Subsequently, the increased use of molecular testing and improved clinical assessment of patients in the modern era generally demonstrate either molecular or clinical evidence of Peutz-Jeghers syndrome in these individuals. In other words, solitary Peutz-Jeghers polyps are highly likely to reflect an underlying heritable condition and should be considered a *forme*

fruste of Peutz-Jeghers syndrome until proven otherwise (79).

Gastric Peutz-Jeghers polyps contain lobules of non-neoplastic mucosal elements in the mucosa and submucosa, intimately associated with slender aggregates of smooth muscle cells; these lesions can be difficult to distinguish from sporadic hyperplastic polyps of the gastric mucosa (fig. 2-37) (80). Peutz-Jeghers polyps of the small bowel classically contain lobules of non-neoplastic mucosal elements separated by arborizing bundles of smooth muscle cells emanating from the abnormally prominent muscularis mucosae (fig. 2-38). Up to 10 percent of small bowel lesions are associated with mural abnormalities; aggregates of epithelium and lamina propria can be seen in the muscularis propria, or even the subserosa (fig. 2-39). Polyps of the colon contain abundant smooth muscle, but a less pronounced arborizing pattern (fig. 2-40). Dysplasia is detected in approximately 10 percent of Peutz-Jeghers polyps and is more commonly encountered in colorectal and small intestinal polyps (fig. 2-41). Carcinomas develop in either polypoid or nonpolypoid mucosa and are of intestinal type, similar to sporadic carcinomas.

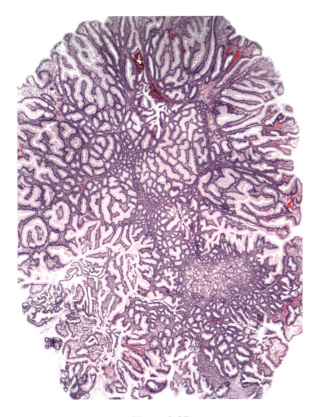

Figure 2-37

GASTRIC PEUTZ-JEGHERS POLYP

This lesion displays foveolar hyperplasia with a vaguely lobular architecture; gastric polyps generally lack arborizing aggregates of smooth muscle cells.

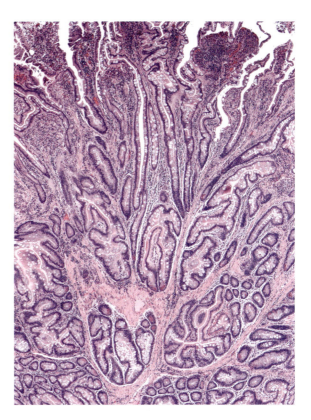

Figure 2-38

SMALL INTESTINAL PEUTZ-JEGHERS POLYP

Small bowel hamartomas contain lobular aggregates of nondysplastic epithelium and lamina propria surrounded by arborizing bundles of smooth muscle cells.

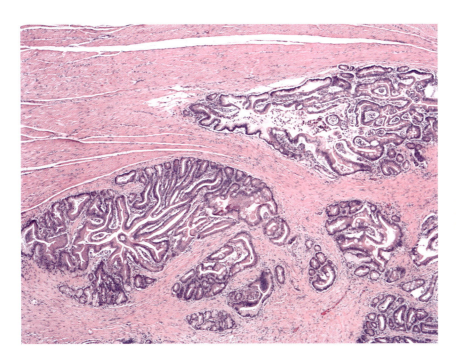

Figure 2-39

**SMALL INTESTINAL
PEUTZ-JEGHERS SYNDROME**

Lobules of mucosal elements are present in the muscularis propria subjacent to a Peutz-Jeghers polyp.

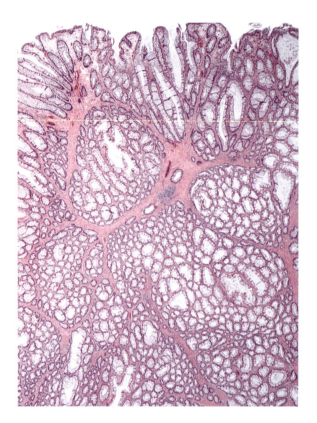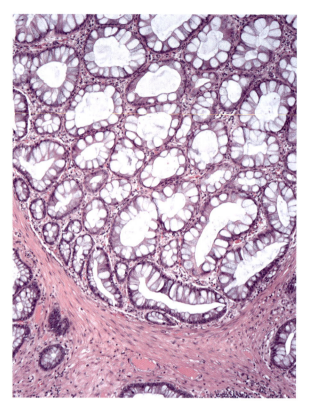

Figure 2-40

PEUTZ-JEGHERS HAMARTOMA OF THE COLON

Left: Sweeping fascicles of smooth muscle cells emanate into the polyp head and completely surround lobules of mucosal elements.

Right: A lobule consisting of normal-appearing crypts is supported by the lamina propria.

Molecular Genetic Findings. Peutz-Jeghers syndrome is associated with germline mutations in *STK11* (*LKB1*) located on chromosome 19p13.3; these abnormalities are detected in more than 90 percent of patients with clinical manifestations of the disease (44,81,82). The gene encodes serine/threonine kinase 11, which is important for maintenance of cell polarity. This protein also has a tumor suppressor function: it inhibits cell proliferation by regulating adenine monophosphate-activated protein kinase (AMPK). Patients with truncating *STK11* mutations generally have more severe disease manifestations than do individuals with missense mutations (83).

Differential Diagnosis. Peutz-Jeghers polyps of the small intestine are readily recognized due to the characteristic tree-like pattern of proliferating smooth muscle cells. Gastric and colonic polyps, however, may be problematic because they tend to show less prominent arborizing bundles of smooth muscle cells. Most Peutz-Jeghers polyps of the stomach show a lesser degree of gland dilation compared to juvenile polyps, and usually contain more smooth muscle toward the head of the polyp. The lamina propria is normal, whereas hyperplastic polyps and juvenile polyps generally show a greater degree of edema and inflammation. Occasional colonic Peutz-Jeghers polyps show stromal edema with inflammation and mucosal cysts that cannot be differentiated from juvenile polyps.

Peutz-Jeghers polyps can simulate mucosal prolapse polyps, adenomas with misplaced epithelium, and invasive adenocarcinomas. Prominent bundles of smooth muscle cells are common in mucosal prolapse polyps, but these lesions often show other inflammatory changes, such as erosions, crypt regeneration and hyperplasia, and surface ischemic injury.

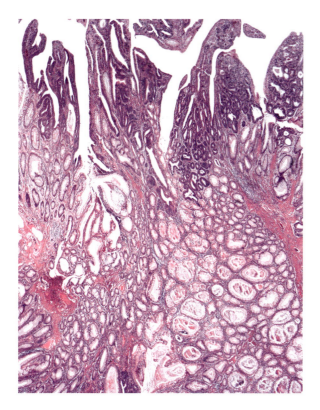 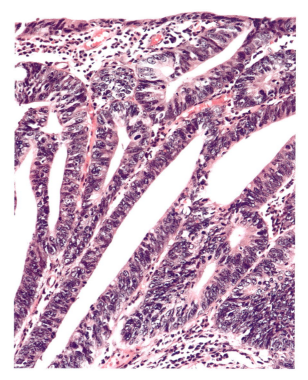

Figure 2-41

SMALL INTESTINAL PEUTZ-JEGHERS POLYP WITH DYSPLASIA

Left: Lobules of nondysplastic epithelium are present in the deep polyp, although the surface contains a crowded proliferation of villi and crypts lined by atypical cells.

Right: The intestinal-type dysplasia in this Peutz-Jeghers polyp is similar to that seen in adenomas of the colorectum and small bowel. Crowded, neoplastic cells contain large, hyperchromatic nuclei with occasional conspicuous nucleoli and mitotic figures.

Adenomas with misplaced epithelium contain lobules of dysplastic epithelium surrounded by lamina propria, similar to Peutz-Jeghers polyps. However, the former also display hemosiderin deposits, extruded mucin, hemorrhage, fibrosis, and other features of trauma. Hamartomatous elements in the submucosa may simulate invasive adenocarcinoma, especially when they contain dysplastic epithelium. Features of a hamartomatous polyp include the lobular arrangement of benign, often non-neoplastic epithelium intimately associated with the lamina propria.

Treatment and Prognosis. Patients with Peutz-Jeghers syndrome are at high risk for malignant complications of their disease: more than 90 percent develop some type of malignancy by 65 years of age. The estimated lifetime risk for colorectal cancer is nearly 40 percent, followed by breast cancer (24 to 54 percent), pancreatic cancer (11 to 36 percent), gastric cancer (29 percent), ovarian neoplasia (21 percent), cervical adenocarcinoma (10 to 23 percent), small bowel carcinoma (13 percent), testicular neoplasia (9 percent), and uterine carcinoma (9 percent) (44,78,84). In addition to mucinous neoplasms of the ovary, female patients may develop distinctive gynecologic tumors, namely, ovarian sex cord tumors with annular tubules and adenoma malignum of the cervix. Men may develop large cell calcifying Sertoli cell tumors.

Surveillance guidelines include complete endoscopic evaluation of the gastrointestinal tract at 8 years of age followed by repeat examination every 3 years if polyps are found and at 18 years of age if polyps are not identified (81,85). Removal of all detectable polyps is preferable, if possible. The value of polyp chemoprevention with COX-2 and mTOR (mammalian target of rapamycin) inhibitors is currently under investigation (86,87). Other recommendations include magnetic resonance or ultrasonographic imaging of the pancreas beginning at age 30, annual self-examination of the breast beginning at age 18 followed by annual imaging beginning at age 25, pelvic ultrasound and examination beginning at age 25, and regular testicular examinations beginning in childhood (47).

MALAKOPLAKIA

Definition. *Malakoplakia* was described over 100 years ago by Michaelis and Guttmann (referenced by Detlefsen [88]) and is a disorder in which collections of histiocytes containing degenerated bacteria present as a mass-like lesion, most commonly in the genitourinary tract. The term malakoplakia derives from Greek: "malaks" refers to "soft" and "plakos" to "plaque." The lesions consist of friable yellow nodules of varying sizes, the accumulation of coliforms in macrophage cytoplasm (Von Hansemann bodies), and large calcified spheres showing a laminated concentric appearance (Michaelis-Guttmann bodies) (89).

General Features. Most cases of malakoplakia (75 percent) are found in the genitourinary tract and the disease was first described in the bladder (88), but examples have been reported in anatomic sites throughout the body. Gastrointestinal examples are believed to account for about 10 percent of cases (88–90). The prevailing hypothesis is that affected patients have defective lysosomal function of their macrophages and chronic bacterial infections, so that engulfed bacteria are incompletely digested in histiocytes, resulting in the accumulation of amorphous material and the mineralized spherules.

Clinical Features. There is a female predominance for malakoplakia arising in the bladder but there seems to be no such predominance at other sites. In the gastrointestinal tract, most examples are found in the sigmoid colon, and patients may present with mass lesions, but malakoplakia is often detected as an inflammatory polyp sampled in the course of screening colonoscopy. Malakoplakia is more likely to arise in patients with a history of immunosuppression due to lymphoma, diabetes mellitus, renal transplantation, or the use of long-term systemic corticosteroids.

Gross Findings. Colorectal malakoplakia lesions tend to be friable polyps with a yellowish appearance, often with erosions/ulcers. Occasional examples can form large masses.

Microscopic Findings. The histiocytes of malakoplakia are brightly eosinophilic with dense cytoplasm, often in clusters in the midst of lymphoid aggregates (fig. 2-42). The nuclei of the histiocytic cells are round and have smooth nuclear membranes. Finding Michaelis-Guttmann bodies is key to the diagnosis. These are intracytoplasmic phagolysosomes that contain iron and calcium salt deposits. These deposits are highlighted with the von Kossa stain, which helps confirm the diagnosis.

Immunohistochemical Findings. The histiocytes express CD68 but not S-100 protein, CD1a, or langerin.

Differential Diagnosis. The differential diagnosis of gastrointestinal tract malakoplakia is essentially with any condition that results in collections of histiocytes. In the intestines, this includes chronic granulomatous disease (which does not produce a mass), and Langerhans cell histiocytosis (fig. 2-43), extranodal Rosai-Dorfman disease (figs. 2-44, 2-45), Erdheim-Chester disease, and tuberculosis, all of which may produce masses. Whipple disease manifests as histiocytes laden with bacteria but the histiocytes are pale and contain many periodic acid–Schiff (PAS)-reactive bacteria (figs. 2-46, 2-47).

Whereas gastrointestinal Langerhans cell histiocytosis tends to present as a diffuse lethal condition in infants and children, it often manifests as an incidental colorectal polyp in adults, detected during screening colonoscopy (91); polypectomy is essentially curative and the lesions are equivalent to eosinophilic granulomas. The lesions express S-100 protein, CD1a, and langerin, and some examples have *BRAF* mutations and are thus amenable to treatment with vemurafanib (92–96). Rosai-Dorfman disease rarely arises in the colon or small bowel. It is a poorly understood condition characterized by the proliferation of S-100 protein-reactive non-Langerhans cell histiocytes that characteristically show emperipolesis (ingestion of cells without destroying them). It tends to be localized and treated by excision but some patients have systemic disease and require immunomodulation therapy. It lacks *BRAF* mutations.

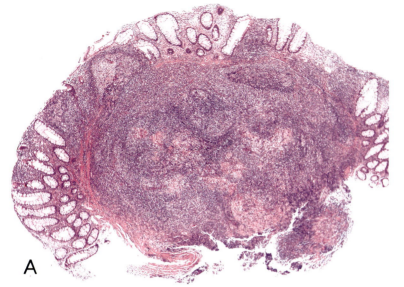

A

Figure 2-42

MALAKOPLAKIA

A: This example presented as a colorectal polyp detected at the time of screening colonoscopy. The lesional histiocytes are brightly eosinophilic, even evident at low magnification.

B: There is a Michaelis-Guttmann body in the center of the field in a pink histiocyte.

C: The von Kossa stain shows the Michaelis-Guttmann bodies to advantage. They have a target-like appearance.

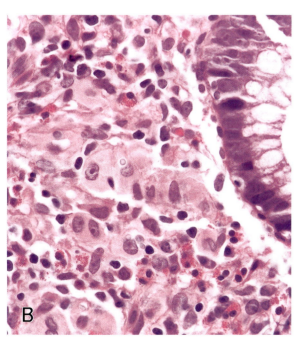

B

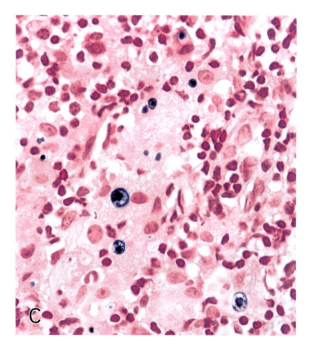

C

Treatment and Prognosis. For colorectal lesions, polypectomy or resection is often performed but for lesions in inaccessible sites, treatment with antibiotics, bethanechol, and ascorbic acid has proven effective (97). Some patients require prolonged antibiotic treatment. There are many isolated case reports of neoplasms arising in patients with malakoplakia (98–109), which may be either coincidental, since such persons tend to have numerous biopsies, or a result of immune issues.

MUCOSAL PROLAPSE POLYPS AND SIMILAR LESIONS

Cap Polyposis

This unusual condition is often included with prolapse syndromes but is not necessarily related to mucosal prolapse. *Cap polyposis* is a rare benign colorectal condition in which patients have numerous polyps in the distal colorectum that are covered by an inflammatory "cap" of

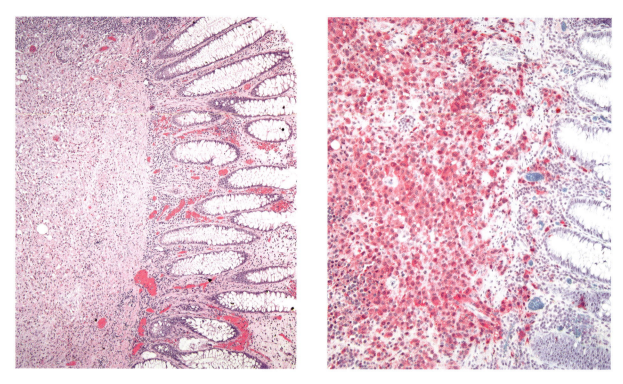

Figure 2-43

LANGERHANS CELL HISTIOCYTOSIS OF THE COLON

Left: The lesion is centered in the submucosa. Eosinophils are prominent.
Right: S-100 protein stains the lesion.

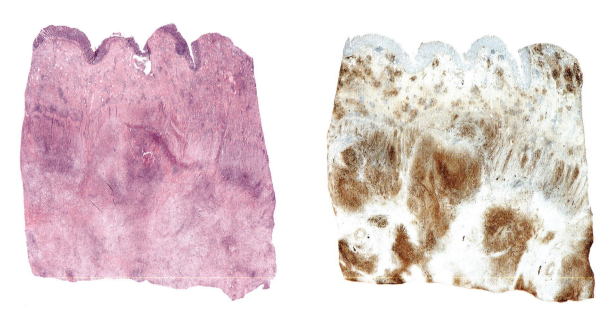

Figure 2-44

EXTRANODAL ROSAI-DORFMAN DISEASE INVOLVING THE COLON

Left: The lesion is pale compared to the scattered lymphoid aggregates distributed throughout.
Right: S-100 protein stains the lesion.

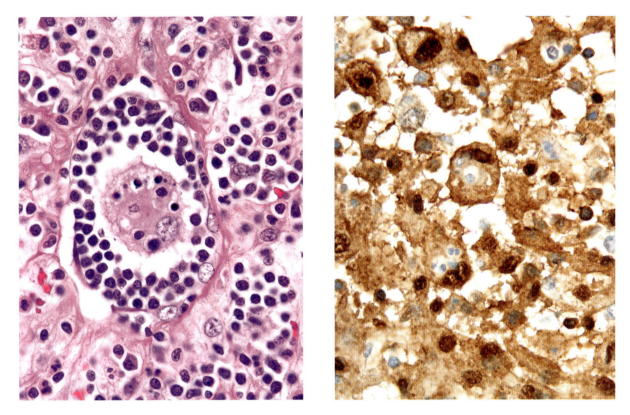

Figure 2-45

EXTRANODAL ROSAI-DORFMAN DISEASE INVOLVING THE COLON

Left: Emperipolesis is seen in the center of the field.

Right: A cell in the center left shows both cytoplasmic and nuclear labeling with S-100 protein but the lymphoid cells that are in the cell's cytoplasm by emperipolesis do not label. At the center is an unlabeled cell with a bilobed nucleus.

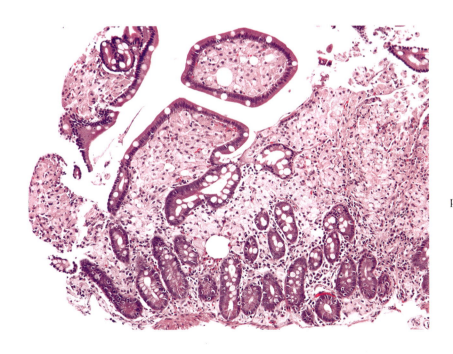

Figure 2-46

WHIPPLE DISEASE

The villi are stuffed with macrophages.

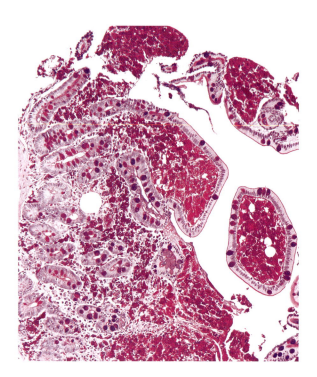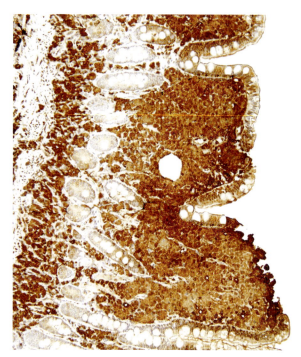

Figure 2-47

WHIPPLE DISEASE

Left: With a PAS/alcian blue stain, the bacteria-laden macrophages are bright pink.
Right: An immunohistochemical preparation for *T. whipplei*.

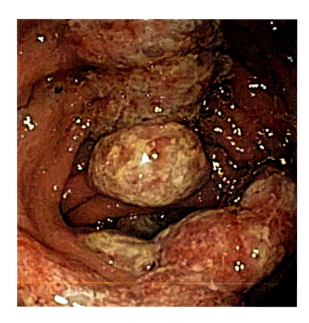

Figure 2-48

CAP POLYPOSIS

The rectal polyps have a "cap" of exudate. (Courtesy of Drs. H. Venbrux and D. Mize, Camp Hill, PA.)

granulation tissue with normal intervening mucosa (110,111).

Most patients are adults with a median age in their early 50s but pediatric cases have been reported. There seems to be a female predominance. Patients present with mucous diarrhea, rectal bleeding, and tenesmus. This can be sufficiently severe to result in a protein-losing colopathy with peripheral edema. Many patients have long-standing constipation and straining to defecate.

On colonoscopy, patients have 1 to over 100 distal polyps covered with thick purulent exudates (fig. 2-48). Some authors show images with the appearance of prolapse polyps (110), but the original report showed peculiar polyps with hyperplastic epithelium, abundant mucus production, and surface exudates with pristine intervening mucosa. Generally, the polyps show dilated glands that are more narrow toward the base, with minimal crypt distortion, but the eye-catching feature is the cap of thick mucin on the surface (fig. 2-49). A case with colitis cystica profunda type changes has been reported (112).

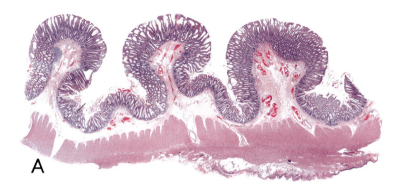

Figure 2-49

CAP POLYPOSIS

A: A resection was performed to alleviate debilitating mucoid diarrhea. This is not an intrinsically inflammatory lesion but each polyp tends to be coated with a cap of exudate.

B: A polypectomy sample shows corkscrew-shaped glands and a surface rind of exudate.

C: Higher magnification of the lesion shown in B.

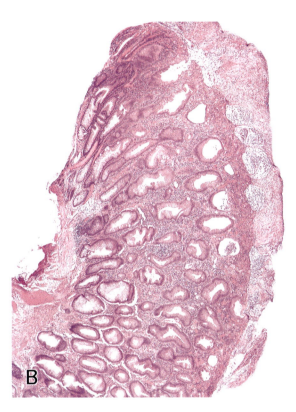

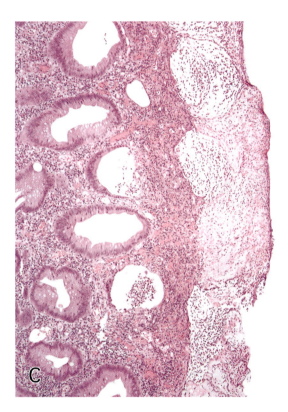

In some instances, the protein loss and symptoms are sufficient to warrant distal colectomy. Some patients have rectal prolapse (113). Various authors have reported clinical response to immunomodulation, *Helicobacter pylori* eradication, and straining avoidance while defecating (110,111,113–119).

Solitary Rectal Ulcer Syndrome

Solitary rectal ulcer syndrome describes a pattern of mucosal changes (encompassing polyps lacking ulceration) that is localized to the terminal rectum and caused by mucosal prolapse. It occurs at all ages, with a peak incidence between 20 and 40 years of age. The classic history is of a young woman who strains when defecating. There may be hematochezia, pain, tenesmus, and sometimes lower abdominal pain. Inability to evacuate the rectum, or a "foreign body" sensation, is described. At endoscopy, ulcers are seen in 20 to 70 percent of patients, usually on the anterior or anterolateral rectal wall, but a mass-like lesion can also be found, which raises the possibility of a neoplasm. Sometimes defecation studies are used to evaluate these patients because they are believed to have difficulty coordinating the smooth muscle during the defecation process, so that the puborectalis sling does not relax at the proper time.

Figure 2-50

SOLITARY RECTAL ULCER SYNDROME/MUCOSAL PROLAPSE LESION

Strands of smooth muscle extend between the glands. This differs from the lobules of glands separated by cords of smooth muscle in the Peutz-Jeghers polyps shown in figures 2-37 through 2-41.

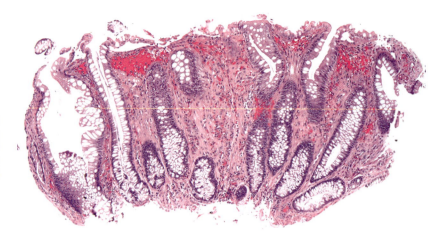

The pathologic changes on biopsies consist of hypertrophy of the muscularis mucosae, with splaying of the fibers that course into the mucosa and are seen throughout the lamina propria (figs. 2-50, 2-51). The proliferated smooth muscle is accompanied by variable fibrosis, and the glands become entrapped and distorted. As the process continues, there is surface ulceration and glands can herniate into the submucosa, accompanied by wisps of lamina propria (a theme in adenomas as well) (120–124). Thus, lesions can have a "polypoid phase" or an ulcerated phase. Often crypts become "diamond-shaped" (125,126).

Frequently, these polyps have serrated features, which has resulted in confusion with sessile serrated adenomas (SSA)/polyps. Studies published when the molecular underpinnings of SSA were poorly understood included attempts to seek evidence of mismatch repair defects in prolapse polyps (127) (such studies are negative but SSAs have intact mismatch repair proteins so their results are misleading in the first place). Since prolapse polyps are typically left sided (in contrast to SSA) and feature prominent smooth muscle proliferation, most cases can be assigned to one or the other category. In general, SSAs lack smooth muscle proliferation in the lamina propria, although some examples have associated perineuriomas/benign fibroblastic polyps in their lamina propria.

A caveat in diagnosing mucosal prolapse polyps is that the mucosal prolapse changes adjacent to carcinomas are the same as those of isolated mucosal prolapse (128), so we suggest multiple biopsies of large "solitary rectal ulcers" to exclude sampling error. *Colitis cystica* profunda is part of

the same spectrum of disease and implies that glands have prolapsed into the submucosa or muscularis propria. Occasional patients with prominent distal rectal mucosal prolapse can present with an apparent polyposis (129).

Inflammatory Cloacogenic Polyp

Inflammatory cloacogenic polyp is a mucosal prolapse polyp arising at the anorectal transition, thus having both squamous and columnar mucosa (fig. 2-52) (123,130). Patients with such polyps present with hematochezia. The polyps are typically found on the anterior wall of the anal canal.

These polyps display a tubulovillous growth pattern, with surface ulceration, displaced clusters of crypts into the submucosa, and abundant fibromuscular stroma that extends into the mucosa. They are essentially the anal form of solitary rectal ulcer, discussed above. Occasionally, anal intraepithelial neoplasia is encountered in the squamous epithelium overlying these polyps (fig. 2-53).

Filiform Polyps (Postinflammatory Polyps)

Filiform polyps (also called *postinflammatory polyps*) are pseudopolyps associated with prior mucosal injury. They are not unusual in patients with inflammatory bowel disease (fig. 2-54) and are found in patients who have had any type of prior ulceration. In patients with inflammatory bowel disease, there may be a dramatic gross appearance, simulating a neoplasm and termed *filiform polyposis* or *giant filiform polyposis*. They are not a reflection of mucosal prolapse.

Filiform polyps consist of finger-like projections of submucosa covered by mucosa on all

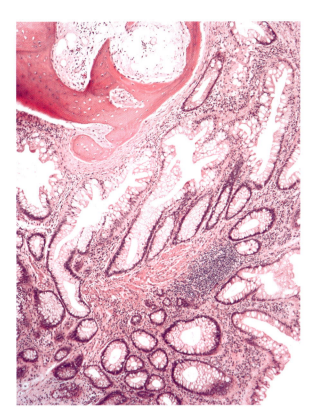
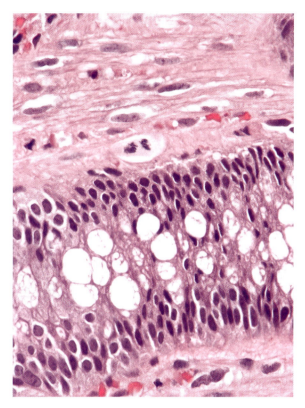

Figure 2-51

SOLITARY RECTAL ULCER SYNDROME/MUCOSAL PROLAPSE LESION

Left: Smooth muscle is present between the glands to the right. This lesion has been present for a long time and has ossified. The glands show serrations but these lesions lack the genetic alterations that characterize the serrated colorectal group of polyps.

Right: Detail of the strands of smooth muscle between the glands shows delicate longitudinal striations in the smooth muscle cells at the top of the image.

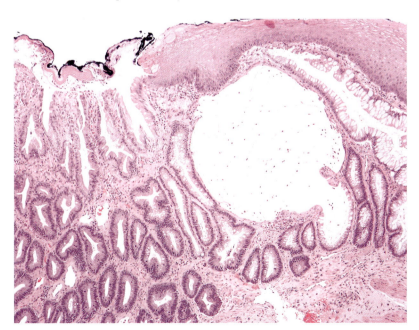

Figure 2-52

INFLAMMATORY CLOACOGENIC POLYP/MUCOSAL PROLAPSE LESION

An entrapped gland with inspissated mucin is seen at the right. There is a coating of anal squamous epithelium at the upper right.

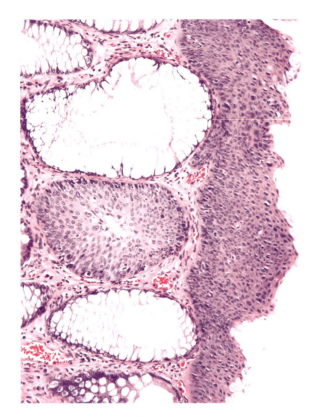

Figure 2-53

**INFLAMMATORY CLOACOGENIC
POLYP/MUCOSAL PROLAPSE LESION**

Anal intraepithelial neoplasia is seen at the right.

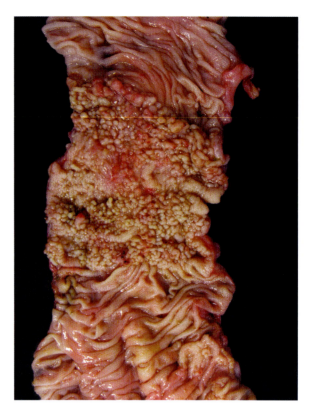

Figure 2-54

FILIFORM POLYPS

This is a dramatic example of postinflammatory polyps in a patient with ileal Crohn disease.

sides. They reflect the healing of undermined mucosal and submucosal remnants and ulcers, and are typically multiple. To the endoscopist, they appear as long, thin, cylindrical projections (131). They are diagnosed by noting their composition (fig. 2-55): two protruding layers of mucosa plastered together with only one intervening layer or no intervening layer of muscularis mucosae. This construction reflects regrowth of mucosa over an area of ulcer that has damaged the muscularis mucosae.

Differential Diagnosis of Mucosal Prolapse Polyps

The differential diagnosis of all the mucosal prolapse polyp types is essentially with one another and with Peutz-Jeghers polyps. To separate Peutz-Jeghers from mucosal prolapse polyps is theoretically simple, but in some instances, Peutz-Jeghers polyps show mucosal prolapse change themselves and are thus difficult to distinguish.

This applies especially in the distal colon and stomach (79,80). In mucosal prolapse polyps, delicate smooth muscle fibrils proliferate in the lamina propria between crypts whereas in Peutz-Jeghers polyps, cords of smooth muscle cordon off groups of crypts that retain their normal lamina propria.

An important differential diagnostic consideration of postinflammatory polyps and part of the same kind of pathology is so-called diaphragm disease (132), associated with use of nonsteroidal anti-inflammatory drugs (NSAIDs). It generally arises in the small bowel and is associated with other pseudotumors that result from many cycles of damage and repair due to NSAID-related erosions and ulcers (133). In diaphragm disease, the repair of erosions at the tips of small bowel folds results in submucosal fibrosis that causes concentric ridges that appear as mucosal ledges/diaphragms macroscopically (fig. 2-56). These require surgical resection to relieve obstruction.

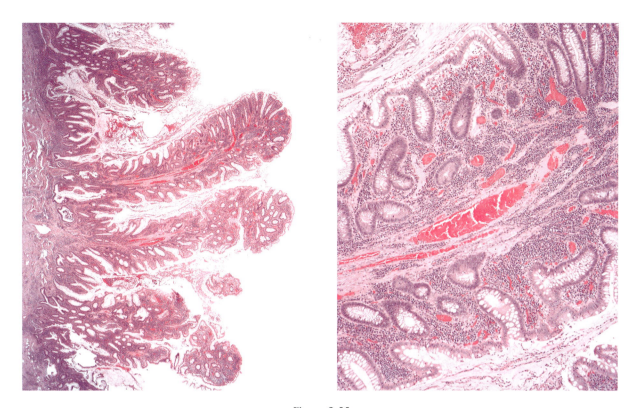

Figure 2-55

FILIFORM POLYPS

Left: Each inflammatory polyp is long, slender, and finger-like.
Right: At high magnification, the disorganized smooth muscle at the core of the polyp is seen.

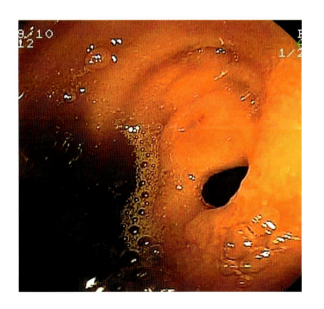
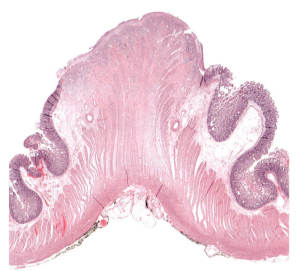

Figure 2-56

DIAPHRAGM DISEASE

Left: Such mucosal diaphragms result in small bowel obstruction.
Right: The surface ulceration and submucosal fibroinflammatory changes resulted in a protuberance.

REFERENCES

1. Kim K, Jang SJ, Song HJ, Yu E. Clinicopathologic characteristics and mucin expression in Brunner's gland proliferating lesions. Dig Dis Sci 2013;58:194-201.
2. Levine JA, Burgart LJ, Batts KP, Wang KK. Brunner's gland hamartomas: clinical presentation and pathological features of 27 cases. Am J Gastroenterol 1995;90:290-294.
3. Akino K, Kondo Y, Ueno A, et al. Carcinoma of duodenum arising from Brunner's gland. J Gastroenterol 2002;37:293-296.
4. Dixon CF, Lichtman AL, et al. Malignant lesions of the duodenum. Surg Gynecol Obstet 1946;83:83-93.
5. Dorandeu A, Raoul JL, Landemore G, et al. [Adenocarcinoma of Brunner's glands: an entity exceptionally described. Report of a case.] Ann Pathol 1995;15:211-215. [French]
6. Itsuno M, Makiyama K, Omagari K, et al. Carcinoma of duodenal bulb arising from the Brunner's gland. Gastroenterol Jpn 1993;28:118-125.
7. Kawamoto K, Motooka M, Hirata N, et al. Early primary carcinoma of the duodenal bulb arising from Brunner's glands. Gastrointest Endosc 1994;40(Pt 1):233-236.
8. Kushima R, Stolte M, Dirks K, et al. Gastric-type adenocarcinoma of the duodenal second portion histogenetically associated with hyperplasia and gastric-foveolar metaplasia of Brunner's glands. Virchows Arch 2002;440:655-659.
9. Shimizu N, Tanaka S, Morikawa J, et al. [Early duodenal cancer of the bulb—report of a case.] Gan no Rinsho 1989;35:100-106. [Japanese]
10. Shorrock K, Haldane JS, Kersham MJ, Leach RD. Obstructive jaundice secondary to carcinoma arising in Brunner's glands. J R Soc Med 1986;79:173-174.
11. Suzuki T, Ito A, Takayasu H, et al. [A case of duodenal Brunner's gland hyperplasia associated with in situ carcinoma.] Nihon Shokakibyo Gakkai Zasshi 1995;92:1189-1193. [Japanese]
12. Zanetti G, Casadei G. Brunner's gland hamartoma with incipient ductal malignancy. Report of a case. Tumori 1981;67:75-78.
13. Poeschl EM, Siebert F, Vieth M, Langner C. Pyloric gland adenoma arising in gastric heterotopia within the duodenal bulb. Endoscopy 2011;43(Suppl 2) UCTN:E336-337.
14. Vieth M, Kushima R, Borchard F, Stolte M. Pyloric gland adenoma: a clinico-pathological analysis of 90 cases. Virchows Arch 2003;442:317-321.
15. Vieth M, Montgomery EA. Some observations on pyloric gland adenoma: an uncommon and long ignored entity! J Clin Pathol 2014;67:883-890.
16. Matsubara A, Ogawa R, Suzuki H, et al. Activating GNAS and KRAS mutations in gastric foveolar metaplasia, gastric heterotopia, and adenocarcinoma of the duodenum. Br J Cancer 2015;112:1398-1404.
17. Sakurai T, Sakashita H, Honjo G, Kasyu I, Manabe T. Gastric foveolar metaplasia with dysplastic changes in Brunner gland hyperplasia: possible precursor lesions for Brunner gland adenocarcinoma. Am J Surg Pathol 2005;29:1442-1448.
18. Wang Y, Shi C, Lu Y, Poulin EJ, Franklin JL, Coffey RJ. Loss of Lrig1 leads to expansion of Brunner glands followed by duodenal adenomas with gastric metaplasia. Am J Pathol 2015;185:1123-1134.
19. Cronkhite LW Jr, Canada WJ. Generalized gastrointestinal polyposis; an unusual syndrome of polyposis, pigmentation, alopecia and onychotrophia. N Engl J Med 1955;252:1011-1015.
20. Slavik T, Montgomery EA. Cronkhite-Canada syndrome six decades on: the many faces of an enigmatic disease. J Clinl Pathol 2014;67:891-897.
21. Bettington M, Brown IS, Kumarasinghe MP, de Boer B, Bettington A, Rosty C. The challenging diagnosis of Cronkhite-Canada syndrome in the upper gastrointestinal tract: a series of 7 cases with clinical follow-up. Am J Surg Pathol 2014;38:215-223.
22. Burke AP, Sobin LH. The pathology of Cronkhite-Canada polyps. A comparison to juvenile polyposis. Am J Surg Pathol 1989;13:940-946.
23. Greene AD, Lang SA, Kendziorski JA, Sroga-Rios JM, Herzog TJ, Burns K. Endometriosis: where are we and where are we going? Reproduction 2016;152:R63-78.
24. Anglesio MS, Papadopoulos N, Ayhan A, et al. Cancer-associated mutations in endometriosis without cancer. N Engl J Med 2017;376:1835-1848.
25. Guadagno A, Grillo F, Vellone VG, et al. Intestinal endometriosis: mimicker of inflammatory bowel disease? Digestion 2015;92:14-21.
26. Parr NJ, Murphy C, Holt S, Zakhour H, Crosbie RB. Endometriosis and the gut. Gut 1988;29:1112-1115.
27. Yantiss RK, Clement PB, Young RH. Endometriosis of the intestinal tract: a study of 44 cases of a disease that may cause diverse challenges in clinical and pathologic evaluation. Am J Surg Pathol 2001;25:445-454.
28. Misdraji J, Lauwers GY, Irving JA, Batts KP, Young RH. Appendiceal or cecal endometriosis with intestinal metaplasia: a potential mimic of appendiceal mucinous neoplasms. Am J Surg Pathol 2014;38:698-705.

29. Donnez J, Squifflet J. Complications, pregnancy and recurrence in a prospective series of 500 patients operated on by the shaving technique for deep rectovaginal endometriotic nodules. Hum Reprod 2010;25:1949-1958.

30. Rimal D, Thapa SR, Munasinghe N, Chitre VV. Symptomatic gastric heterotopic pancreas: clinical presentation and review of the literature. Int J Surg 2008;6:e52-54.

31. Bini R, Voghera P, Tapparo A, et al. Malignant transformation of ectopic pancreatic cells in the duodenal wall. World J Gastroenterol 2010;16:1293-1295.

32. Ginori A, Vassallo L, Butorano MA, Bettarini F, Di Mare G, Marrelli D. Pancreatic adenocarcinoma in duodenal ectopic pancreas: a case report and review of the literature. Pathologica 2013;105:56-58.

33. Kinoshita H, Yamaguchi S, Shimizu A, et al. Adenocarcinoma arising from heterotopic pancreas in the duodenum. Int Surg 2012;97:351-355.

34. Assimakopoulos SF, Kourea HP, Gogos CA, Thomopoulos KC. Gastrointestinal: a rare cause of anal pain: gastric heterotopia of the rectum. J Gastroenterol Hepatol 2013;28:1432.

35. Iacopini F, Gotoda T, Elisei W, et al. Heterotopic gastric mucosa in the anus and rectum: first case report of endoscopic submucosal dissection and systematic review. Gastroenterol Rep 2016;4:196-205.

36. Jiang K, Stephen FO, Jeong D, Pimiento JM. Pancreatic and gastric heterotopia with associated submucosal lipoma presenting as a 7-cm obstructive tumor of the ileum: resection with double balloon enteroscopy. Case Rep Gastroenterol 2015;9:233-240.

37. Ruiz Marin M, Candel Arenas MF, Parra Banos PA, et al. Gastric heterotopia in the rectum: a rare cause of rectal bleeding. Am Surg 2011;77:659-662.

38. Francis A, Kantarovich D, Khoshnam N, Alazraki AL, Patel B, Shehata BM. Pediatric Meckel's diverticulum: report of 208 cases and review of the literature. Fetal Pediatr Pathol 2016:35:199-206.

39. Kotha VK, Khandelwal A, Saboo SS, et al. Radiologist's perspective for the Meckel's diverticulum and its complications. Br J Radiol 2014;87:20130743.

40. Park JJ, Wolff BG, Tollefson MK, Walsh EE, Larson DR. Meckel diverticulum: the Mayo Clinic experience with 1476 patients (1950-2002). Ann Surg 2005;241:529-533.

41. Kotecha M, Bellah R, Pena AH, Jaimes C, Mattei P. Multimodality imaging manifestations of the Meckel diverticulum in children. Pediatr Radiol 2012;42:95-103.

42. Poulsen KA, Qvist N. Sodium pertechnetate scintigraphy in detection of Meckel's diverticulum: is it usable? Eur J Pediatric Surg 2000;10:228-231.

43. Giardiello FM, Hamilton SR, Kern SE, et al. Colorectal neoplasia in juvenile polyposis or juvenile polyps. Arch Dis Child 1991;66:971-975.

44. Schreibman IR, Baker M, Amos C, McGarrity TJ. The hamartomatous polyposis syndromes: a clinical and molecular review. Am J Gastroenterol 2005;100:476-490.

45. Gupta SK, Fitzgerald JF, Croffie JM, et al. Experience with juvenile polyps in North American children: the need for pancolonoscopy. Am J Gastroenterol 2001;96:1695-1697.

46. Chow E, Macrae F. A review of juvenile polyposis syndrome. J Gastroenterol Hepatol 2005;20:1634-1640.

47. Syngal S, Brand RE, Church JM, et al. ACG clinical guideline: genetic testing and management of hereditary gastrointestinal cancer syndromes. Am J Gastroenterol 2015;110:223-262; quiz 263.

48. Baert AL, Casteels-Van Daele M, Broeckx J, Wijndaele L, Wilms G, Eggermont E. Generalized juvenile polyposis with pulmonary arteriovenous malformations and hypertrophic osteoarthropathy. AJR Am J Roentgenol 1983;141:661-662.

49. Offerhaus GJ, Howe JR. Juvenile Polyposis. In: Bosman FT, Carneiro F, Hruban RH, Theise ND, eds. WHO Classification of tumours of the digestive system, 4th ed. Lyon: ??? 2009:166-167.

50. Gallione CJ, Repetto GM, Legius E, et al. A combined syndrome of juvenile polyposis and hereditary haemorrhagic telangiectasia associated with mutations in MADH4 (SMAD4). Lancet 2004;363:852-859.

51. Heiss KF, Schaffner D, Ricketts RR, Winn K. Malignant risk in juvenile polyposis coli: increasing documentation in the pediatric age group. J Pediatr Surg 1993;28:1188-1193.

52. Jarvinen H, Franssila KO. Familial juvenile polyposis coli; increased risk of colorectal cancer. Gut 1984;25:792-800.

53. Howe JR, Sayed MG, Ahmed AF, et al. The prevalence of MADH4 and BMPR1A mutations in juvenile polyposis and absence of BMPR2, BMPR1B, and ACVR1 mutations. J Med Genet 2004;41:484-491.

54. Delnatte C, Sanlaville D, Mougenot JF, Stoppa-Lyonnet D. [Contiguous gene deletion within chromosome arm 10q is associated with juvenile polyposis of infancy, reflecting cooperation between the BMPR1A and PTEN tumor-suppressor genes.] Med Sci (Paris) 2006;22:912-913. [Fremcj]

55. Reardon W, Zhou XP, Eng C. A novel germline mutation of the PTEN gene in a patient with macrocephaly, ventricular dilatation, and features of VATER association. J Med Genet 2001;38:820-823.

56. Aytac E, Sulu B, Heald B, et al. Genotype-defined cancer risk in juvenile polyposis syndrome. Br J Surg 2015;102:114-118.

57. Howe JR, Mitros FA, Summers RW. The risk of gastrointestinal carcinoma in familial juvenile polyposis. Ann Surg Oncol 1998;5:751-756.

58. Ngeow J, Yu W, Yehia L, et al. Exome sequencing reveals germline SMAD9 mutation that reduces phosphatase and tensin homolog expression and is associated with hamartomatous polyposis and gastrointestinal ganglioneuromas. Gastroenterology 2015;149:886-889.

59. Murday V, Slack J. Inherited disorders associated with colorectal cancer. Cancer Surv 1989;8:139-157.

60. DiLiberti JH. Inherited macrocephaly-hamartoma syndromes. Am J Med Genet 1998;79:284-290.

61. Nelen MR, Kremer H, Konings IB, et al. Novel PTEN mutations in patients with Cowden disease: absence of clear genotype-phenotype correlations. Eur J Hum Genet 1999;7(3):267-273.

62. Nelen MR, Padberg GW, Peeters EA, et al. Localization of the gene for Cowden disease to chromosome 10q22-23. Nat Genet 1996;13:114-116.

63. Zbuk KM, Eng C. Cancer phenomics: RET and PTEN as illustrative models. Nat Rev Cancer 2007;7:35-45.

64. Bannayan GA. Lipomatosis, angiomatosis, and macrencephalia. A previously undescribed congenital syndrome. Arch Pathol 1971;92:1-5.

65. Gorlin RJ, Cohen MM Jr, Condon LM, Burke BA. Bannayan-Riley-Ruvalcaba syndrome. Am J Med Genet 1992;44:307-314.

66. Ruvalcaba RH, Myhre S, Smith DW. Sotos syndrome with intestinal polyposis and pigmentary changes of the genitalia. Clin Genet 1980;18:413-416.

67. Butler MG, Dasouki MJ, Zhou XP, et al. Subset of individuals with autism spectrum disorders and extreme macrocephaly associated with germline PTEN tumour suppressor gene mutations. J Med Genet 2005;42:318-321.

68. Zhou XP, Marsh DJ, Morrison CD, et al. Germline inactivation of PTEN and dysregulation of the phosphoinositol-3-kinase/Akt pathway cause human Lhermitte-Duclos disease in adults. Am J Hum Genet 2003;73:1191-1198.

69. Pilarski R, Burt R, Kohlman W, Pho L, Shannon KM, Swisher E. Cowden syndrome and the PTEN hamartoma tumor syndrome: systematic review and revised diagnostic criteria. J Natl Cancer Inst 2013;105:1607-1616.

70. Perriard J, Saurat JH, Harms M. An overlap of Cowden's disease and Bannayan-Riley-Ruvalcaba syndrome in the same family. J Am Acad Dermatol 2000;42(Pt 2):348-350.

71. Minaguchi T, Waite KA, Eng C. Nuclear localization of PTEN is regulated by Ca(2+) through a tyrosil phosphorylation-independent conformational modification in major vault protein. Cancer Res 2006;66:11677-11682.

72. Bayley JP. Succinate dehydrogenase gene variants and their role in Cowden syndrome. Am J Hum Genet 2011;88:674-675; author reply 676.

73. Starink TM, van der Veen JP, Arwert F, et al. The Cowden syndrome: a clinical and genetic study in 21 patients. Clin Genet 1986;29:222-233.

74. Pilarski R, Eng C. Will the real Cowden syndrome please stand up (again)? Expanding mutational and clinical spectra of the PTEN hamartoma tumour syndrome. J Med Genet 2004;41:323-326.

75. Wirtzfeld DA, Petrelli NJ, Rodriguez-Bigas MA. Hamartomatous polyposis syndromes: molecular genetics, neoplastic risk, and surveillance recommendations. Ann Surg Oncol 2001;8:319-327.

76. Jeghers H, McKusick VA, Katz KH. Generalized intestinal polyposis and melanin spots of the oral mucosa, lips and digits; a syndrome of diagnostic significance. N Engl J Med 1949;241:1031-1036.

77. Amos CI, Keitheri-Cheteri MB, Sabripour M, et al. Genotype-phenotype correlations in Peutz-Jeghers syndrome. J Med Genet 2004;41:327-333.

78. van Lier MG, Mathus-Vliegen EM, Wagner A, van Leerdam ME, Kuipers EJ. High cumulative risk of intussusception in patients with Peutz-Jeghers syndrome: time to update surveillance guidelines? Am J Gastroenterol 2011;106(5):940-945.

79. Burkart AL, Sheridan T, Lewin M, Fenton H, Ali NJ, Montgomery E. Do sporadic Peutz-Jeghers polyps exist? Experience of a large teaching hospital. Am J Surg Pathol 2007;31:1209-1214.

80. Lam-Himlin D, Park JY, Cornish TC, Shi C, Montgomery E. Morphologic characterization of syndromic gastric polyps. Am J Surg Pathol 2010;34:1656-1662.

81. Beggs AD, Latchford AR, Vasen HF, et al. Peutz-Jeghers syndrome: a systematic review and recommendations for management. Gut 2010;59:975-986.

82. Aretz S, Stienen D, Uhlhaas S, et al. High proportion of large genomic STK11 deletions in Peutz-Jeghers syndrome. Hum Mutat 2005;26:513-519.

83. Volikos E, Robinson J, Aittomaki K, et al. LKB1 exonic and whole gene deletions are a common cause of Peutz-Jeghers syndrome. J Med Genet 2006;43:e18.

84. McGarrity TJ, Kulin HE, Zaino RJ. Peutz-Jeghers syndrome. Am J Gastroenterol 2000;95:596-604.

85. Giardiello FM, Trimbath JD. Peutz-Jeghers syndrome and management recommendations. Clin Gastroenterol Hepatol 2006;4:408-415.

86. Udd L, Katajisto P, Rossi DJ, et al. Suppression of Peutz-Jeghers polyposis by inhibition of cyclooxygenase-2. Gastroenterology 2004;127:1030-1037.

87. Wei C, Amos CI, Zhang N, et al. Suppression of Peutz-Jeghers polyposis by targeting mammalian target of rapamycin signaling. Clin Cancer Res 2008;14:1167-1171.

88. Detlefsen S, Fagerberg CR, Ousager LB, et al. Histiocytic disorders of the gastrointestinal tract. Hum Pathol 2013;44:683-696.

89. Cipolletta L, Bianco MA, Fumo F, Orabona P, Piccinino F. Malacoplakia of the colon. Gastrointest Endosc 1995;41:255-258.

90. McClure J. Malakoplakia of the gastrointestinal tract. Postgrad Med J 1981;57:95-103.

91. Singhi AD, Montgomery EA. Gastrointestinal tract langerhans cell histiocytosis: a clinicopathologic study of 12 patients. Am J Surg Pathol 2011;35:305-310.

92. Alayed K, Medeiros LJ, Patel KP, et al. BRAF and MAP2K1 mutations in Langerhans cell histiocytosis: a study of 50 cases. Hum Pathol 2016;52:61-67.

93. Badalian-Very G, Vergilio JA, Degar BA, et al. Recurrent BRAF mutations in Langerhans cell histiocytosis. Blood 2010;116:1919-1923.

94. Haroche J, Cohen-Aubart F, Emile JF, Donadieu J, Amoura Z. Vemurafenib as first line therapy in BRAF-mutated Langerhans cell histiocytosis. J Am Acad Dermatol 2015;73:e29-30.

95. Johnson WT, Patel P, Hernandez A, et al. Langerhans cell histiocytosis and Erdheim-Chester disease, both with cutaneous presentations, and papillary thyroid carcinoma all harboring the BRAF mutation. J Cutan Pathol 2016;43:270-275.

96. Roden AC, Hu X, Kip S, et al. BRAF V600E expression in Langerhans cell histiocytosis: clinical and immunohistochemical study on 25 pulmonary and 54 extrapulmonary cases. Am J Surg Pathol 2014;38:548-551.

97. Fudaba H, Ooba H, Abe T, et al. An adult case of cerebral malakoplakia successfully cured by treatment with antibiotics, bethanechol and ascorbic acid. J Neurol Sci 2014;342:192-196.

98. Asiyanbola B, Camuto P, Mansourian V. Malakoplakia occurring in association with colon carcinoma. J Gastrointest Surg 2006;10:657-661.

99. Darvishian F, Teichberg S, Meyersfield S, Urmacher CD. Concurrent malakoplakia and papillary urothelial carcinoma of the urinary bladder. Ann Clin Lab Sci 2001;31:147-150.

100. Edmund L, Mohammed W. Colonic carcinoma associated with malakoplakia. West Indian M J 2014;63:664-666.

101. Kocarslan S, Dokumaci DS, Karakas EY, Boyaci FN, Ulas T. Urothelial carcinoma concomitant with malakoplakia in non-functioning nephrolithic kidneys. Folia Med 2015;57:78-79.

102. Lee SL, Teo JK, Lim SK, Salkade HP, Mancer K. Coexistence of Malakoplakia and papillary urothelial carcinoma of the urinary bladder. Int J Surg Pathol 2015;23:575-578.

103. Lew S, Siegal A, Aronheim M. Renal cell carcinoma with malakoplakia. Eur Urol 1988;14:426-428.

104. Liu S, Christmas TJ, Kirby RS. Malakoplakia and carcinoma of the prostate. Br J Urol 1993;72:120-121.

105. McCormick M, Timme AH. Malakoplakia of the nasopharynx associated with carcinoma. J Laryngol Otol 1982;96:737-742.

106. Ngadiman S, Hoda SA, Campbell WG, Gardner T, May M. Concurrent malakoplakia and primary squamous cell carcinoma arising in long-standing chronic cystitis. Br J Urol 1994;74:801-802.

107. Pattnaik S, Banerjee M, Jalan R, et al. Malakoplakia simulating rectal carcinoma. Indian J Pathol Microbiol 1991;34:52-56.

108. Pillay K, Chetty R. Malakoplakia in association with colorectal carcinoma: a series of four cases. Pathology 2002;34:332-335.

109. Thrasher JB, Donatucci CF. Malakoplakia and carcinoma of the prostate. Br J Urol 1994;74:263.

110. Ng KH, Mathur P, Kumarasinghe MP, Eu KW, Seow-Choen F. Cap polyposis: further experience and review. Dis Colon Rectum 2004;47:1208-1215.

111. Williams G, Bussey H, Morson B. Inflammatory "cap" polyps of the large intestine. Br J Surg. 1985;72:S133.

112. Arana R, Flejou JF, Parc Y, El-Murr N, Cosnes J, Svrcek M. Cap polyposis and colitis cystica profunda: a rare association. Histopathology 2014;64:604-607.

113. Daniel F, Atienza P. Rectal prolapse and cap polyposis: the missing link. Dis Colon Rectum 2005;48:874-875; author reply 875.

114. Kim ES, Jeen YT, Keum B, et al. Remission of cap polyposis maintained for more than three years after infliximab treatment. Gut Liver 2009;3:325-328.

115. Konishi T, Watanabe T, Takei Y, Kojima T, Nagawa H. Confined progression of cap polyposis along the anastomotic line, implicating the role of inflammatory responses in the pathogenesis. Gastrointest Endosc 2005;62:446-447; discussion 447.

116. Konishi T, Watanabe T, Takei Y, Kojima T, Nagawa H. Cap polyposis: an inflammatory disorder or a spectrum of mucosal prolapse syndrome? Gut 2005;54:1342-1343.

117. Maunoury V, Breisse M, Desreumaux P, Gambiez L, Colombel JF. Infliximab failure in cap polyposis. Gut 2005;54:313-314.

118. Nakagawa Y, Nagai T, Okawara H, et al. Cap polyposis (CP) which relapsed after remission by avoiding straining at defecation, and was cured by Helicobacter pylori eradication therapy. Intern Med 2009;48:2009-2013.

119. Oiya H, Okawa K, Aoki T, Nebiki H, Inoue T. Cap polyposis cured by Helicobacter pylori eradication therapy. J Gastroenterol 2002;37:463-466.

120. Bogomoletz WV. Solitary rectal ulcer syndrome. Mucosal prolapse syndrome. Pathol Annu 1992;27(Pt 1):75-86.

121. Britto E, Borges AM, Swaroop VS, Jagannath P, DeSouza LJ. Solitary rectal ulcer syndrome. Twenty cases seen at an oncology center. Dis Colon Rectum 1987;30:381-385.

122. Rutter KR. Solitary rectal ulcer syndrome. Proc R Soc Med 1975;68:22-26.

123. Saul SH. Inflammatory cloacogenic polyp: relationship to solitary rectal ulcer syndrome/mucosal prolapse and other bowel disorders. Hum Pathol 1987;18:1120-1125.

124. Saul SH, Sollenberger LC. Solitary rectal ulcer syndrome. Its clinical and pathological underdiagnosis. Am J Surg Pathol 1985;9:411-421.

125. Warren BF, Dankwa EK, Davies JD. 'Diamond-shaped' crypts and mucosal elastin: helpful diagnostic features in biopsies of rectal prolapse. Histopathology 1990;17:129-134.

126. Warren BF, Davies JD. Prolapse-induced inflammatory polyps of the colorectum and anal transition zone. Histopathology 1994;24:201-202.

127. Ball CG, Dupre MP, Falck V, Hui S, Kirkpatrick AW, Gao ZH. Sessile serrated polyp mimicry in patients with solitary rectal ulcer syndrome: is there evidence of preneoplastic change? Arch Pathol Lab Med 2005;129:1037-1040.

128. Li SC, Hamilton SR. Malignant tumors in the rectum simulating solitary rectal ulcer syndrome in endoscopic biopsy specimens. Am J Surg Pathol 1998;22:106-112.

129. Brosens LA, Montgomery EA, Bhagavan BS, Offerhaus GJ, Giardiello FM. Mucosal prolapse syndrome presenting as rectal polyposis. J Clin Pathol 2009;62:1034-1036.

130. Lobert PF, Appelman HD. Inflammatory cloacogenic polyp. A unique inflammatory lesion of the anal transitional zone. Am J Surg Pathol 1981;5:761-766.

131. Buck JL, Dachman AH, Sobin LH. Polypoid and pseudopolypoid manifestations of inflammatory bowel disease. Radiographics 1991;11:293-304.

132. Lang J, Price AB, Levi AJ, Burke M, Gumpel JM, Bjarnason I. Diaphragm disease: pathology of disease of the small intestine induced by non-steroidal anti-inflammatory drugs. J Clin Pathol 1988;41:516-526.

133. Cortina G, Wren S, Armstrong B, Lewin K, Fajardo L. Clinical and pathologic overlap in nonsteroidal anti-inflammatory drug-related small bowel diaphragm disease and the neuromuscular and vascular hamartoma of the small bowel. Am J Surg Pathol 1999;23:1414-1417.

3
EPITHELIAL NEOPLASTIC (PREMALIGNANT) POLYPS AND HYPERPLASTIC POLYPS OF THE LARGE INTESTINE

Epithelial neoplastic (premalignant) polyps are a group of benign epithelial lesions with the ability to develop into colorectal carcinoma. *Hyperplastic polyps* are a group of epithelial proliferative lesions not considered to be premalignant but they are included in this chapter because of their histologic similarity to premalignant serrated polyps.

Up until the past decade, the only generally recognized category of epithelial neoplastic (or premalignant) polyps of the large intestine was the colorectal "adenoma" (1). This lesion was believed to be the precursor lesion for essentially all colorectal carcinomas up until the identification of the sessile serrated adenoma/polyp (SSA/P) in 2003 (2). *Adenomas* (now referred to as *conventional adenomas*) were defined histologically by what has become known as "dysplasia," a term that refers to cytologically abnormal cells, presumably immature, demonstrating hyperchromasia, pseudostratification of nuclei, and easily identified mitotic activity. As is discussed below, this category of lesions is now considered to be the precursor lesion for the approximately 60 to 70 percent of colorectal carcinomas that arise via the "adenoma-carcinoma" sequence described by Fearon and Vogelstein in 1990 (1,3). This pathway begins with a mutation of the *APC* gene, leading to unregulated cell growth and hence unfettered proliferation of these undifferentiated dysplastic cells which, through the accumulation of additional mutations, become malignant.

In recent years, the concept of a premalignant epithelial polyp that is not cytologically dysplastic has been advanced as the precursor lesion to CpG island methylation (CIMP)-high carcinomas, both microsatellite stable (MSS) and unstable (MSI), and accounts for approximately 30 to 40 percent of colorectal carcinomas (1,4).

The term *sessile serrated adenoma*, coined in 2003, was originally applied to emphasize the premalignant and hence presumably "neoplastic" nature of these lesions. The use of the term adenoma in this context has been problematic for pathologists wishing to retain the term only for lesions with cytologic dysplasia, and the alternative terms of *sessile serrated polyp* and, more recently in Europe, *sessile serrated lesion*, have been offered as synonyms.

This multitude of terms for the same lesion has led to considerable confusion in the literature and among some pathologists and clinicians. In 2011, the World Health Organization (WHO) suggested a compromise terminology by allowing both sessile serrated adenoma and sessile serrated polyp to be used as synonyms with local preferences determining which term to use in daily practice (5). The combined term sessile serrated adenoma/polyp (or SSA/P) is often used in the current literature to allow for this difference and hopefully avoid confusion. SSA/P in a majority of cases is characterized by an activating *BRAF* mutation in its early development, with extensive methylation of numerous genes leading to the eventual development of carcinoma.

There is a third premalignant polyp, referred to as the *traditional serrated adenoma* (TSA), which appears to be unrelated or only marginally related to SSA/P and conventional adenoma by molecular and demographic criteria. In its early form, it does not have the conventional cytologic dysplasia as seen in *APC*-mutated conventional adenomas but rather often has a type of atypical epithelium that is eosinophilic and mitotically inert (and usually does not express MIB-1) (6). This epithelium is considered by some as dysplastic (sometimes referred to as low-grade serrated dysplasia), allowing the term "adenoma" to be used with less controversy

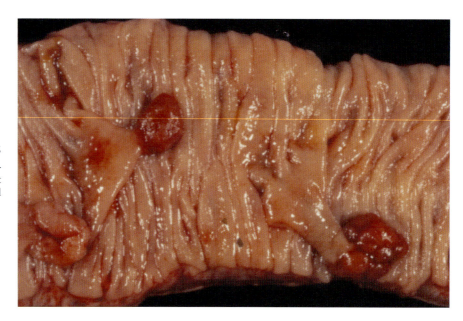

Figure 3-1

PEDUNCULATED TUBULOVILLOUS ADENOMAS

These characteristic pedunculated adenomas are present on a stalk lined with normal mucosa.

than for SSA/P, although others believe that this epithelium is metaplastic and senescent, and hence quite different from the dysplasia seen in *APC*-mutated conventional adenomas. This is discussed in more detail below. The precise mechanism for the development of carcinoma in TSA is currently unknown, although *APC* mutations do not appear to be part of the process and, although some TSAs demonstrate *BRAF* mutations (and others demonstrate *KRAS* mutations), the pathway to carcinoma appears different than that of SSA/P.

As recommended by the WHO, this Fascicle uses the term conventional adenoma for those lesions that are most likely *APC*-mutated precursors to CIMP low-MSS and CIMP low-MSI carcinomas in Lynch syndrome, sessile serrated adenoma/polyp (SSA/P) for the typically *BRAF*-mutated precursor lesion for CIMP-high carcinomas, and traditional serrated adenoma (TSA) for the third category of neoplastic/premalignant polyps. In addition to these premalignant polyps, other polyps usually considered to be hamartomatous may develop into malignancies, particularly in the context of polyposis syndromes, including juvenile polyposis and Peutz-Jeghers syndrome, which are further discussed in chapter 4.

CONVENTIONAL ADENOMAS

Definition. *Conventional adenomas* are clonal tumors composed of cytologically dysplastic epithelium. The terms *tubular adenoma* (*adenoma-*

tous polyp), *tubulovillous adenoma* (*villoglandular polyp*), and *villous adenoma* are used for subtypes of conventional adenomas. These lesions typically demonstrate *APC* mutations.

Gross Findings. Conventional adenomas have a variety of gross/endoscopic appearances depending on their histology and possibly their location. They are subcategorized as tubular (TA), tubulovillous (TVA), or villous (VA) by their histologic growth pattern (as described below). They typically have a red appearance different from the background mucosa, which is thought to be caused by the loss of mucin leading to transparency and allowing the underlying vasculature to be visualized. They can be flat, sessile (or plaque like), or pedunculated (i.e., growing on an identifiable stalk composed of normal mucosa), and hence are not always true "polyps" (figs. 3-1, 3-2). Flat adenomas are usually tubular and most plaque-like sessile lesions are villous or tubulovillous in overall microscopic configuration. Pedunculated lesions are usually tubular or tubulovillous. Their size ranges from millimeters to several centimeters. Lesions that are malignant may show ulceration or may be fixed to the underlying submucosa.

Microscopic Findings. The defining histologic feature of conventional adenoma is the presence of cytologically atypical cells, commonly referred to as dysplastic (fig. 3-3). It is somewhat challenging to define dysplastic, and with the recognition of the serrated pathway

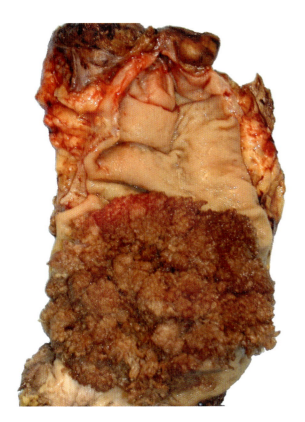

Figure 3-2

VILLOUS ADENOMA OF THE RECTUM

These lesions are characteristically sessile.

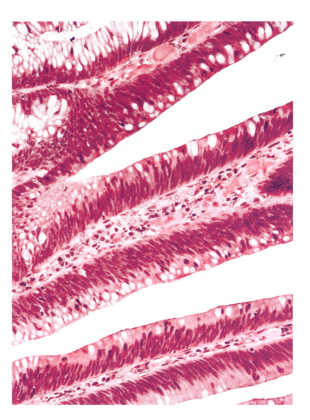

Figure 3-3

VILLOUS ADENOMA

Dysplasia is a defining feature of conventional adenoma. Dysplastic cells have elongated hyperchromatic nuclei with abundant mitotic activity. Low-grade dysplasia, as seen here, has fairly uniform cells showing pseudostratification and uniform nuclear chromatin without prominent nucleoli. Dysplastic cells often have less mucin than normal mucosa.

to colorectal carcinoma, dysplasia has been expanded to include so-called conventional dysplasia (i.e., the type seen in conventional *APC*-mutated adenomas) and serrated dysplasia. The term dysplasia is perhaps an unfortunate one for a cytologic feature, since the derivation of the term indicates that it means "abnormal growth," which is obviously not a cytologic issue but rather an architectural one. Nevertheless, the term is deeply embedded in the parlance of gastrointestinal tract pathology and is not likely to disappear any time soon.

Conventional cytologic dysplasia is usually characterized by cells with elongated, hyperchromatic nuclei and readily identified mitotic activity (fig. 3-3). Typically in low-grade dysplasia, the nuclei are uniform in size with fairly homogeneous, smudged chromatin and no or small nucleoli. They appear unevenly arranged and stratified, but each cell itself sits on the basement membrane and hence, while the nuclei are stratified, the cells themselves are not mul-

tilayered and are not truly stratified (therefore, these cells are referred to as "pseudostratified"). Less commonly, and more often as the degree of dysplasia increases, the nuclei become more rounded, with prominent nucleoli and more vesicular chromatin, and eventually there is true stratification or multilayering of cells. Nuclear pleomorphism also increases (fig. 3-4).

Most dysplastic cells have decreased or absent mucin, although occasionally, the cells retain their mucin or even become hypermucinous (fig. 3-5). When the cells become hypermucinous, the lesion may falsely appear architecturally complex if tangentially sectioned (fig. 3-6). Metaplasia to other cell types also occurs. Conventional adenomas can contain squamous cells or morules (which some observers term "microcarcinoids" since there can be prominent

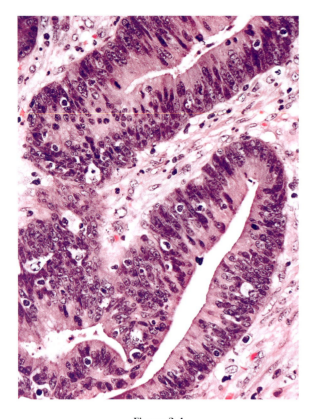

Figure 3-4

**TUBULAR ADENOMA WITH
HIGH-GRADE CYTOLOGIC DYSPLASIA**

High-grade dysplasia is characterized cytologically by rounder nuclei that are truly stratified. Nucleoli are focally prominent, and often, mitotic activity is more robust than in low-grade dysplasia.

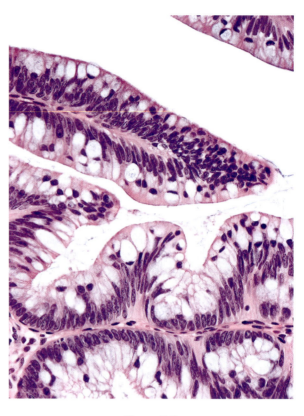

Figure 3-5

TUBULOVILLOUS ADENOMA WITH RETAINED MUCIN

Occasional conventional adenomas retain mucin, which may lead them to simulate hyperplastic polyps. The dysplasia is recognized by the elongated hyperchromatic nuclei with a minor degree of pseudostratification.

Figure 3-6

**TUBULAR ADENOMA WITH
RETAINED MUCIN SIMULATING
HIGH-GRADE DYSPLASIA**

A somewhat cribriform pattern is created by mucinous cytoplasm filling up the lumen of the crypt.

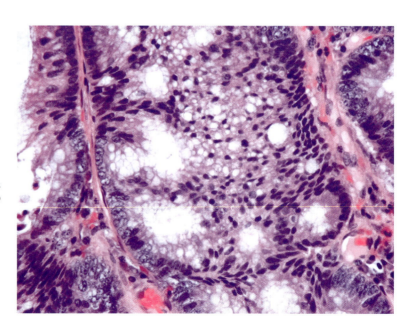

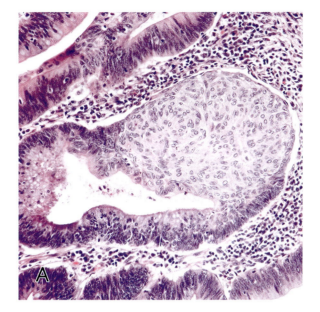

Figure 3-7

TUBULAR ADENOMA

A: Tubular adenoma with morule formation.

B: Tubular adenoma with Paneth cell metaplasia.

C: Tubular adenoma with clear cell change is present on the right. On the left, the dysplastic cells have clear foamy cytoplasm

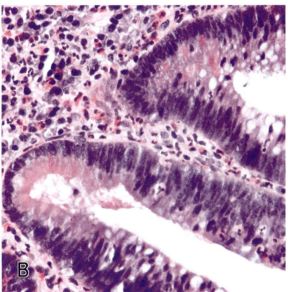

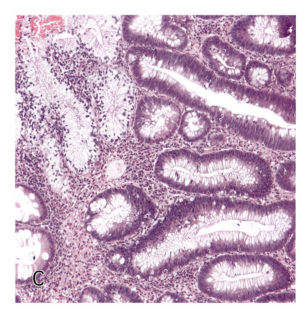

expression of endocrine markers (7,8), Paneth cells, and clear cells (fig. 3-7) (9–12). Scattered neuroendocrine cells are common, and occasional conventional adenomas have cells with enteric metaplasia of the type most commonly seen in TSA (described below) (fig. 3-8). These different cell types have little known clinical significance, although one recent study suggested that the presence of Paneth cells was associated with metachronous development of additional adenomas (10). It has been suggested that colonic squamous cell carcinomas arise from squamous metaplasia in an adenoma and that clear cell

carcinomas arise from tubular adenomas with clear cell change (12–14). Extensive necrosis of individual cells, resembling the single cell necrosis seen in graft versus host disease, is very common in adenomas (fig. 3-9) (15). This necrosis may represent a cell-mediated reaction against "foreign" antigens on the tumor cells.

By definition, all conventional adenomas are dysplastic, but the degree of dysplasia varies. It has been the convention for most pathologists, therefore, not to mention low-grade (mild and moderate) dysplasia in reports, but rather to report only high-grade dysplasia as present or

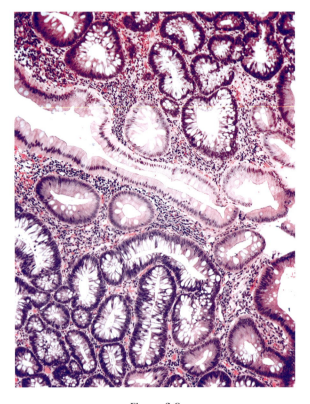

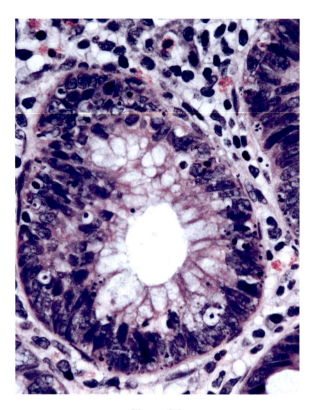

Figure 3-8

TUBULAR ADENOMA WITH ENTERIC METAPLASIA

This is similar to that seen commonly in traditional serrated adenomas (see fig. 3-42).

Figure 3-9

SINGLE CELL NECROSIS (APOPTOSIS) IN A TUBULAR ADENOMA

Extensive karyorrhectic debris and scattered necrotic epithelial cells simulate the changes seen in graft versus host disease.

absent. The criteria for high-grade dysplasia have not been clearly defined, however, resulting in poor interobserver agreement (with kappa values in the range of 0.26 to 0.5) (16,17).

Observational data clearly indicate that cytologic and architectural progression occurs during the transition from conventional early adenoma through advanced adenoma to carcinoma. The cytologic progression includes rounding of nuclei, which become more vesicular and often have prominent nucleoli, and the development of pleomorphism and true stratification of cells. At the upper end of the scale (marked stratification and architectural complexity with significant nuclear pleomorphism), it is easy to recognize these changes as malignant but not invasive (fig. 3-4). Where in the progression one chooses to diagnose a lesion with high-grade dysplasia, however, has not been well defined. Architecturally, progression manifests as papillary tufting and the development of a cribriform

pattern, easy to recognize in a fully developed form but more difficult to define in the transitional stages (fig. 3-10). In addition, tangential sectioning of crypts can lead to a false appearance of cribriform architecture, and lesions with abundant cytoplasmic mucin also often impart a false cribriform appearance (fig. 3-6). Therefore, neither cytologic nor architectural high-grade dysplasia is highly reproducible, which may account for the variable clinical significance of these lesions and the development of metachronous lesions between studies. In a meta-analysis, high-grade dysplasia was not shown to have any significance as a predictor (18).

The earliest dysplasia in the development of conventional adenomas is seen at the luminal surface of the crypts, with a single dysplastic crypt budding into the lamina propria from the surface (fig. 3-11). The process then develops in a top-to-bottom growth fashion (19). Small

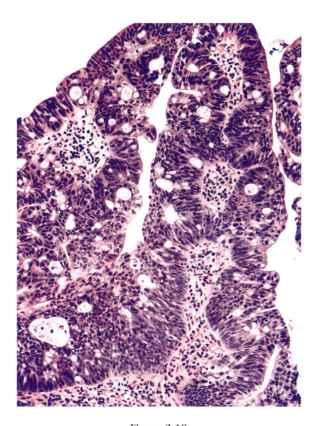

Figure 3-10

**TUBULOVILLOUS ADENOMA
WITH HIGH-GRADE DYSPLASIA**

The piling up of the epithelium forms a cribriform or sieve-like pattern.

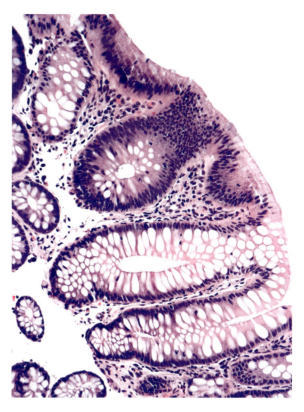

Figure 3-11

EARLY-STAGE TUBULAR ADENOMA

The adenoma consists of a single dysplastic crypt. The dysplasia is present at the luminal surface of the crypt.

lesions typically recapitulate the normal crypt architecture of the mucosa, with tubules of dysplastic cells growing in a downward fashion into the lamina propria (the tubular adenoma) (fig. 3-12). The proliferation of cells leads to the development of a sessile polyp, which with time, may develop a stalk and become pedunculated. Some lesions also develop a villiform architecture, in which the lamina propria appears to grow in an upward fashion, with dysplastic cells lining the outside of finger-like projections of lamina propria (fig. 3-13).

The development of villi may correlate with the progression of disease (or at least with the size of the polyp) and also correlates with *KRAS* mutations (20–22). It is not totally clear whether villous lesions always arise from nonvillous (i.e., tubular) lesions. If villous lesions indeed derive from tubular lesions (which would seem logical since there are many lesions with features of both, the tubulovillous adenomas), the factors driving the development of villi, aside from the possible *KRAS* mutation mentioned above, are not known. Why some adenomas become pedunculated as they grow and others remain sessile is also unknown. It seems unlikely that all tubular adenomas are capable of becoming villous lesions, since large sessile villous adenomas are most often located in the rectosigmoid in a distribution considerably different from that of smaller adenomas. Some rectosigmoid lesions diagnosed as villous adenomas may in fact be TSAs with extensive conventional dysplasia, a possibility discussed later with TSAs.

Conventional adenomas are reported as tubular, tubulovillous, or villous, depending on the degree of villous architecture. These categories are usually arbitrarily defined as less than 25 percent villous, 25 to 75 percent villous, and more than 75 percent villous, respectively,

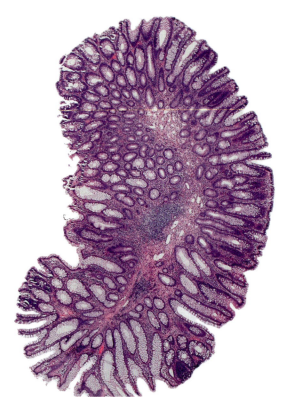

Figure 3-12

TUBULAR ADENOMA

Regularly arranged straight crypts are similar to those of normal colonic mucosa.

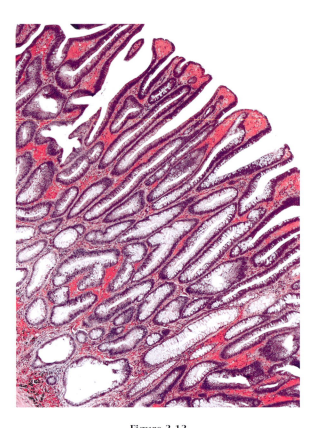

Figure 3-13

**CONVENTIONAL ADENOMA
WITH EXTENSIVE VILLOUS GROWTH**

Long finger-like projections are lined with dysplastic epithelium.

although other arbitrary figures have also been used (23). Villi are not always easy to define. In general, a villous structure is a finger-like projection with the epithelium on the surface and stroma and vascular structures in the center. This differs from a tubular architecture in which the epithelial cells line tubules and the stroma surrounds the tubules (hence recapitulating normal mucosa). This difference is not always readily recognized, and in some cases, adenomas show a tubular architecture in the deeper portions of the polyp, with short villi on the surface, which is different from lesions in which villi extend from the base to the lumen (figs. 3-14, 3-15). This difficulty in defining a villous structure is probably responsible in large part for the suboptimal reproducibility in the distinction of tubular versus tubulovillous versus villous adenoma, with a reported kappa in the range of 0.21 to 0.5 (16,17).

Data indicate that lesions with a greater percentage of villous architecture have higher rates of high-grade dysplasia and invasive carcinoma, when corrected for size, than lesions without villous architecture (23). Hence, lesions with villous architecture are considered "advanced," as are lesions greater than 1 cm and those with high-grade dysplasia. The breakdown of lesions with a villous component by percentage involvement is itself rife with problems, including lack of a definition of what 25 percent of a polyp actually is (i.e., 25 percent of the surface area or 25 percent of the volume), as well as the fact that the assessment considers components of a three dimensional polyp in two dimensions, which adds considerable error to the calculation. Perhaps for this reason, most studies do not distinguish between tubulovillous and villous adenomas but rather consider any lesion with a "significant" villous component, usually

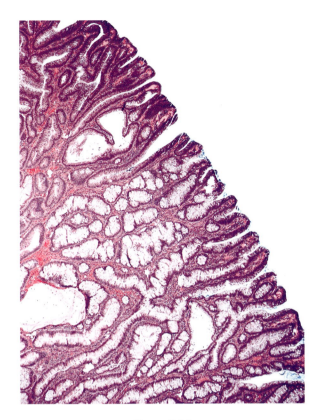

Figure 3-14

LARGE CONVENTIONAL ADENOMA

There is an overall tubular configuration but with short stumpy villous projections on the surface. Polyps like this raise a question regarding how long such projections need to be considered "villi."

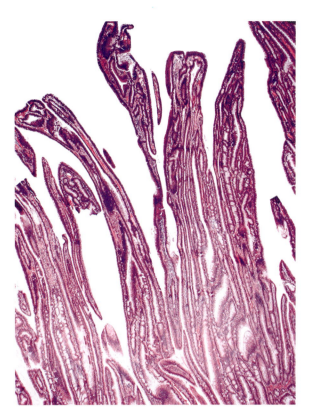

Figure 3-15

VILLOUS ADENOMA WITH LONG VILLI

These villi extend nearly the entire thickness of the lesion and are easy to recognize as true villi.

defined as 25 percent or more of the polyp, as being "advanced" or "high risk."

The concept of "advanced adenoma" has been incorporated into decisions regarding surveillance intervals after screening colonoscopy. Patients with advanced conventional adenomas are assumed to have a greater risk for the development of metachronous adenoma, and therefore undergo colonoscopy at shorter intervals than those patients with adenomas without advanced features. Data supporting this use of the term advanced are, however, not strong. Major risk factors for metachronous adenomas include age and gender of the patient and the presence of three or more adenomas (18). An adenoma over 1 cm is also a risk factor, but is not as strong as the other factors. Evidence regarding the effect of villous architecture is weak, and villous architecture may correlate best with

the development of metachronous advanced adenomas. It is not clear whether high-grade dysplasia carries any significance.

Development of Carcinoma in Conventional Adenomas

Sixty to 70 percent of all colorectal adenocarcinomas arise in conventional adenomas, including those associated with familial adenomatous polyposis, most, but perhaps not all, arising in Lynch syndrome, and most, if not all, sporadic carcinomas developing along the so-called suppressor pathway (also known as chromosomal instability, or *APC*-mutation related, pathway). In all of these categories, the tumors are unassociated with a high level of CpG island methylation (i.e., they are CIMP-L [for low]), they rarely demonstrate mutation of the *BRAF* gene, and with the exception of those arising in Lynch syndrome, they are microsatellite stable. Rarely, conventional adenomas, in particular villous adenomas, are the site of origin of high-grade neuroendocrine carcinomas ("small cell carcinoma"), although grades 1 and 2 neuroendocrine tumors of the large intestine (i.e., carcinoid tumors) are only rarely associated with adenomas (24).

The speed at which conventional adenomas progress to carcinoma seems to be slow, and it has been estimated that removal of 100 adenomas is required to prevent one carcinoma (25). Data from a variety of sources indicate that the time from the development of an adenoma until it progresses to carcinoma is approximately 20 years (26,27), which presumably is the rationale behind the usual recommendation for 10-year screening intervals if a colon is free of adenomas.

High-grade dysplasia is considered to become an adenocarcinoma once it has invaded into and through the muscularis mucosae. Invasion into the lamina propria above the muscularis mucosae can occur, and when it is identified, it can be reported as intramucosal carcinoma, although there appears to be no clinical or prognostic distinction between high-grade dysplasia and intramucosal carcinoma since neither is likely to spread to regional lymph nodes. For this reason reporting intramucosal carcinoma is not universally recommended.

By traditional convention, a tumor is not considered truly malignant in terms of potential for metastatic spread until the muscularis mucosae is breeched. The importance of the muscularis mucosae as a landmark in the colon is that the lamina propria of the mucosa has a very poor lymphatic supply, with lymphatic vessels penetrating from the submucosa only to the base of the crypts. Until the tumor invades into the muscular mucosae, there is essentially no lymphatic access and hence no risk of lymphatic metastasis. It is often stated that invasion through the muscularis mucosae is necessary in order to consider a tumor "invasive" (28). The rationale for this is that in the past lymphatic vessels were believed not to penetrate into the lamina propria. Early ultrastructural studies, as well as more recent studies using immunohistochemical staining for D2-40, have shown that lymphatics are present in the lamina propria, especially in inflamed or neoplastic colonic mucosa (29).

A confounding factor in using penetration through the muscularis mucosae as the gold standard is that, in many adenomas, the muscularis mucosae becomes splayed and thickened, making it difficult to determine when the tumor has actually passed through its complete thickness as opposed to only invading into it (fig. 3-16). Invasion into but not necessarily through the muscularis mucosae would seem adequate to allow a diagnosis of invasion, but the current staging criteria use submucosal invasion as a criterion for T1 invasion, as further discussed in chapter 4. Even when tumors invade through the muscularis mucosae the risk of lymph node metastasis is very small until the tumor extends through the submucosa into the muscularis propria. The risk of metastasis is higher when there is lymphovascular invasion, or if the tumor is high grade or has a high degree of tumor budding or other risk factors further described in the section on adenocarcinoma of the colon in chapter 4. These factors influence the prognosis and management of malignant polyps, and are an important component when reporting these lesions, discussed below.

For large polyps, it is important to section them through the resection site if possible to allow evaluation of the resection margin, particularly in cases with focal adenocarcinoma in the head of a polyp. It is recommended that the margin be inked and that most polyps be only bisected rather than serial sectioned since bisection will assure resection margins in both halves of a specimen. If the polyp is too large to simply bisect, it should first be bisected to achieve two sections with adequate visualization of the margins and then any excess polyp can be trimmed from the outside of these bisections to allow the polyp to be properly cassetted.

Pseudoinvasion (Glandular Displacement in Neoplastic Polyps)

Occasionally, otherwise benign conventional adenomas demonstrate glandular elements in the submucosa, simulating invasive adenocarcinoma (30,31). This happens most often in pedunculated polyps and is a frequent finding in sigmoid colon adenomas. This displacement of glands is thought most likely to be due to intermittent torsion of the polyps, with ischemia, ulceration, and secondary healing over of the ulcer. Typically these glandular elements have a mucinous appearance, consisting of pools of

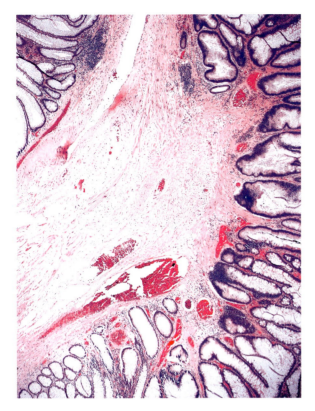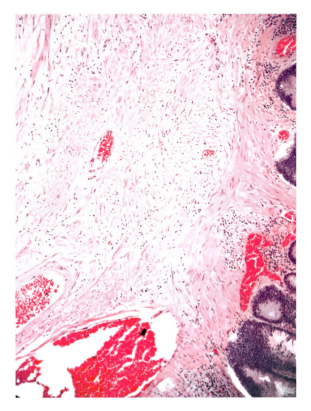

Figure 3-16

TUBULAR ADENOMA WITH SPLAYING OF THE MUSCULARIS MUCOSAE

Left: The muscularis mucosae consists of numerous intertwined bundles of smooth muscle and does not constitute a simple layer of smooth muscle 3 or 4 cells thick.

Right: At higher magnification, the thickened muscularis mucosae is evident.

mucin often devoid of epithelial cells or with a partial lining by epithelial cells that, in general, are very bland and without cytologic features of malignancy, although of course they are dysplastic since they are entrapped adenomatous epithelium (fig. 3-17).

Since these lesions arise following torsion, there is usually evidence of that prior torsion, including hemosiderin deposition and patchy chronic inflammation, and sometimes fibrosis, which should not be mistaken for a desmoplastic reaction to invasive carcinoma. Most of the time this change occurs in adenomas that otherwise have no high-grade dysplasia in the overlying mucosa, in distinction to true invasive adenocarcinomas, which usually do have overlying high-grade dysplasia. This phenomenon is usually easily recognized by the associated findings and lack of high-grade dysplasia. In rare cases in which high-grade dysplasia is iden-

tified, caution is warranted, and in some cases an absolute distinction of pseudoinvasion from carcinoma cannot be made (31). In such cases, the lesion should be reported as "equivocal" and in most cases can be managed by repeat endoscopy to assure complete removal of any residual lesion and by a second endoscopy at a shortened interval (e.g., 1 year) to assure that there is no regrowth of the lesion.

Recommendations on Reporting Conventional Adenomas

Although reporting of conventional adenomas has been codified by current screening recommendations, it is not without controversy. The main controversy revolves around the value of reporting the degree of the villous component and high-grade dysplasia (32,33). Conventional wisdom holds that these factors are predictors of future occurrence of polyps

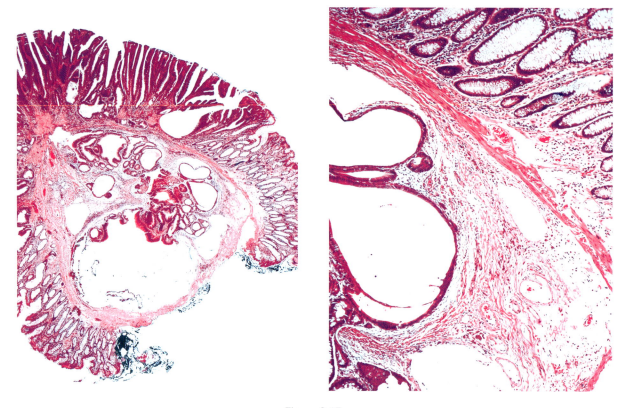

Figure 3-17

PSEUDOINVASION IN AN ADENOMA

Left: This polyp shows extensive displacement of glandular epithelium into the submucosa, simulating invasive adenocarcinoma.

Right: At higher power, the glandular epithelium does not have cytologic features of malignancy and there is abundant hemosiderin deposition in the stroma adjacent to the displaced glands, which are invested in their lamina propria, indicative of prior torsion and hemorrhage in this area.

and hence are of value in determining screening intervals. Countering this is the well-recognized fact that the reproducibility of these features is poor, and management of the current lesion requires complete removal regardless of the presence or absence of these features, and therefore these features are only of value in determining screening intervals and are probably not very good at that.

The more powerful predictors of metachronous lesions are number and size of the adenomas, along with clinical features (age, gender, family history) and colonoscopic-specific factors (e.g. adequacy of preparation, completeness of removal of lesion). It is thought by many that when size is taken into consideration, histologic variables add little to the equation since most adenomas with over 25 percent villous architecture or high-grade dysplasia are greater than 1

cm, and are considered advanced or high risk even without histologic evaluation. For these reasons some authors have recommended that reporting of villous architecture and degree of dysplasia is not necessary (32,33).

In the end, the decision of what to report is mainly driven by requirements of professional societies and by communication between the pathologist and clinician about what information in the local setting is considered of value. Since current screening guidelines recommend screening intervals that are based on histologic features, adequate reporting should include subtyping the lesion by the degree of the villous component and a statement about the presence or absence of high-grade dysplasia (34). Obviously if an adenocarcinoma is present, it should also be reported. In general, size is not reportable from a pathology specimen unless it is a surgical resection. For endoscopy-derived cases, polyp size is based on the endoscopist's assessment, and is not generally part of the pathology report.

For lesions containing invasive adenocarcinoma, additional features should be reported. These vary depending on whether the lesion is sessile or pedunculated, and most require an intact excision of the polyp (rather than a piecemeal excision) to be adequately reported. These features include: grade and histologic type of invasive tumor, depth of invasion, presence or absence of lymphovascular invasion, presence of a high degree of tumor budding, and adequacy of excision (35–37). There are numerous ways that depth of invasion can be reported, and this reporting should be tailored to the needs and understanding of local clinicians. One convenient shorthand is the Haggitt system, which applies numerical designations to the various levels of invasion (38). Another approach is to simply report the depth of invasion descriptively (39). Although initially much was made of different levels of growth, the major factors affecting recurrence of tumor are the status of the resection margin, along with the presence of lymphovascular invasion, tumor budding, and poor differentiation of the tumor. These factors determine whether polypectomy is an adequate excision of the lesion or if additional surgical excision is recommended. The measured depth of invasion, from the base of the muscularis mucosae into the submucosa, may also be important (39).

Technical Issues with the Biopsy Diagnosis of Conventional Adenomas

There are some technical issues with the diagnosis of conventional adenoma that need to be recognized in order to avoid over- or underdiagnosis. One common issue involves a polypectomy specimen that on initial review shows only normal mucosa or a lymphoid aggregate but no adenoma or other type of mucosal polyp. Sometimes, if additional tissue levels are examined, a small polyp will be identified (either neoplastic or hyperplastic) and will allow a correct diagnosis. Therefore, in any case in which the endoscopist identifies a "polyp," it is worthwhile to cut and review additional sections prior to assuming that no lesion is pres-

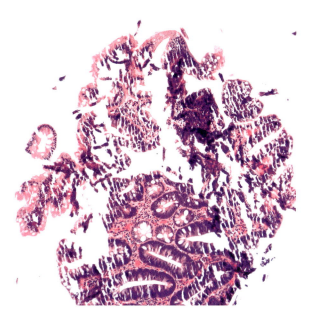

Figure 3-18

SMALL TUBULAR ADENOMA

The technical artifact ("chatter") can mask a small area of dysplastic glands. In this case, adenoma is apparent adjacent to the chatter.

ent. Studies have demonstrated that doing this will reveal an adenoma in at least 10 percent of cases, although personal experience would suggest that the true number may be higher than this (40).

Another common technical issue with small conventional adenomas is "masking" of the adenoma by the technical artifact of chattering, or shattering, of the section in the area of the adenoma. This is common, and may have to do with excessive dehydration of the tissue during processing. It is presumed that a lack of mucin in the neoplastic epithelium results in dehydration and hence the tissue is prone to chattering during microtomy (fig. 3-18). If sections are only examined at low power, the dysplastic epithelium may be overlooked. Therefore, careful examination at high power of all areas of chatter is recommended to exclude a small area of dysplastic epithelium.

A third issue is that the edges of conventional adenomas are slightly hypermucinous, with elongated crypts, resembling a small goblet cell-rich hyperplastic polyp (GCHP). Often, cutting additional levels of lesions that are suggestive of,

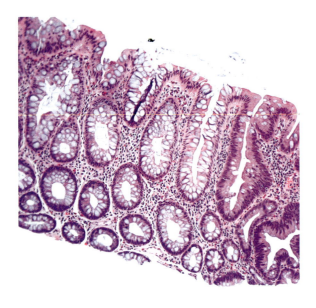

Figure 3-19

TUBULAR ADENOMA AND HYPERPLASIA

Biopsy of tubular adenoma (on the right) with adjacent mucosal hyperplasia simulating a goblet cell-rich hyperplastic polyp (on the left). Occasionally, only the hyperplastic area is identified in initial sections of such a lesion and the conventional adenoma can be missed.

but not diagnostic of, GCHP reveals an adjacent conventional adenoma (fig. 3-19).

Finally, occasionally distinguishing "dysplastic" from "reactive atypical" epithelium can be difficult, similar to the situation in patients with inflammatory bowel disease. This occurs most often when there is ulceration, often in patients with prolapsed hemorrhoids or simple mucosal prolapse syndrome. Usual clues that atypical epithelium is reactive include the presence of inflammation or ulceration in the specimen and the presence of adjacent mucosa with clearly reactive changes (fig. 3-20). True dysplasia should appear to be a clonal process, with dysplastic epithelium directly adjacent to normal epithelium, without any intervening atypical cells. If there is an apparent transition from normal to reactive to "dysplastic," it is probable that the "dysplastic-appearing" epithelium is reactive as well.

Rarely, endometriosis presents as a colonic lesion and can be misinterpreted as an adenoma. Recognition of the background stroma as endometrial allows recognition of endometriosis, a diagnosis that is confirmed with

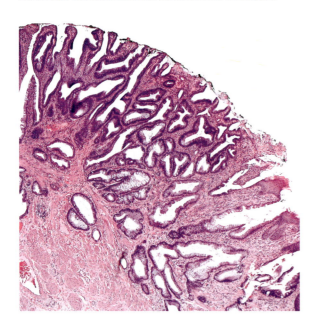

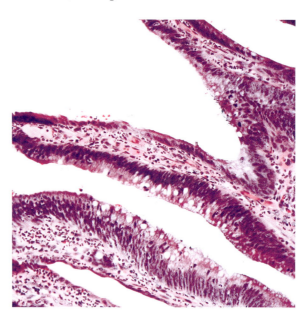

Figure 3-20

PROLAPSED HEMORRHOID DEMONSTRATING MARKED REACTIVE ATYPIA

Left: There is erosion of the surface epithelium with marked reactive atypia that can be misinterpreted as dysplasia (adenoma).

Right: At higher power, the features that allow distinction of dysplasia from reactive change include a prominent neutrophilic infiltrate and adjacent areas of clearly reactive epithelium characterized by cuboidal cells with round uniform nuclei, small prominent nucleoli, and eosinophilic cytoplasm.

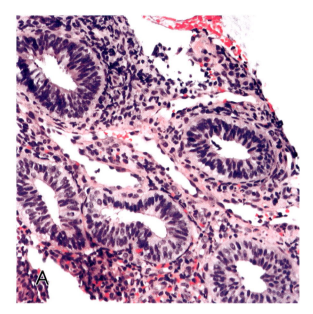

Figure 3-21

ENDOMETRIOSIS MISINTERPRETED AS RECTAL TUBULAR ADENOMA

A: Although the epithelium is atypical, it is not pseudo-stratified or mitotically active, and the background stroma resembles endometrial stroma, not colonic lamina propria.

B: Cytokeratin (CK) 7 marks the epithelium. CK20 was negative.

C: CD10 marks the stroma.

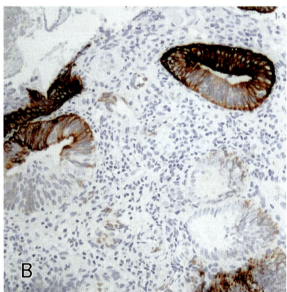

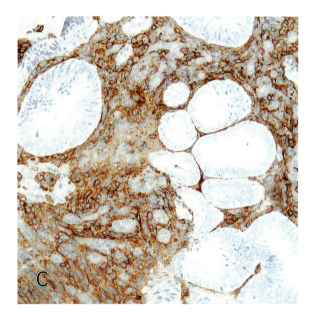

immunohistochemical staining, which shows expression of cytokeratin (CK) 7 but not 20, and CD10-reactive stroma (fig. 3-21).

In many institutions, multiple polyps from separate sites are often submitted in one formalin container. If this is the case, and any of the polyps are large enough to require sectioning, then the polyps should be inked different colors to allow identification on the slide just in case one of more of the lesions contains malignancy. This allows accurate identification of how many malignant polyps there are. In addition, if there is a mixture of serrated and conventional

adenomas in a specimen, it will allow SSA/P with cytologic dysplasia to be distinguished from SSA/P and conventional adenomas (see discussion below).

SERRATED POLYPS AND THE SERRATED PATHWAY TO ADENOCARCINOMA

Until 1990, essentially all serrated lesions of the large intestine were considered benign hyperplastic polyps. In 1989, however, Urbanski et al. (41) reported a case of adenocarcinoma arising in a lesion interpreted as a mixed hyperplastic-adenomatous polyp and suggested that

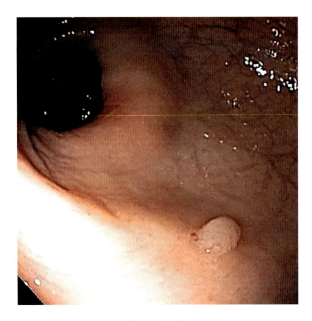

Figure 3-22

HYPERPLASTIC POLYP

At endoscopy, these are characteristically small, sessile, pearly white lesions. They may occur as clusters in the rectum.

hyperplastic polyps might not be as "benign" as previously thought, challenging the conventional wisdom about them. A year later, Longacre and Fenoglio-Preiser (42) introduced the term serrated adenoma to describe lesions fitting the general description of a serrated lesion with cytologic dysplasia, although the definition of this lesion at that time was not totally clear and it now appears that this publication encompassed at least two different types of polyps, now known as traditional serrated adenoma (TSA) and sessile serrated adenoma/polyp with cytologic dysplasia (SSA/PCD).

The lesion now known as SSA/P was first described in 1996 in a study of patients with the syndrome formerly known as hyperplastic polyposis (now renamed serrated polyposis), although the term SSA itself was not coined until a follow-up study of sporadic serrated lesions in 2003 (2,43). It was at that point that the distinction between TSA and SSA/P was first recommended. SSA/P is by far the more common of these two premalignant serrated lesions, and the one about which the most is currently known, despite its relatively recent introduction.

Hyperplastic Polyps

Definition. *Hyperplastic polyps* (HPs) are epithelial polyps characterized by *BRAF* or *KRAS* mutations and decreased apoptosis, leading to the development of a serrated architecture as the cells accumulate. There is no cytologic dysplasia in these lesions and they are not considered immediate precursors to malignancy. Aside from the accumulation of fairly normal cells, the overall architecture of these lesions is normal, which distinguishes them from other serrated polyps. They are included in this chapter because of their similarity to SSA/P.

Gross Findings. HPs are usually small (less than 5 mm), sessile polyps that appear white at endoscopy (fig. 3-22). They are most commonly located in the left colon, although a significant number of lesions, particularly of the microvesicular subtype, are located in the right colon.

Microscopic Findings. The decreased apoptosis resulting from mutations of the *BRAF* or *KRAS* gene causes accumulation of hypermature epithelial cells in the crypts (44). Accumulation of these cells results in a piling up of epithelium, which gives the lesions an overall serrated configuration (fig. 3-23). Since the proliferative zone remains in its normal location at the base of the crypts, which is narrow and lined with immature cells, the crypts are straight and the serrations develop in the upper portions of the crypts (fig. 3-24). The superficial epithelium may appear hypermature, with increased numbers of goblet cells, or may develop an abnormal microvesicular mucin content (fig. 3-25). Occasionally, mucin is decreased or absent. Mitoses are confined to the lower third of the crypts (with staining for MIB-1 also confined to this area). There is no cytologic dysplasia, although reactive atypia may be seen in the mucin-poor variant (see below). In some cases the surface basement membrane may be thickened but this is of little diagnostic value. Neuroendocrine cells may be increased in these lesions in comparison to normal mucosa (figs. 3-24, 3-26).

HPs are subdivided based on the type of mucin present (2). If the lesion has microvesicular mucin (fig. 3-25) it is called a *microvesicular hyperplastic polyp* (MVHP). This is the most common type and the most easily recognized. Serrations tend to be most prominent in this variant. About 80

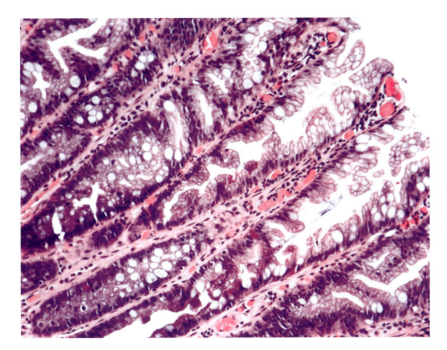

Figure 3-23

MICROVESICULAR HYPERPLASTIC POLYP (MVHP)

All hyperplastic polyps are characterized by variable degrees of serration of the epithelium, as seen in this example. This is thought to result from decreased apoptosis.

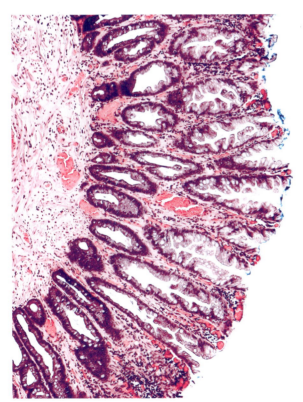

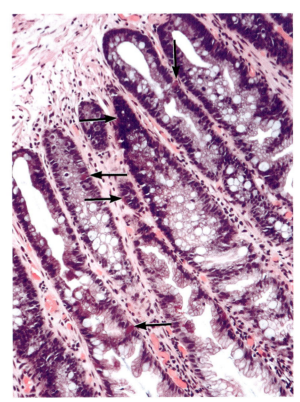

Figure 3-24

MICROVESICULAR HYPERPLASTIC POLYP

Left: The crypts are straight, with uniform narrow bases and increased serration toward the luminal surface.

Right: The bases of the crypts are narrow, with little evidence of differentiation. Mitotic activity and MIB-1 (Ki-67) staining occur in this area. Scattered eosinophilic neuroendocrine cells (Kulchitsky cells) are present (arrows).

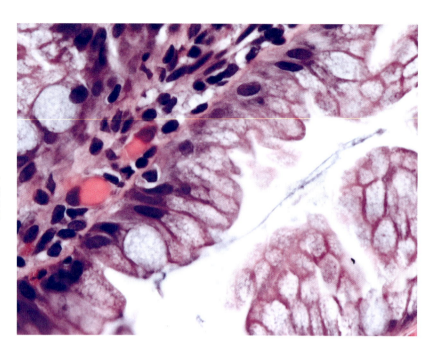

Figure 3-25

**MICROVESICULAR
HYPERPLASTIC POLYP**

The surface shows prominent serrations and epithelial cells containing small droplet (microvesicular) mucin with variable numbers of interspersed goblet cells.

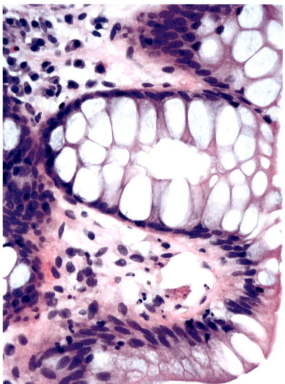

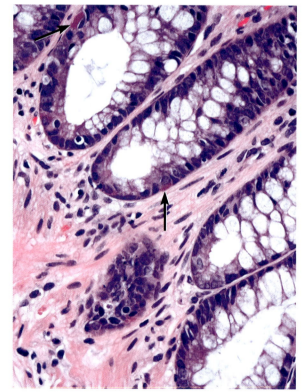

Figure 3-26

GOBLET CELL-RICH HYPERPLASTIC POLYP

Left: The superficial portion of GCHPs show subtle serrations and epithelium that consists exclusively of goblet cells without microvesicular cells.

Right: The base of the crypts are narrow, as in MVHP. Goblet cells can extend deeply into the crypts. Several prominent neuroendocrine cells (arrows) are present.

percent of MVHPs demonstrate *BRAF* mutations. If the lesion has purely goblet cell mucin, without any microvesicular mucin, it is referred to as a *goblet cell-rich hyperplastic polyp* (GCHP) (fig. 3-27). These lesions have less prominent serrations than the MVHPs and are mainly identified in the left colon, often as clusters of diminutive polyps. These lesions are mainly *KRAS* rather than *BRAF* mutated. Some HPs contain little or no mucin. These are referred to as *mucin-poor* (MPHP). They are rare and may represent MVHPs that have been damaged. They are often inflamed and demonstrate reactive atypia, which can suggest a neoplastic polyp (fig. 3-28). They have not been characterized molecularly. At the current time, subtyping of HPs is considered optional since there are no known behavior differences between the subtypes.

Treatment and Prognosis. HPs of all types are generally regarded as indolent lesions and are not considered at risk for the development of malignancy; patients only require more careful

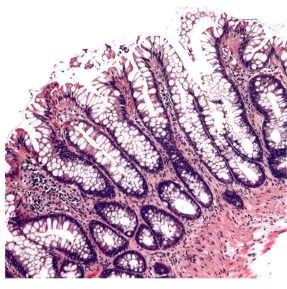

Figure 3-27

GOBLET CELL-RICH HYPERPLASTIC POLYP

Although the crypts are elongated, the degree of serration is less than that of MVHP.

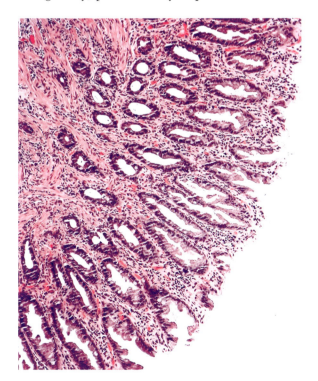
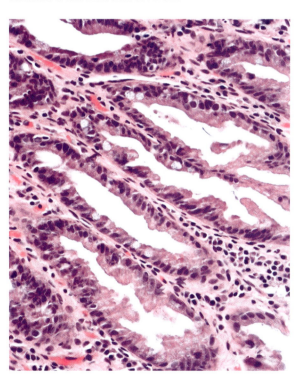

Figure 3-28

MUCIN-POOR HYPERPLASTIC POLYP (MPHP)

Left: This lesion resembles a MVHP in that there is significant serration toward the luminal surface. The lesion has a hyperchromatic appearance, however, because of the lack of mucin.

Right: At higher magnification little mucin is present, mainly in the form of goblet cells. The cells are cuboidal to low columnar and the nuclei are rounded with prominent nucleoli.

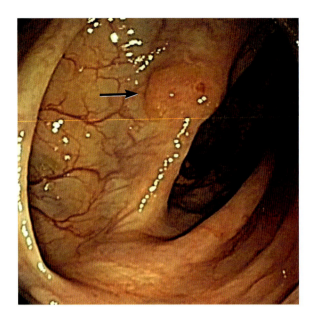

Figure 3-29

SESSILE SERRATED ADENOMA/POLYP (SSA/P)

Endoscopically, these lesions are often similar in color to the background mucosa and slightly elevated. They often have adherent mucin or stool.

surveillance than patients with no lesions. However, since many SSA/Ps demonstrate areas resembling HP, all lesions diagnosed as HP should be removed completely since a biopsy can incorrectly classify a SSA/P as a HP (discussed below). This is particularly true for lesions of the right colon.

Patients with clusters of diminutive polyps in the rectosigmoid colon do not need to have all lesions removed since these are invariably all small HPs. The general recommendation for these cases is to sample the largest polyps for histologic evaluation and if they are HP then the remaining small lesions can be left in place.

Sessile Serrated Adenoma/Polyp

Definition. *Sessile serrated adenoma/polyp* (SSA/P) is a premalignant epithelial polyp characterized by excessive serration of the overall architecture, with abnormal localization of the proliferative zone leading to abnormal architecture and growth. SSA/P is not cytologically dysplastic although cytologic dysplasia may develop as the lesion progresses. Typically, these lesions demonstrate *BRAF* mutations and a high degree of methylation (44). Synonyms for SSA/P include *sessile serrated lesion* and *serrated polyp with abnormal proliferation*.

Gross Findings. SSA/P is typically a very ill-defined, flat, sessile lesion (fig. 3-29). It may be difficult to identify at endoscopy unless the endoscopist is familiar with the lesion and makes a concerted effort to identify it (45). These lesions often extrude excess mucin, resulting in the formation of an overlying mucus cap, which then obscures the underlying SSA/P. Residual fecal material is often adherent to this mucus material. Both the presence of the mucus cap and residual feces act as clues to the presence of an underlying lesion. Careful washing to remove the stool and mucus may make the polyp more visible. These lesions are visible with routine endoscopy and it is unclear whether other technologies such as narrow band imaging or chromoendoscopy necessarily improve the detection rate (46). The difficulty in visualizing and totally resecting these lesions is likely to account for many cases of interval carcinoma.

SSA/Ps have a predilection for the right colon, although they arise the left colon as well. They are often large, particularly compared to HPs, and account for a majority of lesions that used to be diagnosed as giant HPs based on a size greater than 1 cm. Nevertheless, many small examples exist, including lesions well under 1 cm in diameter, that contain invasive carcinoma. Thus, small SSA/Ps cannot be ignored. Given the obscure and subtle appearance of these lesions, they are often biopsied rather than resected, which needs to be taken into account when diagnosing serrated lesions and when making management recommendations.

Microscopic Findings. The basic pathogenesis of SSA/P appears to be a loss of normal localization of the proliferative zone of the crypts, leading to the architectural abnormalities that are the most diagnostic feature (1,6). By definition, uncomplicated SSA/P does not have the type of cytologic dysplasia seen in conventional adenomas. The proliferative zone is often located on the side of the crypt rather than in its usual location at the base, and as cells differentiate and mature, they migrate both toward the lumen of the colon and toward the base. Since the maturing cells, upon reaching the muscularis mucosae, cannot move further downward, they move laterally, leading to dilated, irregular crypt bases (often described as L-shaped, boot shaped, or anchor shaped) lined with mature cells (fig. 3-30). These may be goblet cells or they may demonstrate a gastric phenotype with the appearance of gastric foveolar cells (fig. 3-31). This distorted crypt architecture and the presence of mature cells at the base of the crypts is the major feature that distinguishes SSA/P from HP. This change is often focal, however, and variable proportions of many SSA/Ps have areas with narrow bases showing immature cells nearly identical to those seen in HPs (fig. 3-32).

In order to diagnose a lesion as SSA/P, only a single convincing abnormal crypt is needed. Therefore, small biopsies of large lesions may suggest the incorrect diagnosis of HP. For this reason, complete excision of all serrated lesions is recommended, particularly in the right colon, even if, on biopsy, the lesion resembles a HP.

Neuroendocrine cells are generally reduced in number in SSA/P, compared to HP, and are often absent. Although there is no conventional cytologic dysplasia, as seen in conventional adenomas, there may be subtle nuclear atypia with enlarged nuclei with prominent nucleoli, and occasional cells showing enteric metaplasia, sometimes referred to as serrated dysplasia. Mitoses may be seen at any level of the crypt due to the alterations in the proliferative zone, although overall mitotic activity is not increased significantly over that of the normal mucosa.

These changes are reflected in the location of mature colonocytes expressing CK20, which may be located not only on the surface as they are in normal mucosa, but also at the base of the crypts, or may replace entire crypts (6). Similarly, MIB-1 reactivity may be seen at any level of the crypt and may overlap with CK20 staining, a pattern not seen in any other lesion or in normal mucosa. The serrations may be exaggerated compared with HPs, and most prominent near the dilated base of the crypts (fig. 3-33) in distinction from HPs in which the primary location of the serration is near the luminal aspect of the crypts.

Other features often seen in SSA/P include herniation of epithelium through the muscularis mucosae into the submucosa ("inverted" growth pattern) and a prominent submucosal fat pad, which may lead to a pale endoscopic

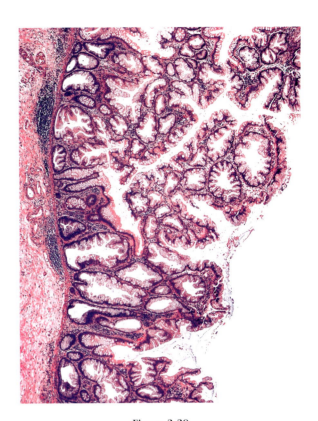

Figure 3-30

SESSILE SERRATED ADENOMA/POLYP

As opposed to the typical hyperplastic polyp, SSA/P is characterized by abnormal distorted crypts that often demonstrate boot- or anchor-shaped bases. There is also often exaggerated serration, including serration near the base of the crypts. Abundant mucin adheres to the surface, which corresponds to what is often seen at endoscopy.

appearance (fig. 3-34). Neither of these features is specific for SSA/P, both being occasionally seen with HPs, although they are much more common in SSA/Ps.

With progression of disease, SSA/P can develop cytologic dysplasia, which may be histologically identical to that seen in conventional adenomas or may be composed of more cuboidal cells with eosinophilic cytoplasm and round vesicular nuclei with prominent nucleoli, known as serrated dysplasia (fig. 3-35). This more obvious type of serrated dysplasia must be distinguished from the enteric metaplasia sometimes also referred to as "serrated dysplasia" often seen in TSA, which has bland oval nuclei without mitotic activity and should not be considered as true dysplasia (fig. 3-36). These more advanced lesions are termed SSA/P with cytologic dysplasia (SSA/PCD).

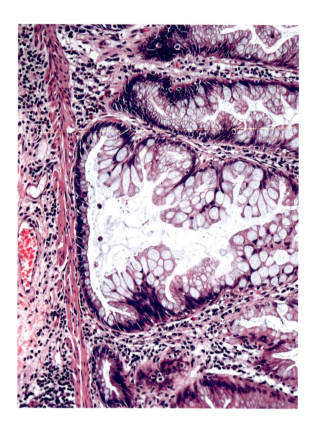 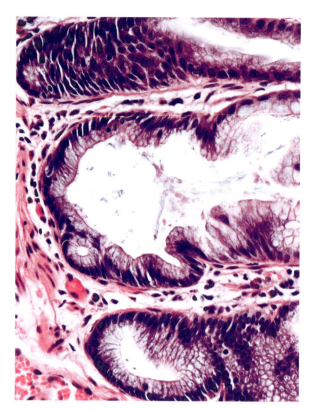

Figure 3-31

SESSILE SERRATED ADENOMA/POLYP

Left: This anchor-shaped crypt base contains mature goblet cells. MIB-1 (Ki-67) would demonstrate no proliferation in this area.

Right: This dilated crypt base is lined with gastric foveolar-type cells.

Figure 3-32

SESSILE SERRATED ADENOMA/POLYP

Significant areas with narrow crypt bases resemble MVHP. A small biopsy of this lesion could be misinterpreted as MVHP if the entire lesion was not removed.

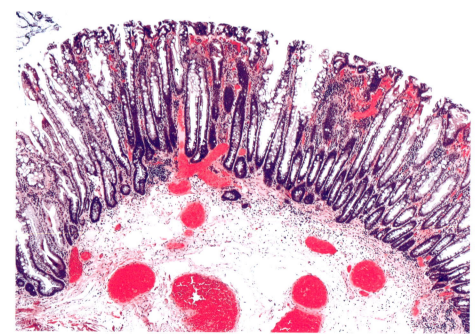

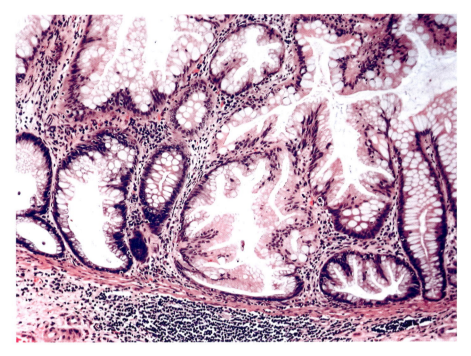

Figure 3-33

SESSILE SERRATED ADENOMA/POLYP

Prominent serration is seen near the base of a crypt.

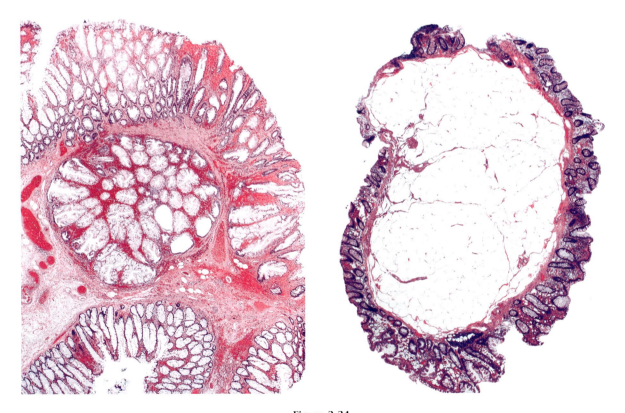

Figure 3-34

SESSILE SERRATED ADENOMA/POLYP

Left: Herniation of the epithelium into the submucosa creates an "inverted" growth pattern, common in large SSAs.
Right: Prominent lipoma-like fat pads often underlie SSA/P.

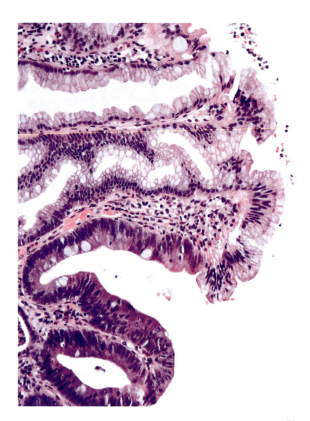
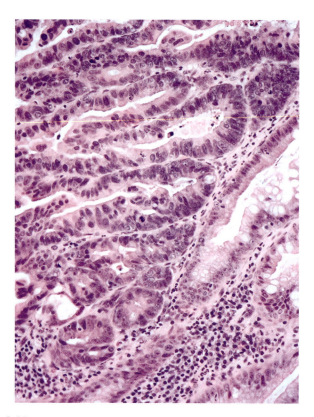

Figure 3-35

SESSILE SERRATED ADENOMA/POLYP WITH CYTOLOGIC DYSPLASIA (SSA/PCD)

Left: This SSA/P shows an area of cytologic dysplasia resembling that of conventional adenoma. The transition from SSA/P at the top to dysplasia at the bottom is sharp.

Right: This SSA/P demonstrates cytologic dysplasia characterized by cuboidal to low columnar cells with round nuclei containing prominent nucleoli and abundant eosinophilic cytoplasm (i.e., serrated dysplasia). These features are similar to those seen in serrated adenocarcinoma.

Figure 3-36

SESSILE SERRATED ADENOMA/ POLYP WITH ENTERIC METAPLASIA

The left side of the crypt shows the typical mucinous epithelium of the SSA, and the right side shows cells resembling small intestinal absorptive epithelium, enteric metaplasia. There is no cytologic atypia or mitotic activity. This type of epithelium does not represent cytologic dysplasia and does not indicate that this lesion is a traditional serrated adenoma.

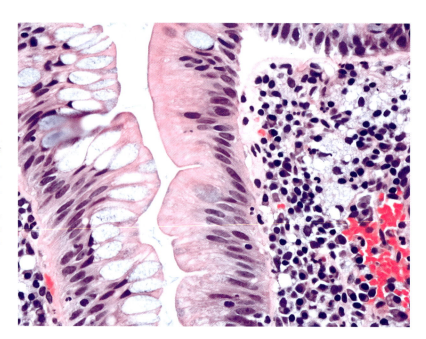

In the past, SSA/PCD was often diagnosed as mixed HP-tubular adenoma, however, such terminology is discouraged because from a molecular and prognostic viewpoint, the dysplastic epithelium is very different from that of conventional adenoma. Whereas conventional adenomas are *APC* mutated and do not express a CIMP-H phenotype or *BRAF* mutation, SSA/PCD are *BRAF* mutated (in at least 80 percent of cases), are CIMP-H, and are potentially prone to rapid progression due to microsatellite instability.

In SSA/PCD, the mitotic activity is generally increased in the cytologically dysplastic areas. The development of cytologic dysplasia correlates in some cases with inactivation of the *MLH1* mismatch repair gene by hypermethylation in those lesions progressing toward MSI carcinoma, and at that point the dysplastic epithelium may be MSI as well (47,48). Cytologic dysplasia also occurs in those lesions progressing to CIMP+MSS carcinoma, although the molecular alterations leading to the development of this dysplasia are unknown. Needless to say, in the pathway to MSS carcinoma, this dysplastic epithelium is not MSI. The reason that SSA/Ps show a high level of methylation is unknown, although it is tempting to tie this phenomenon to the *BRAF* mutations that are common in these lesions, with resultant inhibition of normal apoptosis and increased aging of the cells, which correlate with increased methylation (49).

Adenocarcinomas arise from the cytologically dysplastic epithelium of SSA/PCD, even when the dysplasia is considered low grade if encountered in a conventional adenoma. It is recommended that the cytologic dysplasia not be graded, since low-grade dysplasia is often the only dysplasia present adjacent to carcinoma, and the use of this term might be construed as of less importance and analogous to the situation in conventional adenomas. Since this dysplastic epithelium often has MSI, any cytologic dysplasia in SSA/P is considered an advanced feature in the progression of these polyps.

Cytologic dysplasia and carcinoma may develop when these lesions are very small, in some cases less than 5 mm, hence these polyps are very unpredictable. It would appear that the methylation of the *MLH1* gene leading to the development of MSI occurs on a random basis,

or may never occur, and these lesions can grow to be very large without becoming malignant, but they can become malignant while very small. The fact that carcinoma can presumably develop rapidly once MSI develops may also be part of the reason that these lesions produce carcinomas in the interval between routine colonoscopies (in addition to the fact that they are hard to detect and may be missed and not removed).

Immunohistochemical Findings. Immunohistochemical staining is useful for understanding the pathogenesis of serrated lesions but has not generally been used for diagnosis. Double staining with MIB-1 and CK20 has shown distinctive patterns of proliferation and maturation in the family of serrated lesions, which has been useful in understanding the development of these lesions(6). Although in theory these stains might be useful for diagnosis, that possibility has not been rigorously tested.

There has been some interest in mucin staining of these lesions. Early studies showed increased expression of MUC6 almost exclusively in SSA/P, with little or no staining in HP and TSA (50). Subsequent studies, however, did not confirm such a clear dichotomous staining pattern although essentially all studies demonstrate enhancement of MUC6 expression in SSA/P when compared with HP and TSA (51,52). Although this has been widely interpreted as meaning that MUC6 is not of value in distinguishing these lesions, MUC6 may be a better discriminator than hematoxylin and eosin (H&E) histology alone, which has variable reproducibility. Given the lack of a true gold standard for diagnosis, the variation in expression of MUC6 in different studies may reflect variability in the diagnosis of SSA/P by different pathologists rather than poor reproducibility of the MUC6 expression. Nevertheless, at the current time MUC6 expression has not been demonstrated to be a useful diagnostic tool.

Other markers have been studied to assess expression on the different types of serrated lesions. These include survivin, hedgehog protein, COX2, p504s, p53, and annexin 10 (53–57). Most of these studies (with the possible exception of annexin 10) find HP and SSA/P to demonstrate similar expression of proteins and to be different from TSA (which, if anything, tends to mark more like conventional adenoma when included in the testing, as for COX2). Annexin 10 has been suggested as a potentially useful marker for differentiating SSA/P from both MVHP and TSA, although there is some overlap with MVHP (56), and the stain is not used in daily practice.

Advanced and High-Risk SSA/P

It is clear that SSA/PCD represents an advanced stage of disease in the serrated pathway in that such lesions are closer to developing carcinoma than SSA/P without cytologic dysplasia. Although it is often presumed that large lesions are more likely to develop into carcinoma, and hence lesions over a certain size could be considered "advanced," there are no data suggesting what that size cutoff should be. A size of 1 cm (as is used for conventional adenoma) has been regarded as advanced by some authors, but there are no data to support that presumption. The fact that lesions smaller than 1 cm can develop carcinoma, and that there are many SSA/Ps larger than 1 cm that do not develop carcinoma, casts doubt on any absolute size parameter at this time.

Regarding features indicating a high risk of metachronous lesions, little is known. As a general rule, the simple finding of a single SSA/P is a harbinger of the presence of synchronous or metachronous SSA/Ps. There are even some data indicating that the presence of an SSA/P predicts the current or future presence of conventional adenoma (58). There are also data suggesting that having multiple SSA/Ps indicates greater risk, and that having synchronous high risk adenomas and SSA/P carries a greater risk (59). It is not totally clear, however, whether metachronous lesions are truly the result of a field effect or if some represent incomplete resection of the initial lesion, since there is compelling evidence that the frequency of incomplete resection is very high for SSA/P (60).

There is evidence that the simultaneous presence of conventional adenomas with SSA/P indicates a higher risk of malignancy, both in sporadic lesions and in patients with serrated polyposis (61,62). Although some of these conventional adenomas could be SSA/P with near total replacement by cytologic dysplasia, evidence from the serrated polyposis cases indicates that this is not always the case and that most conventional adenomas in serrated polyposis are, based on an absence of *BRAF* mutations, not SSA/PCD (61).

Management of SSA/P

There is no unanimity of opinion on the most appropriate management of sessile serrated adenomas. A recent consensus paper and task force guidelines suggest that management decisions need to be based on the number, size, and location of polyps; the presence of cytologic dysplasia; and the likelihood that the lesion was completely resected at initial identification (34,45). SSA/PCD deserves careful scrutiny and follow-up since there is a significant chance of microsatellite instability and potential for rapid progression to carcinoma. Any residual lesion potentially conveys high risk; therefore, unless the endoscopist is certain of complete removal, reexamination at a short interval, looking for residual growth, is prudent. Even after presumed complete excision, repeat endoscopy at 1 year is appropriate.

For single or multiple SSA/Ps, the general recommendation has been for a 3-year surveillance interval, assuming that the initial lesion was completely excised. If complete excision is not a practical possibility, then surgical excision may be considered, versus annual repeat endoscopies with generous biopsy of the lesion to assess for cytologic dysplasia. If cytologic dysplasia develops, then complete excision is mandatory unless there are serious clinical contraindications to surgery.

Given that there may be issues with diagnostic accuracy for SSA/P versus HP in the right colon, some authors have recommended that any serrated lesion in the right colon greater than 1 cm in diameter be treated as an SSP/P regardless of the histologic diagnosis. Since several studies have demonstrated that on second review the majority of such cases are reclassified as SSA/P, this suggestion may be a reasonable practical route (63).

Reactive Lesions Resembling SSA/P

Occasionally, reactive conditions create a serrated pattern resembling SSA/P. This can occur, for example, in rectal prolapse (fig. 3-37) or in mucosal prolapse polyps (see chapter 2). We have encountered diffuse colonic mucosal

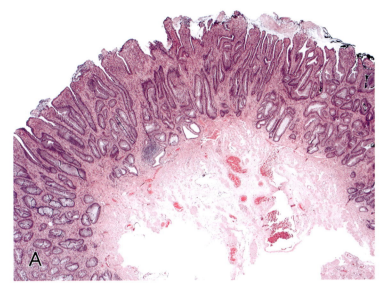

Figure 3-37

MUCOSAL PROLAPSE RESEMBLING SSA/P

A: There is obvious distortion of the mucosa. The surface shows extensive erosion.

B: The base of the crypts are distorted, although with dilated crypts and mature cells. There is also splaying of the muscularis mucosae into the lamina propria, characteristic of mucosal prolapse.

C: The surface shows the extensive erosion characteristic of prolapse.

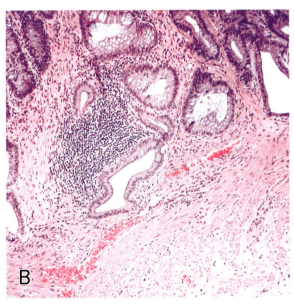

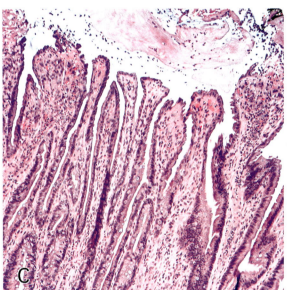

hyperplasia in cytomegalovirus colitis with similar features. Such SSA/P-like changes also occur in active inflammatory bowel disease.

Technical Issues with the Biopsy Diagnosis of Serrated Lesions

There are a number of technical issues that affect the ability of the pathologist to accurately diagnose sessile serrated lesions. Foremost among these are issues related to orientation of the specimen and artifact induced by cautery. Since it is necessary to see the base of the crypts in order to distinguish SSA/P from

HP, the diagnosis generally cannot be made in biopsies that are tangentially sectioned. This actually may be more of a problem with large submucosal one-piece resections compared to piecemeal excisions because in the latter cases the base of crypts may be seen in some of the fragments. Large submucosal resections, unless cross sectioned and oriented perpendicular to the surface, almost always orient themselves in processing in a tangential orientation. If the lesion is tangentially oriented, cutting additional step sections often reveals the base of the crypts and the true nature of the lesion. If a definitive diagnosis of SSA/P cannot be made on a tangential biopsy, then the lesion should be diagnosed as a serrated polyp, unclassified, with an explanation of why a diagnosis cannot be made. If the lesion is located in the right colon, and particularly if the lesion is large, the diagnosis of SSA/P is favored. If the lesion is small and left sided, HP is favored.

As noted in the microscopic description, all serrated lesions that are biopsied and not resected need to be resected, if possible, for both treatment (if the lesion is an SSA/P) and for diagnosis if the biopsy appears to be an HP. Since areas of SSA/P can be histologically identical to HP, a biopsy of a large lesion showing features of only HP is not sufficient to exclude SSA/P.

Cautery artifact can cause two problems for diagnosis. First, distortion caused by the cautery may cause HPs to resemble SSA/Ps. Second, the spindling of the nuclei caused by cautery may resemble cytologic dysplasia. Issues related to cautery should be addressed in any report of these types of lesions.

Traditional Serrated Adenoma

Definition. *Traditional serrated adenoma* (TSA) is a premalignant epithelial lesion characterized by excess serration and often with extensive enteric metaplasia of the surface epithelium. The presence of ectopic crypts has been recommended as a defining feature of this lesion, although this recommendation has not been universally accepted. TSAs may be *BRAF* or *KRAS* mutated and do not necessarily demonstrate conventional cytologic dysplasia.

General Features. Perhaps no neoplastic polyp has been more controversial in recent years than TSA. Much of the controversy revolves around differences in diagnostic criteria, which have hindered a full understanding of this uncommon lesion. The term TSA was proposed to recognize the most characteristic of several types of serrated lesion first termed serrated adenomas by Longacre and Fenoglio-Preiser in 1990 (42). This terminology suggestion occurred after the recognition of SSA/P in 1996 and 2003 (2,43). At the time of the identification of SSA/P in 1996 (although the term was SSA was coined later), it was believed that this lesion was related to the lesion called serrated adenoma by Longacre and Fenoglio-Preiser but differed from their most

characteristic lesion by being flat as opposed to the more protuberant (although still sessile) character of the lesion now known as TSA. We now recognize that these lesions (SSA/P and TSA) are not part of the same pathway to carcinoma. TSA, as defined below, is not a required step in the progression of SSA/P to carcinoma, although recent evidence suggests that some TSAs may arise from SSA/P and progress to *BRAF*-mutated MSS carcinomas (64). It is clear, however, that TSAs do not play a role in the development of MSI carcinomas. Different studies have identified lesions interpreted as SSA/P and HP adjacent to TSA, although there is no general consensus on the frequency of these adjacent lesions or if they are truly precursor lesions.

TSA is a rare lesion, constituting less than 1 percent of all polyps identified in most series. It is located predominantly in the rectum or sigmoid colon. With refined criteria, some lesions previously diagnosed as rectal villous adenomas may actually be advanced TSA, so the actual incidence may be higher than 1 percent (discussed in more detail below). Although it is clear that TSAs may become malignant, the mechanism of their malignant transformation, the rate of the transformation, and the type of carcinoma they produce is not currently known. What is clear is they are not part of the common pathway to sporadic CIMP-H MSI carcinomas.

Gross Findings. TSA is typically an elevated plaque-like or villous sessile lesion located in the rectosigmoid colon or rectum, although it can manifest throughout the colon (fig. 3-38). Rare cases of flat TSA have been reported (64). A few reports in the literature indicate that endoscopically these are usually sessile, although 30 percent in one series appeared pedunculated (65).

Microscopic Findings. TSA is usually a lesion with an overall very villiform configuration at low magnification (which, when exaggerated, has led to the term filiform serrated adenoma [66] for a subset of these lesions) (fig. 3-39). The villi are often expanded at their tips, creating a tennis racquet-like appearance (fig. 3-40). These polyps have a very "busy" look, with exaggerated serrations and often with numerous small crypts budding into the sides of the villi, so called ectopic crypts (fig. 3-41). These ectopic crypts are generally considered an integral and essential feature of the diagnosis and may be a

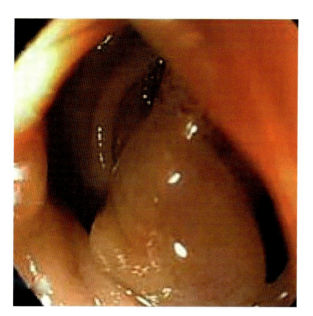

Figure 3-38

TRADITIONAL SERRATED ADENOMA (TSA)

This endoscopic photo shows a large protuberant but sessile, well-circumscribed mass in the sigmoid colon.

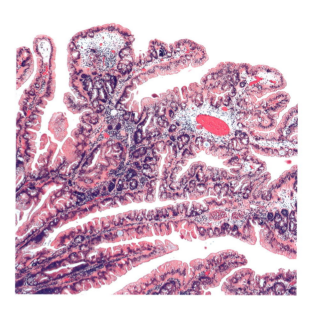

Figure 3-39

TRADITIONAL SERRATED ADENOMA

At low-power, most TSAs have a very villiform configuration. Many have brightly eosinophilic surface epithelial cells and prominent serrations. This case has prominent luminal serrations caused by the presence of enteric-type cells.

reflection of the biology creating these lesions (1,6). Their specificity for the diagnosis has been challenged, although since there is no "gold standard" for the diagnosis of TSA other than its histologic features, to some extent this becomes a matter of opinion (64,67). Even in series that do not require the presence of ectopic crypts for inclusion, however, greater than 90 percent of cases reportedly contain ectopic crypts (64).

The cells lining the villi of TSAs may consist predominantly of goblet cells, although the more characteristic but not universal cytologic finding is the presence of elongated pencillate cells with eosinophilic cytoplasm, often with an identifiable brush border resembling that found in duodenal absorptive cells (fig. 3-42). These cells are generally mitotically inert (with mitotic figures being exceedingly rare and showing no or little marking for the proliferation marker MIB-1). Although sometimes referred to as "dysplastic cells" or "serrated dysplasia," these cells are nondividing, suggesting that they do not share physiological characteristics with the more traditional dysplastic cells seen in conventional adenomas. There are data suggesting that these cells represent a form of enteric metaplasia,

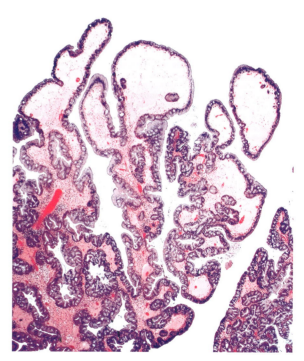

Figure 3-40

TRADITIONAL SERRATED ADENOMA

The tips of some of the villi are expanded and edematous.

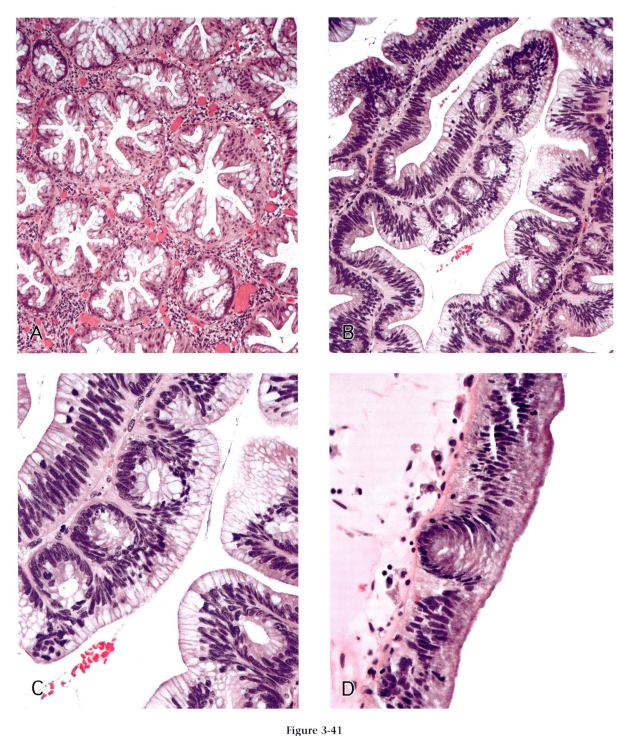

Figure 3-41

TRADITIONAL SERRATED ADENOMA

A: Exaggerated serrations are sometimes seen.

B: Ectopic crypts characteristic of TSA consist of small buds that appear to be miniature crypts extending from the surface into the villi.

C: At higher power, these well-formed ectopic crypts consist of small outpouchings with regenerative compartments and maturation. MIB-1 (Ki-67) staining demonstrates proliferation at the base of these ectopic crypts.

D: An abortive ectopic crypt.

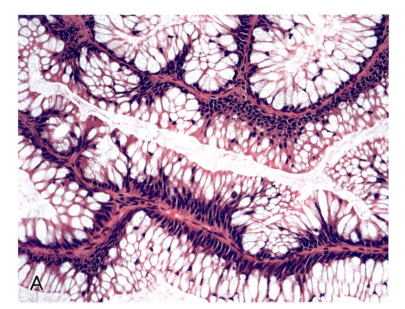

Figure 3-42

TRADITIONAL SERRATED ADENOMA

A: This example is composed almost exclusively of goblet cells.

B: These eosinophilic cells are characteristic but not diagnostic of TSA. They can also be seen in most other polyp types and even in non-neoplastic inflamed mucosa.

C: At higher power, the pencillate eosinophilic cells have elongated but not hyperchromatic nuclei and rarely manifest mitotic activity. They appear to have a brush border and are histologically similar to small intestinal absorptive cells. Some authors consider them a form of serrated dysplasia.

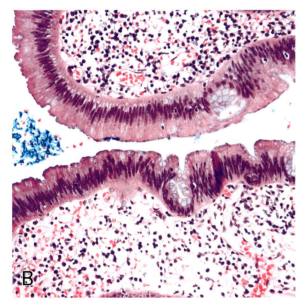

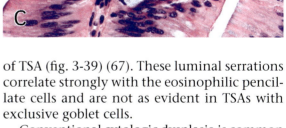

including electron microscopic observations showing abundant mitochondria and a brush border with tight junctions (68). Although these cells are commonly found in TSA, they are not unique to this lesion, being often seen as small foci in SSA/P and occasionally in conventional adenomas or even in non-neoplastic inflamed colonic mucosa. Therefore, although helpful for the diagnosis in the correct context, they are not a diagnostic feature of these lesions, and some TSAs lack this type of cell.

So-called luminal serrations have been suggested by some as the most diagnostic feature of TSA (fig. 3-39) (67). These luminal serrations correlate strongly with the eosinophilic pencillate cells and are not as evident in TSAs with exclusive goblet cells.

Conventional cytologic dysplasia is common in TSA and presumably is a prerequisite to the development of carcinoma in these lesions (fig. 3-43). Since the dysplasia can be widespread, it may be that many lesions in the rectum diagnosed as villous adenomas but having focal areas of ectopic crypt formation or villi lined with eosinophilic pencillate cells are in actuality TSAs with extensive conventional dysplasia,

Figure 3-43

TRADITIONAL SERRATED ADENOMA WITH CONVENTIONAL DYSPLASIA

A: The TSA on the left sharply transitions to an adenoma having the appearance of a villous adenoma (right).

B: Conventional dysplasia can have an appearance similar to that of a conventional adenoma, or it can have serrated dysplasia similar to that seen in some cases of SSA/PCD (see "C" and figure 3-35). It can be low or high grade and should be reported as such.

C: High-grade serrated dysplasia.

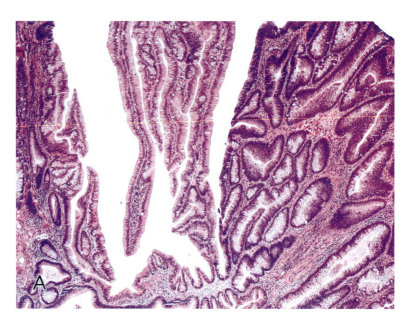

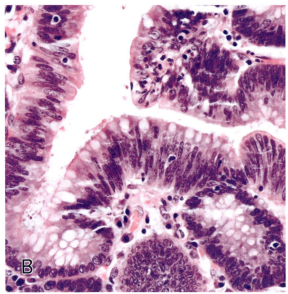

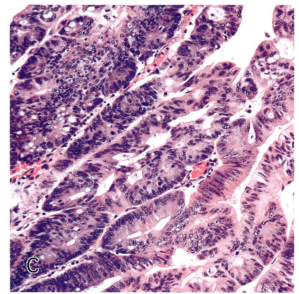

although this finding has been used to challenge the specificity of ectopic crypts (67). Determining the correct interpretation requires refined molecular characterization of these lesions.

Since the mechanism of development of carcinoma in TSA is currently not well understood, it is unclear whether there are significant management issues for patients with TSA versus conventional villous adenomas. Occasionally, TSA can be difficult to distinguish from SSA/P with extensive enteric metaplasia although the distinction is usually not an issue except in "flat" TSAs.

High-Risk Features and Management. At the current time little is known about rate of conversion of TSA to carcinoma, or the type of carcinoma that develops, although there have been suggestions that MSI-L carcinoma may develop as a result of inactivation of the *MGMT* gene. It is clear that MSI-H carcinomas are rarely, if ever, associated with TSA (64). Carcinomas presumably develop in the face of dysplasia morphologically resembling that of conventional adenomas, including high-grade dysplasia; therefore, the presence of conventional cytologic dysplasia should be considered an advanced feature in the development of carcinoma. Small TSAs with invasive carcinoma have not been described, which is different from SSA/Ps in which invasive carcinoma in lesions less than 1 cm is well documented. This suggests that conversion to carcinoma in these lesions is a slow process, more like conventional adenomas than SSA/P.

It has been suggested that there may be two pathways of development of carcinoma from TSA, with *BRAF*-mutated TSAs developing into *BRAF*-mutated MSS carcinomas, often in the right colon, and with *KRAS*-mutated TSAs being responsible for the development of *KRAS*-mutated MSS carcinomas in the rectum (64). Given the very villiform appearance of most TSAs, it may be that *KRAS*-mutated lesions interpreted in the past as villous adenomas may in fact be TSAs with extensive conventional dysplasia. This could explain the association between *KRAS* mutations and "villous adenomas" (20,21).

The frequency of synchronous or metachronous lesions is unknown, thus developing specific guidelines for follow-up is not possible. At the current time there is no documented reason to suspect a high rate or speed of conversion of TSA to malignancy nor a high rate of metachronous lesions, so management guidelines should probably mirror those for conventional adenomas, although since most TSAs are greater than 1 cm they would be considered "advanced" by that criterion. Closer surveillance may also be warranted for TSA with conventional dysplasia, at least to assure complete excision and no local recurrence.

Other Polyps that Occasionally Lead to Colon Carcinoma

Rarely, adenocarcinoma can develop in lesions that are generally not considered premalignant, including most commonly juvenile polyps in juvenile polyposis, and occasionally hamartomatous polyps in Peutz-Jeghers syndrome (69,70). In both of these cases areas of conventional dysplasia develop prior to the development of malignancy, although the pathogenesis of the cancer is not necessarily via the usual *APC*-mutated pathway of the more common adenoma-carcinoma sequence (69,71). HPs do not directly become malignant, although it is in theory possible that some SSA/Ps derive from microvesicular HPs. This possibility remains controversial, however, and has not been demonstrated to the extent that MVHPs themselves should be considered premalignant.

REFERENCES

1. Snover DC. Update on the serrated pathway to colorectal carcinoma. Hum Pathol 2011;42:1-10.
2. Torlakovic E, Skovlund E, Snover DC, Torlakovic G, Nesland JM. Morphologic reappraisal of serrated colorectal polyps. Am J Surg Pathol 2003;27:65-81.
3. Fearon ER, Vogelstein B. A genetic model for colorectal tumorigenesis Cell 1990;61:759-767.
4. Jass JR. Serrated adenoma of the colorectum and the DNA-methylator phenotype. Nat Clin Pract Oncol 2005;2:398-405.
5. Bosman FT, World Health Organization, International Agency for Research on Cancer. WHO classification of tumours of the digestive system, 4th ed. Lyon: International Agency for Research on Cancer; 2010.
6. Torlakovic EE, Gomez JD, Driman DK, et al. Sessile serrated adenoma (SSA) vs. traditional serrated adenoma (TSA). Am J Surg Pathol 2008;32:21-29.
7. Lin J, Goldblum JR, Bennett AE, Bronner MP, Liu X. Composite intestinal adenoma-microcarcinoid. Am J Surg Pathol 2012;36:292-295.
8. Salaria SN, Abu Alfa AK, Alsaigh NY, Montgomery E, Arnold CA. Composite intestinal adenoma-microcarcinoid clues to diagnosing an underrecognised mimic of invasive adenocarcinoma. J Clin Pathol 2013;66:302-306.
9. Domoto H, Terahata S, Senoh A, Sato K, Aida S, Tamai S. Clear cell change in colorectal adenomas: its incidence and histological characteristics. Histopathology 1999;34:250-256.
10. Pai RK, Rybicki LA, Goldblum JR, Shen B, Xiao SY, Liu X. Paneth cells in colonic adenomas: association with male sex and adenoma burden. Am J Surg Pathol 2013;37:98-103.
11. Pantanowitz L. Colonic adenoma with squamous metaplasia. Int J Surg Pathol 2009;17:340-342.
12. Shi C, Scudiere JR, Cornish TC, et al. Clear cell change in colonic tubular adenoma and corresponding colonic clear cell adenocarcinoma is associated with an altered mucin core protein profile. Am J Surg Pathol 2010;34:1344-1350.
13. Soga K, Konishi H, Tatsumi N, et al. Clear cell adenocarcinoma of the colon: a case report and review of literature. World J Gastroenterol 2008;14:1137-1140.
14. Williams GT, Blackshaw AJ, Morson BC. Squamous carcinoma of the colorectum and its genesis. J Pathol 1979;129:139-147.
15. AbdullGaffar B, Hotait H, Gopal P, Al-Awadhi S, Bamakhrama K, ElFaki B. The prevalence and importance of crypt apoptosis, focal active cryptitis, and neutrophilic infiltrate of the lamina propria in colorectal adenomas. Int J Surg Pathol 2013;21:247-256.
16. Mahajan D, Downs-Kelly E, Liu X, et al. Reproducibility of the villous component and high-grade dysplasia in colorectal adenomas <1 cm: implications for endoscopic surveillance. Am J Surg Pathol 2013;37:427-433.
17. Osmond A, Li-Chang H, Kirsch R, et al. Interobserver variability in assessing dysplasia and architecture in colorectal adenomas: a multicentre Canadian study. J Clin Pathol 2014;67:781-786.
18. Martinez ME, Baron JA, Lieberman DA, et al. A pooled analysis of advanced colorectal neoplasia diagnoses after colonoscopic polypectomy. Gastroenterology 2009;136:832-841.
19. Shih IM, Wang TL, Traverso G, et al. Top-down morphogenesis of colorectal tumors. Proc Natl Acad Sci U S A 2001;98:2640-2645.
20. Barry EL, Baron JA, Grau MV, Wallace K, Haile RW. K-ras mutations in incident sporadic colorectal adenomas. Cancer 2006;106:1036-1040.
21. Maltzman T, Knoll K, Martinez ME, et al. Ki-ras proto-oncogene mutations in sporadic colorectal adenomas: relationship to histologic and clinical characteristics. Gastroenterology 2001;121:302-309.
22. Yadamsuren EA, Nagy S, Pajor L, Lacza A, Bogner B. Characteristics of advanced- and non advanced sporadic polypoid colorectal adenomas: correlation to KRAS mutations. Pathol Oncol Res. 2012;18:1077-1084.
23. Shinya H, Wolff WI. Morphology, anatomic distribution and cancer potential of colonic polyps. Ann Surg 1979;190:679-683.
24. Mills SE, Allen MS Jr, Cohen AR. Small-cell undifferentiated carcinoma of the colon. A clinicopathological study of five cases and their association with colonic adenomas. Am J Surg Pathol 1983;7:643-651.
25. Ladabaum U, Song K. Projected national impact of colorectal cancer screening on clinical and economic outcomes and health services demand. Gastroenterology 2005;129:1151-1162.
26. Jones S, Chen WD, Parmigiani G, et al. Comparative lesion sequencing provides insights into tumor evolution. Proc Natl Acad Sci U S A 2008;105:4283-4288.
27. Muto T, Bussey HJ, Morson BC. The evolution of cancer of the colon and rectum. Cancer 1975;36:2251-2270.

28. Washington MK, Berlin J, Branton P, et al. Protocol for the examination of specimens from patients with primary carcinoma of the colon and rectum. Arch Pathol Lab Med 2009;133:1539-1551.

29. Kenney BC, Jain D. Identification of lymphatics within the colonic lamina propria in inflammation and neoplasia using the monoclonal antibody D2-40. Yale J Biol Med 2008;81:103-113.

30. Muto T, Bussey HJ, Morson BC. Pseudo-carcinomatous invasion in adenomatous polyps of the colon and rectum. J Clin Pathol 1973;26:25-31.

31. Pascal RR, Hertzler G, Hunter S, Goldschmid S. Pseudoinvasion with high-grade dysplasia in a colonic adenoma. Distinction from adenocarcinoma. Am J Surg Pathol 1990;14:694-697.

32. Appelman HD. Con: High-grade dysplasia and villous features should not be part of the routine diagnosis of colorectal adenomas. Am J Gastroenterol 2008;103:1329-1331.

33. Rex DK, Goldblum JR. Pro: Villous elements and high-grade dysplasia help guide post-polypectomy colonoscopic surveillance. Am J Gastroenterol 2008;103:1327-1329.

34. Lieberman DA, Rex DK, Winawer SJ, et al. Guidelines for colonoscopy surveillance after screening and polypectomy: a consensus update by the US Multi-Society Task Force on Colorectal Cancer. Gastroenterology 2012;143:844-857.

35. Aarons CB, Shanmugan S, Bleier JI. Management of malignant colon polyps: current status and controversies. World J Gastroenterol 2014;20:16178-16183.

36. Hassan C, Zullo A, Risio M, Rossini FP, Morini S. Histologic risk factors and clinical outcome in colorectal malignant polyp: a pooled-data analysis. Dis Colon Rectum 2005;48:1588-1596.

37. Yasuda K, Inomata M, Shiromizu A, Shiraishi N, Higashi H, Kitano S. Risk factors for occult lymph node metastasis of colorectal cancer invading the submucosa and indications for endoscopic mucosal resection. Dis Colon Rectum 2007;50:1370-1376.

38. Haggitt RC, Glotzbach RE, Soffer EE, Wruble LD. Prognostic factors in colorectal carcinomas arising in adenomas: implications for lesions removed by endoscopic polypectomy. Gastroenterology 1985;89:328-336.

39. Kawachi H, Eishi Y, Ueno H, et al. A three-tier classification system based on the depth of submucosal invasion and budding/sprouting can improve the treatment strategy for T1 colorectal cancer: a retrospective multicenter study. Mod Pathol 2015;28:872-879.

40. Wu ML, Dry SM, Lassman CR. Deeper examination of negative colorectal biopsies. Am J Clin Pathol 2002;117:424-428.

41. Urbanski SJ, Kossakowska AE, Marcon N, Bruce WR. Mixed hyperplastic adenomatous polyps-an underdiagnosed entity. Report of a case of adenocarcinoma arising within a mixed hyperplastic adenomatous polyp. Am J Surg Pathol 1984;8:551-556.

42. Longacre TA, Fenoglio-Preiser CM. Mixed hyperplastic adenomatous polyps/serrated adenomas. A distinct form of colorectal neoplasia. Am J Surg Pathol 1990;14:524-537.

43. Torlakovic E, Snover DC. Serrated adenomatous polyposis in humans. Gastroenterology 1996;110:748-755.

44. Yang S, Farraye FA, Mack C, Posnik O, O'Brien MJ. BRAF and KRAS Mutations in hyperplastic polyps and serrated adenomas of the colorectum: relationship to histology and CpG island methylation status. Am J Surg Pathol 2004;28:1452-1459.

45. Rex DK, Ahnen DJ, Baron JA, et al. Serrated lesions of the colorectum: review and recommendations from an expert panel. Am J Gastroenterol 2012;107:1315-1329; quiz 1314, 1330.

46. Rex DK, Clodfelter R, Rahmani F, et al. Narrow-band imaging versus white light for the detection of proximal colon serrated lesions: a randomized, controlled trial. Gastrointest Endosc 2016;83:166-171.

47. Goldstein NS. Small colonic microsatellite unstable adenocarcinomas and high-grade epithelial dysplasias in sessile serrated adenoma polypectomy specimens: a study of eight cases. Am J Clin Pathol 2006;125:132-145.

48. Sheridan TB, Fenton H, Lewin MR, et al. Sessile serrated adenomas with low- and high-grade dysplasia and early carcinomas: an immunohistochemical study of serrated lesions "caught in the act." Am J Clin Pathol 2006;126:564-571.

49. Issa JP, Ottaviano YL, Celano P, Hamilton SR, Davidson NE, Baylin SB. Methylation of the oestrogen receptor CpG island links ageing and neoplasia in human colon. Nat Genet 1994;7:536-540.

50. Owens SR, Chiosea SI, Kuan SF. Selective expression of gastric mucin MUC6 in colonic sessile serrated adenoma but not in hyperplastic polyp aids in morphological diagnosis of serrated polyps. Mod Pathol 2008;21:660-669.

51. Bartley AN, Thompson PA, Buckmeier JA, et al. Expression of gastric pyloric mucin, MUC6, in colorectal serrated polyps. Mod Pathol 2010;23:169-176.

52. Fujita K, Hirahashi M, Yamamoto H, et al. Mucin core protein expression in serrated polyps of the large intestine. Virchows Arch 2010;457:443-449.

53. Kiedrowski M, Mroz A, Kraszewska E, et al. Cyclooxygenase-2 immunohistochemical expression in serrated polyps of the colon. Contemp Oncol (Pozn) 2014;18:409-413.

54. Ngo NT, Tan E, Tekkis P, Peston D, Cohen P. Differential expression of p53 and p504s in hyperplastic polyp, sessile serrated adenoma and traditional serrated adenoma. Int J Colorectal Dis 2010;25:1193-1200.

55. Parfitt JR, Driman DK. Survivin and hedgehog protein expression in serrated colorectal polyps: an immunohistochemical study. Hum Pathol 2007;38:710-717.

56. Gonzalo DH, Lai KK, Shadrach B, et al. Gene expression profiling of serrated polyps identifies annexin A10 as a marker of a sessile serrated adenoma/polyp. J Pathol 2013;230:420-429.

57. Wiland HO 4th, Shadrach B, Allende D, et al. Morphologic and molecular characterization of traditional serrated adenomas of the distal colon and rectum. Am J Surg Pathol 2014;38:1290-1297.

58. Pai RK, Hart J, Noffsinger AE. Sessile serrated adenomas strongly predispose to synchronous serrated polyps in non-syndromic patients. Histopathology 2010;56:581-588.

59. Pereyra L, Zamora R, Gomez EJ, et al. Risk of metachronous advanced neoplastic lesions in patients with sporadic sessile serrated adenomas undergoing colonoscopic surveillance. Am J Gastroenterol 2016;111:871-878.

60. Pohl H, Srivastava A, Bensen SP, et al. Incomplete polyp resection during colonoscopy-results of the complete adenoma resection (CARE) study. Gastroenterology 2013;144:74-80 e71.

61. Rosty C, Buchanan DD, Walsh MD, et al. Phenotype and polyp landscape in serrated polyposis syndrome: a series of 100 patients from genetics clinics. Am J Surg Pathol 2012;36:876-882.

62. Vu HT, Lopez R, Bennett A, Burke CA. Individuals with sessile serrated polyps express an aggressive colorectal phenotype. Dis Colon Rectum 2011;54:1216-1223.

63. Singh H, Bay D, Ip S, et al. Pathological reassessment of hyperplastic colon polyps in a city-wide pathology practice: implications for polyp surveillance recommendations. Gastrointest Endosc 2012;76:1003-1008.

64. Bettington ML, Walker NI, Rosty C, et al. A clinicopathological and molecular analysis of 200 traditional serrated adenomas. Mod Pathol 2015;28:414-427.

65. Kim MJ, Lee EJ, Suh JP, et al. Traditional serrated adenoma of the colorectum: clinicopathologic implications and endoscopic findings of the precursor lesions. Am J Clin Pathol 2013;140:898-911.

66. Yantiss RK, Oh KY, Chen YT, Redston M, Odze RD. Filiform serrated adenomas: a clinicopathologic and immunophenotypic study of 18 cases. Am J Surg Pathol 2007;31:1238-1245.

67. Hafezi-Bakhtiari S, Wang LM, Colling R, Serra S, Chetty R. Histological overlap between colorectal villous/tubulovillous and traditional serrated adenomas. Histopathology 2015;66:308-313.

68. Yokoo H, Usman I, Wheaton S, Kampmeier PA. Colorectal polyps with extensive absorptive enterocyte differentiation: histologically distinct variant of hyperplastic polyps. Arch Pathol Lab Med 1999;123:404-410.

69. van Hattem WA, Langeveld D, de Leng WW, et al. Histologic variations in juvenile polyp phenotype correlate with genetic defect underlying juvenile polyposis. Am J Surg Pathol 2011;35:530-536.

70. Giardiello FM, Brensinger JD, Tersmette AC, et al. Very high risk of cancer in familial Peutz-Jeghers syndrome. Gastroenterology 2000;119:1447-1453.

71. Gruber SB, Entius MM, Petersen GM, et al. Pathogenesis of adenocarcinoma in Peutz-Jeghers syndrome. Cancer Res 1998;58:5267-5270.

4 CARCINOMAS OF THE SMALL AND LARGE INTESTINES (EXCLUDING NEUROENDOCRINE NEOPLASMS)

Colorectal carcinoma is a malignant epithelial lesion occurring as a primary tumor in the colon or rectum. These neoplasms are considered malignant only after they gain access to the lymphatic circulation, which is not present within the superficial lamina propria; hence, invasion at least into the muscularis mucosae is required for this diagnosis, although most guidelines use submucosal invasion as definitional.

EPIDEMIOLOGY AND RISK FACTORS

Colorectal carcinoma (CRC) has a widespread distribution, and in the United States is the third most common malignancy and the third most common cause of death due to malignancy in this country (1). Most cases are adenocarcinomas, and most epidemiologic studies relate only to adenocarcinoma. For 2016, approximately 135,000 people in the United States are estimated to have a new diagnosis of colorectal carcinoma, with approximately 49,000 deaths (1).

There is considerable geographic, gender, and racial variation in the incidence and mortality from colorectal carcinoma (1). With modern screening techniques for the disease, the incidence and mortality rates among screened populations have decreased in recent years, particularly for carcinoma of the left colon in older patients. These screening programs, however, have had little effect on right-sided colorectal carcinoma (for reasons to be described in the section on epithelial preneoplastic polyps), and in certain groups the incidence of colorectal carcinoma seems to be increasing, including young patients (2).

The risk factors for colorectal cancer include geographic and personal factors (age, gender, and race), as well as a number of other genetic and environmental factors. Some of these factors are under the control of patients, such as dietary factors, and hence provide a possible mechanism for primary prevention of this disease.

Worldwide, colorectal carcinoma is most common in Western, "developed" countries (3). Individuals who immigrate to these countries tend to develop colorectal carcinoma at a rate similar to that of their new country, and hence environmental factors are thought to play a major role in development. Colorectal carcinoma is most common in older male patients, with the highest incidence and mortality in black males. Most (90 percent) cases occur in patients older than 50 years. The incidence and mortality in African-American patients (male and female) are 20 percent and 45 percent higher than for non-Hispanic whites, with most other ethnic groups having lower rates than whites. There are also considerable geographic differences that may reflect diet and other environmental factors as well as ethnic mix and availability of screening. For example, the incidence among Native Americans (including Alaska natives) is approximately five times higher for those living in Alaska versus those living the southwest United States (4).

Genetics plays an important role, not only for patients with a defined syndrome (familial adenomatous polyposis and Lynch syndrome, described below), but also for patients with just one or two relatives with colorectal carcinoma. In these latter cases, it may be difficult to determine whether this is a risk associated with genetic abnormalities or associated with a common exposure to high-risk behavior (such as diet), although both probably play a role. Inflammatory bowel disease and diabetes also increase risk.

Diet has been a topic of much interest since it is something that most individuals can control (5,6). A great deal of research has gone into this topic, often with contradictory results. Much of the variation in results comes from the type of study performed. Most initial data come from population-based case-controlled epidemiological studies that often point to possible factors that may, in and of themselves, be related to colorectal carcinoma, or may act as markers for other factors that are the true determining factor. More directed studies, such as cohort studies or interventional trials, often result in less definitive results than initially anticipated.

Another potential but largely unexplored factor confounding the results of nutritional studies is that different types of colorectal carcinoma (e.g., microsatellite stable versus unstable carcinoma, right- versus left-sided versus rectal carcinoma, CpG island methylation phenotype high versus low carcinoma) are influenced by different factors and in essence require separate studies to prevent dilution of results by type of tumors not affected by the trial agent. This has been shown to be the case for rectal versus nonrectal carcinomas and some risk factors (7). Since subdividing carcinomas reduces the number of cases available for study, this type of division reduces the power of most studies. In addition, molecular studies (or even careful histologic review) are often not available to epidemiological researchers.

Studies of diet and carcinoma are essentially case controlled and cohort studies; interventional trials directed solely at colorectal carcinoma incidence are impractical. Interventional studies are often directed at assessing the effect of interventional substances on the development of conventional adenomas in high-risk populations (usually patients with a prior history of adenomas or patients with familial adenomatous polyposis) (8). The presumption is that prevention of precursor lesions will prevent colon carcinoma. However, since conventional adenomas are not the only precursor to colorectal carcinoma (accounting for perhaps 60 to 70 percent of all colorectal carcinomas), these studies only examine a subset of carcinomas (albeit the largest subset). In addition, studies directed at the prevention of conventional adenomas do not evaluate factors that might prevent the progression of adenoma to carcinoma. Given the low rate of conversion of conventional adenoma to carcinoma (less than 1 percent are estimated to become carcinoma), preventing progression may be more important and easier than preventing the occurrence of adenomas to begin with.

Because the end point for most interventional studies is adenoma development, caution should be used when interpreting negative results for interventional substances, which have a strong epidemiological basis, with carcinoma as the end point. For example, studies showing no effect of vitamins C, D, and E on the development of recurrent adenomas are generally interpreted in the lay press as showing that these vitamins have no effect on the development of colon cancer. This is not necessarily an appropriate conclusion, however, since carcinoma was not the end point of the study and it is possible that these vitamins might prevent progression of adenoma to carcinoma (9).

A few factors have stood the test of time and are generally recognized as being of some importance. In general, consumption of red meat, processed meat, and alcohol is associated with increased risk of carcinoma, and consumption of calcium and milk with lower risk. High fat and low fiber diets have also been associated with increased risk in many case-controlled studies, although data are inconsistent, and in cohort and interventional trials the effect of fat and fiber appears minimal. The reason for this may be that intake of fiber is associated with intake of other substances (e.g., folate) that may have protective effects, and different types of fiber may have different effects. In some experimental model systems with carcinogen-induced tumors in mice, some types of fiber decreased the rate of development of carcinoma whereas other fiber types had either no effect or even increased the rate of development (10). This may be important when recommending dietary fiber supplements. In one human interventional study of the effect of fiber supplementation on recurrence of adenomas, one type of fiber, ispaghula husk, increased the risk of recurrent adenomas (11).

Smoking is associated with increased risk and physical activity is associated with a lower risk of colon carcinoma (12,13). The intake of certain vitamins and minerals has also been associated with variation of incidence, and has formed the backbone of potential nutritional intervention as part of primary prevention. Folate, vitamin B6, calcium, selenium, vitamin D, antioxidant vitamins, and others are potentially useful intervention agents. Calcium initially was shown, in a prospective trial, to have a modest effect on adenoma formation and hence was suggested as a potentially useful supplement, however, a follow-up study by the same group failed to show a reduction in adenoma formation with calcium (8).

Overall food intake and the result of that intake, obesity or metabolic syndrome, also affect the risk of colorectal carcinoma (6). Obesity and diabetes have a positive correlation with colorectal carcinoma (13). The effect of obesity and diabetes may be related to increased insulin production, which affects proliferation and apoptosis in the colon. As with so many diseases of Western society, adherence to a healthy diet and lifestyle may be key for the primary prevention of colorectal carcinoma.

Among other agents considered candidates for primary prevention, COX2 inhibitors have been a focus of much attention. Aspirin, particularly in low dose, has been shown to have a modest effect in preventing recurrence of advanced adenomas (14). Other nonsteroidal anti-inflammatory drugs decrease adenoma occurrence in patients with familial adenomatous polyposis. Curcumin has also shown some promise as a potential inhibitor of adenoma formation (15).

PRECURSOR LESIONS

Most adenocarcinomas of the large intestine arise in a precursor lesion (see chapter 3 and the sections below on hereditary colorectal carcinomas). Most commonly, these precursors are conventional adenomas (approximately 65 percent of colorectal carcinomas), sessile serrated adenomas/polyps (SSA/P) (approximately 35 percent), or traditional serrated adenomas (TSA) (less than 1 percent). Occasional cases arise in other types of polyps, particularly in the setting of polyposis syndromes.

Hamartomatous polyps of various types may develop carcinoma, with the most common being carcinomas arising in the colon in patients with juvenile polyposis. It appears that there is a transitional stage in which the hamartoma develops cytologic dysplasia, resembling that of a conventional adenoma. Carcinoma has also been reported arising in hamartomatous polyps in the small intestine and colon of patients with Peutz-Jeghers syndrome.

Cases of colorectal carcinoma have been reported in patients with Cowden syndrome (multiple hamartoma syndrome), however, it is unclear whether this condition is truly associated with an increased risk of colorectal cancer. Other polyposis syndromes are rarely if ever associated with carcinoma. Adenocarcinoma may also arise from apparently nonpolypoid mucosa, most commonly in the setting of inflammatory bowel disease.

The possible occurrence of "de novo" carcinoma, meaning adenocarcinoma arising from flat mucosa without the presence of a preexisting adenoma, is controversial and is of little practical significance. If such a process did exist, however, it could account for some interval cancers that occur in screening programs. This has been hypothesized in Japan in particular, where it is reported that small flat adenocarcinomas without precursor lesions are common (16). The most likely scenario in which de novo carcinoma might arise is in patients with Lynch syndrome, in which it is, in theory, possible that inactivation of the second allele for the missing mismatch repair enzyme might randomly occur in nonadenomatous mucosa, leading to the development of microsatellite instability and the development of carcinoma from morphologically "normal" mucosa. Proving this possibility, however, is improbable since by the time a carcinoma develops it is impossible to absolutely prove that there was not a preexisting lesion that was either destroyed by the carcinoma or is just not seen in the plane of section available for review. Therefore, the existence of de novo carcinoma will remain, for practical purposes, an untestable hypothesis.

CLASSIFICATION

Up until recently, essentially all colorectal carcinomas were believed to arise from a single pathway, the "suppressor" pathway first delineated by Fearon and Vogelstein in 1990 (17). We now know, however, that there are a number of pathways to colorectal carcinoma having different precursor lesions, different baseline mutations, and different rates of progression and prognoses. Colorectal carcinoma can therefore be classified in multiple ways based on location, growth pattern, histologic appearance, precursor lesion, and molecular pathway of development (18,19). These classifications are not mutually exclusive, and the molecular pathway is reflected to some degree by the precursor lesion, location of tumor, and histologic pattern. The molecular characteristics of the tumor affect the prognosis and play an increasing role in management, including decisions regarding appropriate adjuvant therapy. The nature of the precursor lesion has a major effect on screening strategies, including screening intervals.

Current molecular testing and classification usually begin with testing for microsatellite instability (20). Tumors are classified as microsatellite stable (MSS) or unstable (MSI) based on the expression of mismatch repair proteins by immunohistochemistry or, less commonly, by assessing directly for evidence of MSI by polymerase chain reaction (PCR) analysis. MSS tumors (which account for approximately 85 percent of all colon carcinomas) tend to be left sided whereas MSI tumors tend to be right sided and often have characteristic histologic features (e.g., tumor infiltrating lymphocytes and mucinous or medullary morphology). This classification is important for determining the risk of the patient having Lynch syndrome, the most common inherited syndrome leading to colon carcinoma, and also has some bearing on prognosis and treatment. Determining microsatellite status is currently recommended for grading mucinous carcinomas and may influence decisions regarding chemotherapy in patients with stage II disease (21). Nevertheless, microsatellite stability classification is often interpreted as though MSS and MSI are homogeneous categories, which is not the case.

MSS tumors arise from at least two pathways. Most commonly, they arise via the suppressor or "chromosomal instability" pathway, initiated by mutation of the *APC* gene; however, some tumors with a high degree of CpG island methylation (CIMP-H carcinomas) without *APC* mutations are also MSS. For MSS CIMP-L (low) tumors, the precursor lesion in most cases is the conventional adenoma; however, for CIMP-H carcinomas the precursor lesion appears to be the SSA/P or possibly a subset of TSA (22,23). MSI tumors arise either from conventional adenomas as part of Lynch syndrome (MSI-CIMP-L) or from SSA/Ps when they are sporadic and CIMP-H (19,24). These factors are important when designing screening programs and are also useful in determining whether an MSI carcinoma is sporadic or inherited, since if there is an adjacent SSA the carcinoma is most

likely sporadic but if the tumor is clearly arising in a conventional adenoma it is more likely to represent Lynch syndrome.

GROSS AND ENDOSCOPIC FINDINGS

Grossly, most adenocarcinomas of the colon appear as mass lesions, which can be plaque like, exophytic, polypoid, or circumferential, all with or without ulceration (fig. 4-1). Circumferential carcinomas can obstruct the colonic lumen.

Carcinomas, particularly in the rectum, are often deeply ulcerated when they grow to a large size. They typically have rolled edges, with flattening of the mucosa caused by tumor undermining adjacent normal mucosa, and are usually not difficult to identify grossly or endoscopically. Despite being grossly apparent, endoscopic biopsies of apparent carcinomas may obtain only normal mucosa or ulcer debris and not tumor, and be nondiagnostic even with lesions that grossly are obvious carcinomas. Therefore, correlation of biopsy with endoscopic findings is always important, and even with a negative biopsy, a grossly worrisome lesion cannot be ignored. It has been argued that biopsy of obvious carcinoma is not warranted for this reason; however, depending on the clinical circumstances, biopsy may be of value in determining the extent of surgery because it provides tissue for screening for Lynch syndrome (i.e., if it is determined that the patient has Lynch syndrome based on the biopsy, more extensive surgery is usually warranted).

Not all lesions that are "obvious" carcinoma prove to be carcinoma. Rare cases of fungal infection in immunosuppressed patients (e.g., *Histoplasma* infection in patients taking antitumor necrosis factor alpha or with acquired immunodeficiency syndrome [AIDS]) can grossly mimic carcinoma. Biopsy in these cases may forestall surgery if the underlying infection can be treated.

With current screening programs, large obstructing or deeply ulcerated tumors are becoming less common. Conversely, occasional cases are now being identified in which there is no obvious mass lesion but only an area of erythema or a small nonspecific ulceration. This seems to happen most commonly with small carcinomas arising in SSA/Ps, which, in and of themselves, can be difficult to identify endoscopically. Many MSI carcinomas arising

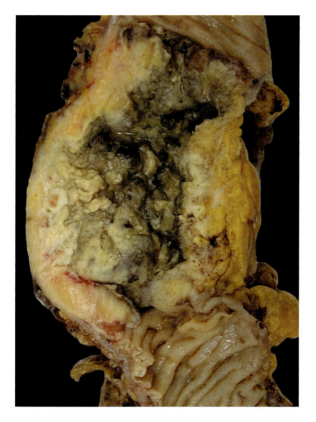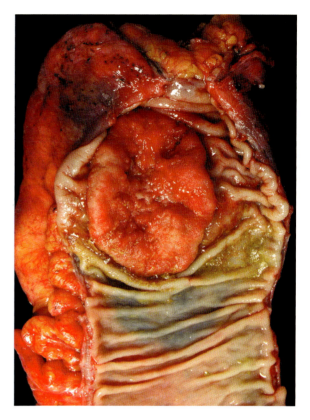

Figure 4-1

COLON CARCINOMA

Left: A circumferential growth pattern is seen. This growth pattern is often associated with obstructive symptoms.
Right: The pattern is plaque like.

in SSA/P are less than 1 cm in diameter but clearly invasive (fig. 4-2) (25–27). These tumors raise significant questions about the ability of colonoscopic screening to ever eliminate the risk of carcinoma development and it is these types of lesions that no doubt play a role in the occurrence of "interval cancers," although they are probably not the only cause.

Identifying carcinoma grossly within a preexisting adenoma can be very difficult if the carcinoma is small. However, sometimes carcinoma can be suspected if the adenoma is ulcerated or, in the case of a sessile lesion, if it appears immobile due to infiltration into the underlying submucosa.

HISTOLOGIC FINDINGS

Adenocarcinoma of the colon may have a variety of histologic appearances, although most have characteristic features ("classic pattern"), which allow some degree of identification in metastases even without the use of special staining. Some of the histologic subtypes have prognostic significance (medullary, mucinous, and signet ring subtypes in particular) and reflect the molecular makeup of the carcinoma (identification of MSI tumors and Lynch syndrome) (28,29).

While many of the patterns of colorectal adenocarcinoma are reported as specific types of carcinoma (e.g., micropapillary carcinoma), several of these "subtypes" are histologic variations of the classic pattern. Also, it is not unusual to see multiple patterns within one tumor. It is best to designate these patterns as prognostic features (similar to tumor budding) rather than as separate subtypes. Categories that are sufficiently unique to be considered as true subtypes include pure signet ring carcinoma and medullary carcinoma. By tradition

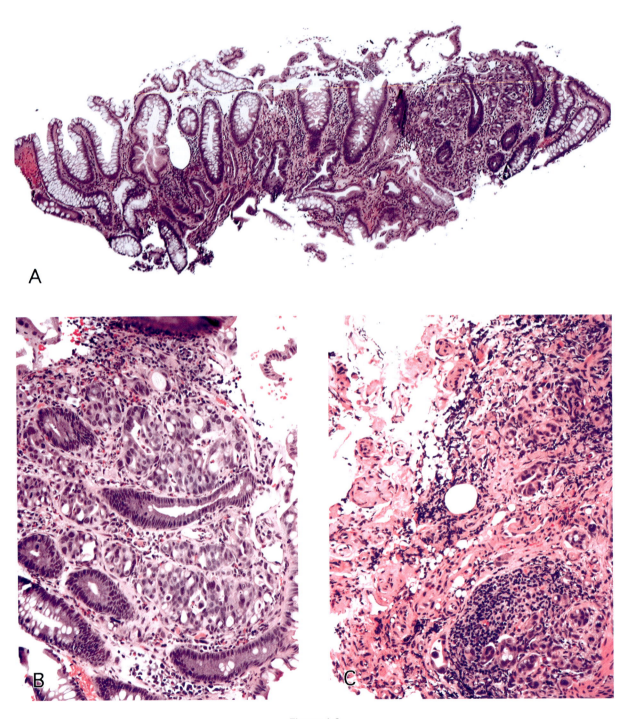

Figure 4-2

ADENOCARCINOMA ARISING IN 4-MM SESSILE SERRATED ADENOMA/POLYP (SSA/P)

A: An area of intramucosal carcinoma is seen near the right end of the biopsy.

B: Intramucosal carcinoma is evident. The surrounding glands show low-grade dysplasia characteristic of SSA/P with cytologic dysplasia.

C: Submucosal invasion.

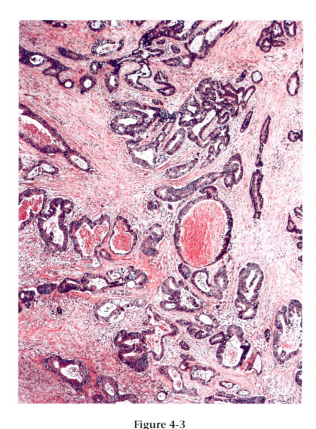

Figure 4-3

ADENOCARCINOMA OF THE COLON, NOT OTHERWISE SPECIFIED (NOS)

This low-grade adenocarcinoma demonstrates more than 50 percent glandular formation. In this case there is an intermixture of cribriform and single glands, some containing dirty necrosis.

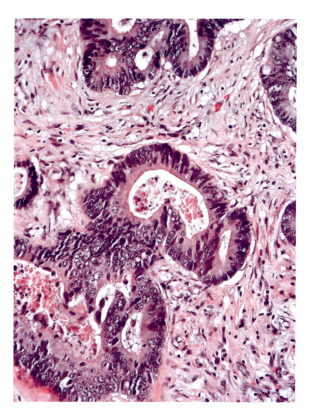

Figure 4-4

ADENOCARCINOMA OF THE COLON, NOS

Typical colonic adenocarcinoma consists of tall columnar cells with elongated, hyperchromatic nuclei, which may have nucleoli.

mucinous carcinoma is also retained as a separate category although with the realization that the distinction of mucinous carcinoma from "adenocarcinoma with mucinous features" is an arbitrary one.

Classic Pattern (Adenocarcinoma, Not Otherwise Specified [NOS])

The *classic pattern* consists of well-formed single glands or tumor cells growing in a cribriform architecture (fig. 4-3). The individual cells that make up the glands tend to be elongated, have hyperchromatic nuclei without a great deal of overt nuclear pleomorphism, and show pseudostratification or true stratification (fig. 4-4). Mitoses are generally easy to identify. These tumors tend to be better differentiated near the colonic lumen and often become less differentiated at the leading invasive edge. In

some cases, this loss of differentiation results in an infiltrative growth pattern or the formation of small tumor buds (tumor budding), which have prognostic significance (fig. 4-5). Other cases invade across a broad front in a pushing pattern (fig. 4-6).

Necrosis is common, especially "dirty necrosis." This term implies necrosis within a nest of tumor cells or within the lumen of glandular spaces with abundant nuclear debris present, rendering the "dirty" appearance (fig. 4-7). Dirty necrosis is typically a feature of tumors with MSI.

Classic pattern adenocarcinoma is typically well or moderately differentiated (low-grade) (see description of grading, below), although most cases of poorly differentiated (high-grade) adenocarcinoma have some areas of lower-grade adenocarcinoma present, which allows identification as adenocarcinoma rather than as undifferentiated carcinoma. The grading of

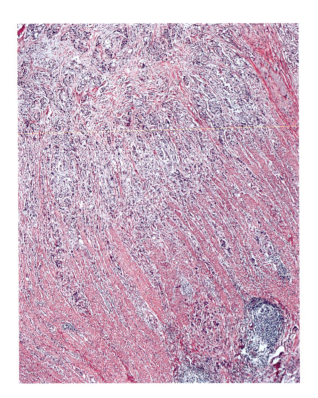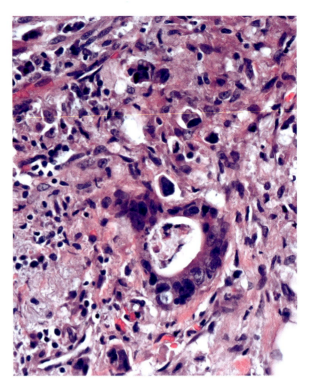

Figure 4-5

LEADING INVASIVE EDGE OF ADENOCARCINOMA, NOS

Left: There is diffuse irregular infiltration of the muscularis propria by cords of tumor cells.
Right: There are individual cells and small clusters of less than five cells, characteristic of tumor budding.

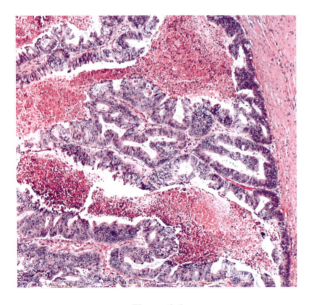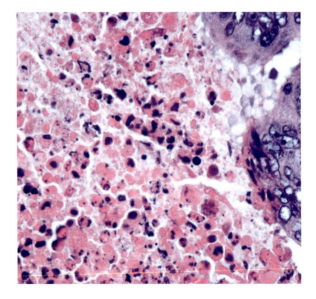

Figure 4-6

**LEADING INVASIVE EDGE
OF ADENOCARCINOMA, NOS**

There is noninfiltrative "pushing" invasion across a broad border.

Figure 4-7

DIRTY NECROSIS IN ADENOCARCINOMA, NOS

The lumen of the gland contains necrotic cells and debris intermixed with neutrophils. This necrosis is characteristic of microsatellite stable (MSS) tumors.

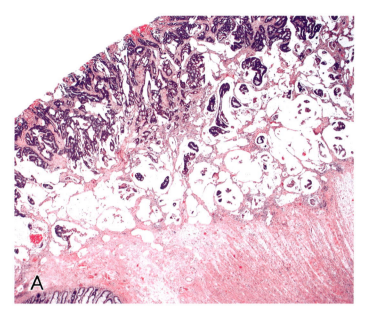

Figure 4-8

MUCINOUS ADENOCARCINOMA

A: The luminal aspect of the tumor on the upper surface does not manifest the mucinous features seen deeper. The mucinous component may be missed on a small superficial biopsy.

B: The invasive portion of the tumor is composed of greater than 50 percent mucin pools containing clusters of tumor cells, many floating freely in the mucin.

C: A tumor cell is seen in the mucin. In this case, the cells have the general appearance of adenocarcinoma, NOS.

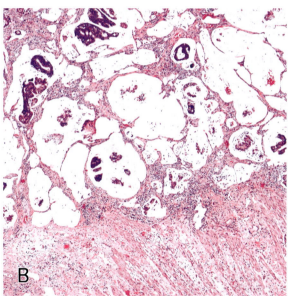

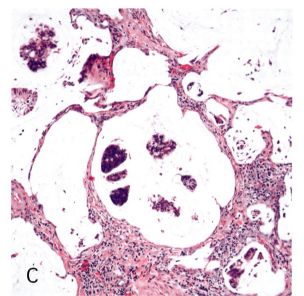

colonic adenocarcinoma, as described below, relates mainly to this pattern of tumor. The prognosis depends on the grade along with stage and other features that may or may not be seen in association with adenocarcinoma NOS.

Mucinous Carcinoma

Mucinous carcinoma is characterized by dilated glandular spaces filled with mucin, usually with additional pools of mucin that may contain nests of tumor cells (fig. 4-8). Although signet ring cells may be present, by definition, the majority of the mucin must be extracellular (fig.

4-9). The presence of signet ring cells should be reported, however, since it may have an effect on prognosis (30). Many adenocarcinomas of the colon have small areas manifesting mucinous differentiation, but a tumor is not classified as "mucinous" type unless at least 50 percent of the invasive tumor volume is mucinous (in the past figures as high as 75 percent were required although in recent years the 50 percent figure has been recommended by the World Health Organization [WHO] and is generally accepted). Despite the arbitrary definition of mucinous carcinoma, this diagnosis does

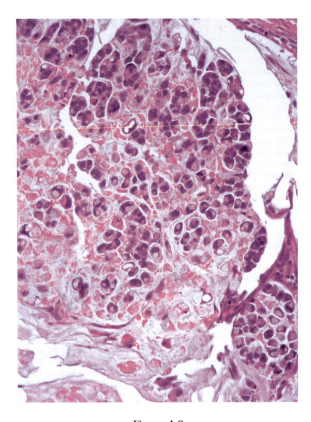

Figure 4-9

**MUCINOUS ADENOCARCINOMA
WITH SIGNET RING FEATURES**

Signet ring cells are present both in clusters and singly. Most of the mucin is extracellular, however. If less than 50 percent of the tumor cells are signet ring, this is considered a mucinous carcinoma with signet ring cells.

termixed with the classic pattern. Many cases of serrated adenocarcinoma, described below, have a considerable mucinous component and could be categorized as both mucinous and serrated, which may lead to some confusion about which specific term is best applied in some cases.

Typically, the luminal surface of mucinous carcinoma does not have a mucinous appearance but rather has the appearance of adenocarcinoma NOS, with the mucinous component more prominent in the deeper aspects of the tumor (fig. 4-8A). A small superficial biopsy may miss the mucinous component. Tumor budding is less common than in nonmucinous carcinomas. When these tumors metastasize, they often maintain their mucinous character.

There has been controversy about the prognostic significance of mucinous carcinoma. For many years it was regarded as more aggressive than nonmucinous adenocarcinoma, particularly in the rectum, where late local recurrence was commonly fatal (31–33). Some of this difference in prognosis was ascribed to the higher stage at which these tumors present, although in the rectum this did not appear to explain the entire picture. Most recent literature, however, suggests that stage for stage, the prognosis of mucinous carcinoma is similar to that of nonmucinous tumors.

An additional complicating factor is that mucinous carcinomas are not a homogeneous group. Mucinous carcinomas are over-represented in the right colon and have a higher incidence of MSI than nonmucinous carcinomas, and are more likely to be CIMP-H. Rectal mucinous carcinomas tend to be MSS and are not CIMP-H (34). MSI mucinous tumors have a better prognosis than both adenocarcinoma NOS and MSS mucinous tumors (21,35). Therefore, the WHO has suggested that mucinous carcinomas cannot be graded unless the microsatellite status is known, with MSI mucinous carcinoma considered low-grade tumors and MSS mucinous carcinomas considered high-grade tumors despite the fact that based on histologic criteria alone, most of these tumors would be graded as low grade as they display a high degree of gland formation. The microsatellite and CIMP status may also affect response to chemotherapy, particular with fluorouracil-based treatment regimens (33,36,37).

have some clinical significance. Tumors with lesser degrees of mucinous differentiation are considered to have focal mucinous differentiation, which is worthy of mention in a report since the presence of any mucinous component, no matter how small, is suggestive of MSI and is used as a marker of Lynch syndrome in the Bethesda guidelines.

Mucinous carcinomas may develop in conventional adenomas, particularly in the rectum, and in the context of Lynch syndrome, whereas sporadic mucinous carcinomas, particularly in the right colon, are often associated with SSA/P as the precursor lesion. As with many of the "subtypes" of colorectal carcinoma, whether mucinous carcinoma is truly a specific "type" or just a morphologic growth pattern is debatable, since the mucinous component is almost always in-

Signet Ring Carcinoma

Signet ring carcinoma is another type of carcinoma with abundant mucin, but with a considerably different prognostic implication than mucinous carcinoma (33,37). It is much less common than mucinous carcinoma, accounting for less than 1 percent of primary colorectal carcinomas. By WHO criteria, greater than 50 percent of the tumor cells should be signet ring cells in order to make this diagnosis, although any significant number of signet ring cells may affect the prognosis and should be reported (30).

The individual tumor cells show minimal pleomorphism although they may be hyperchromatic. Using the 50 percent signet ring cell definition of signet ring carcinoma, these tumors may have both extracellular and intracellular mucin or intracellular mucin alone. These patterns have different prognostic significance, and it may be more appropriate to consider the former mucinous carcinoma with abundant signet ring cells and the latter pure signet ring carcinoma (also referred to as mucin-poor signet ring carcinoma) (38). In mucin-poor signet ring carcinoma, the mucin is exclusively intracellular without extracellular mucin pools, and the tumor cells invade in a diffuse fashion similar to that of gastric diffuse or signet ring carcinoma (fig. 4-10). Given this growth pattern, these tumors grow in a linitis plastica fashion, creating a plaque or wall thickening without a protruding mass or ulceration. On small biopsies the tumor cells may be mistaken for inflammatory cells. These tumors have a propensity to develop in the right colon, and the precursor lesion has not been well defined since a precursor lesion is often not seen.

Most signet ring carcinomas present at advanced stage and the patient prognosis, stage for stage, is worse than that for any other type of colonic adenocarcinoma. Since signet ring carcinomas are more common in the stomach than in the colon, many cases found in the colon are drop metastases from the stomach. It is generally recommended that a signet ring carcinoma identified in the colon not be considered a primary tumor unless gastric carcinoma has been excluded with appropriate upper endoscopic studies and biopsy.

Metastatic lobular breast carcinoma can simulate primary signet ring carcinoma. Several studies have shown that signet ring carcinoma often has *BRAF* mutations and is MSI, however, a study that separated mucinous carcinoma with abundant signet ring cells (i.e., mucin-rich signet ring carcinoma) from carcinoma without abundant mucin demonstrated *BRAF* mutations and MSI predominantly in the tumors with abundant extracellular mucin, supporting the suggestion that these be considered mucinous carcinomas (38,39).

Medullary Carcinoma

Medullary carcinoma (also known as *medullary adenocarcinoma* and *large cell carcinoma with minimal differentiation*) is a tumor composed of poorly differentiated large tumor cells growing in sheets or syncytia without significant glandular formation (fig. 4-11A–C) (40–42), similar to medullary carcinoma of the breast. The cells are large, with vesicular nuclei and often prominent nucleoli. A key feature is the presence of large numbers of lymphocytes infiltrating into and around the tumor (fig. 4-11). Presumably this inflammation is a reaction to the tumor, since medullary carcinoma is associated with a better prognosis than other types of colorectal carcinoma.

Although medullary carcinoma may exist in pure form, it is often admixed with other patterns characteristic of MSI tumors, including mucinous and serrated components. This "heterogeneous" appearance suggests that a tumor has MSI (28,29). The usual precursor lesion is the SSA/P, although medullary carcinoma may arise in conventional adenomas, particularly in patients with Lynch syndrome.

On a purely morphologic basis, this tumor would be considered "poorly differentiated" because of its lack of gland formation. However, the prognosis of these patients is better than that for those with other forms of adenocarcinoma. The WHO recommends not grading this tumor but considering it low grade in behavior (21).

Serrated Adenocarcinoma

Serrated adenocarcinoma refers to an invasive tumor having histologic features of serration or other features commonly seen in the context of otherwise clearly serrated lesions, such as cytoplasmic eosinophilia or a mucinous component (43,44). Diagnostic criteria include a serrated pattern of growth showing papillae without

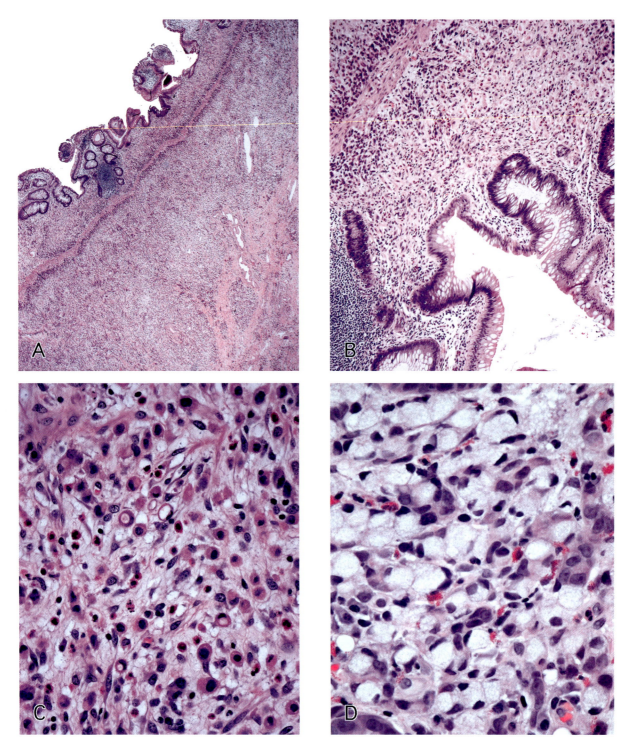

Figure 4-10

SIGNET RING CARCINOMA (MUCIN-POOR TYPE)

A: The tumor infiltrates throughout the wall in a diffuse fashion without forming cohesive glands.

B: The tumor cells have an appearance that can be mistaken for inflammation on superficial biopsy.

C: The infiltrating cells include an intermixture of small single cells without mucin along with classic signet ring cells.

D: The tumor cells have foamy mucin-containing cytoplasm, which can be mistaken for muciphages.

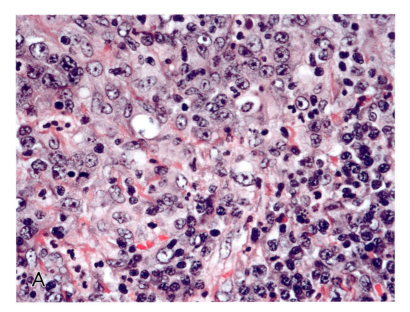

Figure 4-11

MEDULLARY CARCINOMA

A: The large tumor cells with vesicular nuclei and prominent nucleoli are growing in sheets with no glandular formation. There is an aggregate of lymphocytes in addition to tumor-infiltrating lymphocytes.

B: The cytologic features are similar to those in A, but the tumor cells are growing in cords rather than sheets, with no glandular formation. Numerous tumor-infiltrating lymphocytes are evident.

C: There is diffuse infiltration by small mature lymphocytes.

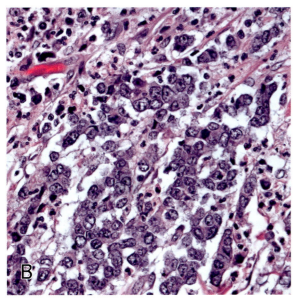

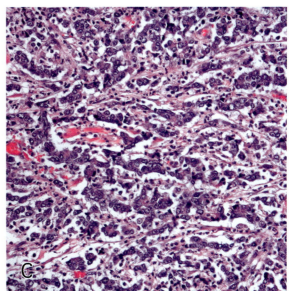

fibrovascular cores and lining cells showing abundant eosinophilic cytoplasm and vesicular nuclei (fig. 4-12).

These tumors often have dilated glandular spaces filled with mucin and lined with cells showing serrated features, including cytoplasmic eosinophilia, but otherwise resembling mucinous carcinoma (fig. 4-13). A mucinous pattern has been reported in more than 40 percent of serrated carcinomas, with the remainder having a more conventional growth pattern (fig. 4-14). It may be that some mucinous carcinomas are serrated adenocarcinomas with flattening

and loss of the serrated pattern caused by compression of the tumor cells. The association of both serrated adenocarcinoma and mucinous carcinoma with MSI and the serrated pathway to carcinoma demonstrates that the relationship holds at a molecular level as well. Nevertheless, to designate a mucinous carcinoma as a serrated adenocarcinoma requires that the cytologic features of the serrated pattern (the eosinophilic cytoplasm and vesicular nuclei) remain. It may be that this serrated pattern accounts to some degree for the apparent dichotomous behavior of mucinous carcinomas described above.

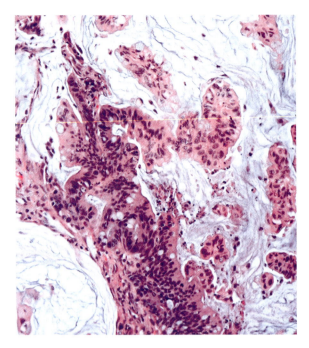

Figure 4-12

SERRATED ADENOCARCINOMA

Typical cases of serrated adenocarcinoma are characterized by large cells with eosinophilic, abundant cytoplasm and open nuclei with prominent nucleoli. Typically, they grow in a papillary fashion.

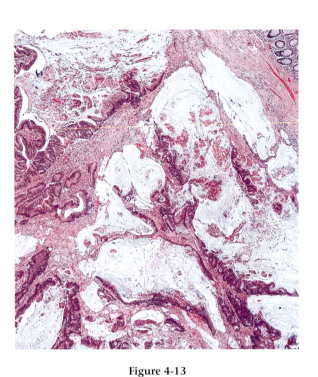

Figure 4-13

SERRATED ADENOCARCINOMA

Many cases of serrated adenocarcinoma are mucinous, as in this case.

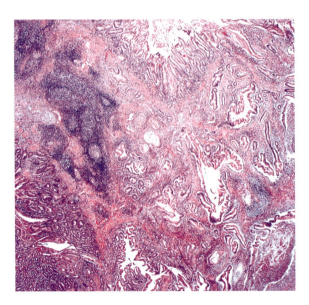

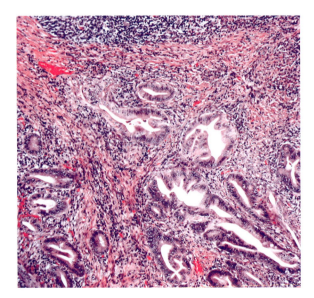

Figure 4-14

SERRATED ADENOCARCINOMA

Left: This tumor, which is arising in a patient with Crohn disease, is conventional, without a mucinous component. A somewhat papillary growth pattern can be seen at this power.

Right: At higher power, the abundant eosinophilic cytoplasm and papillary growth pattern characteristic of serrated adenocarcinoma are seen.

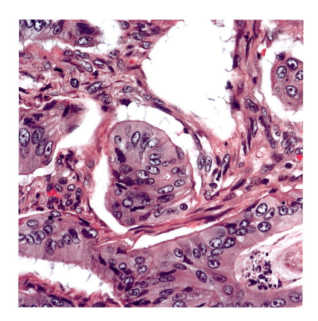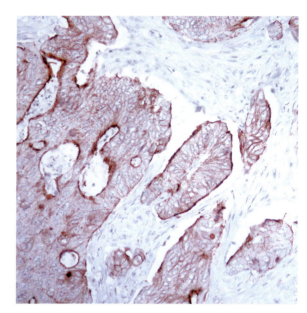

Figure 4-15

MICROPAPILLARY CARCINOMA

Left: Typically, there is a clear space surrounding a cluster of tumor cells without a lumen. In some cases, a brush border indicating differentiation can be seen on the external surface of the micropapillae.

Right: The epithelial membrane antigen (EMA) stain marks the outer surface of the micropapillae rather than the lumen, as in conventional adenocarcinoma NOS.

It has been suggested that serrated adenocarcinomas in the right and left colons behave differently, with right-sided lesions (which are probably derived from SSA/P) conferring a better prognosis and tending to have MSI whereas those in the rectum may derive from TSA and demonstrate a low level of MSI or are MSS (43). The relationship of serrated and mucinous adenocarcinomas to the CIMP-H phenotype also remains to be elucidated. Molecular studies have shown a characteristic gene expression profile for serrated adenocarcinomas (45).

Micropapillary Carcinoma

The term *micropapillary carcinoma* is applied in the colon to tumors showing a micropapillary pattern of growth in at least 5 percent of the tumor volume (46). The background colon carcinoma in which this micropapillary pattern arises is usually classic adenocarcinoma, NOS. Carcinomas showing a pure micropapillary pattern are almost never encountered, and hence, as is the situation with mucinous carcinoma and some other subtypes, whether the micropapillary pattern represents a distinct subtype

of colorectal carcinoma or rather represents a growth pattern within an otherwise garden variety colorectal carcinoma (similar to tumor budding, for example) is debatable. The significance of the micropapillary pattern of growth is that it is associated with a very high probability of lymph node metastases (46,47). Most published series of cases report that this pattern is found in 10 to 20 percent of all colorectal carcinomas and may be more common than other variants.

The micropapillary pattern is defined by the presence of small clusters of tumor cells typically sitting in spaces, suggesting lymphatic or vascular invasion (fig. 4-15, left). The cells often have eosinophilic cytoplasm and are not pleomorphic, and thus have features in common with serrated carcinoma. These "micropapillae" do not have fibrovascular cores, and seem to show an "inverted" growth pattern in that the surface of the cells, as demonstrated with epithelial membrane antigen (EMA), MUC1, or villin staining, is on the outside of the clusters, not in the inner surface as is seen with more typical gland formation in colorectal carcinoma (fig. 4-15, right).

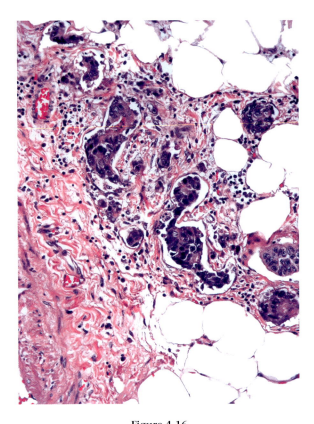

Figure 4-16

**LYMPHATIC INVASION SIMULATING
A MICROPAPILLARY PATTERN**

Although there is a peripheral space similar to that seen in figure 4-15, left, the tumor cells are not organized into a micropapillary pattern.

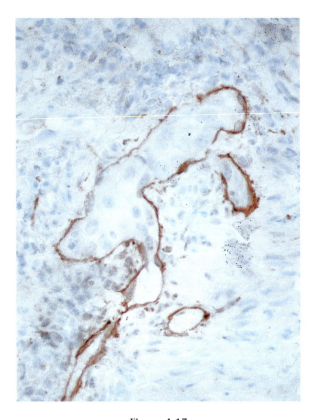

Figure 4-17

**LYMPHATIC INVASION SIMULATING
A MICROPAPILLARY PATTERN**

A D2-40 stain highlights the surrounding lymphatic endothelium.

Although only 5 percent of the tumor volume needs to be micropapillary in order for the carcinoma to be considered "micropapillary," most tumors show a 5 to 30 percent micropapillary pattern; if this pattern is present in at least 5 percent of cells, the frequency of lymph node metastases is approximately 80 percent. Micropapillae must be distinguished from lymphatic invasion, artifactual retraction, and tumor budding (figs. 4-16, 4-17). Tumor budding involves smaller clusters of cells (less than 5 per cluster) and the cells are not surrounded by a clear space. Artifactual retraction is distinguished by the lack of "reverse polarity" of the cells. Lymphatic invasion also does not show reverse polarity of cells and the spaces are lined with endothelial cells that may be marked with the immunostain D2-40 (fig. 4-17).

Although one publication suggests that micropapillary carcinoma has a right-sided and female predominance, this study excluded rectal carcinoma (48). Most other publications have shown that the gender, age of onset, and location of this tumor is similar to those of patients with colorectal carcinoma. Since the micropapillary pattern is associated with a high risk of lymph node metastases, it has been suggested that a micropapillary pattern within a polyp with invasive carcinoma warrants a more aggressive surgical approach, and that a micropapillary pattern might be included in indications for follow-up resections in malignant polyps (47). An increased probability of CK7 staining in these tumors (along with the usual CK20 positivity) has been reported (49), although this feature did not reach statistical significance and was not noted in another study (46). Tumors with a micropapillary pattern are also less likely to have MSI than the usual colorectal carcinomas (49).

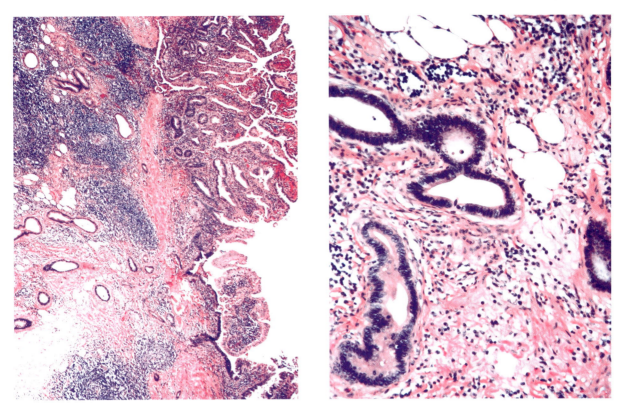

Figure 4-18

TUBULOGLANDULAR CARCINOMA

Left: Individual infiltrating glands can be seen in the submucosa of a patient with ulcerative colitis.

Right: The infiltrating glands are lined with hyperchromatic, elongated cells, simulating low-grade dysplasia. Only their infiltrative nature indicates their malignant potential.

Low-Grade Tubuloglandular Carcinoma

Low-grade tubuloglandular carcinoma is characterized by extremely well-formed single glands that infiltrate with minimal tissue reaction (fig. 4-18) (50,51). The cells forming the glands are bland, having nuclear features similar to those of low-grade dysplasia. Diagnosis is based on knowledge of the invasive nature of the glands, since taken out of context they are often mistaken for simple dysplastic glands. Since this tumor occurs almost exclusively in the context of chronic inflammatory bowel disease (IBD) (11 percent of all IBD cases in one study [51]), in which dysplasia is common, a biopsy diagnosis can be challenging. In many cases the low-grade tubuloglandular pattern is seen in conjunction with other more easily recognizable patterns including mucinous and poorly differentiated carcinomas, obviating errors in diagnosis.

The more poorly differentiated patterns are most often seen in the deeper portions of the tumor, therefore, biopsy diagnosis may be a significant problem. The presence of more poorly differentiated patterns heralds a poorer prognosis in comparison with tumors that are purely low-grade tubuloglandular. This tumor type has a prevalence of MSI due to loss of MLH1 of at least 55 percent in one study.

Rare and Unusual Tumor Types

There are a number of unusual or rare carcinomas that arise in the large intestine. These include squamous and adenosquamous carcinomas, rhabdoid carcinoma, lymphoepithelial-like carcinoma, adenocarcinoid, clear cell carcinoma, and giant cell carcinoma. In addition, melanoma may arise in the colon and mimic carcinoma.

Squamous Cell Carcinoma. Pure squamous cell carcinoma arising as a primary tumor of the

115

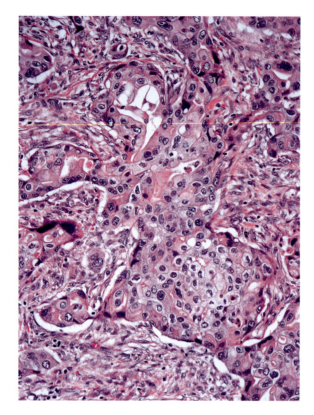

Figure 4-19

ADENOSQUAMOUS CARCINOMA

This tumor shows areas of intermixed glandular and squamous differentiation.

large intestine is rare (52–56). Cases have been described in the colon and rectum; however, in all cases it is important to exclude metastatic carcinoma or direct extension of carcinoma from the adjacent anus or cervix. In the rectum, squamous cell carcinoma may be more common in women and associated with cervical dysplasia, and therefore, with human papillomavirus (HPV) infection, although definitive results of studies for HPV are lacking (52,57). Cases have been described in patients with ulcerative colitis as well as with intestinal parasitic infestations.

Adenosquamous Carcinoma. Squamous differentiation may be a minor component of tumors that would otherwise be considered conventional adenocarcinomas of the large intestine, especially at the leading edge. These tumors are designated as adenosquamous carcinoma (fig. 4-19) (54,58,59). How much squamous differentiation is needed to designate a

tumor as adenosquamous has not been defined but may be important in determining the prognosis. It is unclear whether these tumors differ from pure squamous cell carcinoma, although several authors have suggested that they do not differ significantly, assuming that carcinomas extending into the rectum from the anus are excluded. Unfortunately, the reported case series is small, and there are significant differences in the reported most common site and prognosis.

Lymphoepithelial-Like Carcinoma. Lymphoepithelial carcinomas (LEC) are tumors thought histologically to resemble LEC of the upper airway (60–62). These tumors are characterized by a poorly differentiated carcinoma component with a heavy intratumoral infiltrate of lymphocytes. The tumor cells often nest, are poorly differentiated, and are considered adenocarcinomas although in the upper airway they are often considered to be variants of squamous cell carcinoma. The tumor cells are pleomorphic, with large vesicular nuclei and prominent nuclei.

Many of these features are identical to what is now better known as medullary carcinoma in the colon. Although some authors distinguish medullary carcinoma as showing less pleomorphism and having a less infiltrative border, it is unlikely that LEC truly represents a separate entity and it should probably be subsumed under medullary carcinoma in the colorectum. Among other reasons for this is that LEC in many organs is associated with Epstein-Barr virus (EBV) infection whereas in the colon that is not the case.

Rhabdoid Carcinoma. Rhabdoid carcinomas histologically similar to malignant rhabdoid tumor of the kidney and soft tissue have now been described in a number of locations including all parts of the gastrointestinal tract (63–66). Histologically, these tumors are characterized by large discohesive cells with abundant eosinophilic cytoplasm and large vesicular nuclei (fig. 4-20). The cytologic features are superficially similar to those of medullary and serrated carcinomas. In rhabdoid carcinoma, however, the nucleus is eccentric, and other features, such as a heavy lymphoid infiltrate or serrated architecture, are not present. Many cases have a pure rhabdoid morphology although they can be intermixed with more conventional forms

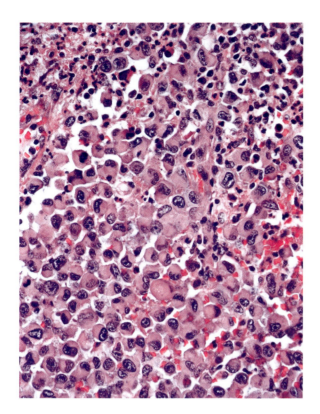

Figure 4-20

RHABDOID CARCINOMA

These tumors have discohesive large cells with abundant eosinophilic cytoplasm, resembling rhabdoid tumors of other organ systems.

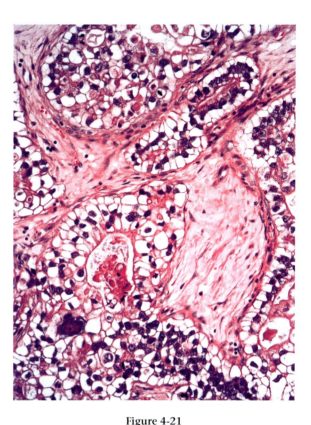

Figure 4-21

CLEAR CELL CARCINOMA

This tumor is composed of nests of clear cells histologically similar to clear cell tumors of the lung or female genital tract.

of colorectal carcinoma (in up to 33 percent of gastrointestinal cases), indicating that they should be considered rhabdoid carcinomas and not rhabdoid tumors.

The major entity in the differential diagnosis is metastatic melanoma, which can have a similar appearance, as well as rhabdoid tumors metastatic from other sites. Rhabdoid carcinoma cells mark with broad spectrum cytokeratins such as AE1/AE3 and are negative for CK7 and CK20 (64). They are strongly vimentin positive, and show nuclear loss of INI1 (SMARB1) or BRG1 (SMARCA4) in some cases.

Prognosis is poor regardless of site. MSI with loss of MLH1 and *BRAF* mutation has been reported, suggesting that rhabdoid carcinomas may arise via the serrated pathway (63–65).

Adenocarcinoid (Goblet Cell Carcinoid; Crypt Cell Carcinoma) Tumor. Tumors showing both glandular and neuroendocrine differentiation similar to goblet cell carcinoids occur

rarely in the gastrointestinal tract, including the colon (67). In all cases, it is necessary to exclude an appendiceal primary prior to regarding the tumor as extra-appendiceal. These lesions are discussed in detail in chapter 5.

Clear Cell Carcinoma. Approximately 16 cases of colonic adenocarcinoma with clear cell features have been reported in the literature (68–71). These include cases in which the clear cell features are admixed with other areas of more conventional histology, cases in which the tumor has well-formed glands lined with clear cells, and tumors with a solid clear cell growth pattern (fig. 4-21). All cases that have been stained have shown typical a CK20(+)/CK7(-) phenotype typical of colorectal carcinoma, and have also stained with CDX2. Although the numbers are small, the demographic features are similar to CIMP-L, MSS carcinomas arising in conventional adenomas: more common in men and in the left colon. Cases are reported that have arisen in

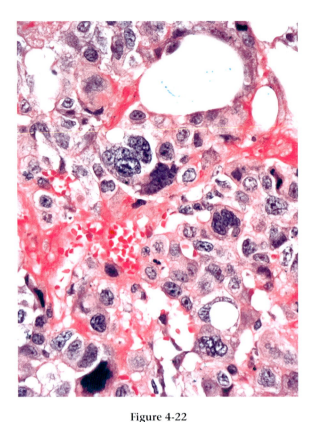

Figure 4-22

GIANT CELL CARCINOMA

Large pleomorphic cells and scattered bizarre multinucleated tumor cells are seen.

conventional adenomas with clear cell change (72–74). Given the small number of cases, it cannot be determined how the prognosis compares to that of other types of colorectal carcinoma.

In addition to these cases, gynecologic clear cell carcinoma has been reported arising in colonic endometriosis (75). These cases, not surprisingly, occur in young women and express a phenotype characteristic of tumors of mullerian origin, being positive for CK7 and negative for CK20 and CDX2. Clear cell carcinomas from other sites, such as kidney, can also metastasize to the colon and need to be distinguished with appropriate immunohistochemical studies.

Giant Cell Carcinoma. Giant cell carcinoma of the colon has been occasionally reported, in some cases with an accompanying sarcomatoid component and in other cases with an appearance similar to that of giant cell carcinoma of the lung (fig. 4-22) (72,73). The latter case expressed granulocyte colony stimulating factor

and was characterized by a heavy neutrophilic infiltrate and emperipolesis of neutrophils by tumor cells (73). This tumor stained only for AE1/AE3 and was negative for CK7, CK20, and CDX2. Some cases in the older literature reported as giant cell carcinomas may represent rhabdoid carcinomas based on more modern staining techniques and terminology.

Sarcomatoid Carcinoma. Fewer than 10 cases of colorectal sarcomatoid carcinoma (carcinosarcoma) have been reported. These tumors are biphasic, with a generally well-differentiated adenocarcinomatous component and malignant stromal components, which can be undifferentiated spindle cell sarcoma, osteosarcoma, or chondrosarcoma (76,77). Some cases have lacked an obvious epithelial component, however, and have had a giant cell component (72). Given the small number of reported cases, it is difficult to draw any conclusions regarding behavior, although most reported patients have done poorly.

Secondary Carcinomas. Not uncommonly, tumors arising outside the colon present as possible primary colorectal tumors. This includes direct invasion of the colon by adenocarcinoma arising in the prostate gland, adenocarcinoma or squamous cell carcinoma arising in the cervix, adenocarcinoma of the ovary, adenocarcinoma of the appendix, and urothelial carcinoma arising in the bladder (which can have glandular differentiation or be purely adenocarcinoma) (fig. 4-23). Similarly, metastatic carcinoma or melanoma from a variety of sites can present in the large intestine. Signet ring carcinoma, as mentioned above, characteristically arises in the stomach and spreads through the abdomen to the colon. The colon is also commonly involved with intraperitoneal spread of ovarian carcinomas and carcinomas from distant sites such as lung or breast. Endometrioid and clear cell adenocarcinomas developing in endometriosis in the wall of the intestine can mimic primary colorectal carcinoma.

Paramount to diagnosing these tumors is remembering that they occur, applying appropriate immunostains, and obtaining additional clinical history when a tumor does not show features characteristic of primary colorectal carcinoma. Clues to an extracolonic source for tumors include absence of preexisting adenoma and an epicenter of tumor that appears to be in the colonic wall or outside the colon rather than

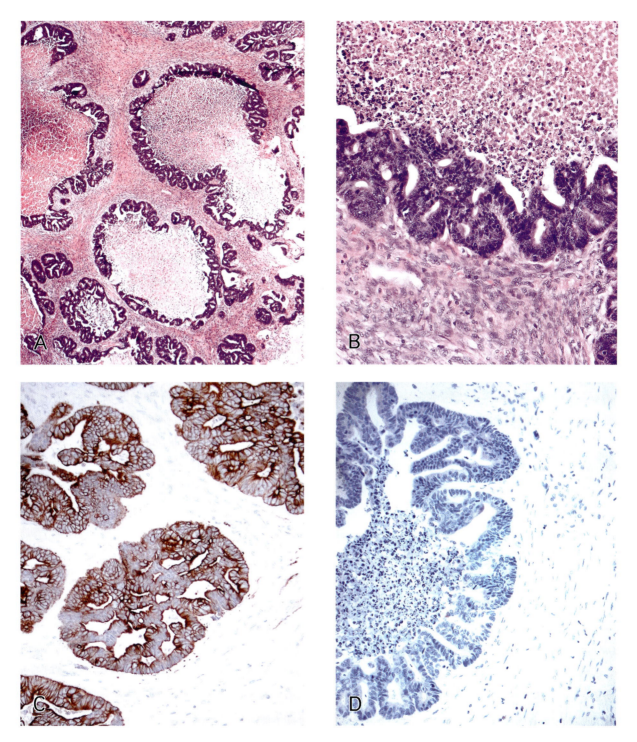

Figure 4-23

CARCINOMA METASTATIC FROM OVARY TO COLON

A: This tumor, found in the colon wall, has a somewhat cribriform pattern, with dirty necrosis that could be mistaken for colon carcinoma.

B: Higher power view.

C: Uniform staining with a cytokeratin (CK) 7 stain.

D: CK20 is negative. This staining pattern is not consistent with a primary colorectal carcinoma.

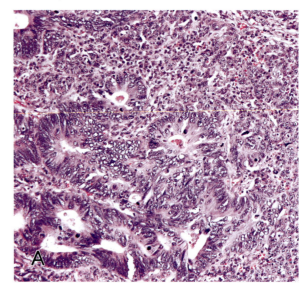

Figure 4-24

**NEUROENDOCRINE CARCINOMA
ARISING IN CONVENTIONAL ADENOMA**

A: Residual adenoma is seen at the left. The tumor shows the typical features of a neuroendocrine carcinoma, with sheets of uniform hyperchromatic cells.

B: A higher-power view demonstrates small cells with scant cytoplasm and abundant mitotic activity.

C: Synaptophysin is uniformly positive, characteristic of neuroendocrine carcinomas.

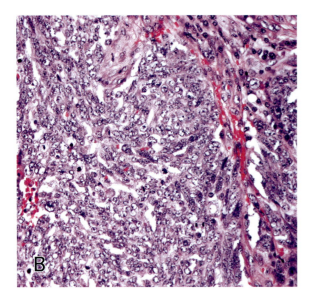

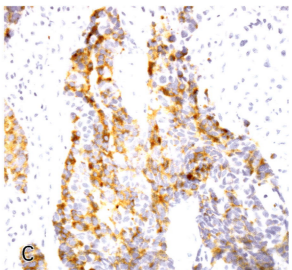

in the mucosa. Since the epicenter of a tumor cannot be ascertained on a biopsy, correlation with radiologic findings may be useful if the pathologist is suspicious that a tumor is not primary. Typically, biopsies show tumor undermining normal mucosa, although if there is ulceration over the tumor this may not be the case. Occasionally, metastatic tumors overgrow the surface of the colon, mimicking a preexisting adenoma.

Another important clue to the diagnosis is that the tumor does not have the typical morphology of colorectal carcinoma. Any tumor showing a solid growth pattern without well-formed glands, or that lacks columnar cells with pseudostratification should lead to some

concern about the primary site. Any tumor that is not clearly adenocarcinoma (i.e., squamous cell carcinoma, adenosquamous carcinoma, clear cell carcinoma, papillary carcinoma, or melanoma) is likely to be secondary rather than primary.

High-Grade Neuroendocrine Carcinoma (Small and Large Cell Types). Neuroendocrine carcinomas having morphologic characteristics similar to those in the lung occur throughout the colon (78) and are further discussed in chapter 7. Small cell neuroendocrine carcinomas are composed of moderately pleomorphic small cells with angular hyperchromatic nuclei that mold into each other (fig. 4-24). Geographic necrosis is often present and mitotic activity is high. These tumors often arise at the base of conventional adenomas, typically villous adenomas, and hence do not seem to be directly related to low-grade neuroendocrine (carcinoid) tumors, which rarely develop in this context.

The major diagnostic issue with small cell neuroendocrine carcinoma is distinction from lymphoma, which is usually not a problem with immunohistochemical staining. Large cell neuroendocrine carcinomas need to be differentiated from large cell lymphoma and also from undifferentiated carcinoma (non-neuroendocrine) and poorly differentiated adenocarcinoma, especially on biopsy specimens. These distinctions are also usually easily made with appropriate immunohistochemical staining.

Many cases of non-neuroendocrine carcinoma of the large intestine, including low-grade adenocarcinomas, have a significant component of neuroendocrine cells, which represents neuroendocrine differentiation within the adenocarcinoma and not a true neuroendocrine tumor. Studies have shown that a small component of neuroendocrine differentiation, as demonstrated with immunohistochemical stains, does not affect the prognosis of colonic adenocarcinoma. For this reason, the WHO recommends not diagnosing a tumor as having a neuroendocrine component unless more than 30 percent of the tumor cells mark with neuroendocrine markers (21).

GRADING OF ADENOCARCINOMA

Adenocarcinoma of the colon has traditionally been graded based on the degree of glandular formation by the tumor. The traditional method of grading these tumors was a three-tier system (well, moderate, and poorly differentiated). However, reproducibility of the distinction between well and moderately differentiated tumors has been poor, and studies of prognosis generally have shown a difference between poorly differentiated tumors and those considered well and moderately differentiated but not between well and moderately differentiated tumors. Thus, for practical purposes, the well and moderately differentiated categories are combined into the "low-grade" grouping. Using the glandular criteria, low-grade tumors have 50 percent or more gland formation and high-grade tumors less than 50 percent (figs. 4-3, 4-25) (79).

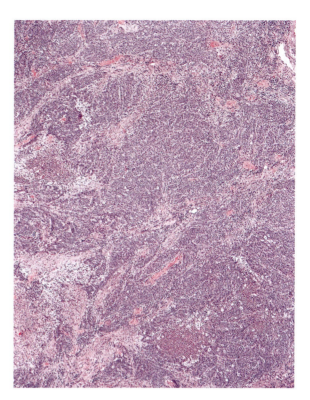

Figure 4-25

HIGH-GRADE ADENOCARCINOMA

In this example, less than 50 percent of the tumor is glandular. The differential diagnosis for a tumor with this appearance includes a neuroendocrine carcinoma. In this case, stains for chromogranin and synaptophysin were negative.

Grading mainly applies to tumors in the classic adenocarcinoma, NOS category. Most other types of non-neuroendocrine carcinoma carry their own inherent grade. For example, medullary carcinoma has a good prognosis and is considered low grade despite the fact that most cases have no glandular formation. For mucinous carcinomas, the prognosis, and hence functional grade, depends on the microsatellite status, with MSS tumors having a worse prognosis than adenocarcinoma, NOS, and MSI tumors a better prognosis. Signet ring carcinomas are all by definition high grade.

SPECIAL STAINS IN THE DIAGNOSIS AND MANAGEMENT OF COLORECTAL CARCINOMA

Immunohistochemistry can be very valuable in diagnosing colorectal tumors, particularly when trying to determine the primary site of metastatic lesions identified in other sites such as the lung or liver (80). In addition, as mentioned above, tumors secondarily involving the colon can be identified with appropriate staining. Staining is essential for identifying neuroendocrine tumors. It is also used to assess mismatch repair enzymes as part of screening for Lynch syndrome and to assess tumors for MSI, which may help determine prognosis and play a role in appropriate patient management (20). The discussion here is limited mainly to staining patterns of primary colorectal lesions and the use of stains to facilitate their staging. Extensive discussion of staining patterns of noncolorectal tumors is beyond the scope of this Fascicle, however, staining of neuroendocrine tumors and the diagnosis of Lynch syndrome is discussed below and in chapter 5.

Most primary colorectal carcinomas of the usual type (i.e., adenocarcinoma NOS) have a characteristic and almost pathognomonic staining pattern: strongly positive for CK20 and CDX2, and negative for CK7. Very few other tumors share this staining pattern. Some cases of mucinous carcinoma of the ovary may express CK20 in addition to CK7, and also may express CDX2, however, the CK20 and CDX2 patterns are typically patchy and weak in comparison to those of most colorectal carcinomas, whereas the CK7 is stronger and more uniform than that of most colorectal carcinomas (81). CK7 can be expressed in some cases of colorectal carcinoma but it is usually very patchy, although it may be strong in the cells expressing it. Mucinous ovarian carcinoma is distinguished from colorectal carcinoma by AMACR (p504s), which marks about 30 percent of colorectal carcinomas, but not ovarian mucinous carcinomas, and PAX8, which is reported to mark 50 percent of ovarian but not colorectal carcinomas (81).

Not all colorectal carcinomas show this typical CK20(+)/CK7(-) profile. Some, particularly MSI tumors and undifferentiated carcinomas, are negative for both CK7 and CK20, which leads to another differential diagnostic grouping, although most metastatic tumors that fail to express either CK7 or CK20 are not likely to be confused histologically with colorectal carcinoma (e.g., hepatocellular and renal cell carcinomas).

Approximately 5 percent of colorectal carcinomas are negative for CDX2, and loss of CDX2 has been cited as a possible marker of poor prognosis, which may be important for management of patients with stages II and III disease (82–84). Loss of CDX2 correlates with lack of CK20 expression, CIMP-H status, MSI, *BRAF* mutation, poor differentiation, and advanced stage. Most of these features, with the exception of MSI, also are associated with a poorer prognosis, hence the significance of CDX2 as a marker is confounded. Nevertheless, CDX2 staining is quicker and less expensive than CIMP or *BRAF* mutation analysis, and thus it may be a reasonable surrogate. Although MSI generally portends a better prognosis than MSS status in CIMP-H tumors, there is some evidence that loss of CDX2 may carry a somewhat worse prognosis within the subset of cases with MSI (85).

Signet ring carcinoma differs somewhat from most colon carcinomas in that CK7 may be diffusely positive in some cases, and approximately 20 percent of cases do not express CK20 or do so only focally and weakly. However, gastric signet ring carcinoma often shows a CK7(+)/CK20(-) profile, and this profile in a colorectal signet ring carcinoma should strongly raise the possibility of metastasis from the stomach (80,86).

Immunochemical and immunohistochemical stains are occasionally useful for staging carcinoma. Stains may assess lymphovascular invasion (elastic, CD34, and D2-40), aid in identification of tumor budding (pancytokeratin), and search for small metastatic deposits in lymph nodes (pancytokeratin). None of these techniques is considered standard.

A number of studies have evaluated the use of elastic stains as an adjunct to identifying vascular invasion (87–91). Mainly, this technique confirms that suspected vascular invasion is actually that and not just retraction artifact. As such, this staining is of limited utility, particularly since the reported prognostic significance of vascular invasion is mainly based on hematoxylin and eosin (H&E) analysis and may not be relevant in cases of vascular invasion identified with special techniques. There appears to be no question that the use of elastic stains increases the identification of the number of cases with vascular invasion. However, since most studies of vascular invasion using elastic stains do not compare survival based on method of detection, it is unclear whether such identification is as significant as finding it by H&E techniques alone.

Some studies have not shown significance to the finding of vascular invasion by elastic stains (88), although others have (90,91). D2-40 and CD34 are also used to evaluate lymphatic and venous invasion (90,92). Although these stains are useful to confirm invasion, it is questionable whether they provide much additional information over H&E techniques.

Several studies have used cytokeratin staining to identify tumor buds, and with this technique the number of tumor buds identified is increased over those identified only with H&E (93–95). Tumor budding identified by cytokeratin staining does have prognostic significance, although studies evaluating this parameter by H&E techniques also show prognostic significance. A recent analysis comparing H&E with cytokeratin identification demonstrated, in multivariate analysis, that identification by H&E was more significant than identification by cytokeratin staining, which may be over sensitive (94). It is thus unclear whether using cytokeratin actually improves patient care. It does increase the cost of examination, and does delay reporting of cases, and thus, is not likely to become common practice. In some cases with equivocal budding, this technique may be useful. The importance of tumor budding is discussed in detail below.

Finally, a number of studies have assessed the utility of cytokeratin staining to identify isolated tumor cells and micrometastases in lymph nodes, including "sentinel" lymph nodes (96–100). While this technique increases the yield of positive nodes, it is unclear whether these micrometastases have any prognostic significance or should influence therapy, and thus the use of cytokeratin to identify metastases is not recommended as routine practice. Several publications do suggest that micrometastases may influence prognosis, so this view may change over time (96). At of this writing, however, nodal metastases smaller than 0.2 mm are considered N0 (i+) for staging purposes (79).

ROUTINE MOLECULAR TESTING OF COLORECTAL CARCINOMA

Although a number of molecular markers have been evaluated to assess prognosis and response to specific therapies, only a few have been determined to be sufficiently reproducible for routine use (101). As noted elsewhere in this chapter, testing for microsatellite status is considered routine for all newly diagnosed colorectal cancer cases regardless of stage. This testing is useful for evaluating the possibility of Lynch syndrome as well as for determining the need for neoadjuvant chemotherapy. Patients with MSI tumors have a better prognosis than those with MSS tumors, and they may not benefit from fluorouracil-based chemotherapy.

BRAF mutational analysis is useful in determining whether patients with loss of the MLH1 protein have Lynch syndrome or if such loss is caused by methylation of the promoter of the gene. Since 80 percent of cancers with methylation of MLH1 have a mutation of the V600E codon of *BRAF*, identification of this mutation argues strongly against Lynch syndrome. Methylation analysis may be a more cost effect test, however, since it detects nearly 100 percent of sporadic cases. *BRAF* mutation may also occur in MSS carcinomas, and in that setting it is associated with a poor prognosis and lack of response to anti-EGFR therapies, similar to *KRAS*-mutated tumors.

Patients with stage IV colon carcinoma who are going to receive chemotherapy should be tested for mutations of the *KRAS* and *NRAS* genes since certain mutations of these genes are associated with a lack of response to anti-EGFR-based therapies (101). Analysis of other markers, such as *PIK3CA* and *PTEN* are not recommended for routine testing.

BIOPSY DIAGNOSIS OF COLORECTAL CARCINOMA

There are a number of issues related to the biopsy of colorectal carcinoma, including whether it is even necessary if there is an obvious tumor at endoscopy that requires resection regardless of the histologic findings on biopsy. An argument can be made that biopsy provides no benefit to the clinician or patient in most cases, and can be misleading for a variety of reasons detailed below. On the other hand, in certain patients, most notably those who might have Lynch syndrome, biopsy does provide a determination of the mismatch repair status of the tumor prior to resection. Patients with known Lynch syndrome generally undergo a more extensive resection than others since their residual colonic tissue is at increased risk for the development of metachronous carcinoma.

Therefore, for any patient in whom making a diagnosis of Lynch syndrome is reasonably likely and for whom the surgeon would base a surgical decision on the knowledge of the mismatch repair status of the tumor, biopsy and mismatch repair testing are recommended.

Biopsy is not without some risk, however, and not every carcinoma is amenable to biopsy. Sometimes biopsy can be misleading since it is only a small sample of the total tumor. In some cases, either due to poor colonic preparation or to the nature of the tumor and surrounding mucosa, it is not possible to obtain lesional tissue. Biopsies of lesions that are difficult to reach may show only normal mucosa, or may show mucosa that is reactive or ulcerated. It is important for the pathologist to know the circumstance of the biopsy in order to make an appropriate comment in the report.

Sometimes only precursor lesion (i.e., adenoma), with or without high-grade dysplasia, is sampled but not the underlying carcinoma. Knowing that the biopsy is of a large probable carcinoma allows the pathologist to comment on the superficiality and size of the biopsy and to note that the findings do not exclude the possibility of carcinoma. It is because of this potential sampling error that complete excision of all precursor lesions (i.e., conventional adenomas, SSA/P, and traditional serrated adenomas) is recommended, along with the fact that the residual precursor may become malignant at a later time, even if it is not malignant at the time the biopsy is performed.

Particularly vexing are cases in which there is an obvious tumor but a biopsy obtains small fragments of tissue showing high-grade dysplasia but not invasive carcinoma. In these cases, the pathologist typically "knows" that there must be a carcinoma present but doesn't want to overdiagnose a lesion. Rather than simply diagnose "tubulovillous adenoma with high-grade dysplasia," a diagnosis of "tubulovillous adenoma with high-grade dysplasia/carcinoma in situ (cannot rule out invasive carcinoma, see description)" can be offered. Although the term "carcinoma in situ" is generally not recommended in the diagnosis of adenomas in the large intestine, use of the term in conjunction with "high-grade dysplasia" allows the pathologist to alert the clinician to the probability of

a more advanced lesion than is present in the available biopsy material.

Another issue that arises is that of classification and grading of tumors on biopsy. Typically, the superficial portions of a carcinoma are the best differentiated portions and if there is a mucinous component or poorly differentiated component present it is often at the deeper leading edge of the tumor and thus not represented in a biopsy. Therefore, one could argue that tumors should not be graded based on biopsy findings.

Finally, biopsy can be misleading in regard to primary versus metastatic tumor. If carcinoma can be seen arising in an unequivocal preexisting precursor lesion, then the lesion is very likely to be primary. Conversely, if tumor is noted only in the submucosa beneath normal mucosa, then the possibility of metastatic carcinoma should be more seriously considered.

PATHOLOGIC EXAMINATION OF RESECTED COLORECTAL CARCINOMA

Pathologic examination of the resected specimen provides prognostic information and guides therapy. Pathologic findings relate to the tumor itself (grade, histologic type, stage, response to any neoadjuvant treatment) and to the surgery (adequacy of margins, adequacy of nodal removal). Examination and the prognostic information it provides vary with the type of resection (i.e., right hemicolectomy and low anterior left colon resections are treated somewhat differently than abdominal perineal resections for removal of lower rectal carcinoma).

Evaluation of colorectal carcinoma as of 2017 follows the guidelines of the 7th edition of the American Joint Committee on Cancer (AJCC) manual for staging of malignancies, which is recapitulated by the American College of Pathologists (CAP) as a series of protocols and checklists (79,102). As of January 1, 2018, the 8th edition will be in effect (103). The staging guidelines contain mandatory and optional elements, the use of the latter being driven by considerations of what might be the most useful, or desirable, parameters for clinicians. Close communication with colorectal surgeons and oncologists regarding their preferences is important. Some aspects of the AJCC and CAP protocols are controversial and some are detailed below. In

Table 4-1

GROSS DESCRIPTION OF RESECTED SPECIMEN

1. Size of specimen and portions of intestine included; the appendix should be described if the specimen includes the cecum, along with the extent (length from colon to mesenteric surgical margin) of any included mesocolon

2. Presence of any tattoo dye marking prior polypectomy

3. Location of the tumor with measurements to the resection margins
   a. for nonrectal tumor this includes proximal and distal mucosal margins as well as to the mesenteric margin and for some resections (e.g., tumors of the ascending, hepatic flexure, and descending colon) to the free retroperitoneal margin if it can be identified
   b. for rectal tumors this includes proximal and distal mucosal margins as well as the circumferential soft tissue (radial) margin. Part of this assessment should be a statement about the completeness of the mesorectal envelope resection (see description below)

4. Designate location of the tumor in relationship to the mesentery (i.e., mesenteric or antimesenteric) and the relationship of the tumor to the free peritoneal surface (including in the rectum if it is partially peritonealized)

5. Estimate size of tumor

6. Estimate depth of invasion of tumor and, for tumors in a subserosal location, the distance of the tumor from the free serosal surface

7. Note whether the tumor invades other structures or organs

8. Estimate the number of dissected nodes and describe the range of size of the nodes identified

9. Mention any additional mucosal lesions or other tumors

---

addition, changes introduced in the 8th edition are reviewed where appropriate.

Gross Examination

Examination of the specimen begins with a good description and dissection of the gross specimen. Developing an adequate gross description obviously requires familiarity with information relevant to staging and with the normal anatomy of the large intestine and rectum. Elements that are required in the gross description of the resected specimen are outlined in Table 4-1.

Gross Anatomy of the Normal Large Intestine. The large intestine begins at the ileocecal valve and extends to the anus. Most of the large intestine is in the peritoneal cavity and is at least partly invested in peritoneum. The rectum is extraperitoneal and is directly surrounded by soft tissue and other organs (bladder and prostate in men, vagina and uterus in women). The colon, for the most part, is separated from the retroperitoneum by a mesocolon, although portions of both the right and left colons are retroperitoneal. Proper assessment of what constitutes a surgical "margin" depends in large part on the exact location of the tumor and the extent of its resection.

The entire transverse colon is located on a mesocolon. For a transverse colectomy, the resection margins are the proximal and distal colonic margins and the cut edge of the mesocolon. There is no radial, circumferential, or retroperitoneal margin in the transverse colon. The cecum is usually totally intraperitoneal, with a short mesocolon, although portions may be retroperitoneal and there may be a radial or retroperitoneal soft tissue surgical margin. This is generally difficult to positively identify in a surgical specimen, however.

Most of the ascending colon is retroperitoneal with a retroperitoneal margin. A defined mesocolon can be found in approximately 30 percent of patients. The hepatic flexure has a free retroperitoneal surface in contact with the right kidney. The splenic flexure and descending colon typically have a free retroperitoneal surface that constitutes a margin. The sigmoid colon is completely invested in peritoneum with a mesocolon.

The rectum is outside of the peritoneal cavity and differs considerably from the remainder the colon in its surgical aspects as well as in terms of pathologic assessment. The upper portion of the rectum may have peritoneum on the lateral and anterior surfaces where it transitions from the sigmoid colon.

The serosa overlying the tumor should be inked to allow identification of the free serosal surface, and if any of the resection margins are close to the tumor, those should be inked as well. Sampling of the specimen traditionally includes sections of all surgical margins (proximal and distal mucosal margins and the mesenteric or circumferential soft tissue margin), although assessment of widely distant mucosal margins is almost never revealing. If margins are close to the tumor they should be inked and sections taken perpendicular to the free margin. Sections of the tumor closest to the free peritoneal surface should also be taken if the tumor is located underlying the free peritoneal surface. There should be least three additional full-thickness sections of the tumor (ideally with one including adjacent mucosa with any residual grossly identifiable precursor lesion [i.e., adenoma] and two or more sections of the deepest extent of tumor), and sections of any additional noted lesions and lymph nodes.

Adequacy of Mesorectal or Mesenteric (Mesocolonic) Excision. The adequacy of the mesorectal envelope excision is a major factor in determining the risk of local recurrence for rectal carcinoma (104–107). It is recommended that the examining pathologist provide such an assessment of the adequacy. The degree of excision is assessed as follows: incomplete (muscularis propria plane)—little bulk to the mesorectum, defects down to the muscularis propria, very irregular circumferential margin; nearly complete (intramesorectal plane)—moderate bulk to the mesorectum, irregularity to the mesorectal surface with defects greater than 5 mm in depth, not extending to the muscularis propria and no areas of visible muscularis propria (with the exception of the insertion of the levator muscles); and complete (mesorectal plane)—intact bulky mesorectum, with a smooth surface with only minor irregularities and no surface defects greater than 5 mm in depth.

In recent years there has been a movement toward a more complete mesenteric excision, sometimes down to the retroperitoneal wall (108–110). Data supporting this degree of excision are less compelling than for complete mesorectal excision in rectal carcinomas and hence this is not a universal practice. Most treatment failures for colonic adenocarcinoma are not local recurrences in the mesenteric stump, in distinction from the frequent rate of local recurrence for rectal carcinoma.

Nevertheless, for surgeons attempting more complete excisions, the determination of the adequacy of mesenteric excision, similar to that used for mesorectal excision, has been proposed as follows (110): poor plane of surgery (muscularis propria plane)—little bulk to mesocolon, disruptions extending into the muscularis propria; moderate plane of surgery (intramesocolic plane)—moderate bulk to mesocolon, irregularity to the margin but incisions not extending down to the muscularis propria; and good plane of surgery (mesocolic plane)—intact mesocolon with smooth peritoneal-lined surface, smooth intact resection margin.

Microscopic Examination

Size and Radial Margins. The size of the tumor is a gross determination, however, the status of the margins is based on microscopic examination. The distal and proximal mucosal margins for all operations except low anterior resections are rarely positive for carcinoma, nor is the typical mesocolonic margin. However, for rectal excisions, the status of the radial (circumferential) margin is very important to the determination of recurrence and the radial margin should be examined carefully. The general recommendation is to prepare sections perpendicular to the margin, especially the closest margin (for documentation if clearly negative) or of all visibly close margins.

For rectal carcinomas, the specimen should be fixed intact and serial cross sections made to allow optimal assessment of all margins. Unfortunately, in daily practice in most settings such a delay may not be practical. Nevertheless, the longer the specimen is fixed prior to sectioning the better. Even without prior fixation, cross sectioning should allow good visualization of the status of the margin and allow appropriate sectioning to be undertaken.

What Constitutes a Positive Margin? If tumor is located at a margin, that obviously represents margin involvement. However, according to the AJCC protocol, circumferential margins (i.e., the mesorectal envelope in rectal carcinoma cases and the retroperitoneal margin in resections of colon with retroperitonal free margins) are considered positive if the tumor is within 0.1 cm (1 mm) of the margin. This number is supported by a reported rate of local recurrence of 55 percent with a positive margin and 28 percent with tumor within 1 mm of the margin (105). Local recurrence diminishes markedly at 1.1 mm and greater.

STAGING OF COLORECTAL CARCINOMAS

Colorectal carcinoma staging follows the guidelines of the AJCC, currently in the 7th edition through 2017 and will be replaced by the 8th edition in 2018, and CAP (79,103). Areas of controversy, however, are included in the discussion below.

T Stages: General Features

The depth of tumor invasion, or T stage, is fairly straightforward. pTX represents cases in which the primary tumor cannot be assessed for technical reasons, which includes cases in which the primary tumor is not resected. pT0 refers to cases in which upon resection there is no evidence of primary tumor. This may represent a successful response to neoadjuvant therapy or may be the result of an incorrect diagnosis of malignancy on biopsy (a false positive biopsy). It may also represent complete resection of the tumor by the biopsy procedure. In the latter case, however, staging may be performed using the biopsy and resection specimen together if the biopsy is available.

pTis represents high-grade dysplasia or carcinoma confined to the lamina propria of the mucosa, known as intramucosal carcinoma. These tumors are considered to have no ability to metastasize. Although in the past the term "carcinoma in situ" was applied to this category (hence the designation Tis), there is general consensus to avoid the term carcinoma if possible and high-grade dysplasia is the preferred term. In the 8th edition of the AJCC manual tumors invading into but not through the muscularis mucosae are also considered to be Tis because of their "negligible risk of metastasis."

pT1 represents tumor that has invaded through the muscularis mucosae into submucosa without invasion of the muscularis propria.

pT2 represents tumor that invades into but not through the muscularis propria. pT3 represents tumor that invades through the muscularis propria but without invasion of adjacent structures, penetration of the serosa or, in the rectum, invasion of pelvic muscles

beyond the external anal sphincter. pT4a is invasion through the intestine wall to involve the serosal surface. This is discussed in detail below. pT4b is invasion into adjacent structures. The T4b designation is applied when direct tumor Invasion of the adjacent structure is identified, or when tumor invades adhesions to an adjacent organ. Inflammatory adhesions between the carcinoma and adjacent structures without microscopic evidence of tumor in the adjacent structure also constitute pT4b. In the rectum, invasion of pelvic muscles beyond the external anal sphincter, such as the levator ani, is considered pT4b disease.

T-Stage Controversies

T staging is straightforward as far as pT2 (into the muscularis propria) and pT3 (through the muscularis propria) are concerned. Issues regarding pT1 and pT4 that have been problematic although these are addressed in the 8th edition staging manual.

Regarding T1, the standard diagnosis has been that a lesion is considered T1 only when it has penetrated through the muscularis mucosae into the submucosa. The rationale for this is based on the concept that lymphatic vessels are not present in the mucosa and hence a tumor does not have access to lymphatics until the muscularis mucosae is breached. However, electron microscopic data and immunohistochemical studies as well as daily observations indicate that lymphatic vessels are indeed present in the lamina propria, extending through the muscularis mucosae to the base of the crypts of Lieberkuhn (111). This indicates, therefore, that tumors that invade into the muscularis mucosae have access to lymphatics and are, in theory, capable of metastastazing to regional lymph nodes. This is often evident at the edge of colorectal carcinomas with lymphatic invasion, where it is common to see tumor emboli in lymphatics at the base of the crypts and above the muscularis mucosae (fig. 4-26).

The fact that the muscularis mucosae in polyps underlying carcinomas is often hyperplastic and splayed also complicates interpretation since tumor can often extend some distance into the muscularis mucosae without traversing its entire thickness. Thus, tumors invading into the muscularis mucosae might be considered

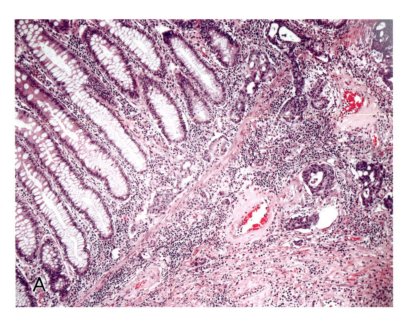

Figure 4-26

CARCINOMA IN INTRAMUCOSAL LYMPHATICS

A: Colon carcinoma can be clearly seen in lymphatic vessels at the base of the mucosa, above the muscularis mucosae.

B: Non-neoplastic mucosa near a colon carcinoma with intramucosal lymphatic invasion.

C: D2-40 stain of the area seen in figure A confirms the presence of lymphatic vessels in the lamina propria above the muscularis mucosae.

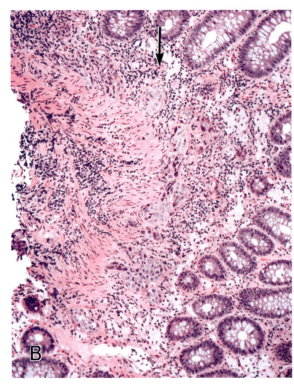

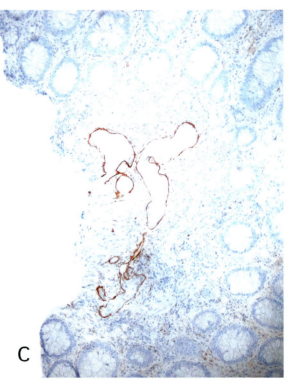

T1 lesions based on the possibility that they could invade lymphatics and spread, but in reality there are no data that support such a modification to the existing staging schemes. Some observers offer a comment indicating that the tumor technically does not meet the criteria for submucosal invasion and is not T1, but that it does have access to lymphatic vessels such that it may be biologically equivalent to an early T1 lesion.

The 7th edition of the AJCC guidelines for staging does not specifically address this issue since it states that tumors should be considered pTis if they grow "up to but not through the muscularis mucosae (intramucosal carcinoma)" and that "tumor extension through the muscularis mucosae into the submucosa is classified as T1," without discussion of tumors into but not through the muscularis mucosae. This deficiency has been addressed in the 8th edition, which states that tumors invading into but not through the muscularis mucosae should be considered Tis.

The major current issue of T4 colon carcinoma revolves around the significance of the distinction of tumor that grows through the colon or rectal wall and involves adjacent organs (currently considered T4b) from tumors that grow through peritonealized portions of the large intestine to involve the peritoneal surface (currently considered T4a).

Regarding serosal involvement, the serosal surface of the colon does not constitute a margin, although sometimes it is mistakenly inked and reported as such. The peritoneal surface is very important to prognosis, however. It is identified by either mesothelial cells or by the presence of ink placed on the surface at the time of gross examination. There has been some variation in past staging protocols in what is considered a "positive" serosal surface, and also in categorizing a positive serosal margin as T4a or T4b.

The most widely cited study (112) regarding definitions of serosal penetration described three patterns of involvement: the presence of a mesothelial inflammatory and/or hyperplastic reaction with tumor close to, but not at, the serosal surface; tumor present at the serosal surface with inflammatory reaction, mesothelial hyperplasia, and/or erosion/ulceration; and free tumor cells on the serosal surface (in the peritoneum) with underlying ulceration of the visceral peritoneum. Those authors found that the latter two situations were probably more significant and associated with poorer clinical outcomes (fig. 4-27).

Tumors with positive serosal surfaces were, in the 6th edition of the AJCC staging manual, classified as T4b, based on data indicating that the prognosis in patients with serosal involvement was worse than invasion of adjacent organs, which was therefore classified as T4a (113). The 7th edition of the manual defines a positive serosal surface as tumor growing into or sitting on the surface. However, detection of serosal involvement can be challenging because the inflammatory reaction elicited by tumoral

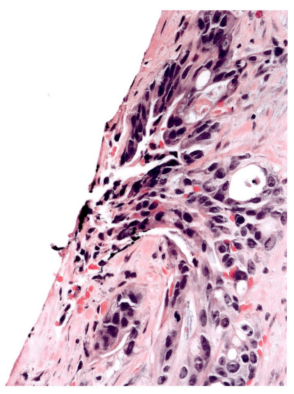

Figure 4-27

CARCINOMA AT FREE PERITONEAL SURFACE

Tumor cells can be seen on ink at the surface. This constitutes T4a disease.

penetration can mask the presence of mesothelial cells in the vicinity of tumor cells. For this reason, any type of fibroinflammatory reaction at the serosal surface in close proximity to the tumor should prompt careful examination, potentially with submission of more tissue sections. Penetration of the visceral peritoneum is often more evident in the clefts between lobules of peritoneal fat (fig. 4-28). Detection of serosal penetration can be enhanced through the use of serosal cytology preparations obtained from the resection specimen (114). Some authors have found elastin stains to enhance detection of serosal penetration by demonstrating tumoral penetration of the subserosal elastic lamina (115). New to the 8th edition of the staging manual is the additional concept that tumors with perforation in which tumor cells are contiguous with the serosal surface through inflammation are also considered T4a even if the tumor cells themselves are not seen on the surface of the inflammation (103).

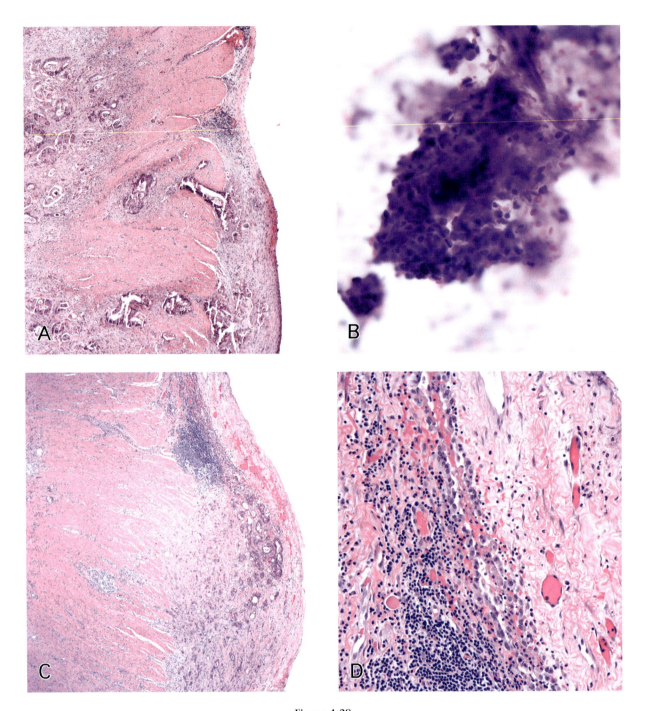

Figure 4-28

SEROSAL PENETRATION BY COLONIC CARCINOMA

A: Tumor cells are present within 1 mm of the serosal surface. They are associated with a dense fibroinflammatory reaction that expands the subserosal connective tissue compared to the normal serosa on the left.

B: Although this tumor may be staged as T3 because tumor cells are not present at the serosal surface, a cytology smear prepared from the serosa of the specimen contains tumor cells, supporting T4a classification.

C: Another deeply invasive carcinoma is associated with expansion of the subserosa with deposition of collagen at the peritoneal surface.

D: Tumor cells are not present on the peritoneal surface, but closer examination demonstrates entrapment of mesothelial cells within the inflammatory reaction.

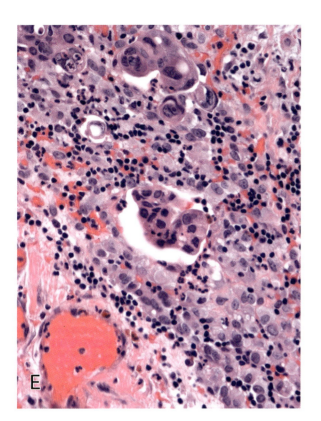
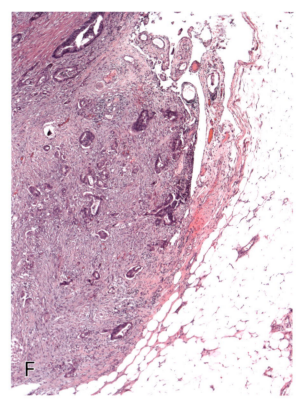

Figure 4-28, continued

E: Malignant cells are commingled with mesothelial cells; the pathologic stage is T4a.

F: Peritoneal penetration is often detected upon examination of mesocolic fat. Tumor cells are present in association with mesothelial hyperplasia in the clefts between fat lobules.

The 7th and 8th editions also classify serosal involvement as T4a rather than T4b, citing one large study as indicating that the prognosis of patients with serosal involvement is actually better with direct invasion into adjacent organs (102,116). This conclusion is in contrast with earlier studies and has been challenged by another, albeit smaller, subsequent study that did not show a survival difference between the T4a and T4b groupings (112,117,118). Although the recent study showing a better prognosis for T4a is very large, being based on the Surveillance, Epidemiology, and End Results (SEER) data, the quality of the diagnosis of T4a is compromised by a lack of central validation of the pathologic findings. This leaves considerable room for error in diagnosis, which is influenced by the changing definition of T4a (i.e., requiring actual tumor cells on the surface and not just desmoplasia) since the data set was taken from 1992 to 2004, a time period prior to the 7th edition definition of a positive margin, and by institutional variation in reporting. Needless to say, T4b (i.e., direct invasion of adjacent organs) has had a much more uniform definition and is not subject to much interpretive variation.

Earlier smaller studies with more carefully controlled analysis of pathologic features demonstrated that peritoneal involvement carried a worse prognosis than involvement of adjacent organs (i.e., T4a as currently defined is worse than T4b) and a second study by the same group demonstrated that peritoneal involvement but not involvement of adjacent organs was an independent prognostic factor in multivariate analysis (119). In univariate analysis, both were significant and the 5-year survival rate was slightly better for those with peritoneal involvement than for those with adjacent organ involvement, similar to the recent Korean studies (118,120). At the current time the issue of the prognostic difference of

T4a and T4b is not firmly established and will require continued study.

In the rectum, the T4b category is complicated by the relationship of the external anal sphincter and other pelvic muscles to the rectum. Involvement of the external sphincter is considered T3 disease; involvement of other pelvic muscles, in particular the levator ani, is considered T4b.

Lymph Node Involvement

The lymph node stage (pN) is fairly straightforward. pNX implies no nodes were submitted for examination. If any nodes are retrieved and they are all negative, the tumor is staged pN0. A single positive lymph node is staged as pN1a; 2 or 3 lymph nodes as pN1b; 4 to 6 as pN2a; and 7 or greater as pN2b. In the 7th edition of the staging manual a new category of pN1c was created to address non-nodal tumor deposits. If there are no unequivocal positive lymph nodes but tumor deposits, then the tumor is given a pN1c designation. Issues with this designation are discussed in detail below.

The number of lymph nodes involved is a well-documented predictor of outcome for colorectal carcinoma. Examination of lymph node status begins with an adequate excision of the colon with regional nodes, and with a complete dissection to identify and remove as many nodes as possible. Dissection techniques may involve identification of the nodes by touch (i.e., palpating the fat to identify possible nodes), by visual inspection of thin sections of mesentery or perirectal adipose tissue, or visual inspection aided by clearing fixative to highlight the nodes. The number of nodes identified can be influenced by a number of factors including the size of the surgical procedure, age of the patient, presence of complicating inflammatory processes which may increase the size of nodes (e.g., inflammatory bowel disease), use of presurgical neoadjuvant therapy which will decrease the size and number of nodes, and the diligence of the person performing the gross dissection.

N-Stage Controversies

There has been considerable controversy about how many lymph nodes should routinely be retrieved from resection specimens, and about the significance of variance in the number of harvested lymph nodes. Identification of a larger number of lymph nodes is associated with a better outcome, at least for stage I and II colon carcinomas (i.e., tumors without lymph node involvement) (121,122). Data for stage III, however, are less clear. Some studies find that even for stage III disease, the total number of lymph nodes retrieved affects survival, and a number of studies find that the lymph node ratio (i.e., the number of positive lymph nodes divided by the total harvested number of nodes) is a better predictor of outcome than total number of positive lymph nodes alone, although this is not universally true (122,123).

There are two major theories for the fact that finding more nodes is associated with a better outcome. A commonly stated reason is that obtaining more nodes leads to more accurate staging, and many cases with small numbers of identified nodes, all negative for tumor, actually harbor undiagnosed metastases. This was a significant contributing factor in the past when lymph node retrieval often was less than 10 (121,124). A second theory, however, is that patients with more robust immune systems have larger and more easily identified lymph nodes and hence the identification of larger numbers of nodes is a marker of immune tumor resistance. This may be a more important factor now that most pathology laboratories diligently assure that at least 12 nodes are examined. This second theory is harder to prove and remains speculative, although there are data suggesting that the finding of larger negative nodes alone is a predictor of better prognosis, a finding that would support the "active immune system" hypothesis (125).

Data indicating that understaging is true exist mainly in the form of documentation that over time labs have been identifying larger numbers of nodes, and concurrently, the proportion of stage III cases is increasing. A few direct studies have, however, challenged the premise that more nodes always leads to upstaging of the case, leading to the question of how many nodes is enough to prevent understaging. Several studies of the relationship between the number of retrieved nodes and the percentage of stage III cases over time have failed to show a relationship, indicating that the improved survival associated with increased lymph node counts is not because of understaging (126–128).

The only well-documented studies in which clearing and reexamination are statistically likely to result in significant upstaging of disease involve cases of rectal carcinoma resected after neoadjuvant therapy (128). The minimum number of 12 lymph nodes is generally adopted and is recommended in most guidelines, although there are publications suggesting that both smaller and larger numbers are needed. There is no definitive answer to this question and the best advice is to attempt to obtain as many nodes as possible in all cases. Regardless of the reason for the importance of node counts, given the current recommendation to attempt to identify at least 12 nodes in each case, if less than 12 negative nodes are identified, reexamination for additional nodes should be performed and a comment or addendum report issued to document this search regardless of the results. Generally, the use of a clearing fixative to aid in identification of small nodes is warranted if fewer than 12 nodes are identified on initial sampling.

If a large number of positive nodes (greater than 4) are identified, additional information from searching for additional nodes to reach a preset number (i.e., 12) is minimal and it may not be necessary to look further simply to fulfill a staging requirement. In some circumstances, nodes are difficult to identify, with the most difficult cases being rectal carcinoma in elderly patients who have been treated with preoperative cytoreductive therapy. In these cases, fewer nodes are acceptable after a thorough search.

Isolated Tumor Cells

By definition, tumor in a lymph node is considered a metastasis if it is greater than 0.2 mm in maximum dimension. Lymph nodes containing a collection of tumor cells measuring less than 0.2 mm are not considered positive nodes for staging purposes since the significance of these so called isolated tumor cells (ITCs) is unknown (79). Such deposits are given the designation pN0(i+) when staging the tumor. In the AJCC 7th edition, deposits between 0.2 mm and 2.0 mm are considered micrometastases and designated pN1(mic) if they are the only deposits present, and are simply considered to represent positive lymph nodes if accompanied by lymph nodes that contain larger tumor deposits. The number of lymph nodes involved with ITCs or micrometastases should be recorded in the report.

Although older studies have not shown an effect of ITCs on survival, recent data suggest that ITCs may predict tumor recurrence and survival (96,129,130). Micrometastases have also been associated with disease recurrence (99). The 8th edition of the staging manual recommends considering any tumor deposit less than or equal to 2 mm as a lymph node metastasis and suggests that the term pN1 (mic) is optional but perhaps not necessary. Although the 8th edition does recognize recent data showing a potential adverse effect of ITCs, it continues to classify deposits smaller than 0.2 mm as pN0.

Non-nodal Tumor Deposits (Discontinuous Extramural Extension)

Non-nodal tumor deposits are nodules of tumor in pericolorectal adipose tissue that do not have evidence of residual lymph node (figs. 4-29–4-31). Typically, they are irregular in shape and have an infiltrative appearance. The exact significance and classification of non-nodal tumor deposits have been and remain controversial, although many deposits represent vascular or perineural invasion (figs. 4-30, 4-31) (131–135). There seems to be little debate that the presence of these deposits predicts a worse outcome than unequivocal lymph node metastases alone.

The perceived origin and definition of these deposits changes with each new edition of the staging guidelines. In the 5th edition of the AJCC staging manual, mesenteric deposits were considered as discontinuous tumor extension (i.e., part of the T stage) if they were less than 3 mm in diameter and as lymph node metastases (part of the N stage) if they were greater than 3 mm. In the 6th edition they were considered lymph node metastases if they had a smooth contour resembling a lymph node totally replaced by tumor (fig. 4-29, left). Irregular, stellate tumor deposits were not considered lymph node metastases but rather a manifestation of vascular invasion (fig. 4-29, right).

In the 7th edition, the distinction of the histologic subtypes is somewhat ambiguous since tumor deposits are described as "irregular discrete tumor deposits in pericolic or perirectal fat……showing no evidence of residual lymph node tissue" whereas in the section entitled

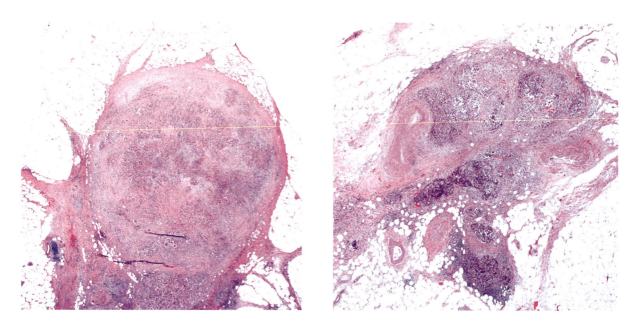

Figure 4-29

NON-NODAL TUMOR DEPOSIT

Left: The deposit is round or oval, with a regular contour, and probably is a lymph node totally replaced by tumor.

Right: The outline of the deposit is irregular with a small tumor nest next to the larger deposit. This pattern often is associated with vascular or perineural invasion and does not represent a totally replaced lymph node. There was no defined vascular or perineural invasion.

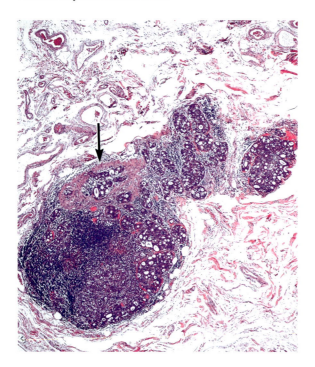
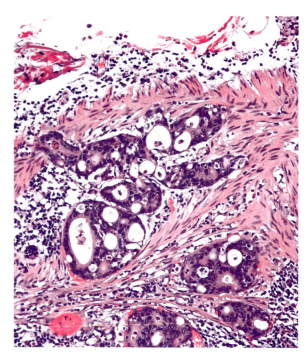

Figure 4-30

NON-NODAL TUMOR DEPOSIT WITH VASCULAR INVASION

Left: Venous invasion was identified in this lesion (arrow).

Right: At higher power, the tumor is seen within a small vein.

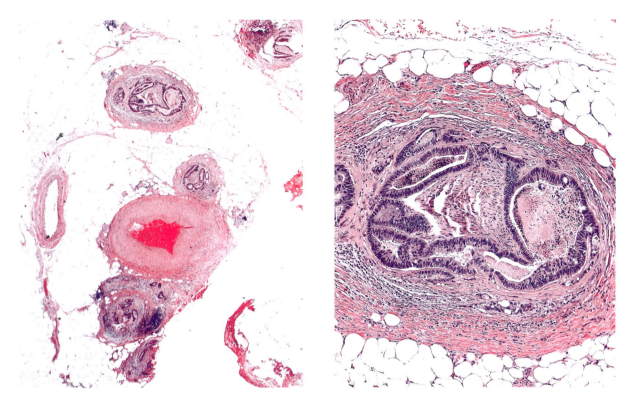

Figure 4-31

NON-NODAL TUMOR DEPOSIT WITH PERINEURAL INVASION

Left: Tumor is present in several nerves.
Right: Higher-power view shows clear perineural tumor.

"Lymph nodes replaced by tumor," a tumor deposit is defined as "a tumor nodule in the peri-colonic/perirectal fat without histologic evidence of residual lymph node" without mention of shape (102). The intent is that any tumor deposit without unequivocal residual lymph node tissue is reported separately and included as part of the "N" staging if there are no other bone fide lymph node metastases (staged as pN1c). In practice, including these deposits in the "N" category changes the stage of cancers with only non-nodal deposits from II to III, and may result in patients receiving chemotherapy using 7th edition criteria as opposed to being considered stage II and not given chemotherapy using the 6th edition criteria. Since non-nodal tumor deposits appear to have prognostic significance over and above the effect of lymph node metastases alone, it is important to report them separately as well.

As noted above, non-nodal tumor deposits represent totally replaced lymph nodes (i.e., nodal metastases with extranodal extension, which has

an adverse effect on prognosis), soft tissue extension of tumor from pre-existing vascular spaces, lymphatic channels, or perineural invasion, and discontinuous growth from the primary tumor (136,137). In the 8th edition of the staging manual, examples that can be recognized as vascular or perineural invasion are not considered in the category of non-nodal tumor deposits, and are reported only as small or large vessel invasion or as perineural invasion, all of which have prognostic significance as discussed below. One issue of this decision that is not addressed is that of how much effort should be put into identifying these features in non-nodal deposits. It is clear that if these lesions are entirely sectioned that the likelihood of finding vascular or perineural invasion increases. Therefore, if only a single section of non-nodal tumor deposits is examined it is highly likely that cases that would not be considered to have non-nodal tumor deposits but rather vascular or perineural invasion will be misclassified. It may be that with adequate sectioning

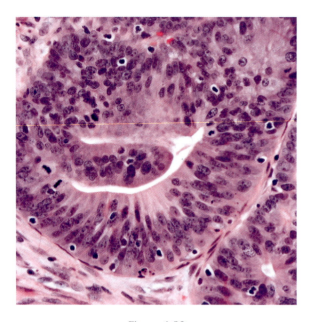

Figure 4-32

**TUMOR-INFILTRATING LYMPHOCYTES
IN LOW-GRADE ADENOCARCINOMA**

In a patient with Lynch syndrome there are many more than 4 intraepithelial lymphocytes per high-power field.

most non-nodal tumor deposits, particularly those with irregular outlines, would be reclassified. According to the 8th edition guidelines, tumor deposits should be further quantified as 1 to 4 or 5 or more isolated deposits.

Nonregional Lymph Node Metastases

From a staging perspective, it is important to remember that metastases to lymph nodes that are not regional (e.g., periaortic or common iliac nodes) are considered a manifestation of distant metastasis. They are included as M1, not as part of the N category.

ADDITIONAL PROGNOSTIC FACTORS NOT INCLUDED IN THE STAGE

Tumor-Infiltrating Lymphocytes and a Crohn-Like Tumoral Reaction

Tumor-infiltrating lymphocytes (TILs) and a Crohn-like reaction are typical features of MSI carcinomas and have long been demonstrated to predict a more favorable outcome (138,139). However, the definition of these processes is not standardized. Different definitions of TILs impact the predictive value of this marker.

TILs are usually defined by the number of lymphocytes seen between tumor cells per high-power field (figs. 4-11C, 4-32). The greater the number used to define TILs, the more sensitive the marker is for MSI, at a cost of decreased specificity. Balance is generally maintained between the two, and a figure of 4 TILs per high-power field has been accepted by many as a reasonable number (138).

Since the purpose of identifying TILs is in part to predict which cancers should be tested for MSI, the general trend toward universal testing for MSI has made this parameter less meaningful. Nevertheless, TILs reportedly do impact prognosis and have also been reported to predict PD-L1 positivity in colon carcinoma (139,140).

Vascular Space Invasion

Vascular space infiltration by tumor has long been considered an important prognostic factor in a number of malignancies, although its use has been beset with many technical issues, least of which is the definition and identification of vascular invasion. This is particularly a problem for lymphatic invasion, which is notoriously difficult to distinguish from tumor retraction from the surrounding stroma.

Another issue is the significance of the location of the invasion. Is vascular invasion within the bed of a tumor of the same significance as vascular invasion outside the tumor? Does it make a difference if large or small vessels are involved, and if those vessels are outside of any particular layer of the bowel?

Data supporting a relationship of lymphatic invasion to prognosis are limited and somewhat contradictory. Most data agree that lymphatic invasion predicts the presence of lymph node metastases and is perhaps most useful in assessing polyps with carcinoma and the need for colonic excision for these polyps (141–143). It may also predict lymph node metastases in stage II disease (92,144–147), although its prognostic impact is less clear, especially in patients with documented lymph node metastases (144,145,148,149).

While identifying lymphatic invasion can be challenging, attention to the location of the potential lymphatic invasion to adjacent structures can be helpful. While lymphatic vessels permeate all stroma, the efferent lymphatic vessels accompany and run parallel to neurovascular bundles; therefore, if tumor is located in a vascular space adjacent to an artery and vein as part of a bundle, then true lymphatic invasion rather than retraction is almost assured (fig. 4-33). On the other hand, if the putative lymphatic invasion is present only in areas with abundant tumor, and particularly if there are many areas that look like lymphatic invasion, it probably is retraction artifact. The use of D2-40 immunostaining has been advocated as an adjunct for the identification of true lymphatic invasion and is useful in suspicious cases (see fig. 4-17).

Blood vessel invasion is usually easier to identify because of the obvious nature of the vessels, although it is often difficult to be sure whether tumor within a blood vessel is true vascular invasion or if the tumor was artifactually pushed into the vessel during the cutting of the tissue. True vascular invasion is assured if the tumor is actually seen growing through the vessel wall into the lumen (a very unusual circumstance) or if the tumor is adherent to the endothelium or overgrown with endothelium (fig. 4-34). The presence of a fibrin clot on the surface of the tumor is also

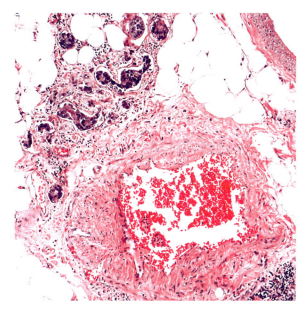

Figure 4-33

LYMPHATIC INVASION

Lymphatic invasion next to an artery outside the bed of the tumor.

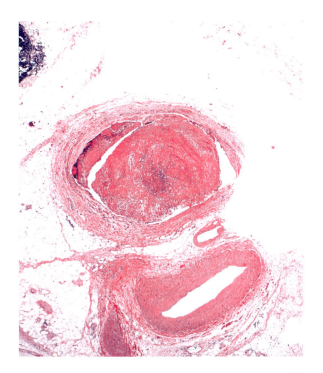
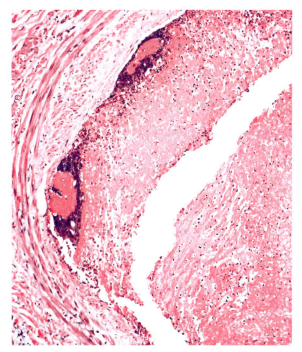

Figure 4-34

VENOUS INVASION

Left: Venous invasion by tumor with extensive necrosis
Right: At higher power, the tumor can be seen adherent to the endothelial surface of the vessel.

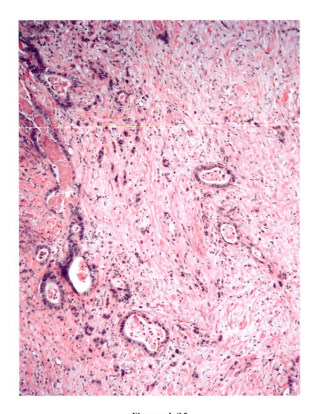

Figure 4-35

**TUMOR BUDDING NEAR
THE LEADING EDGE OF TUMOR**

Numerous small clusters of infiltrating tumor cells are seen.

an indicator of true vascular invasion. The use of elastic staining to identify vascular invasion is often advocated but uncommonly used in routine daily practice (87,150,151).

In part because of the difficulty in identifying true vascular invasion, its prognostic significance has never been totally clear. This difficulty is partly reflected by a wide variation in the reported incidence of vascular invasion, ranging from 30 to 70 percent of colorectal carcinoma cases in different series. Much of the variation depends on the number of tissue blocks examined, the diligence of the examination, and the use of elastic stains. Nevertheless, there is general consensus that vascular invasion in large vessels outside the muscularis propria ("extramural" invasion) carries a bad prognosis, which seems intuitively obvious (152). A number of studies either support this conclusion, support the conclusion that both intramural and extramural vascular invasion are

associated with poor outcome, or conclude that vascular invasion has little effect on prognosis (144,145,153). Problems with these studies include lack of consistency in the definition of vascular invasion, variations in methods used to assess vascular invasion, inclusion of only rectal cases versus colonic cases, and variation in what is considered an adverse outcome. Few studies actually examine survival, relying on recurrence rate or presence of hematogenous metastases as surrogates for prognosis.

It remains uncertain what effect vascular invasion has on prognosis or how it should be reported. It is clear that the use of special stains (usually an elastic stain) increases the detection rate of vascular invasion. However, as suggested by the one article showing no prognostic significance of vascular invasion, it is possible that the use of these techniques identifies many small insignificant vessels that are involved with tumor, diluting out the prognostic effect of an H&E exam only finding more obvious tumor in larger thicker vessels (88). Increasing the sensitivity of a test can result in a reduction in its specificity, which may be the case with the use of special stains. At this time, the use of special stains to assess for vascular invasion cannot be endorsed as a routine procedure although such stains may be used as an adjunct in suspicious cases.

The 8th edition of the AJCC staging manual recommends reporting vascular invasion as large vessel (V) and small vessel (lymphatic and venule) (L). In addition, soft tissue deposits that can be recognized as representing vascular invasion are reported as such; they are no longer considered non-nodal tumor deposits (103).

Tumor Budding

Tumor budding has been well demonstrated to be a significant prognostic factor and indicator of the probability of lymph node metastases, although it is not a mandatory element in the staging of colorectal carcinoma in the 7th edition of the AJCC staging manual (154). Part of the reason for this may be that tumor budding has not been clearly defined. Tumor buds are small clusters of one to five tumor cells extending beyond the invasive front of the tumor (figs. 4-5, right, 4-35). Careful examination of the leading edge of many tumors will identify at least a few "buds," therefore, the simple presence of a tumor bud does not constitute tumor budding.

Several methods have been proposed for identifying a "high degree of" tumor budding, the term used for tumor budding regarded as sufficient to affect prognosis. Several of these methods are time consuming and somewhat tedious, but the use of immunohistochemistry for cytokeratin detection makes identification of tumor buds easier, resulting in improved reproducibility and sensitivity but not specificity (93,155,156). Recent data suggest that H&E identification of tumor budding may actually provide better prognostic information than tumor budding identified by cytokeratin staining (94). For daily use, therefore, using the H&E-stained slide alone is probably preferable to routine cytokeratin staining.

The method of Ueno et al. (154,157) for detecting tumor budding has the advantage of simplicity and has been shown to be prognostically significant. This method identifies the areas of greatest tumor budding and counts the number of buds (single cells or clusters of less than five cells) in a 20X high-power field. More than 10 buds is considered "high budding" and carries a significant risk of poor prognosis and lymph node metastasis. Tumor budding is much more common in MSS tumors than in MSI tumors and its significance in MSI tumors is currently not as well worked out as for MSS tumors (158). Despite the fact that tumor budding is not a required element of reporting in the 7th edition of the AJCC manual, it is recommended that a statement regarding budding be included when reporting colorectal carcinoma.

Perineural Invasion

Perineural invasion is not a required element of reporting and has been considered of variable significance in different studies (fig. 4-31, right). A recent meta-analysis, however, suggests that perineural invasion is a strong prognostic factor, although it is seen less commonly in colonic adenocarcinoma than in rectal carcinoma or carcinomas in many other sites (159).

The 8th edition of the AJCC staging manual recommends including tumor nodules that can be recognized as perineural invasion as representing perineural invasion, rather than non-nodal tumor deposits (103).

Additional Comments on Staging

Pathologic stages are always preceded by the "p" designator (pTX, pNX, pMX) to distinguish them from clinical staging. Recurrent tumors can be staged but require the use of an "r" prefix for recurrent (rpTX, rpNX, rpMX). Tumors following therapy can be staged with the "y" modifier before the staging parameters (ypTX, ypNX, ypMX).

The degree of regression of tumor following preoperative adjuvant chemoradiation therapy should be reported. The system proposed by the CAP is a 4-grade system, with grade 0 representing complete response with no residual tumor, grade 1 representing moderate response with scattered single or small groups of residual cells, grade 2 representing minimal response with residual tumor showing some overgrowth by fibrosis, and grade 3 representing poor response with little obvious tumor kill and extensive residual tumor. Response grading applies only to the primary tumor and not adjacent lymph nodes. Residual pools of mucin without epithelial cells are not considered residual tumor but are categorized as complete tumor response (fig. 4-36).

ADENOMAS AND ADENOCARCINOMAS OF THE SMALL INTESTINE

General Features

Overall, small intestinal neoplasms are rare even though the small intestine accounts for about 90 percent of the length of the tubular gastrointestinal tract (160). Malignancies of the small intestine account for less than 1 percent of all cancers (1). Adenocarcinomas and neuroendocrine tumors comprise the majority of these malignancies. Newer imaging techniques have contributed to increased detection of lesions of the small bowel in recent years (160), as has capsule endoscopy (161,162), and the substantial increase in the incidence of small bowel adenocarcinomas reported between the 1970s and 2004 probably reflects advances in detection (163).

Persons with familial adenomatous polyposis (FAP) or classic Lynch syndrome (160) are prone to small intestinal adenocarcinomas. These are also common in patients with the clinical syndrome of biallelic mismatch repair deficiency, which is likely to be encountered in the setting of consanguity (164).

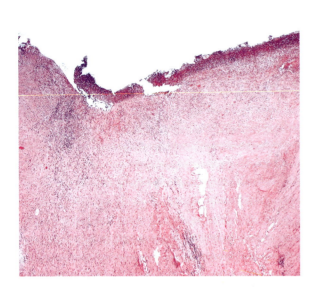
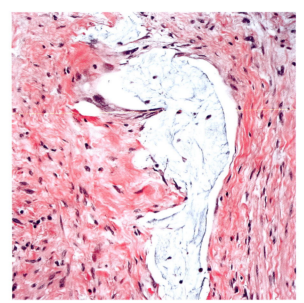

Figure 4-36

RECTAL ADENOCARCINOMA AFTER PREOPERATIVE CHEMORADIATION THERAPY

Left: This is a grade 0 response, with no residual tumor, just an ulcer bed with underlying fibrosis where the tumor had been.
Right: The presence of sterile pools of mucin is not considered residual tumor.

Small Intestinal Adenomas

Definition. *Conventional small intestinal adenomas* with intestinal differentiation, like those that arise in the colorectum, are clonal benign neoplasms composed of cytologically dysplastic epithelium. Like their colon counterparts, those in the small intestine frequently demonstrate *APC* mutations.

General Features. Most small intestinal adenomas are found in the duodenum, and, like their colon counterparts, are of three major histologic types: tubular, tubulovillous, and villous. The exact incidence of adenomas in the jejunum and ileum is not known, but they are uncommon in the duodenum and rare in the jejunum and ileum. In persons undergoing endoscopy, 0.3 to 0.4 percent have duodenal adenomas (165). In data reported from a large commercial laboratory, of 203,277 patients who had both upper tract and lower tract screening, 537 had duodenal adenomas (0.2 percent) (166) while 85,801 had colorectal adenomas (42 percent). Patients with duodenal adenomas were more likely to have colorectal adenomas than patients who did not have duodenal adenomas. The patients with duodenal adenomas had a median age of 65 years and there was no gender prevalence (166).

Most small bowel adenomas occur singly; the presence of multiple small intestinal adenomas in the absence of FAP or another syndrome that predisposes to small bowel adenomas is unusual. The presentation is nonspecific but some present with obstructive symptoms sometimes associated with intussusception (fig. 4-37). Patients with both Peutz-Jeghers syndrome and classic Lynch syndrome with germline mutations in mismatch repair genes have an increased likelihood of developing small bowel adenocarcinomas and adenomas, but these risks are less striking than the risk in patients with FAP (160).

Gross Findings. Small bowel adenomas are endoscopically similar to colorectal adenomas. The configuration is lobulated or fronded, depending on whether there is a prominent villous component. They appear pinkish and can display a cerebriform appearance, with areas of secondary erosion and ulceration. They can protrude from a stalk or be sessile, similar to colorectal lesions.

Microscopic Findings. Small intestinal adenomas have essentially the same morphology as those of the colorectum (fig. 4-38). They often show intestinal differentiation in the form of goblet cells and Paneth cells, and, like their colorectal counterparts, feature elongated hyperchromatic nuclei, prominent apoptosis, and inconspicuous nucleoli. They have disorganized crypt architecture such that the glands lose their orientation to the surface, as described in colorectal adenomas (167). Since they are rarer than colorectal examples, they are far less likely to display the range of variant patterns (clear cell change [74], squamous morules/microcarcinoids [168]) that are occasionally encountered in colorectal examples. In some cases, since the small bowel has underlying villi, it is difficult to determine whether a given lesion is tubular or villous, a distinction of little consequence clinically.

Small intestinal adenomas in syndromic patients have the same appearances as those seen sporadically (fig. 4-39). In patients with FAP, Paneth cells are often a prominent component (fig. 4-38), but they can be numerous in sporadic small intestinal adenomas as well. These patients can also show single crypt adenomas in their small intestinal mucosa (fig. 4-40) as they do in their colorectal mucosa.

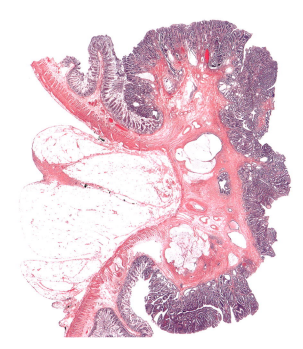

Figure 4-37

SMALL INTESTINAL TUBULAR ADENOMA

This large lesion resulted in intussusception and misplacement of glands into the submucosa and muscularis propria. Other than the small bowel location, this lesion has an appearance identical to that of colorectal adenoma.

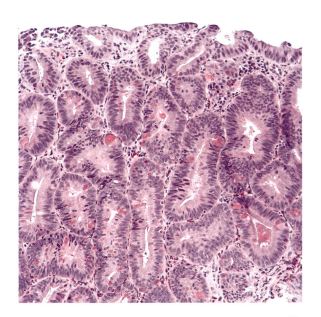 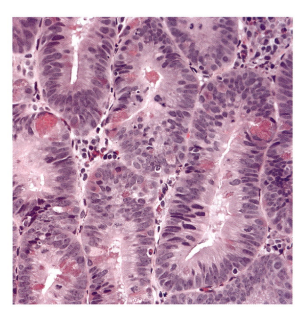

Figure 4-38

SMALL INTESTINAL TUBULAR ADENOMA

Left: This example arose in a patient with familial adenomatous polyposis (FAP). Paneth cells are prominent, a feature of small intestinal adenomas.

Right: At high magnification, the Paneth cell component is clearly seen.

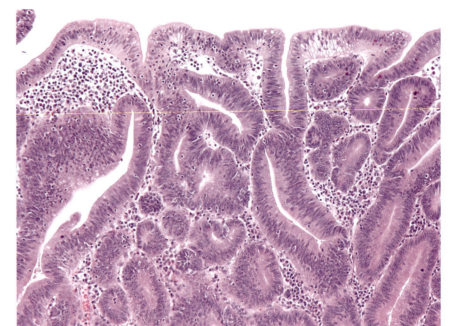

Figure 4-39

**SMALL INTESTINAL
TUBULAR ADENOMA**

This adenoma is from a
patient with FAP and lacks prominent Paneth cells.

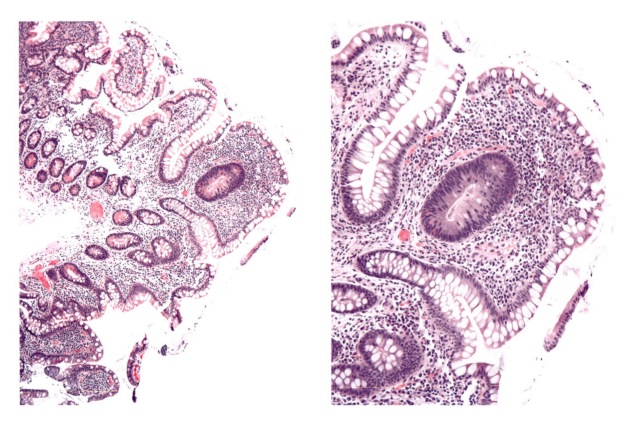

Figure 4-40

SINGLE CRYPT ADENOMA IN FAMILIAL ADENOMATOUS POLYPOSIS

Left: The lesion was present in the flat mucosa near the base of a resected adenoma.
Right: At high power, the single crypt adenoma displays Paneth cells.

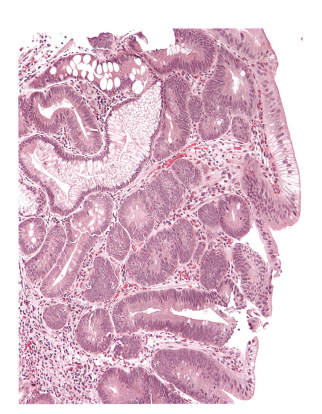
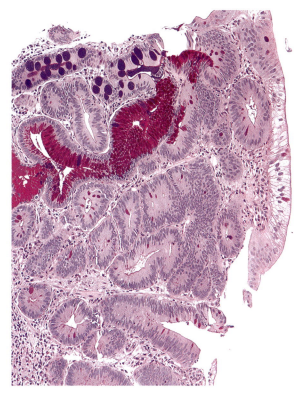

Figure 4-41

TUBULAR ADENOMA: DUODENUM

Left: The surface cells contain lipid. There is also some gastric mucin cell metaplasia at the top of the field.

Right: This periodic acid–Schiff/alcian blue (PAS/AB) stain proved that there is no mucin in the surface adenoma cells and also highlights the gastric mucin cell metaplasia at the top of the image.

Immunohistochemical Findings. Sporadic small bowel adenomas and adenocarcinomas express CDX2 consistently but have atypical CK7 and CK20 profiles, namely, expression of CK7 and absence of CK20 in about a third of cases and a CK7/CK20 double-positive pattern in about two thirds of cases (169). In contrast, normal small intestinal mucosa is CK7 negative and expresses CK20. An important immunolabeling pitfall is that reparative small intestinal and colonic epithelium expresses CK7, so CK7 staining cannot be used to separate small bowel adenomas from reactive lesions, although it sometimes separates primary small intestinal adenocarcinomas from metastases from the colorectum (169).

Molecular Genetic Findings. Most small bowel adenomas harbor *APC* mutations, including those found in patients with FAP. In both Lynch syndrome and biallelic mismatch repair deficiency, a subset of adenomas shows MSI.

Differential Diagnosis. Probably the biggest pitfall in interpreting adenomas in the small bowel is the proclivity of reparative lesions to mimic them. When duodenitis has a nodular configuration, together with marked reactive epithelial changes, it is easily confused with an adenoma. A clue to recognizing reactive duodenal injury is that it often has surface gastric mucin cell metaplasia in the atypical focus. Also, adenomas have their initiation point just beneath the surface epithelium (170), whereas reparative lesions that occur with duodenitis have theirs at the base of the mucosa. Additionally, the surface cells of duodenal adenomas tend to accumulate lipids in the neoplastic enterocytes (fig. 4-41). Presumably, since they are neoplastic, these cells can absorb lipid but then are unable to package it for further digestion so there is often prominent intracytoplasmic lipid at the surface of duodenal adenomas.

143

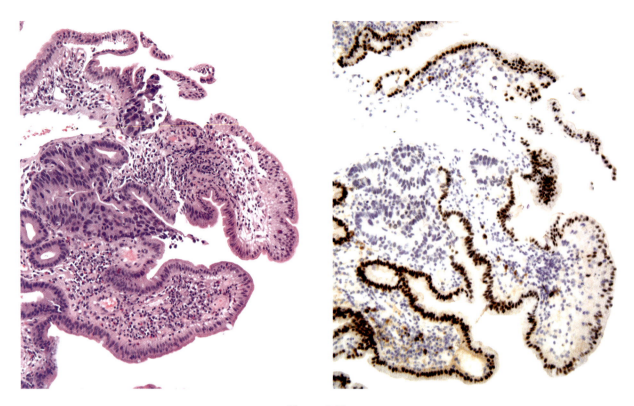

Figure 4-42

PANCREATIC CARCINOMA EXTENDING ONTO DUODENAL SURFACE

Left: This phenomenon can mimic an in situ component.
Right: A CDX2 immunostain is reactive in the enterocytes but not in the carcinoma.

There are some cases for which it is impossible to distinguish adenomas from reparative processes, and the difficulty must be expressed in the report. This distinction is not trivial since there is a precedent for treating large ampullary adenomas with pancreatoduodenectomy, based on their high likelihood of harboring an occult invasive carcinoma (171). When a clearly neoplastic small bowel lesion displays peculiar features, it is always important to consider whether the process is a metastasis or if it extends directly from the pancreatobiliary tree (fig. 4-42).

Treatment and Prognosis. Adenomas should be removed via endoscopic polypectomy for pedunculated tumors and endoscopic mucosal resection or surgical resection for large sessile lesions. Many surgical colleagues manage high-grade dysplasia in these lesions with radical surgery, so the pathologist should exercise caution in diagnosing high-grade dysplasia. Surveillance of both FAP patients and those with Lynch syndrome and its variants with upper endoscopy

or wireless capsule endoscopy is recommended (160,172–174).

Adenomas are benign. Their removal is curative and prevents progression to carcinoma.

Pyloric Gland Adenoma

Definition. *Pyloric gland adenoma* (PGA) is a benign neoplasm that usually arises in the stomach and shows differentiation reminiscent of that of gastric antral (pyloric) glands or gastric cardiac glands. It often arises in zones with pyloric (pseudopyloric) metaplasia.

General Features. Though classically described in the stomach, PGAs are also encountered in the duodenum (175–177). They were first described in 1976 by Kurt Elster (178). They were formally noted as a separate entity in the 1990 WHO classification (179). The German literature also uses the term "gastric differentiated adenoma" for PGAs (180).

Clinical Features. Most PGAs arise in the gastric body, often in patients who have autoimmune

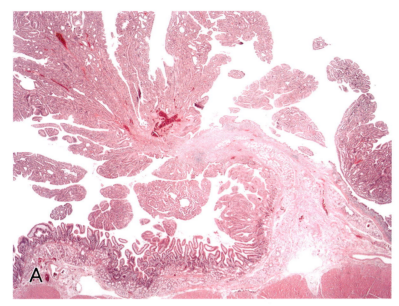

Figure 4-43

PYLORIC GLAND ADENOMA

A: The adenoma is composed of many closely packed tubules. It is less hyperchromatic than tubular adenomas with intestinal differentiation.

B: The closely packed tubules contain basally oriented, round nuclei arranged in a monolayer, with ground-glass cytoplasm without nuclear stratification or prominent nucleoli.

C: High power magnification shows the eosiniphilic ground-glass cytoplasm and round nuclei.

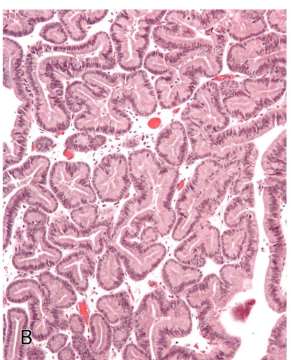

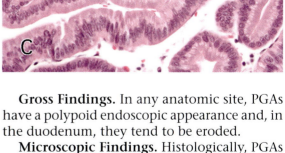

gastritis (with pyloric metaplasia), but even in this setting they are rare (181). Duodenal PGAs account for 10 to 25 percent of all PGAs, depending on the population studied (177). Whereas gastric examples have a female predominance, since they tend to arise in a background of autoimmune gastritis, duodenal lesions have no gender predominance, but all reported cases have been in middle-aged to older adults (175–177).

Gross Findings. In any anatomic site, PGAs have a polypoid endoscopic appearance and, in the duodenum, they tend to be eroded.

Microscopic Findings. Histologically, PGAs are composed of closely packed tubules with cuboidal to low columnar epithelium showing pale or eosinophilic, ground-glass cytoplasm (figs. 4-43–4-45). Their nuclei are round and basally oriented, without prominent nucleoli.

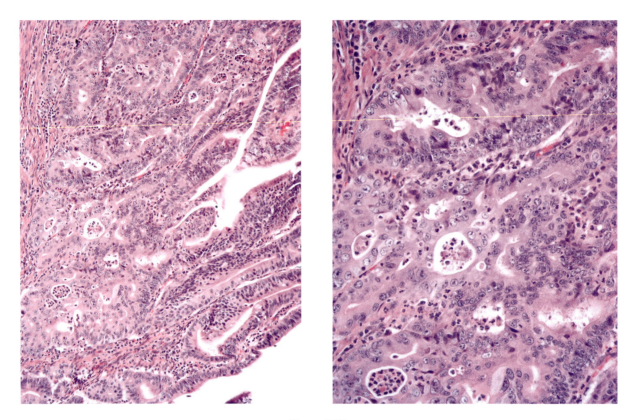

Figure 4-44

INVASIVE CARCINOMA ARISING IN PYLORIC GLAND ADENOMA

Left: High-grade dysplasia is present at the lower right and lamina propria invasion in the center of the field (T1).

Right: The invasive component shows cells with round nuclei and small nucleoli, and retains the ground-glass cytoplasmic appearance.

Figure 4-45

PYLORIC GLAND ADENOMA

This adenoma arose at the junction of the stomach and duodenum. The PAS/AB stain is from the antral aspect. The antral foveolar cells have a magenta appearance with the PAS stain, but the lesion lacks such staining and also lacks goblet cells.

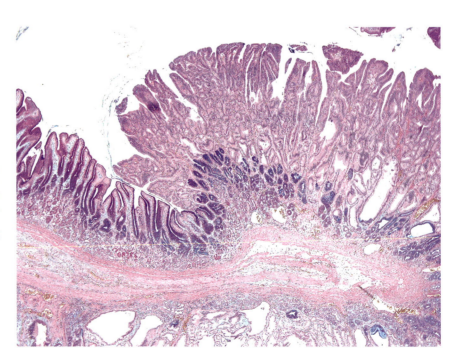

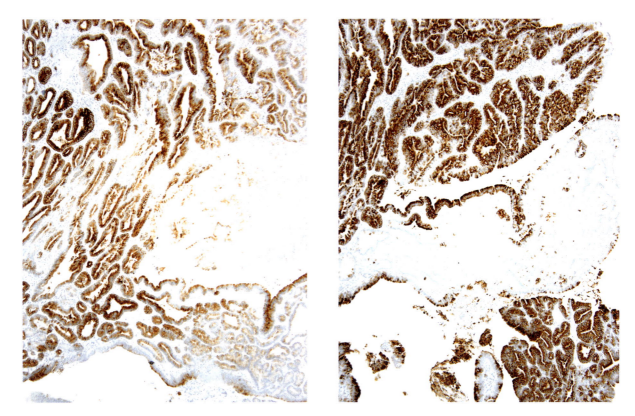

Figure 4-46

PYLORIC GLAND ADENOMA

Left: There is focally intense MUC6 labeling. The Brunner glands also express MUC6.
Right: MUC5 co-labels much of the zone that shows MUC6 expression.

Foci of high-grade dysplasia/carcinoma are commonly encountered.

The criteria for high-grade dysplasia in PGAs differs from that of conventional adenomas since the nuclei of PGAs are far less hyperchromatic. Loss of nuclear polarity and multilayering of the nuclei is sufficient for a diagnosis of high-grade dysplasia. Invasive carcinoma is associated with 12 to 47 percent of the lesions, depending on the authors' criteria for carcinoma (182). In studies published in the United States, the percentage with carcinoma is low compared to Japanese studies since criteria to diagnose carcinoma in Japan differ from those used in the United States (175,176).

Immunohistochemical Findings. PGAs co-express MUC6 (marker of pyloric gland mucin) and MUC5AC (marker of foveolar mucin) (fig. 4-46), and, in their pure form, lack expression of MUC2 (marker of intestinal mucin) and CDX2 (fig. 4-47). Some PGAs, however, show areas with intestinal differentiation and these foci may immunolabel with MUC2 and CD10 (182). Concanavalin A or MUC3 (expressed by pyloric glands, gastric mucous neck cells, and Brunner glands) shows a similar expression pattern to that of MUC6 (182).

Molecular Genetic Findings. *GNAS* and *KRAS* mutations are encountered in both gastric and duodenal PGAs (183). However, since most studies on the molecular features of PGAs have focused on gastric lesions, which arise most typically in patients with autoimmune gastritis, with a subset in patients with FAP (174), the genetics probably differ somewhat from those of small intestinal lesions. Gastric PGAs have also been reported in the setting of Lynch syndrome (184), but review of the illustrations casts some doubt as to whether PGAs were the reported lesions.

Differential Diagnosis. The main entity in differential diagnosis of duodenal PGA is Brunner gland adenoma, a distinction that can

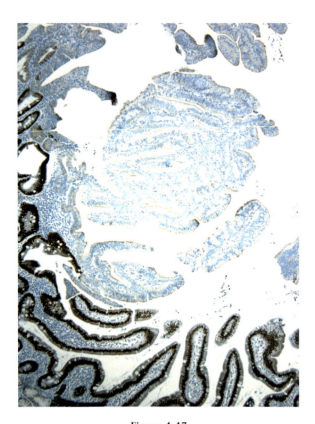

Figure 4-47

PYLORIC GLAND ADENOMA

A CDX2 stain of a small bowel pyloric gland adenoma shows nuclear labeling of the small intestinal mucosa, but not the pyloric gland adenoma.

be difficult since these lesions have overlapping features and both express MUC6. Brunner gland lesions, discussed in chapter 2, feature more abundant frothy cytoplasm and typically lack MUC5 expression.

Treatment and Prognosis. These tumors are benign and polypectomy should be curative. Associated carcinomas are managed as per stage, but most have been associated with a favorable outcome as they tend to be detected at early stage.

Other Adenomas Involving the Small Intestine

Traditional serrated adenomas have been reported in the small intestine, where they are mostly encountered in the duodenum (185,186). These lesions are rare (fig. 4-48). The reported patients are adults with a median age of around 70 years, without a gender predominance. A review of the illustrations of some of the reported lesions casts doubt on whether a homogeneous group of lesions is represented but at least one of the cases reported seems to fulfill the criteria for traditional serrated adenoma (185).

Like their colorectal counterparts, some serrated duodenal adenomas feature eosinophilic cytoplasm and slender long nuclei that are smaller and paler than in conventional adenomas. They also lack the prominent apoptosis encountered in conventional tubular adenomas. Reported lesions (186) have cytologic features that resemble those of conventional colorectal adenomas. They express CDX2, and some show nuclear beta catenin labeling. Some reported tumors have *KRAS* mutations but none have *BRAF* mutations. Some have a methylator phenotype but none have loss of MLH1 on immunolabeling. Brunner gland adenomas are discussed in chapter 2.

Small Bowel Adenocarcinoma

Definition. *Small bowel adenocarcinoma* is a primary adenocarcinoma of the small intestine that arises in association with an intestinal adenoma or enteritis-associated dysplasia (such as associated with celiac disease or inflammatory bowel disease, primarily Crohn disease).

General and Clinical Features. Adenocarcinomas are the most common malignancies of the small intestine (30 to 50 percent of small bowel malignancies). Nevertheless, primary adenocarcinomas are still rare lesions, accounting for 2 percent of gastrointestinal tract tumors and less than 1 percent of gastrointestinal tract cancer deaths (1). The estimated figures for 2016 are 10,090 new cases of small intestinal cancer (with adenocarcinomas accounting for about 45 percent), and 1,330 deaths (1). As noted above, an apparent substantial increase in the incidence of small bowel adenocarcinomas reported between the 1970s and 2004 probably reflects advances in detection (160,187). Small bowel adenocarcinomas present in older adults (median age, 65 to 70 years), have a male predominance, and are more common in African-Americans than Caucasians.

Most cases are sporadic and, like sporadic colorectal adenocarcinomas, share clinical risk factors and development from adenomatous polyps. Alcohol consumption, smoking, and diets rich in refined sugar, refined carbohydrates, red meat, and smoked food are also linked to small

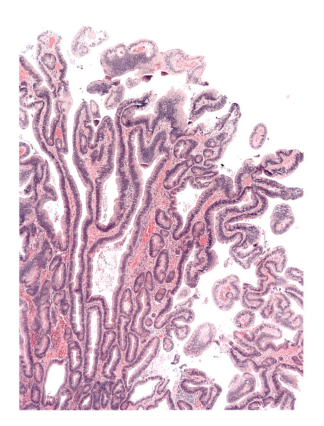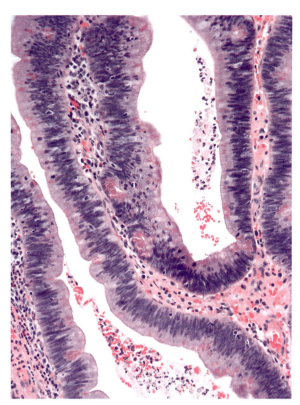

Figure 4-48

SMALL BOWEL TRADITIONAL SERRATED ADENOMA

Left: This small polyp has a markedly serrated appearance.
Right: The surface cells show lipid accumulation and the epithelium has a striking serrated appearance. There are a few ectopic crypts.

intestinal adenocarcinoma (187). Theoretically, the decreased exposure time of any zone of the small bowel to the offending agents compared to colon exposure accounts for the higher prevalence of colorectal carcinomas (187).

The remaining cases arise in patients with polyposis syndromes (primarily FAP, *MUTYH* polyposis, hereditary nonpolyposis colon carcinoma syndrome [HNPCC]/Lynch syndrome, biallelic mismatch repair deficiency syndrome, Peutz-Jeghers syndrome, and juvenile polyposis syndrome) (160,164); Crohn disease; gluten-sensitive enteropathy (GSE); ileostomy; and ileal conduits. The greatest known risk for small intestinal adenocarcinomas is FAP. In these patients, the relative risk of duodenal adenocarcinoma is astonishing (relative risk, 330.82) (173). Curiously, there seems to be only slightly enhanced risk for gastric or nonduodenal small intestinal cancer in FAP patients. The

risk of small intestinal cancer in patients with Crohn disease and celiac disease are each about 50- to 100-fold but since the incidence of small intestinal adenocarcinoma is low, cases are only infrequently encountered.

Both sporadic small intestinal adenocarcinomas and those associated with preexisting conditions are most common in the duodenum, where 65 percent are periampullary, and their prevalence decreases progressively through the rest of the small intestine. The key exception to this proximal location occurs in patients with Crohn disease, in whom 70 percent of adenocarcinomas are ileal, in line with the topography of their inflammatory disease.

Patients with small intestinal adenocarcinomas have nonspecific presentations, the most common being abdominal pain. Some present with symptoms of obstruction. Some patients may have elevated serum carcinoembryonic

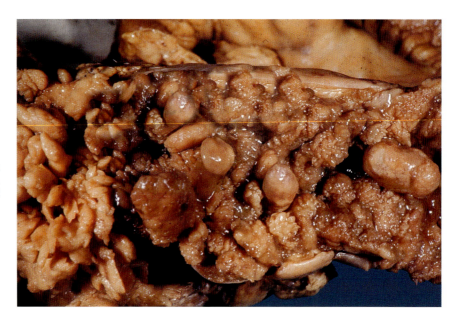

Figure 4-49

SMALL INTESTINAL ADENOCARCINOMA

This lesion arose in the ileum of a patient with Crohn disease. It is a bulky tumor that caused small bowel obstruction.

antigen, but this is not a sensitive or specific test for the detection of these lesions.

Gross Findings. Small intestinal adenocarcinomas have an appearance similar to those that arise in the colorectum. An example of an ileal adenocarcinoma that arose in a patient with Crohn disease is shown in figure 4-49 and an example of Peutz-Jeghers polyposis with an associated adenocarcinoma appears in figure 4-50.

Microscopic Findings. Small bowel adenocarcinomas are similar histologically to colorectal adenocarcinomas (fig. 4-51). Most are moderately differentiated, and one third is poorly differentiated. The degree of differentiation and the histologic subset (mucinous, adenosquamous, sarcomatoid) have little bearing on prognosis and mirror the subtypes encountered in the colorectum. Most small bowel adenocarcinomas have invaded through the bowel wall by the time of diagnosis.

Residual adenomatous epithelium is found accompanying most resected proximal tumors but often cannot be demonstrated with large distal small intestinal adenocarcinomas, presumably due to tumor overgrowth. Adenomatous epithelium is readily mimicked by tumors metastatic to the gastrointestinal mucosa and thus the pathologist should be cautious in reporting an in situ component (188). Adenocarcinomas arising in syndromic settings and in patients with enteritis or enteropathy appear similar to sporadic ones.

Staging. The staging of colorectal carcinomas has been covered in detail above. Staging of small bowel carcinomas is nearly identical except that lamina propria invasion in the small intestine is regarded as T1 rather than Tis as it is in the colon. Invasion of the lamina propria is T1a and submucosal invasion is T1b.

Immunohistochemical Findings. Immunohistochemistry is primarily of value in excluding metastatic disease, specifically metastatic adenocarcinomas (e.g., colon, breast, lung, or mimickers thereof such as melanoma and lymphoma) or direct spread from pancreas cancer. Coordinate labeling for CK7 and CK20, as noted above in the adenoma section, can be helpful in distinguishing small bowel adenocarcinomas from metastatic colon adenocarcinomas. In small intestinal adenocarcinomas, there is expression of CK7 and absence of CK20 in about a third of cases and a CK7/CK20 double-positive pattern in about two thirds of cases (169). Such labeling does not distinguish adenocarcinomas from adjacent sites (such as pancreatobiliary, stomach, lung, ovarian, and endometrial tumors), which may share the same CK7 or CK20 pattern as seen in small bowel adenocarcinomas.

Immunohistochemistry should be tailored to differential diagnostic considerations and can frequently help in cases of poorly differentiated malignancies. The use of DPC4 (SMAD4) antibodies can be helpful in identifying some cases of pancreatic carcinoma because about 60

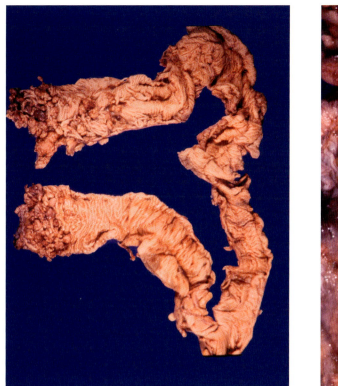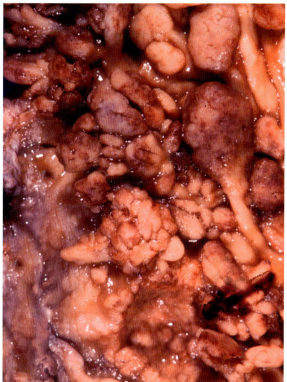

Figure 4-50

SMALL INTESTINAL ADENOCARCINOMA

Left: This carcinoma arose in a patient with Peutz-Jeghers syndrome. The polyps are so large and complex that the carcinoma was difficult to identify.

Right: This is from a patient with Peutz-Jeghers syndrome.

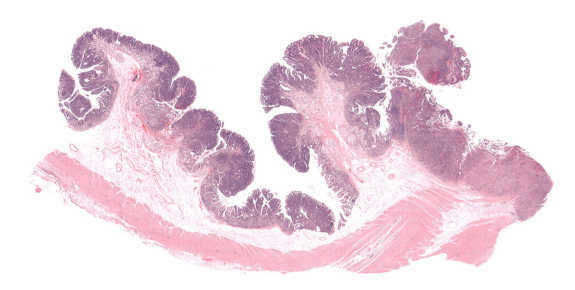

Figure 4-51

SMALL INTESTINAL ADENOCARCINOMA

This patient had FAP. The carcinoma, at the right side of the image, developed in a background of multiple adenomas.

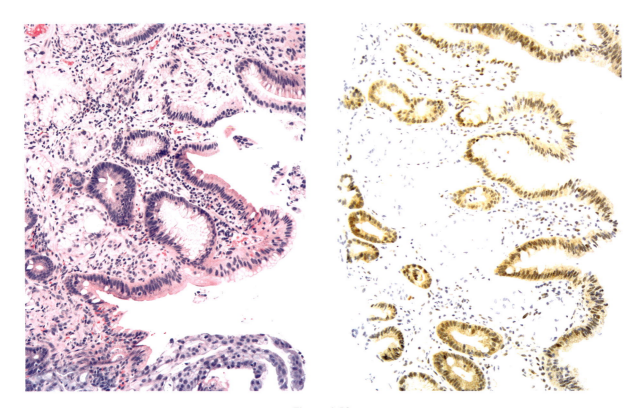

Figure 4-52

PANCREATIC DUCTAL CARCINOMA EXTENDING INTO DUODENAL MUCOSA

Left: The malignant glands consist of cells with voluminous cytoplasm but they are clearly not Brunner glands.
Right: A DPC4/SMAD4 immunstain shows nuclear loss in the malignant cells.

percent of pancreatic carcinomas show loss of this marker in their nuclei (185), an uncommon occurrence in colorectal and small intestinal adenocarcinomas (fig. 4-52).

In persons with suspected Lynch syndrome or its variants, immunolabeling for mismatch repair proteins (MLH1, PMS2, MSH2, MSH6) can be informative. HER2 expression is rare, p53 overexpression is noted in about 40 percent, and abnormal beta-catenin expression in about 20 percent of cases (163).

Molecular Genetic Findings. Overall, the molecular alterations in small bowel adenocarcinomas mirror those of colorectal adenocarcinomas. In one study of 63 small bowel adenocarcinomas, *KRAS* mutations were detected in about 43 percent of cases, *BRAF* V600E in 2.5 percent, and mismatch repair deficiency in 23 percent; about 40 percent of mismatch repair deficiency was attributable to Lynch syndrome (163).

Differential Diagnosis. The key differential diagnostic issue is separating metastatic disease from primary small intestinal adenocarcinoma. Spread from the pancreatobiliary tract, stomach, and lung is common but metastases from essentially any anatomic site can be encountered in the small intestine, mimicking a primary. In young male patients, germ cells tumors can present as primary small bowel adenocarcinomas. Most of these metastases can be separated using judicious immunolabeling. This issue is further addressed in chapter 10.

Treatment and Prognosis. Resection and harvesting of lymph nodes is the treatment for early stage lesions in general. For ampullary tumors, a Whipple procedure is standard.

Adjuvant treatment protocols remain poorly established since small intestinal adenocarcinomas are rare, but treatments that have been offered include radiation therapy and chemotherapy protocols similar to those for colorectal carcinomas (187). Suggested strategies for adjuvant therapy have included the use of oxoliplatin-based therapy with fluoropyrimidine as well as a host of combinations similar to those used for colorectal carcinoma for advanced disease, with only limited success (187). Given the high percentage of Lynch syndrome-associated small intestinal adenocarcinomas, immune therapy exploiting PD1 blockade may be useful in the future (190).

Since patients with small bowel adenocarcinoma have vague symptoms, over half have stage III or IV disease at presentation. The 5-year survival rate is unfavorable: 50 to 60 percent for patients with stage I, 49 to 55 percent for stage II, 10 to 40 percent for stage III, and an abysmal 3 to 5 percent for stage IV (163,187). Based on SEER data, the overall survival rate for all patients with small bowel adenocarcinoma is about 30 percent (21). Patients with mismatch repair deficient neoplasms seem to have an improved outcome over those with MSS lesions (163).

INFLAMMATORY BOWEL DISEASE-ASSOCIATED NEOPLASIA

Risk of Neoplasia. Patients with idiopathic inflammatory bowel disease (IBD) are at increased risk for the development of glandular dysplasia as well as colorectal adenocarcinoma; IBD-related tumors account for 1 to 2 percent of all colorectal carcinomas. The magnitude of cancer risk is related to a variety of factors and increases with both duration and extent of disease (191). The risk is highest among patients with at least 10 years of pancolitis and increases at a rate of 0.5 to 1.0 percent/year thereafter, culminating in a 20 to 30 percent cancer risk 30 years after diagnosis (192,193). However, use of more effective therapies, such as thiopurines, seems to decrease cancer risk, even among patients with longstanding pancolitis (194,195). Cancer risk is also increased among patients who have left-sided colitis, although it is only appreciable after 15 to 20 years of disease.

Other important risk factors include disease onset before 25 years of age, concomitant primary sclerosing cholangitis, colonic pseudopolyps, and a personal history of colorectal dysplasia (196,197). Of these, epithelial dysplasia is probably most important: 80 to 100 percent of patients with IBD-related colorectal cancer have dysplasia in the background mucosa. The risk of colorectal neoplasia is generally higher among

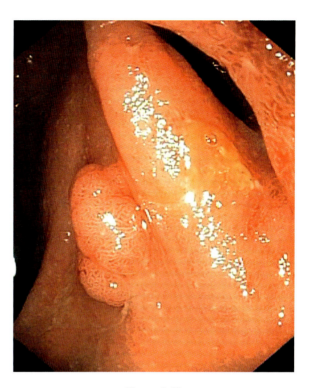

Figure 4-53

POLYPOID VISIBLE DYSPLASIA ASSOCIATED WITH ULCERATIVE COLITIS

Polypoid dysplasia is endoscopically indistinguishable from a sporadic adenoma.

patients with ulcerative pancolitis compared with those with Crohn disease, presumably reflecting a greater surface area of affected mucosa.

Endoscopic Findings. IBD-related dysplasia is classified as visible and invisible based on its endoscopic appearance; flat dysplasia or dysplasia-associated lesion or mass (DALM) are older terms that are no longer encouraged (198). Visible dysplasia is further classified as polypoid (pedunculated or sessile) or nonpolypoid; the latter may appear as a plaque-like mucosal elevation, flat, or depressed mucosal irregularity or ulcer with circumscribed or ill-defined borders (figs. 4-53, 4-54). Invisible dysplasia is, by definition, detected by nontargeted, random biopsies of the mucosa. It comprises less than 5 percent of cases, particularly in an era of magnifying endoscopy, chromoendoscopy, and other enhancing techniques (199). Invisible dysplasia and endoscopically unresectable visible dysplasias are strong indications for colectomy, particularly if multifocal (200).

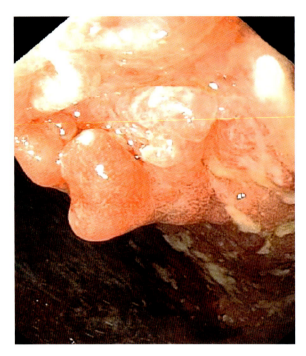

Figure 4-54

**NONPOLYPOID VISIBLE DYSPLASIA
ASSOCIATED WITH ULCERATIVE COLITIS**

A dysplastic focus appears as a multinodular plaque-like elevation.

Surveillance in Chronic Colitis. Patients with longstanding ulcerative colitis are encouraged to undergo regular colonoscopic surveillance, preferably with high-definition endoscopy, chromoendoscopy, or other enhancing techniques (fig. 4-55). Individuals with pancolitis should begin surveillance 8 years after disease onset, whereas those with distal colitis usually begin surveillance 15 years after diagnosis.

The follow-up interval depends upon findings at colonoscopy. Low-risk patients without dysplasia undergo a follow-up examination at 2 to 5 years, whereas patients with primary sclerosing cholangitis, extensive active colitis, or strictures undergo annual surveillance. Those with findings indefinite for dysplasia are treated for disease control and reexamined at a 3- to 6-month interval. Surveillance intervals for patients with dysplasia are variable.

Patients with visible dysplasia may be treated conservatively, provided the lesion is amenable to complete endoscopic excision, whereas those with endoscopically unresectable dysplasia are managed with colectomy (201). Patients with invisible dysplasia are also encouraged to undergo colectomy, although most authorities

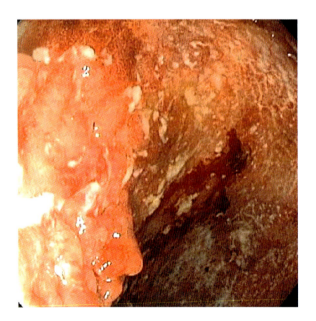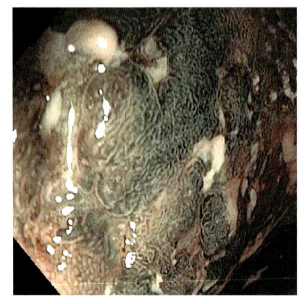

Figure 4-55

NONPOLYPOID VISIBLE DYSPLASIA ASSOCIATED WITH ULCERATIVE COLITIS

Left: A dysplastic focus appears as an irregular nodular area, but its extent is difficult to ascertain.

Right: The extent of dysplasia is more apparent under narrow band imaging. The nodular area visible is one component of a larger plaque that shows an irregular crypt pattern.

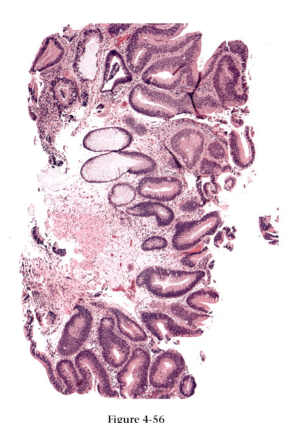

Figure 4-56

INFLAMMATORY BOWEL DISEASE (IBD)-RELATED LOW-GRADE DYSPLASIA

The dysplastic crypts are slightly crowded, without complex architectural abnormalities. Neoplastic crypts are lined by pseudostratified cells with elongated, hyperchromatic nuclei.

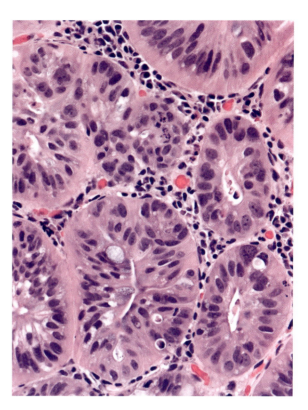

Figure 4-57

IBD-RELATED HIGH-GRADE DYSPLASIA

Crowded crypts contain cells with large, ovoid nuclei and high-grade cytologic features. Nuclear chromatin is open, with peripheral condensation, and nucleoli are readily identified. Many nuclei show no specific relationship to the basement membrane. Apoptotic cells, necrotic cellular debris in lumens, and mitotic figures are readily identified.

recommend a diagnosis of dysplasia to be confirmed by another pathologist with expertise in gastrointestinal pathology prior to definitive therapy. Polypoid lesions can be managed with complete endoscopic removal followed by regular surveillance, regardless of the degree of dysplasia present; patients may develop similar polyps during surveillance, but are not at increased risk for invisible dysplasia or carcinoma (202).

Microscopic Findings. Mucosal biopsy samples obtained from IBD patients are classified as negative for dysplasia, positive for dysplasia, or indefinite for dysplasia. When present, dysplasia is deemed low or high grade based on criteria developed for assessing conventional tubular and villous adenomas of the colon.

Low-grade dysplasia shows mild to moderate cytologic abnormalities in the surface epithelium, with nuclear enlargement, hyperchroma-

sia, nuclear membrane irregularities, increased mitotic activity, and single cell necrosis. Most lesional cells show nuclear pseudostratification, although focal loss of cell polarity may be present (fig. 4-56). Crypts may be normally distributed or slightly crowded.

High-grade dysplasia is defined by the presence of severe cytologic abnormalities. These include complete loss of cell polarity, nucleomegaly with open, peripherally condensed chromatin, and nucleolar prominence (fig. 4-57). The nuclei tend to be ovoid or round; mitotic figures and cellular necrosis are readily identified. Cases of high-grade dysplasia may also show crypt architectural complexity with micropapillary epithelial cell projections, cribriform growth, and fused glands, although these features are not required for diagnosis.

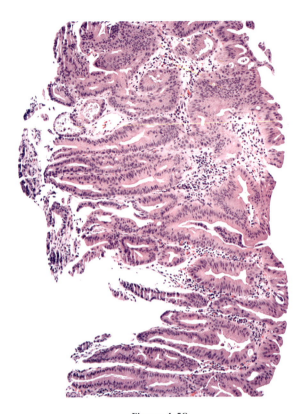

Figure 4-58

SERRATED DYSPLASIA IN PATIENT WITH IBD

A biopsy sample from a plaque in the distal colon contains epithelial cells that display a serrated architecture. Neoplastic cells contain eosinophilic, mucin depleted cytoplasm and enlarged, hyperchromatic nuclei present in the deep mucosa and at the surface.

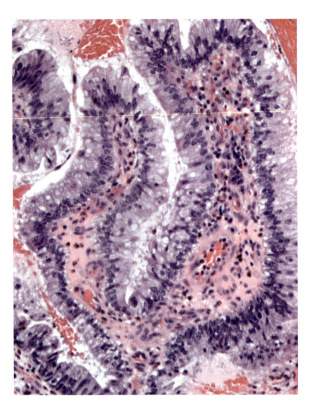

Figure 4-59

IBD-RELATED DYSPLASIA WITH MUCINOUS FEATURES

Proliferative goblet and non-goblet mucinous epithelial cells show low-grade cytologic atypia with nuclear crowding and enlargement. Scattered cells contain prominent nucleoli and apoptotic debris.

Some examples of IBD-related dysplasia show unusual features that may not be readily recognized as neoplastic. Most of these variants have been incompletely studied and thus, their biologic significance and diagnostic criteria are not established. Dysplasias can appear as one or more serrated polyps with variably severe cytologic atypia, and some patients have innumerable serrated polyps, simulating the appearance of serrated polyposis (fig. 4-58) (203). Dysplasias can contain cells with foamy cytoplasm that reflects the presence of numerous, tiny mucin vacuoles, or show mucin-depleted, somewhat eosinophilic cytoplasm (fig. 4-59). Regardless of the cytoplasmic quality, nuclear irregularities and hyperchromasia are uniformly present.

Invasive adenocarcinomas developing in association with IBD are grossly and histologically similar to sporadic colorectal carcinomas, although they are usually associated with atrophy, pseudopolyps, and the variably active inflammation typical of chronic mucosal injury. These cancers can produce intraluminal masses, but often form annular tumors that simulate the appearance of benign strictures (fig. 4-60). Many IBD-related cancers are deeply invasive despite the presence of low-grade mucosal elements that simulate the appearance of an adenoma (fig. 4-61). Infiltrating carcinomas typically show intestinal-type gland formation, although many show high-grade cytologic features including signet ring cell and mucinous differentiation (figs. 4-62, 4-63). Approximately 11 percent of carcinomas developing in IBD are of the low-grade tubuloglandular type (51).

Molecular Genetic Findings. Colorectal adenocarcinomas that develop in association with IBD often show molecular features similar

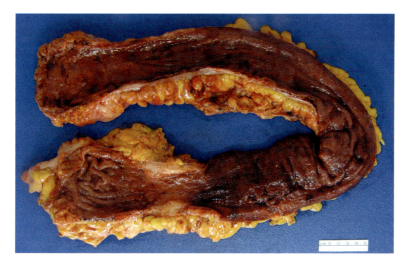

Figure 4-60

INVASIVE ADENOCARCINOMA ARISING IN ASSOCIATION WITH ULCERATIVE COLITIS

A large invasive adenocarcinoma appears as a strictured mass without a prominent luminal component. The background mucosa is granular and erythematous, with loss of transverse mucosal folds.

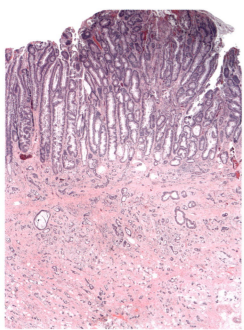
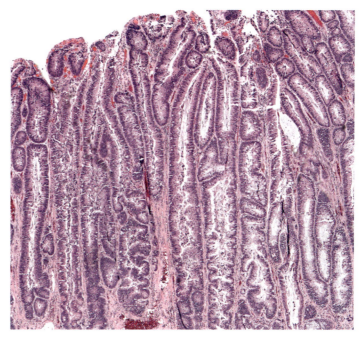

Figure 4-61

INVASIVE ADENOCARCINOMA ARISING IN ASSOCIATION WITH ULCERATIVE COLITIS

Left: A deeply invasive adenocarcinoma infiltrates the colonic wall and penetrates the serosa.

Right: Mucosal changes overlying the invasive adenocarcinoma may be deceptively bland and simulate the appearance of dysplasia in mucosal biopsy samples. In this case, the epithelium has a low-grade adenomatous appearance despite the presence of an underlying cancer that extended to the serosa.

to those of sporadic colorectal carcinomas, and presumably develop via similar mechanisms. Approximately 80 percent of cases harbor abnormalities in Wnt signaling and show chromosomal instability with loss of heterozygosity affecting tumor suppressor genes, including *APC* and *TP53*.

Compared to sporadic colorectal carcinogenesis, these alterations develop at different points in the progression of IBD-related neoplasia. Sporadic colorectal adenomas generally show *APC* mutations and develop *TP53* mutations later in cancer progression (204). On the other hand, *APC* mutations are less frequently observed in

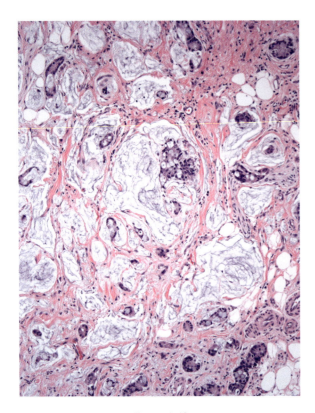

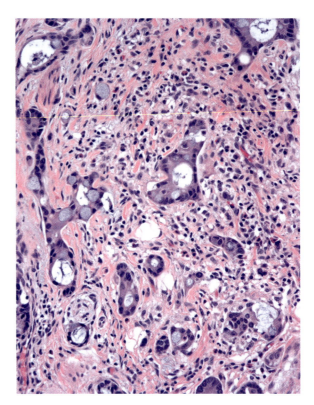

Figure 4-62

**INVASIVE MUCINOUS CARCINOMA
ASSOCIATED WITH ULCERATIVE COLITIS**

The tumor is composed of small, irregular pools of mucin that dissected through the colonic wall. Cellular clusters, glands, and single cells are present within the mucin.

Figure 4-63

**ULCERATIVE COLITIS-ASSOCIATED
ADENOCARCINOMA WITH SIGNET RING CELLS**

Many IBD-related carcinomas show high-grade features including signet ring cell differentiation. This tumor contains strips and clusters of infiltrating tumor cells, as well as abortive gland formation and signet ring cells.

IBD-related dysplasia, whereas *TP53* mutations are identified in over 80 percent of cases (205). In fact, *TP53* mutations may be detected in background colitic mucosae of patients with IBD-related neoplasms, suggesting an important role for this gene in neoplastic progression (206).

Activating *KRAS* mutations are detected at rates comparable to sporadic tumors (207). MSI has been reported in roughly 20 percent of IBD-related colorectal carcinomas, most of which show methylation of the *MLH1* promoter (208). These tumors may show widespread epigenetic DNA hypermethylation and *BRAF* mutations.

Differential Diagnosis. Two main diagnostic issues arise when evaluating biopsy samples from IBD patients for the presence of dysplasia. The first is the distinction between dysplasia and reactive, non-neoplastic atypia and the second is the distinction between sporadic colorectal adenomas and IBD-related neoplasia.

Inflammatory activity in patients with IBD often produces regenerative, or repair-type, changes such as slight nuclear enlargement, increased proliferation, and cytoplasmic depletion. These reactive epithelial cell changes can simulate the features of low-grade dysplasia, particularly in the deep mucosa. Dysplastic foci, however, generally show an abrupt transition between the atypical foci and adjacent, non-neoplastic epithelium, and should be present at the luminal surface. A provisional diagnosis of indefinite for dysplasia may be considered when low-grade atypia in colonic crypts is associated with nondysplastic surface epithelium, or when low-grade cytologic atypia in surface epithelium is limited to areas of neutrophilic inflammation. Most patients with these findings have subsequent samples that are negative for dysplasia. Thus a diagnosis of low-grade dysplasia in the setting of surface maturation, inflammation, or ulcers should be cautiously made.

Several reports describe the value of immunohistochemical stains in distinguishing IBD-related dysplasia from reactive epithelial cell atypia: Ki-67, alpha-methylacyl-CoA racemase (AMACR), and TP53 immunostains all show increased staining in foci of dysplasia compared with nondysplastic epithelia. Ki-67 immunolabeling is normally restricted to the crypt region, but is increased in dysplasia; AMACR and TP53 show staining in high-grade dysplasia, and are usually negative in low-grade dysplasia and non-neoplastic, regenerative epithelium (209). Nevertheless, the added value of these markers to routinely stained sections is limited. Nondysplastic surface epithelia can show Ki-67 staining, especially when severe inflammation or erosions are present (210). Neither AMACR nor TP53 reliably distinguishes between low-grade dysplasia and reactive cytologic atypia, which is often a more relevant differential diagnosis than the distinction between high-grade dysplasia and foci that are negative for dysplasia.

Pathologists may be asked to distinguish between sporadic adenomas and IBD-related dysplasia when endoscopists encounter visible dysplasia with a polypoid appearance. Although this distinction is not always possible, polyps in nondiseased mucosa or in older patients are more likely to be sporadic adenomas, whereas lesions occurring in colitic mucosae of young patients with longstanding IBD are more worrisome for IBD-related dysplasia. Fortunately, pathologic classification of dysplasia may not be as important as its endoscopic appearance and resectability. If visible dysplasia is amenable to complete endoscopic resection, patients can be followed (211). However, dysplasias that are not amenable to endoscopic excision should be surgically managed, even if the biopsy findings are interpreted to be "adenomatous."

HEREDITARY COLORECTAL CARCINOMA

Approximately 35 percent of patients with intestinal adenocarcinoma have a family history of gastrointestinal cancer, although no more than 5 percent of intestinal carcinomas develop in association with heritable polyposis syndromes (212–216). Most heritable disorders are characterized by increased numbers of adenomas and other polyp types throughout the gastrointestinal tract, as well as colorectal and small bowel carcinomas. They usually result from germline alterations in genes that have some type of tumor suppressor function, although not all affected patients have a detectable mutation. Final disease classification often requires collaboration between pathologists and other clinical colleagues.

Lynch Syndrome

Definition. *Hereditary nonpolyposis colorectal cancer* (HNPCC) is a clinical term that encompasses patients who meet Amsterdam I or Amsterdam II clinical criteria based on family cancer history and age of cancer onset. Fifty to 60 percent of patients who meet Amsterdam criteria for HNPCC have *Lynch syndrome*, which is defined as an autosomal dominant disorder resulting from alterations affecting one of several DNA mismatch repair genes (*MLH1*, *MSH2*, *MSH6*, and *PMS2*). Most patients have one defective mismatch repair gene in the germline, and develop a somatic mutation that inactivates the other allele. Lynch syndrome is the most common polyposis syndrome, accounting for 2 to 4 percent of all colorectal carcinomas, with a prevalence of 1 in 5,000 to 10,000 persons (217).

Clinical Features. Lynch syndrome is associated with a lifetime colorectal cancer risk ranging up to 75 percent, depending on the nature of the germline mutation. Patients with colorectal cancer generally come to clinical attention approximately 20 years earlier than do individuals with sporadic tumors, and are also at risk for carcinomas of the endometrium, ovary, renal pelvis and ureter, small intestine, stomach, and hepatobiliary tract (218); 20 to 30 percent of affected patients present with extracolonic malignancies. Two variants describe Lynch syndrome and associated extraintestinal manifestations: *Muir-Torre syndrome* is defined as Lynch syndrome in combination with sebaceous neoplasms and *Turcot syndrome* is characterized by intestinal tumors and glioblastoma multiforme (219).

The Amsterdam criteria are designed to select patients for germline testing based on age at colorectal cancer onset or the presence of a strong family history (220). The revised Bethesda Criteria build on these objectives by

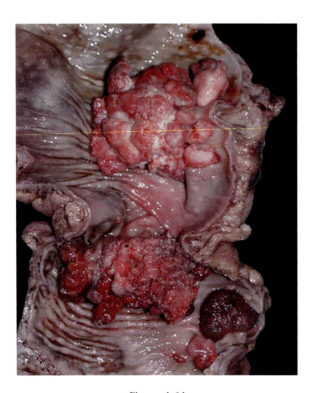

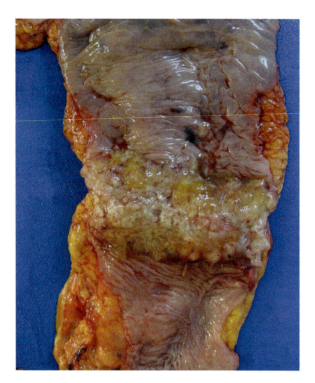

Figure 4-64

HEREDITARY BIALLELIC MISMATCH REPAIR DEFICIENCY (CONSTITUTIONAL MISMATCH REPAIR DEFICIENCY)

This colectomy specimen from a 12-year-old boy contains three polypoid carcinomas. The patient had metastases to regional lymph nodes, as well as glioblastoma multiforme.

Figure 4-65

LYNCH SYNDROME-ASSOCIATED COLON CANCER

A 47-year-old male presented with obstructive symptoms secondary to a circumferential tumor. The carcinoma has a gelatinous appearance owing to an abundance of mucin production by tumor cells. Immunostains showed combined loss of MSH2 and MSH6 staining, reflecting deficient *MSH2*.

incorporating the histologic features suggestive of MSI in the testing criteria (221).

Rare patients carry biallelic germline mutations in mismatch repair genes, which is termed hereditary biallelic mismatch repair deficiency, or constitutional mismatch repair deficiency (222). Biallelic germline deficiencies in *PMS2* and *MSH6* are the most common (66 percent and 21 percent, respectively), possibly because biallelic loss of *MLH1* or *MSH2* is more often lethal in utero (223). Affected patients have a much more severe phenotype than those with one defective germline allele. They develop Lynch syndrome-related cancers in late adolescence or early adulthood, often in combination with gastrointestinal polyposis reminiscent of attenuated FAP (fig. 4-64). Patients also have café au lait spots that mimic those seen in patients with neurofibromatosis and are prone to hematologic malignancies as well as tumors of the central nervous system (223,224). A history of parental consanguinity

can be elicited in over half of affected families (223). Many patients previously diagnosed with the Turcot syndrome (glioblastoma and colorectal adenomatous polyposis) prove to have biallelic mismatch repair deficiency.

Microscopic Findings. Patients with Lynch syndrome develop carcinomas anywhere in the colorectum; most tumors are proximal to the sigmoid colon. They are often large and bulky, or fungating, with a fleshy or gelatinous cut surface, depending on the histologic components of the tumor (fig. 4-65). Most carcinomas appear circumscribed at low magnification, with broad, pushing borders and heterogeneous growth patterns, including medullary, mucinous, or signet ring cell differentiation (figs. 4-66–4-68). Multiple growth patterns in a tumor can be a clue to underlying MSI (225,226). Tumor-infiltrating lymphocytes and peripheral lymphoid aggregates are characteristic (fig. 4-69). They presumably

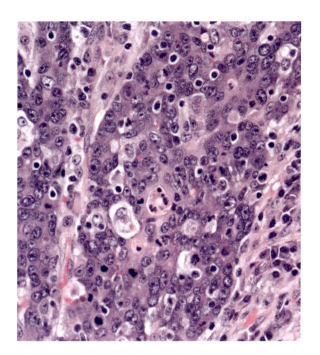

Figure 4-66

**LYNCH SYNDROME-ASSOCIATED
MEDULLARY COLON CANCER**

Tumor cells grow in syncytial sheets with poorly defined cytoplasmic borders. They contain large round or ovoid nuclei with peripheral condensation and prominent nucleoli.

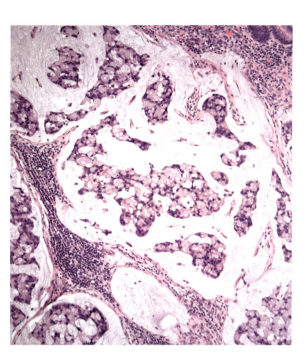

Figure 4-67

**LYNCH SYNDROME-ASSOCIATED
MUCINOUS COLON CANCER**

Lace-like strips and clusters of neoplastic cells freely float in mucin pools. The tumor cells contain large, pale blue cytoplasmic vacuoles that compress the nuclei.

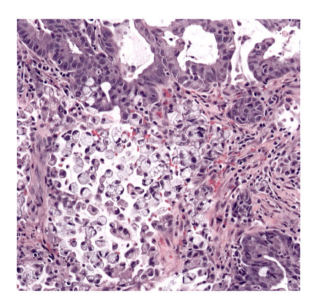

Figure 4-68

LYNCH SYNDROME-ASSOCIATED COLON CANCER

Heterogeneous morphologic features are clues to the presence of microsatellite instability (MSI). Intestinal differentiation is present at the left, but foci of invasive signet ring cell carcinoma are also present.

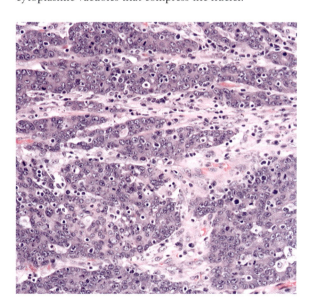

Figure 4-69

**LYNCH SYNDROME-ASSOCIATED
MEDULLARY COLON CANCER**

Nests and cords of tumor cells grow in an inflammatory stroma. Numerous lymphocytes are present in the neoplastic epithelium.

161

reflect a host immune response to neoantigens elaborated by underlying MSI status (227,228).

Patients with Lynch syndrome may have adenomas in the background mucosa, although they tend to be few. Adenomas show tubular or villous morphology; serrated adenomas are uncommon and nondysplastic serrated polyps (i.e., SSA/P) are not a feature of Lynch syndrome. Most adenomas lack intraepithelial lymphocytes, at least when they are small. Larger lesions or those with high-grade dysplasia are more likely to show tumor-infiltrating lymphocytes. Larger lesions are also more likely to show immunohistochemical loss of mismatch repair protein staining, whereas staining may be preserved in smaller adenomas.

Molecular Genetic Findings. As stated above, patients with Lynch syndrome have heritable deficiencies in DNA mismatch repair mechanisms. Most have inactivating mutations in *MLH1* or *MSH2*; mutations in *PMS2* and *MSH6* are less common. Rare patients lack mutations in mismatch repair genes, but have deficiencies resulting from other causes. Some have germline epigenetic hypermethylation (and silencing) of the *MLH1* promoter (229,230). Others have germline deletions in the 3' end of *TACSTD1* (*EPCAM*) that remove its transcription termination site. This gene is directly upstream of *MSH2*, so these mutations result in nonfunctional *EPCAM-MSH2* fusion transcripts (231). Transcriptional read-through of MSH2 causes methylation of its promoter, thereby silencing *MSH2* from transcription (232–234).

The protein products of *MLH1*, *MSH2*, *PMS2*, and *MSH6* form a DNA repair complex composed of two heterodimers. This complex normally corrects base pair mismatches that occur during replication. MSH2 and MSH6 form a heterodimer that binds to mismatched base pairs and subsequently recruits the MLH1/PMS2 heterodimer to correct the error. Deficiencies in mismatch repair protein function result in failure to correct mismatch errors that are propagated in subsequent replicative cycles. These errors occur as single base pair changes throughout the genome. Mismatches take two forms: single base pair mismatches and insertion-deletion loops. Single base pair mismatches lead to point mutations, whereas insertion-deletion loops result in frameshifts in the daughter DNA strand.

Colorectal cancers are evaluated for mismatch repair deficiency using complimentary assays, namely, polymerase chain reaction (PCR) to assess for MSI and immunohistochemistry to evaluate for expression of DNA mismatch repair proteins. The PCR-based assay detects expansion or contraction of microsatellite markers in the tumor relative to nontumor tissue from the same patient (235). Microsatellites are short repetitive nucleotide sequences prone to replicative errors because of a propensity for DNA polymerase to slip, or "misread," the nucleotide sequence. Although the original Bethesda panel consisted of a combination of mononucleotide and dinucleotide repeats, most laboratories now assess for MSI using a panel of five mononucleotide markers (BAT25, BAT26, NR-1, NR-24, MONO-27) because instability in dinucleotide markers is not entirely specific for mismatch repair deficiency (236,237).

Instability at two markers is sufficient to classify a tumor as MSI-H, although most cancers with mismatch repair deficiency show instability at multiple markers (fig. 4-70). Tumors that are stable at all five markers are classified as MSS. Instability at one locus is rarely associated with underlying mismatch repair deficiency and, thus, these cases are considered to be indeterminate. Low-frequency MSI (MSI-L) is a historical term for cases that showed instability at one locus (usually a dinucleotide marker) of the Bethesda panel and generally does not reflect underlying Lynch syndrome.

Immunohistochemical stains for all four DNA mismatch repair proteins are commercially available and widely used to assess for mismatch repair deficiency. Staining patterns reflect the normal physiologic roles of each protein and can be used to identify the defective protein. PMS2 and MSH6 require their binding partners to maintain integrity; PMS2 degenerates in the absence of MLH1; and MSH6 degenerates when MSH2 is defective. Both MLH1 and MSH2 typically maintain their stability regardless of the presence or absence of PMS2 and MSH6. Thus, cancers that harbor defective *MLH1*, generally show loss of MLH1 and PMS2 immunolabeling, whereas those with deficient *PMS2* show isolated PMS2 loss by immunohistochemistry. Tumors with deficient *MSH2* show immmohistochemical loss of both MSH2 and MSH6, and those with

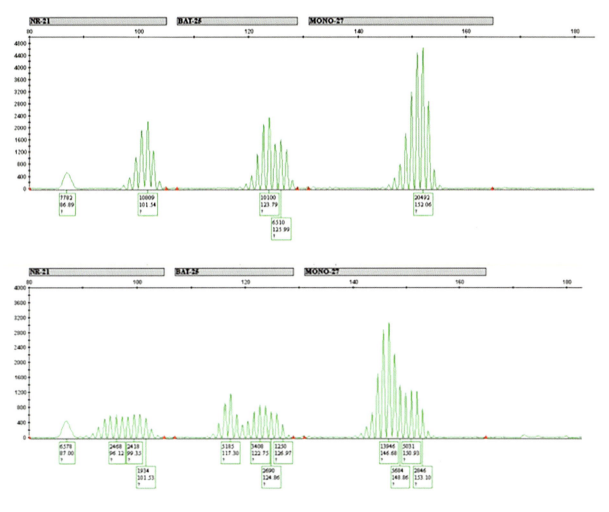

Figure 4-70

DNA ELECTROPHEROGRAM OF MICROSATELLITE UNSTABLE COLON CANCER

Tightly clustered peaks are present at three microsatellite markers (NR-21, BAT-25, MONO-27) in normal tissue (top). A carcinoma with MSI-H shows clusters of additional, shifted peaks at all three markers (bottom).

alterations affecting *MSH6* show isolated loss of MSH6 immunolabeling. Nuclear staining for all four markers is preserved in non-neoplastic proliferating cells, such as lymphocytes and crypt epithelial cells; these elements provide a useful internal control. An absence of staining in non-neoplastic cells, however, does not necessarily imply a technical artifact.

Tumors and even adenomas from patients with hereditary biallelic mismatch repair deficiency show an absence of staining for one or two markers in both tumoral and nontumoral tissues; the pattern of loss depends on the nature of the biallelic mutation (figs. 4-71–4-73). In this

situation, all of the cells in the body lack the associated mismatch repair protein, resulting in an entirely negative preparation (164).

Diagnosis and Genetic Evaluation. Screening for Lynch syndrome among colorectal cancer patients based on clinical and histologic features identifies most, but not all, patients with germline mutations: 10 to 20 percent of patients with Lynch syndrome do not meet criteria for testing. For this reason, most professional organizations in the United States and Europe now endorse universal screening practices and evaluation of all colorectal cancer cases for possible Lynch syndrome (20,238–241). Despite the

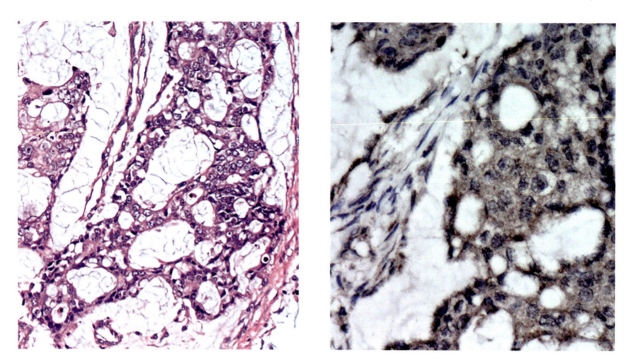

Figure 4-71

HEREDITARY BIALLELIC MISMATCH REPAIR DEFICIENCY (CONSTITUTIONAL MISMATCH REPAIR DEFICIENCY)

Left: Histologic sections reveal mucinous and solid growth patterns typical of MSI-H tumors.
Right: Biallelic *MSH6* germline mutations result in complete loss of staining in both tumor cell nuclei and non-neoplastic fibroblasts.

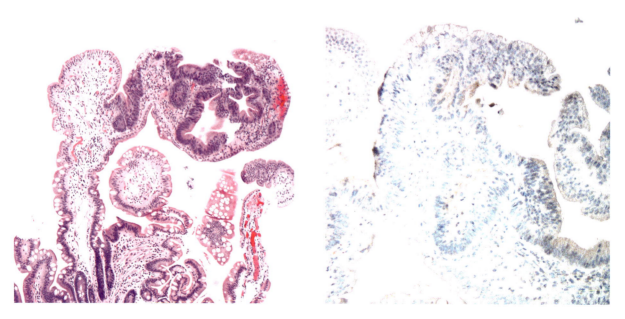

Figure 4-72

ADENOMA IN PATIENT WITH BIALLELIC MISMATCH REPAIR DEFICIENCY

Left: This adenoma appears similar to a sporadic adenoma.
Right: This patient had biallelic mutations in *PMS2* (Trimbath syndrome). The adenoma cells are nonreactive with a PMS2 immunostain, but so is every other cell in the field in a preparation with adequate controls.

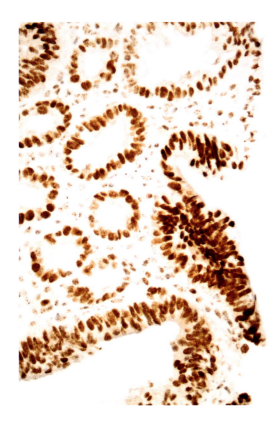

Figure 4-73

ADENOMA IN PATIENT WITH BIALLELIC MISMATCH REPAIR DEFICIENCY

This patient had biallelic mutations in *PMS2* (Trimbath syndrome). This is an MLH1 immunostain. This protein is intact in both the adenoma and the lamina propria constituents. Normally MLH1 and PMS2 are lost together but in this case only PMS2 is affected, resulting in a host of tumors for the patient and a syndrome with café au lait spots, superficially mimicking neurofibromatosis.

intensive nature of this practice, available data suggest that universal testing is cost effective when considering long-term cancer-related morbidity and mortality among patients and potentially affected family members (242).

Ten to 15 percent of sporadic colonic adeno-carcinomas show MSI, most of which develop through methylation and silencing of MLH1. Given that sporadic colorectal carcinoma is much more common than Lynch syndrome, an MSI-H tumor that shows loss of MLH1/PMS2 immunostaining is more likely to be sporadic than Lynch related, particularly in an older patient population. On the other hand, any other positive stain result (e.g., loss of MSH2/

MSH6, isolated loss of PMS2 or MSH6) has been historically considered to be strong evidence of Lynch syndrome. This view has changed in the wake of widespread universal testing; it is now clear that a spectrum of mismatch repair deficiency etiologies may be seen in sporadic MSI-H tumors (243). Sporadic MSI-H colonic carcinomas may develop as a result of somatic alterations affecting any of the mismatch repair genes; this situation has been described as "Lynch-like" carcinoma, as described below. Such terminology is unfortunate and misleading. By definition, acquired biallelic mutations would not be associated with a heritable disorder such as Lynch syndrome. Caution should be used when interpreting immunohistochemical or PCR results and rendering a firm diagnosis of Lynch syndrome based on these methods alone; final classification requires collaboration among clinical colleagues in many cases.

Adenocarcinomas associated with Lynch syndrome are derived from adenomas that show Wnt signaling abnormalities due to inactivation of APC or *CTNNB1* mutations; they develop MSI-H late in their evolution. Screening adenomas for potential Lynch syndrome has a low yield because sporadic adenomas are frequent, even among patients under the age of 40 years. While universal testing of adenomas for Lynch syndrome is not recommended, it is reasonable to evaluate adenomas when there is a strong clinical suspicion for a heritable syndrome. However, more than 20 percent of adenomas removed from patients with Lynch syndrome are MSS, with preserved staining for mismatch repair proteins (244). In other words, failure to detect mismatch deficiency in an adenoma does not necessarily exclude the possibility of Lynch syndrome, whereas the presence of mismatch deficiency in an adenoma is virtually diagnostic of Lynch syndrome. Testing should be performed on the most advanced lesion (i.e., largest polyp with most severe cytologic atypia). There is no value in screening serrated polyps for Lynch syndrome, even if multiple polyps are present.

Differential Diagnosis. Distinguishing Lynch-related colorectal cancer from sporadic MSI-H colorectal cancer can be problematic. Most sporadic MSI-H tumors show combined loss of MLH1/PMS2 immunostaining that results from *MLH1* promoter hypermethylation;

this pattern is indistinguishable from that of *MLH1*-deficient Lynch-related cancers. Fortunately, at least 50 percent of sporadic MSI-H cancers also show *BRAF* V600E mutations, whereas *MLH1*-deficient tumors of Lynch syndrome lack *BRAF* mutations; the presence of a *BRAF* mutation reasonably classifies the tumor as sporadic in nature (245). An immunostain directed against the BRAF V600E mutant protein is commercially available. This stain may be technically challenging to perform and requires familiarity for interpretation (246). Carcinomas that are MLH1/PMS2 deficient can be assessed for *MLH1* promoter methylation, which is present in both *BRAF*-mutant and wild-type sporadic tumors.

Twenty to 30 percent of patients with MSI-H colorectal cancers and suspected Lynch syndrome (i.e., wild-type *BRAF*, or immunohistochemical profile other than loss of MLH1/PMS2) lack detectable germline mutations in mismatch repair genes. Some of these individuals prove to have Lynch syndrome resulting from uncommon types of germline alteration, such as the recently identified inversion of *MSH2* exons 1 to 7, somatic mosaicism, and biallelic *MUTYH* mutations (247–249). Others may have germline mutations that are simply undetectable by currently available methods. Importantly, somatic events simulate features of Lynch syndrome-related carcinomas. In addition to *MLH1* promoter methylation, sporadic tumors can result from biallelic somatic mutations or loss of heterozygosity affecting DNA mismatch repair genes (250). Patients with somatic alterations (and their family members) have a subsequent cancer risk likely comparable to that of patients with sporadic cancers.

The differential diagnosis of Lynch syndrome also includes attenuated FAP and *MUTYH*-associated polyposis, both of which can present with colorectal cancer and colonic adenomas. Polyps, however, tend to be fewer in patients with Lynch syndrome, and associated cancers show morphologic features of underlying MSI, such as medullary, mucinous, or signet ring cell differentiation, or tumor infiltrating lymphocytes. Immunohistochemical stains for mismatch repair proteins are highly sensitive for Lynch syndrome and facilitate its distinction from other polyposis disorders. Rare MSI-H cancers occurring in patients with *MUTYH*-associated polyposis require germline testing for final classification.

Treatment and Prognosis. The lifetime cancer risk among patients with Lynch syndrome depends on the nature of the germline mutation. Patients with *MSH6* or *PMS2* mutations have a lower cumulative lifetime risk for all types of cancer, as well as a slightly older age at cancer onset compared to patients with *MLH1* or *MSH2* mutations (251). Tumors of the ovary, urinary tract, and upper gastrointestinal tract are much more common among patients with *MLH1* and *MSH2* mutations than in those with *MSH6* mutations, and *PMS2* mutations are infrequently associated with cancers at these sites. Indeed, *PMS2* and *MSH6* mutations appear to have a lower phenotypic penetrance than other mismatch repair genes.

General surveillance recommendations vary based on the affected gene. Patients with *MLH1* or *MSH2* mutations should undergo screening colonoscopy at 20 to 25 years of age with subsequent examinations at 1- to 2-year intervals, whereas those with *MSH6* and *PMS2* mutations should have their first colonoscopy by 30 and 35 years of age, respectively. Female patients are encouraged to undergo pelvic examination, endometrial sampling, and transvaginal ultrasound at 30 to 35 years of age. Upper endoscopic examination and urinalysis at 30 to 35 years of age should be considered for mutation carriers. These guidelines should be adjusted so that surveillance of a carrier is initiated 10 years earlier than that of the affected family member at first cancer detection (239).

Most data suggest that patients with MSI-H colorectal carcinomas have a better prognosis than those with stage-matched MSS tumors. Biologic differences are particularly important among patients with stage II (negative regional lymph nodes) cancers: some MSS tumors with "high-risk" features may be treated with adjuvant therapy, whereas chemotherapy has no clear benefit among patients with stage II MSI-H cancers (252). Chemotherapy is generally considered for patients with stage III and IV colorectal carcinomas, regardless of microsatellite status. Microsatellite status is also an important predictor of response to therapeutic agents that act through immune checkpoint blockade of PD-1 and PD-L1, programmed cell death protein-1 (PD-1) and its ligand (190,253).

Familial Colorectal Cancer Type X

Forty to 50 percent of patients who meet the clinical criteria for HNPCC do not have Lynch syndrome; their colorectal cancers are mismatch repair proficient and they seemingly lack germline alterations in DNA mismatch repair genes. These individuals are currently labeled as having *familial colorectal carcinoma type X*. They have a 2-fold increased risk for colorectal carcinoma compared to the general population. Unlike other heritable disorders, affected patients do not seem to be at risk for extracolonic malignancies (254).

Unlike tumors of Lynch syndrome, familial colorectal cancer type X shows no predilection for the proximal colon, and lacks the morphologic features of MSI, such as mucinous histology and tumor-infiltrating lymphocytes (255). The mechanisms underlying tumorigenesis in this setting have not been elucidated, and it is likely that heterogeneous molecular alterations are at play. Preliminary data suggest that genes encoding ribosome-associated proteins may play a role in some cases, whereas alterations in genes regulating cell signaling are important in others (256–259).

Familial Adenomatous Polyposis

Definition. *Familial adenomatous polyposis* (FAP) is an autosomal dominant condition caused by a spontaneous or inherited germline mutation in *APC*. Mutations develop at a rate of 1/10,000 to 15,000 live births, resulting in a disease prevalence of 2.3 to 3.2 per 100,000 individuals (217). Approximately 25 percent of affected patients do not have a family history of gastrointestinal polyposis; they develop either de novo germline mutations or have a parent with germline *APC* mosaicism (260).

Clinical Features. Phenotypic disease manifestations are dependent upon the nature of the *APC* mutation. Truncating mutations lead to innumerable colorectal adenomas and a colorectal cancer risk that approaches 100 percent by 40 years of age; mutations that do not completely abrogate protein function are associated with fewer polyps, lower cancer risk, and delayed cancer onset (i.e., attenuated FAP).

Colorectal polyps begin to appear in late childhood or early adolescence, and progressively increase in size and number. Presenting symptoms are usually related to chronic blood loss and include frank blood in the stool, melena, and iron deficiency anemia. Obstructive symptoms, weight loss, and changing bowel habits herald the development of a cancer.

In addition to adenomatous polyps of the colorectum, patients with FAP develop several types of polyp in the stomach and adenomas of the small intestine. FAP patients who have already undergone colectomy are most likely to die from upper gastrointestinal tract malignancy (172). Most FAP patients develop upper gastrointestinal tract polyps in addition to their colorectal adenomas; those in the gastric antrum and duodenum are usually neoplastic (174). One study documented the occurrence of ileal pouch adenomas in 20 to 25 percent of FAP patients who underwent proctocolectomies. A subset of those patients also had jejunal and ileal adenomas diagnosed by capsule endoscopy (261). Overall, 50 to 90 percent of FAP patients are estimated to have duodenal adenomas (capsule endoscopy studies have estimated that about 90 percent of FAP patients have jejunal or ileal adenomas [238]) of which about 5 percent are believed to progress to carcinoma.

Patients with attenuated FAP and fewer colorectal polyps still have a polyp burden in the upper gastrointestinal tract similar to that of other FAP patients. Common extraintestinal manifestations include osteomas, mesenteric fibromatosis, cutaneous cysts, lipomas, and dental abnormalities. FAP in conjunction with tumors of the central nervous system can result from germline mutations in either *APC* or DNA mismatch repair genes. Germline *APC* mutations are usually associated with medulloblastomas, as first described by Crail in 1949 (262), whereas Turcot (263) reported patients with colorectal polyposis and glioblastoma who later proved to have mismatch repair deficiency and Lynch syndrome. Congenital hyperpigmentation of the retinal pigmented epithelium is usually seen in patients with whole gene deletions or mutations between codons 311 and 1444 (264).

Microscopic Findings. Colectomy specimens from FAP patients often contain hundreds to thousands of adenomas, which carpet

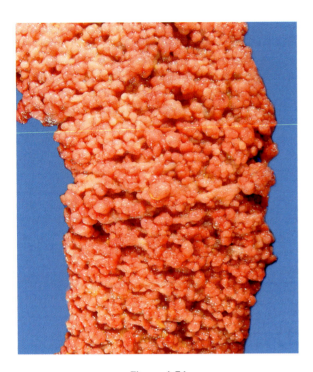

Figure 4-74

FAMILIAL ADENOMATOUS POLYPOSIS

The colonic mucosa is carpeted with innumerable polyps ranging from a few millimeters to more than a centimeter in diameter.

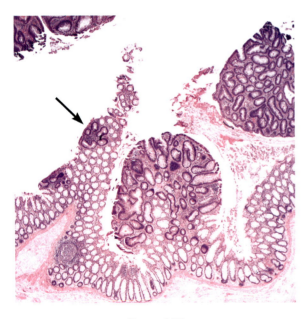

Figure 4-75

FAMILIAL ADENOMATOUS POLYPOSIS

Several tubular adenomas appear as polypoid projections into the lumen. Microscopic adenomas consist of only a few neoplastic crypts with low-grade dysplasia (arrow).

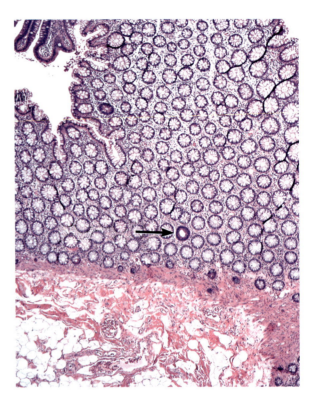

Figure 4-76

FAMILIAL ADENOMATOUS POLYPOSIS

A single neoplastic crypt (arrow) is present in the nonpolypoid mucosa.

the mucosa, although patients undergoing prophylactic colectomy in late adolescence or early adulthood usually have smaller polyps that are fewer in number (fig. 4-74). Colorectal adenomas of FAP show conventional tubular, villous, or tubulovillous features that are indistinguishable from sporadic adenomas (fig. 4-75). Single crypt adenomas in flat, grossly normal mucosae are common (fig. 4-76). When present, invasive adenocarcinomas can be single or multiple (fig. 4-77). Invasive adenocarcinomas are morphologically indistinguishable from sporadic colorectal carcinomas and generally show intestinal-type differentiation (fig. 4-78).

Patients with FAP develop several types of polyp in the upper gastrointestinal tract. Gastric lesions include intestinal- and foveolar-type adenomas, pyloric gland adenomas, and fundic gland polyps, which may be numerous (174). Fundic gland polyps commonly show foveolar-type dysplasia, which tends to be low grade (265). At least 50 percent of FAP patients with

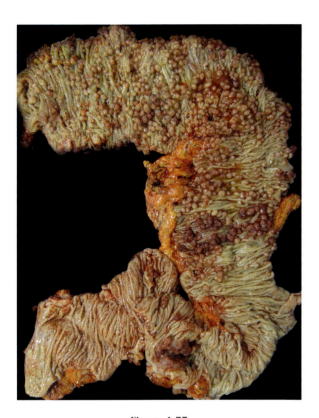

Figure 4-77

FAMILIAL ADENOMATOUS POLYPOSIS AND ADENOCARCINOMA

This patient presented with occult blood loss related to an ulcerated adenocarcinoma in the left colon. The background mucosa displays numerous small, sessile polyps, particularly in the proximal to mid colon.

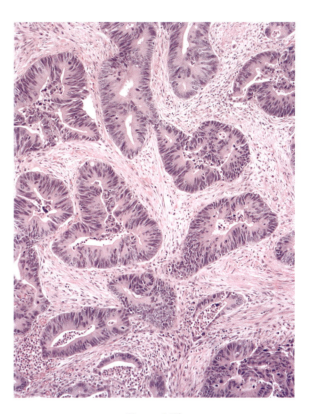

Figure 4-78

FAMILIAL ADENOMATOUS POLYPOSIS-ASSOCIATED ADENOCARCINOMA

This rectal carcinoma developed in a 21-year-old female with FAP. The tumor contains intestinal-type glands enmeshed in desmoplastic stroma, similar to sporadic rectal adenocarcinoma.

fundic gland polyps have some lesions that show dysplasia compared to approximately 1 percent with sporadic fundic gland polyps (fig. 4-79). Pyloric gland adenomas are also surprisingly common in FAP. They contain small crowded glands with pale cytoplasm and little intervening stroma, with or without dysplasia (fig. 4-80). Despite the frequent occurrence of gastric neoplasia in FAP, the overall risk of gastric carcinoma among affected patients is low (less than 1 percent), so patients are usually monitored with surveillance and endoscopic removal of large polyps, rather than prophylactic gastrectomy. Patients with FAP are also prone to developing small intestinal adenomas, particularly in the duodenum and periampullary region (fig. 4-81) (266).

Molecular Genetic Findings. FAP results from biallelic inactivation of *APC*. Patients carry a germline mutation in one allele and develop an inactivating somatic mutation in the other allele (267). The effective result of these alterations is marked suppression of APC production and loss of its tumor suppressor function. Most patients with FAP have nonsense mutations that produce a truncated protein, or frameshifts resulting from insertions or deletions (268).

The phenotypic manifestations of disease are related to the site of the *APC* mutation. Severe colonic polyposis is more common among patients with mutations in codons 1290-1400, whereas adenomas of the small intestine are associated with mutations between codons 976 and 1067. Attenuated FAP results from germline mutations at the extreme 3' (c78-167) or 5' (c1581-2843) ends of the gene, which result in a partially functional protein (269,270). Two subsequent somatic mutations inactivate

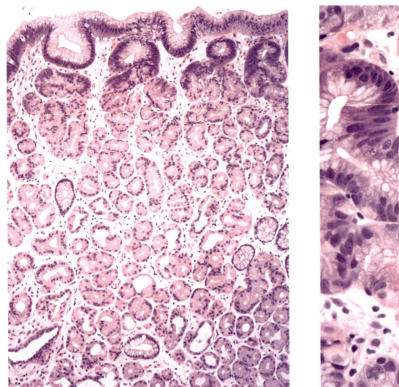
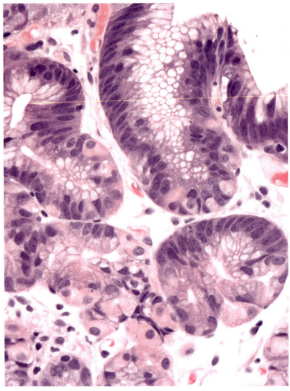

Figure 4-79

FAMILIAL ADENOMATOUS POLYPOSIS-ASSOCIATED FUNDIC GLAND POLYP WITH LOW-GRADE DYSPLASIA

Left: The polyp contains several cystically dilated oxyntic glands in the deep mucosa, as well as crowded foveolar epithelial cells with large, hyperchromatic nuclei at the surface.

Right: Foveolar cells contain elongated, hyperchromatic nuclei; apoptotic nuclear debris is present in the epithelium.

Figure 4-80

FAMILIAL ADENOMATOUS POLYPOSIS-ASSOCIATED PYLORIC GLAND ADENOMA

The lesion is composed of closely apposed tubules with round nuclei and ground glass cytoplasm.

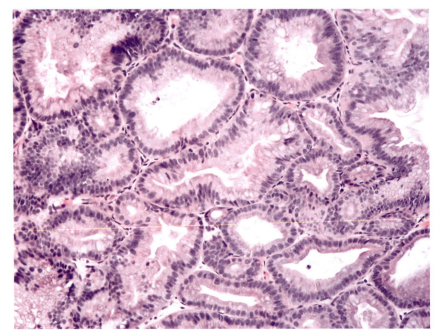

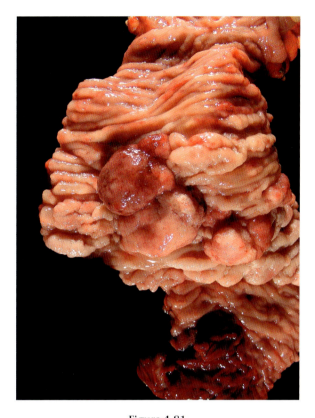

Figure 4-81

FAMILIAL ADENOMATOUS POLYPOSIS-ASSOCIATED AMPULLARY CARCINOMA AND DUODENAL POLYPS

A multinodular mucosa-based tumor is present at the ampulla. Additional adenomas appear as large plaques and nodules on the background mucosa.

the second allele as well as the allele carrying a germline mutation, thereby removing APC function. Thus, tumors from patients with attenuated FAP may show three genetic events affecting *APC*: the initial germline mutation, a second somatic mutation involving the other *APC* allele, and a third mutation on the same allele that carried the germline mutation. Patients with suspected FAP undergo genetic evaluation with full sequencing of *APC* exons and intron-exon boundaries, or linkage analysis if there are multiple affected families members.

Patients with phenotypic FAP may lack detectable *APC* mutations, but show promoter-specific alterations (271). Large deletions around the *APC* promoter 1B may be detected in patients with colonic polyposis as well as numerous gastric polyps. These patients appear to have an increased risk for adenocarcinoma,

similar to the phenotype of gastric adenocarcinoma and proximal polyposis (272,273).

Biallelic inactivation of *APC* occurs through interdependent events; the nature of the germline mutation dictates that of the somatic mutation (274). Germline mutations between codons 1250 and 1450 are usually followed by somatic loss of heterozygosity, with complete loss of *APC* in the other allele. Germline mutations that result in no gene product, or nonfunctional APC protein, are associated with somatic mutations between codons 1250 and 1450 (275). This selection results in a mutant APC protein that retains some of the 20 amino acid sequence required to bind β-catenin, and provides enough Wnt/β-catenin signaling to promote carcinogenesis (276).

The APC protein functions as a tumor suppressor and is normally present in nonproliferative epithelium. It exerts many of its effects by suppressing Wnt-mediated cell proliferation. Active Wnt signaling promotes the tumorigenic effects of β-catenin by preventing its cytoplasmic degradation. As β-catenin accumulates in the cytoplasm, it is transported to the nucleus where it promotes cell proliferation through interactions with T-cell factor and lymphoid enhancer factor. This process is interrupted by APC, which forms a complex with axin and glycogen synthase kinase (GSK)-3, and promotes cytoplasmic degradation of β-catenin by facilitating phosphorylation of serine and tyrosine residues. In addition, the APC protein directly suppresses Wnt signaling through negative interactions with Wnt responsive genes and β-catenin transport out of the nucleus. It also regulates cytoskeletal integrity and mitotic activity by interfering with microtubule dynamics.

Differential Diagnosis. Adenomas and carcinomas that develop in patients with FAP show molecular abnormalities that are indistinguishable from those of sporadically occurring neoplasms and, thus, tissue testing has no role in establishing a diagnosis. A clinical diagnosis of FAP is generally straightforward when patients are identified through family screening programs or have typical disease manifestations. Nevertheless, characteristic abnormalities in the upper gastrointestinal tract can raise the possibility of FAP when the diagnosis is otherwise unsuspected. Any young patient with multiple polyps should be evaluated for a heritable disorder, especially when multiple polyp types or polyps with dysplasia are encountered. Nonampullary adenomas of the duodenum are extremely uncommon in the sporadic setting and, when they occur, are almost always solitary lesions. Detection of multiple duodenal adenomas is strong evidence of an underlying heritable polyposis syndrome, especially FAP.

Multiple lymphomatous polyposis, inflammatory bowel disease, and hamartomatous polyposis syndromes can all simulate the colonoscopic features of FAP, although these disorders are readily distinguishable on biopsy analysis. The differential diagnosis of multiple gastrointestinal adenomas generally includes other polyposis disorders, such as *MUTYH*-associated polyposis, which also manifest with multiple colorectal adenomas and require germline analysis for diagnosis. Patients with Lynch syndrome may have multiple colorectal adenomas, although they are less numerous than those of FAP. Patients with Lynch syndrome can also develop small intestinal and periampullary adenomas that simulate the upper gastrointestinal tract manifestations of FAP. Patients with hereditary biallelic mismatch repair deficiency present with colorectal carcinomas, multiple colonic polyps, café au lait spots, and glial neoplasms, mimicking the phenotypic characteristics of FAP.

Treatment and Prognosis. Virtually 100 percent of patients with FAP and numerous (over 100) colorectal adenomas develop colorectal cancer by the age of 40, whereas those with attenuated FAP have a lifelong colorectal cancer risk of approximately 80 percent, with later cancer onset (40 to 70 years of age). Unfortunately, patients are also at risk for other types of cancer, even if they undergo prophylactic colectomy. Extracolonic tumors occurring in this population include gastric and small bowel adenocarcinoma (0.5 percent and 5 percent, respectively), hepatoblastoma in children (1.5 percent), pancreatic adenocarcinoma (2 percent), and papillary thyroid carcinoma (2 percent), particularly the cribriform morular variant (277,278). Also, patients with FAP develop adrenal cortical adenomas and nasopharyngeal angiofibromas more frequently than do individuals in the general population.

Treatment strategies are designed to prevent cancer development while minimizing disease-related morbidity. Patients undergo colonoscopic examination at 10 to 12 years of age, with subsequent surveillance at 1- to 2-year intervals until a prophylactic colectomy is performed. Ideally, colectomy is deferred until skeletal maturity, although it is advisable when patients have a heavy polyp burden (more than 20 adenomas), large polyps, or high-grade dysplasia (279). Surveillance of the ileal pouch mucosa is continued at 1- to 3-year intervals after ileal pouch-anal anastomosis. Chemoprevention with nonsteroidal anti-inflammatory drugs may be used to decrease polyp burden in the rectum following surgery, or to prevent polyp development in the duodenum (117,280,281). Patients usually undergo examination of the upper gastrointestinal tract by age 25, with surveillance every 1 to 3 years, and children undergo screening for hepatoblastoma. Annual physical examinations include palpation of the thyroid gland, with follow-up ultrasound and fine-needle aspiration biopsy of any nodules (238).

MUTYH-Associated Polyposis

Definition. *MUTYH-associated polyposis* is an autosomal recessive polyposis syndrome that develops as a result of biallelic inactivation of *MUTYH*, a base excision repair gene located on chromosome 1p32-34. The prevalence of heterozygous mutations is estimated to be 2 percent in Caucasian populations, which translates to a disease incidence of approximately 1 in 10,000 persons (282). The disorder is an uncommon cause of colorectal carcinoma, but it is an important consideration when evaluating patients with colorectal polyposis (283). Approximately one third of patients with suspected FAP and wild-type *APC* have *MUTYH*-associated polyposis (284).

Clinical Features. *MUTYH*-associated polyposis shares many clinical features with attenuated FAP, including involvement of the upper gastrointestinal tract (285,286). Patients generally have fewer than 100 colorectal polyps, although rare individuals with hundreds of polyps have been described (fig. 4-82). Adenomas of the small bowel, particularly the duodenum, are detected in nearly 20 percent of affected patients; fundic gland polyps and gastric adenomas are also frequently identified (286,287). Duodenal adenomas occur less frequently than

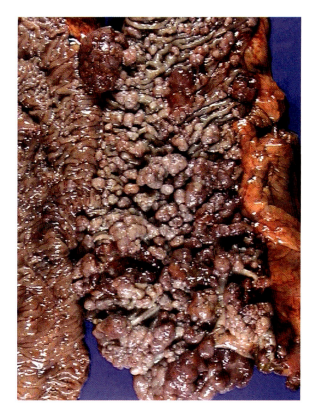

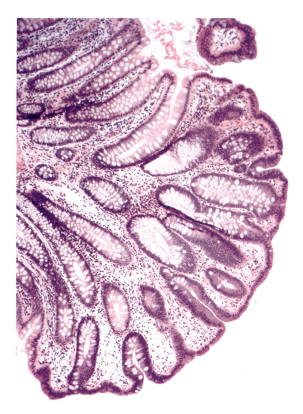

Figure 4-82

MUTYH-ASSOCIATED POLYPOSIS SYNDROME

The colonic mucosa is carpeted by innumerable adenomas, including several large lesions.

Figure 4-83

MUTYH-ASSOCIATED POLYPOSIS SYNDROME

Patients with germline *MUTYH* mutations develop adenomas that are histologically indistinguishable from tubular or villous adenomas that develop in association with FAP.

with FAP (50 to 90 percent of those with classic FAP manifest duodenal polyposis [287]).

The extraintestinal manifestations can mimic either FAP or Lynch syndrome (248,284). Occasional patients have congenital hypertrophy of retinal pigment epithelium, osteomas, or sebaceous tumors, as well as carcinomas of the skin, breast, ovary, and urinary bladder (288). Some patients present with early onset colorectal cancer unassociated with polyposis (289).

Microscopic Findings. Patients with *MUTYH*-associated polyposis generally develop conventional intestinal-type adenomas with tubular or villous architecture, although hyperplastic polyps and SSA/Ps can occur (figs. 4-83, 4-84). Indeed, 15 to 20 percent of patients meet the diagnostic criteria for serrated polyposis and have multiple nondysplastic serrated polyps and adenomas (290).

Cancers are typically intestinal-type adenocarcinomas with features similar to those of spo-radic adenocarcinomas. Some patients develop MSI-H cancers when mismatch repair genes are affected by transversions (291). These tumors may contain infiltrating lymphocytes and show heterogeneous growth patterns similar to other cancers with mismatch repair deficiency.

Molecular Genetic Findings. *MUTYH* encodes MYH glycosylase, which normally corrects oxidative abnormalities that accumulate in guanine. These alterations promote transversion mutations because they facilitate binding of guanine to adenine rather than to cytosine. Patients with biallelic *MUTYH* inactivation accumulate transversions in multiple genes and have a predilection for somatic *APC* mutations, which explains the phenotypic similarities between *MUTYH*-associated polyposis and attenuated FAP. Transversion mutations and spontaneous promoter methylation also occur in *MLH1*, resulting in *MLH1* inactivation and MSI-H (291).

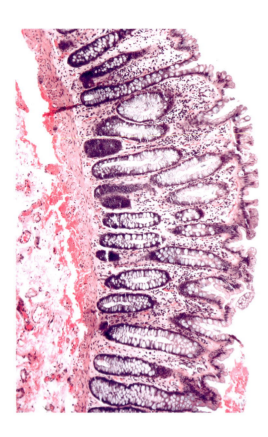 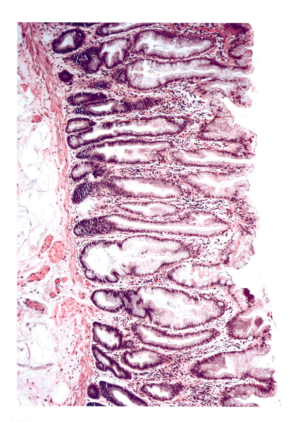

Figure 4-84

MUTYH-ASSOCIATED POLYPOSIS SYNDROME

Left: Some patients have findings simulating the features of serrated polyposis. A polyp contains superficially dilated, slightly serrated crypts typical of a hyperplastic polyp.

Right: The polyps show features of SSA/P with dilated, serrated crypts in the deep mucosa.

Differential Diagnosis. Attenuated FAP, Lynch syndrome, and serrated polyposis can all simulate the phenotype of *MUTYH*-associated polyposis. Germline mutational testing is generally required to conclusively distinguish between these disorders and, thus, *MUTYH*-associated polyposis should be considered in patients with FAP, especially when other disorders are excluded by molecular testing. Patients with attenuated FAP, however, do not develop numerous serrated polyps; if present, they are suggestive of *MUTYH*-associated polyposis. Congenital hypertrophy of retinal pigment epithelium and osteomas have been described in a minority of patients with *MUTYH*-associated polyposis, but these extra-intestinal findings are more typical of FAP.

Some colorectal carcinomas that develop in MUTYH-associated polyposis simulate Lynch syndrome. They may present as early onset solitary cancers, show MSI-H, or occur in combination with other clinical features of Lynch syndrome. MSI-H cancers associated with *MUTYH*-associated polyposis are usually *MLH1* deficient; deficiencies in any other mismatch repair gene suggest Lynch syndrome. Germline testing in these cases can also be illuminating, as patients with *MUTYH*-associated polyposis lack alterations in *MLH1*, *MSH2*, *PMS2*, and *MSH6*.

Treatment and Prognosis. The prognosis and recommended surveillance of patients with *MUTYH*-associated polyposis are comparable to those of patients with attenuated FAP. The lifetime colorectal cancer risk has been reported to be 40 to 100 percent, but is probably near 80 percent, whereas that for duodenal carcinoma is 4 percent (288). Patients with biallelic mutations are predisposed to carcinomas of the urinary

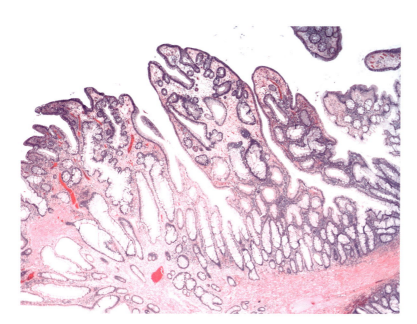

Figure 4-85

JUVENILE POLYP WITH LOW-GRADE DYSPLASIA

Frond-like projections of mucosa contain crypts lined by neoplastic epithelial cells with enlarged, hyperchromatic nuclei. Non-neoplastic, dilated crypts are surrounded by edematous, inflamed lamina propria.

bladder and ovary, as well as other malignancies; the overall lifetime risk of extraintestinal cancer is approximately 38 percent (285,287).

It is recommended that affected individuals undergo a complete colonoscopy at 25 to 30 years of age, with subsequent surveillance every 1 to 2 years thereafter. Residual colorectal mucosa should be examined at 1- to 2-year intervals following colectomy. Initial upper endoscopic examination takes place at 30 to 35 years of age, with follow-up surveillance intervals dependent on the findings. There are some data to suggest that monoallelic *MUTYH* mutation carriers are at increased risk for cancers of the colorectum, hepatobiliary tree, endometrium, and breast, although there are no specific guidelines for this patient group (218,285).

CARCINOMAS IN JUVENILE POLYPOSIS SYNDROME

As previously discussed, *juvenile polyposis syndrome* is an autosomal dominant polyposis disorder that affects 1 in 100,000 persons in the United States (292). It results from alterations affecting TGF-β driven cell signaling; germline *SMAD4* mutations are detected in approximately 20 percent of patients and 20 to 25 percent have *BMPR1A* mutations (293,294).

Patients with juvenile polyposis syndrome develop inflammatory-type polyps throughout the gastrointestinal tract. Polyps with dysplasia contain frond-like projections filled with crowd-

ed, irregularly shaped glands and little intervening stroma (fig. 4-85). Dysplasia is more common among patients with numerous polyps. Small bowel and colorectal polyps show intestinal-type dysplasia with a tubular, villous, or serrated architecture, whereas gastric polyps show foveolar differentiation (figs. 4-86, 4-87).

Patients with juvenile polyposis syndrome have a 70 percent lifetime risk for colorectal carcinoma development. Tumors develop in either polypoid or nonpolypoid mucosa, and are morphologically similar to nonsyndromic adenocarcinomas, although the background mucosa often shows increased inflammation and edema.

CARCINOMAS IN PEUTZ-JEGHERS SYNDROME

Peutz-Jeghers syndrome is an autosomal dominant hereditary hamartomatous polyposis syndrome due to germline *LKB1 (STK11)* mutations that affects 1 in 200,000 persons in the United States. Hamartomatous polyps are most common in the small bowel, but may occur anywhere in the gastrointestinal tract. Dysplasia may develop in polyps at any site, but is most common in lesions of the colorectum, where it is has an intestinal phenotype similar to that of conventional tubular or villous adenomas (fig. 4-88).

Malignant complications are common. The lifetime risk of colorectal cancer is 35 to 40 percent and that of pancreatic cancer and gastric carcinoma is nearly as high; small bowel

175

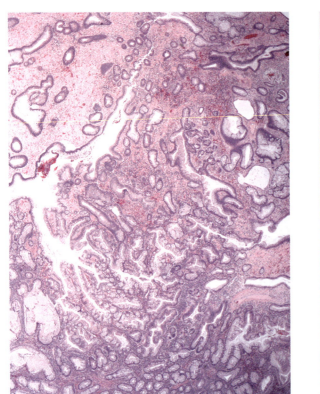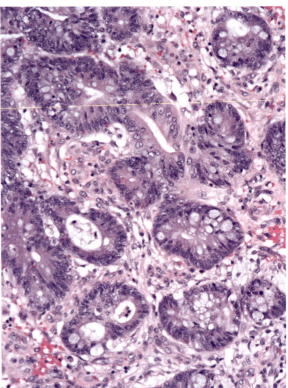

Figure 4-86

JUVENILE POLYP WITH DYSPLASIA

Left: A large, edematous juvenile polyp contains an area of serrated, crowded crypts lined by dysplastic epithelial cells (bottom).

Right: Neoplastic cells contain enlarged, hyperchromatic nuclei, many of which show prominent nucleoli.

Figure 4-87

JUVENILE POLYP WITH LOW-GRADE DYSPLASIA

An irregularly shaped crypt contains neoplastic epithelial cells with elongated, hyperchromatic nuclei and apoptotic nuclear debris.

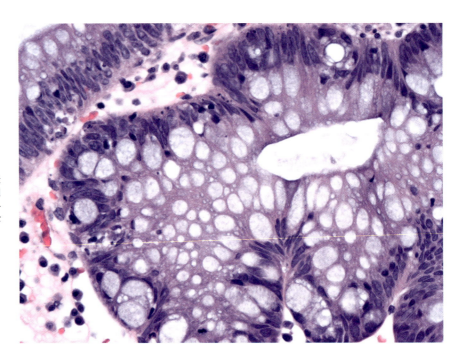

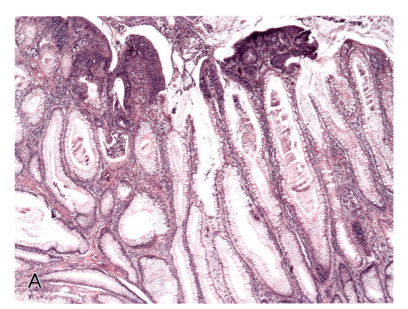

Figure 4-88

PEUTZ-JEGHERS POLYP WITH LOW-GRADE DYSPLASIA

A: Clusters of crowded, mucin depleted crypts are present at the surface of this hamartomatous polyp.

B: Two foci of low-grade dysplasia are present at the surface of a Peutz-Jeghers polyp. Bundles of smooth muscle cells emanate into the polyp head.

C: There is an abrupt transition between non-neoplastic epithelium of the hamartoma and a focus of dysplasia. Crowded neoplastic epithelial cells contain enlarged, hyperchromatic nuclei with irregular contours and increased proliferative activity.

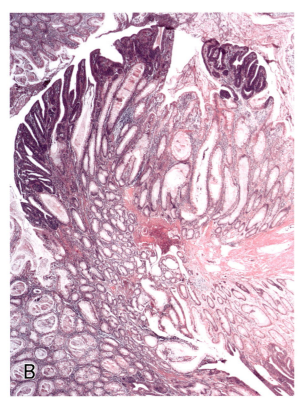

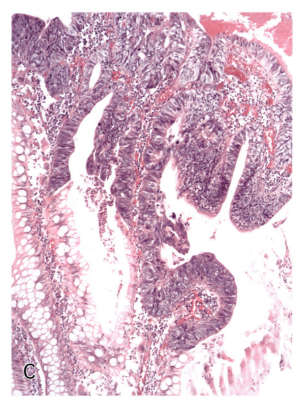

carcinomas are less frequent (lifetime risk of 10 to 15 percent). Intestinal adenocarcinomas develop in either the polypoid or nonpolypoid mucosa and are usually of intestinal type, similar to sporadic adenocarcinomas (fig. 4-89) (295–297).

SERRATED (HYPERPLASTIC) POLYPOSIS

Definition. *Serrated polyposis* is defined by the WHO as the presence of: 1) five or more nondysplastic serrated polyps located proximal to the sigmoid colon, two of which span at least 1 cm; 2) 20 or more hyperplastic polyps of any

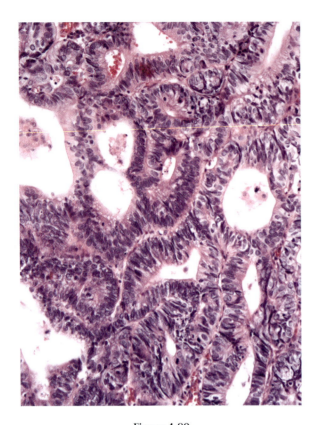

Figure 4-89

ADENOCARCINOMA ARISING IN PEUTZ-JEGHERS POLYP

Confluent aggregates of neoplastic glands infiltrate a Peutz-Jeghers polyp. Malignant glands contain intestinal-type epithelial cells with large, atypical nuclei and luminal necrotic debris.

size distributed throughout the colorectum; or 3) any number of hyperplastic polyps proximal to the sigmoid colon in a first-degree relative of a patient with the disorder (19,298). Multiple large polyps of the abdominal colon are often associated with other polyp types, including SSA/P with dysplasia, conventional adenomas with a tubular or villous morphology, and even invasive adenocarcinoma (299). Many patients with nondysplastic serrated polyps that span at least 2 cm in diameter meet the WHO criteria for serrated polyposis.

Clinical Features. Serrated polyposis occurs with near equal frequency among men and women, and tends to occur in older adults. The polyps are asymptomatic; the condition is usually discovered during screening or surveillance colonoscopy, although some patients present with symptoms related to cancer development. Patients may have small polyps distributed throughout the colon, with the largest lesions showing a predilection for areas proximal to the splenic flexure, particularly the cecum.

The clinical phenotype is variable. Some patients have a few large polyps proximal to the splenic flexure, and others have numerous small polyps located throughout the colorectum. Polyps in the former group show the variably dilated and branching serrated crypts typical of SSA/P, whereas those in the latter group show features of hyperplastic polyps. Serrated polyposis is unassociated with extracolonic manifestations or cancer risk.

Microscopic Findings. Serrated polyposis should be suspected when dealing with resection specimens that contain one or more colonic carcinomas in combination with sessile polyps of the abdominal colon (fig. 4-90, above). Small tumors appear as umbilicated nodules, whereas larger lesions are often bulky with grossly evident mucin (fig. 4-90, left).

A variety of polyp types are seen, often in the same patient. Most nondysplastic serrated polyps show morphologic features that warrant a diagnosis of SSA/P: mucosal expansion by slightly dilated, serrated crypts with branching above the muscularis mucosae; inverted maturation; and an asymmetrically increased proliferative zone. Dysplasia can occur in pre-existing SSA/P, in which case polyps contain mixed populations of nondysplastic serrated epithelium and dysplasia, with either a serrated, tubular, or villous appearance (fig. 4-91). Patients with serrated polyposis can also develop conventional tubular or villous adenomas.

Invasive adenocarcinomas often show high-grade nuclear abnormalities and infiltrative glands with a serrated appearance (fig. 4-92). These tumors may contain heterogeneous cell populations with mucinous or medullary differentiation and tumor-infiltrating lymphocytes that reflect underlying MSI.

Molecular Genetic Findings. Nearly 50 percent of patients with serrated polyposis have a family cancer history, raising the possibility of a heritable component to the disease. Unfortunately, the genetic etiology for disease remains elusive, at least for most patients. Occasional patients with phenotypic serrated polyposis

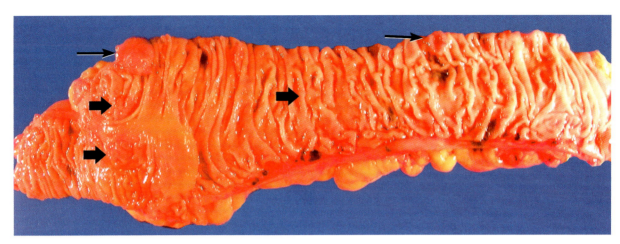

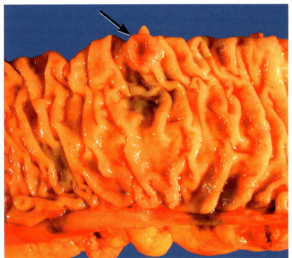

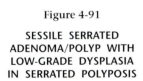

Figure 4-90

SERRATED POLYPOSIS

Above: This older female patient underwent right colectomy following a biopsy diagnosis of colon cancer. The specimen contained two invasive adenocarcinomas (arrows): there was a polypoid cancer near the ileocecal valve and a small, umbilicated tumor in the ascending colon. Scattered SSA/Ps (short arrows) were also present.

Left: A small, ulcerated carcinoma (arrow) is present in the ascending colon and shows adjacent tattoo pigment.

Figure 4-91

SESSILE SERRATED ADENOMA/POLYP WITH LOW-GRADE DYSPLASIA IN SERRATED POLYPOSIS

This polyp contains nondysplastic dilated crypts with serrated convoluted crypts typical of sessile serrated adenoma. Some crypts, however, show cytologic dysplasia with nuclear enlargement and hyperchromasia (arrow).

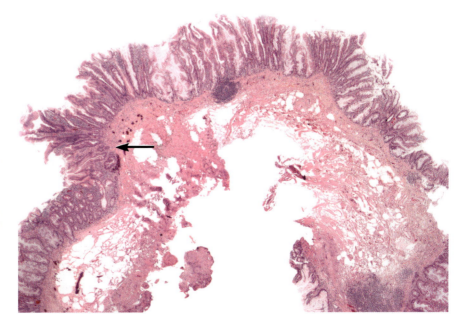

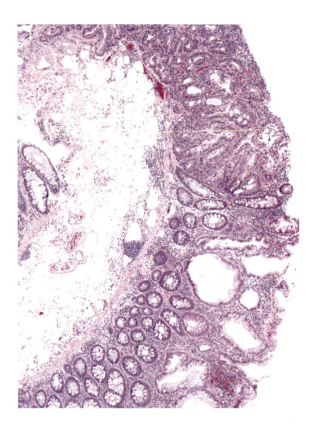 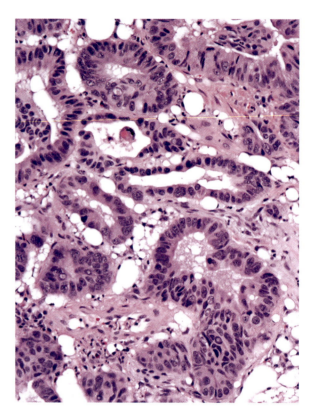

Figure 4-92

SERRATED POLYPOSIS WITH EARLY INVASIVE ADENOCARCINOMA

Left: Nondysplastic serrated crypts are present in association with a crowded proliferation of malignant glands that infiltrate the superficial submucosa (left).

Right: Invasive malignant glands are arranged in irregular aggregates and contain large, hyperchromatic nuclei with heterogeneous chromatin. Luminal necrosis is present.

prove to have *MUTYH*-associated polyposis, as previously described (300).

Treatment and Prognosis. The overall colon cancer risk among patients with multiple tiny polyps is probably not substantially higher than that of individuals in the general population (301). On the other hand, prospective data estimate the cancer risk to be 5 to 10 percent at 7 years among patients with large polyps of the proximal colorectum (302,303). For this reason, patients who have a diagnosis of serrated polyposis are encouraged to undergo colonoscopic surveillance and polyp removal every 1 to 3 years, depending on the number of

polyps present at the time of endoscopic examination. Some clinicians recommend colectomy for patients with multiple large polyps that are not readily amenable to endoscopic resection, although emerging data suggest that these lesions can also be managed conservatively until the onset of dysplasia.

A growing body of evidence suggests that large serrated polyps may represent an increased risk for colonic carcinoma, but that risk is not necessarily related to malignant transformation of the polyp (304). First-degree adult relatives of afflicted patients should probably be offered screening colonoscopy (302,303,305).

REFERENCES

1. Siegel RL, Miller KD, Jemal A. Cancer statistics, 2016. CA Cancer J Clin 2016;66:7-30.
2. Ahnen DJ, Wade SW, Jones WF, et al. The increasing incidence of young-onset colorectal cancer: a call to action. Mayo Clin Proc 2014;89:216-224.
3. Center MM, Jemal A, Ward E. International trends in colorectal cancer incidence rates. Cancer Epidemiol Biomarkers Prev 2009;18:1688-1694.
4. Perdue DG, Perkins C, Jackson-Thompson J, et al. Regional differences in colorectal cancer incidence, stage, and subsite among American Indians and Alaska Natives, 1999-2004. Cancer 2008;113(Suppl):1179-1190.
5. Aune D, Chan DS, Lau R, et al. Dietary fibre, whole grains, and risk of colorectal cancer: systematic review and dose-response meta-analysis of prospective studies. BMJ 2011;343:d6617.
6. Pericleous M, Mandair D, Caplin ME. Diet and supplements and their impact on colorectal cancer. J Gastrointest Oncol 2013;4(4):409-423.
7. Wei EK, Giovannucci E, Wu K, et al. Comparison of risk factors for colon and rectal cancer. Int J Cancer 2004;108:433-442.
8. Baron JA, Barry EL, Mott LA, et al. A trial of calcium and vitamin D for the prevention of colorectal adenomas. N Engl J Med 2015;373:1519-1530.
9. Greenberg ER, Baron JA, Tosteson TD, et al. A clinical trial of antioxidant vitamins to prevent colorectal adenoma. Polyp Prevention Study Group. N Engl J Med 1994;331:141-147.
10. Reddy BS. Dietary fiber and colon cancer: animal model studies. Prev Med 1987;16:559-565.
11. Bonithon-Kopp C, Kronborg O, Giacosa A, Rath U, Faivre J. Calcium and fibre supplementation in prevention of colorectal adenoma recurrence: a randomised intervention trial. European Cancer Prevention Organisation Study Group. Lancet 2000;356:1300-1306.
12. Botteri E, Iodice S, Bagnardi V, Raimondi S, Lowenfels AB, Maisonneuve P. Smoking and colorectal cancer: a meta-analysis. JAMA 2008; 300:2765-2778.
13. Boyle T, Keegel T, Bull F, Heyworth J, Fritschi L. Physical activity and risks of proximal and distal colon cancers: a systematic review and meta-analysis. J Natl Cancer Inst 2012;104:1548-1561.
14. Baron JA, Cole BF, Sandler RS, et al. A randomized trial of aspirin to prevent colorectal adenomas. N Engl J Med 2003;348:891-899.
15. Johnson JJ, Mukhtar H. Curcumin for chemoprevention of colon cancer. Cancer Lett 2007;255:170-181.
16. Goto H, Oda Y, Murakami Y, et al. Proportion of de novo cancers among colorectal cancers in Japan. Gastroenterology 2006;131:40-46.
17. Fearon ER, Vogelstein B. A genetic model for colorectal tumorigenesis. Cell 1990;61:759-767.
18. Jass JR. Classification of colorectal cancer based on correlation of clinical, morphological and molecular features. Histopathology 2007;50:113-130.
19. Snover DC. Update on the serrated pathway to colorectal carcinoma. Hum Pathol 2011;42:1-10.
20. Evaluation of Genomic Applications in Practice and Prevention (EGAPP) Working Group. Recommendations from the EGAPP Working Group: genetic testing strategies in newly diagnosed individuals with colorectal cancer aimed at reducing morbidity and mortality from Lynch syndrome in relatives. Genet Med 2009;11:35-41.
21. Bosman FT, World Health Organization, International Agency for Research on Cancer. WHO classification of tumours of the digestive system, 4th ed. Lyon: International Agency for Research on Cancer; 2010.
22. Jass JR. Serrated adenoma of the colorectum and the DNA-methylator phenotype. Nat Clin Pract Oncol 2005;2:398-405.
23. Bettington ML, Walker NI, Rosty C, et al. A clinicopathological and molecular analysis of 200 traditional serrated adenomas. Mod Pathol 2015;28:414-427.
24. Mecklin JP, Aarnio M, Laara E, et al. Development of colorectal tumors in colonoscopic surveillance in Lynch syndrome. Gastroenterology 2007;133:1093-1098.
25. Goldstein NS. Small colonic microsatellite unstable adenocarcinomas and high-grade epithelial dysplasias in sessile serrated adenoma polypectomy specimens: a study of eight cases. Am J Clin Pathol 2006;125:132-145.
26. Sheridan TB, Fenton H, Lewin MR, et al. Sessile serrated adenomas with low- and high-grade dysplasia and early carcinomas: an immunohistochemical study of serrated lesions "caught in the act." Am J Clin Pathol 2006;126:564-571.
27. Ban S, Mitomi H, Horiguchi H, Sato H, Shimizu M. Adenocarcinoma arising in small sessile serrated adenoma/polyp (SSA/P) of the colon: clinicopathological study of eight lesions. Pathol Int 2014;64:123-132.
28. Truta B, Chen YY, Blanco AM, et al. Tumor histology helps to identify Lynch syndrome among colorectal cancer patients. Fam Cancer 2008;7:267-274.

29. Tuppurainen K, Makinen JM, Junttila O, et al. Morphology and microsatellite instability in sporadic serrated and non-serrated colorectal cancer. J Pathol 2005;207:285-294.

30. Sung CO, Seo JW, Kim KM, Do IG, Kim SW, Park CK. Clinical significance of signet-ring cells in colorectal mucinous adenocarcinoma. Mod Pathol 2008;21:1533-1541.

31. Gao P, Song YX, Xu YY, et al. Does the prognosis of colorectal mucinous carcinoma depend upon the primary tumour site? Results from two independent databases. Histopathology 2013;63:603-615.

32. Kanemitsu Y, Kato T, Hirai T, et al. Survival after curative resection for mucinous adenocarcinoma of the colorectum. Dis Colon Rectum. 2003;46(2):160-167.

33. Kang H, O'Connell JB, Maggard MA, Sack J, Ko CY. A 10-year outcomes evaluation of mucinous and signet-ring cell carcinoma of the colon and rectum. Dis Colon Rectum 2005;48:1161-1168.

34. Park SY, Lee HS, Choe G, Chung JH, Kim WH. Clinicopathological characteristics, microsatellite instability, and expression of mucin core proteins and p53 in colorectal mucinous adenocarcinomas in relation to location. Virchows Arch 2006;449:40-47.

35. Leopoldo S, Lorena B, Cinzia A, et al. Two subtypes of mucinous adenocarcinoma of the colorectum: clinicopathological and genetic features. Ann Surg Oncol 2008;15:1429-1439.

36. Shiovitz S, Grady WM. Molecular markers predictive of chemotherapy response in colorectal cancer. Curr Gastroenterol Rep 2015;17:431.

37. Psathakis D, Schiedeck TH, Krug F, Oevermann E, Kujath P, Bruch HP. Ordinary colorectal adenocarcinoma vs. primary colorectal signet-ring cell carcinoma: study matched for age, gender, grade, and stage. Dis Colon Rectum 1999;42:1618-1625.

38. Hartman DJ, Nikiforova MN, Chang DT, et al. Signet ring cell colorectal carcinoma: a distinct subset of mucin-poor microsatellite-stable signet ring cell carcinoma associated with dismal prognosis. Am J Surg Pathol 2013;37:969-977.

39. Kakar S, Deng G, Smyrk TC, Cun L, Sahai V, Kim YS. Loss of heterozygosity, aberrant methylation, BRAF mutation and KRAS mutation in colorectal signet ring cell carcinoma. Mod Pathol 2012;25:1040-1047.

40. Wick MR, Vitsky JL, Ritter JH, Swanson PE, Mills SE. Sporadic medullary carcinoma of the colon: a clinicopathologic comparison with nonhereditary poorly differentiated enteric-type adenocarcinoma and neuroendocrine colorectal carcinoma. Am J Clin Pathol 2005;123:56-65.

41. Kasapidis P, Grivas E, Papamichail V, Alfaras P. Medullary carcinoma of the colon: an adenocar-

cinoma with better prognosis. Ann Gastroenterol 2015;28(2):289.

42. Thirunavukarasu P, Sathaiah M, Singla S, et al. Medullary carcinoma of the large intestine: a population based analysis. Int J Oncol 2010;37:901-907.

43. Makinen MJ. Colorectal serrated adenocarcinoma. Histopathology 2007;50:131-150.

44. Stefanius K, Ylitalo L, Tuomisto A, et al. Frequent mutations of KRAS in addition to BRAF in colorectal serrated adenocarcinoma. Histopathology 2011;58:679-692.

45. Laiho P, Kokko A, Vanharanta S, et al. Serrated carcinomas form a subclass of colorectal cancer with distinct molecular basis. Oncogene 2007;26:312-320.

46. Kim MJ, Hong SM, Jang SJ, et al. Invasive colorectal micropapillary carcinoma: an aggressive variant of adenocarcinoma. Hum Pathol 2006;37:809-815.

47. Sonoo H, Kameyama M, Inatugi N, Nonomura A, Enomoto Y. Pedunculated polyp of early sigmoid colon cancer with invasive micropapillary carcinoma. Jpn J Clin Oncol 2009;39:523-527.

48. Lino-Silva LS, Salcedo-Hernandez RA, Caro-Sanchez CH. Colonic micropapillary carcinoma, a recently recognized subtype associated with histological adverse factors: clinicopathological analysis of 15 cases. Colorectal Dis 2012;14:e567-572.

49. Verdu M, Roman R, Calvo M, et al. Clinicopathological and molecular characterization of colorectal micropapillary carcinoma. Mod Pathol 2011;24:729-738.

50. Hartman DJ, Binion D, Regueiro M, et al. Isocitrate dehydrogenase-1 is mutated in inflammatory bowel disease-associated intestinal adenocarcinoma with low-grade tubuloglandular histology but not in sporadic intestinal adenocarcinoma. Am J Surg Pathol 2014;38:1147-1156.

51. Levi GS, Harpaz N. Intestinal low-grade tubuloglandular adenocarcinoma in inflammatory bowel disease. Am J Surg Pathol 2006;30:1022-1029.

52. Audeau A, Han HW, Johnston MJ, Whitehead MW, Frizelle FA. Does human papilloma virus have a role in squamous cell carcinoma of the colon and upper rectum? Eur J Surg Oncol 2002;28:657-660.

53. Copur S, Ledakis P, Novinski D, et al. Squamous cell carcinoma of the colon with an elevated serum squamous cell carcinoma antigen responding to combination chemotherapy. Clin Colorectal Cancer 2001;1:55-58.

54. Frizelle FA, Hobday KS, Batts KP, Nelson H. Adenosquamous and squamous carcinoma of the colon and upper rectum: a clinical and histopathologic study. Dis Colon Rectum 2001;44:341-346.

55. Lyttle JA. Primary squamous carcinoma of the proximal large bowel. Report of a case and review of the literature. Dis Colon Rectum 1983;26:279-282.

56. Williams GT, Blackshaw AJ, Morson BC. Squamous carcinoma of the colorectum and its genesis. J Pathol 1979;129:139-147.

57. Bognar G, Istvan G, Bereczky B, Ondrejka P. Detection of human papillomavirus type 16 in squamous cell carcinoma of the colon and its lymph node metastases with PCR and southern blot hybridization. Pathol Oncol Res 2008;14:93-96.

58. Petrelli NJ, Valle AA, Weber TK, Rodriguez-Bigas M. Adenosquamous carcinoma of the colon and rectum. Dis Colon Rectum 1996;39:1265-1268.

59. Cagir B, Nagy MW, Topham A, Rakinic J, Fry RD. Adenosquamous carcinoma of the colon, rectum, and anus: epidemiology, distribution, and survival characteristics. Dis Colon Rectum 1999;42:258-263.

60. Delaney D, Chetty R. Lymphoepithelioma-like carcinoma of the colon. Int J Clin Exp Pathol 2012;5:105-109.

61. Kojima Y, Mogaki M, Takagawa R, et al. A case of lymphoepithelioma-like carcinoma of the colon with ulcerative colitis. J Gastroenterol 2007;42:181-185.

62. Mori Y, Akagi K, Yano M, et al. Lymphoepithelioma-like carcinoma of the colon. Case Rep Gastroenterol 2013;7:127-133.

63. Agaimy A, Rau TT, Hartmann A, Stoehr R. SMARCB1 (INI1)-negative rhabdoid carcinomas of the gastrointestinal tract: clinicopathologic and molecular study of a highly aggressive variant with literature review. Am J Surg Pathol 2014;38:910-920.

64. Pancione M, Di Blasi A, Sabatino L, et al. A novel case of rhabdoid colon carcinoma associated with a positive CpG island methylator phenotype and BRAF mutation. Hum Pathol 2011;42(7):1047-1052.

65. Pancione M, Remo A, Sabatino L, et al. Right-sided rhabdoid colorectal tumors might be related to the serrated pathway. Diagn Pathol 2013;8:31.

66. Remo A, Zanella C, Molinari E, et al. Rhabdoid carcinoma of the colon: a distinct entity with a very aggressive behavior: a case report associated with a polyposis coli and review of the literature. Int J Surg Pathol 2012;20:185-190.

67. Gui X, Qin L, Gao ZH, Falck V, Harpaz N. Goblet cell carcinoids at extraappendiceal locations of gastrointestinal tract: an underrecognized diagnostic pitfall. J Surg Oncol 2011;103:790-795.

68. Barisella M, Lampis A, Perrone F, Carbone A. Clear cell adenocarcinoma of the colon is a unique morphological variant of intestinal carcinoma: case report with molecular analysis. World J Gastroenterol 2008;14:6575-6577.

69. Barrera-Maldonado CD, Wiener I, Sim S. Clear cell adenocarcinoma of the colon: a case report and review of the literature. Case Rep Oncol Med 2014;2014:905478.

70. Soga K, Konishi H, Tatsumi N, et al. Clear cell adenocarcinoma of the colon: a case report and review of literature. World J Gastroenterol 2008;14:1137-1140.

71. Wang W, Li X, Qu G, Leng T, Geng J. Primary clear cell adenocarcinoma of the colon presenting as a huge extracolic mass: A case report. Oncol Lett 2014;8:1873-1875.

72. Serio G, Aguzzi A. Spindle and giant cell carcinoma of the colon. Histopathology 1997;30:383-385.

73. Tajima S, Waki M, Tsuchiya T, Hoshi S. Granulocyte colony-stimulating factor-producing undifferentiated carcinoma of the colon mimicking a pulmonary giant cell carcinoma: a case showing overexpression of CD44 along with highly proliferating nestin-positive tumor vessels. Int J Clin Exp Pathol 2014;7:7034-7041.

74. Shi C, Scudiere JR, Cornish TC, et al. Clear cell change in colonic tubular adenoma and corresponding colonic clear cell adenocarcinoma is associated with an altered mucin core protein profile. Am J Surg Pathol 2010;34:1344-1350.

75. McCluggage WG, Desai V, Toner PG, Calvert CH. Clear cell adenocarcinoma of the colon arising in endometriosis: a rare variant of primary colonic adenocarcinoma. J Clin Pathol 2001;54:76-77.

76. Choi YY, Jeen YM, Kim YJ. Sarcomatoid carcinoma of colon: extremely poor prognosis. J Korean Surg Soc 2011;80(Suppl 1):S26-30.

77. Kim JH, Moon WS, Kang MJ, Park MJ, Lee DG. Sarcomatoid carcinoma of the colon: a case report. J Korean Med Sci 2001;16:657-660.

78. Gaffey MJ, Mills SE, Lack EE. Neuroendocrine carcinoma of the colon and rectum. A clinicopathologic, ultrastructural, and immunohistochemical study of 24 cases. Am J Surg Pathol 1990;14:1010-1023.

79. Edge SB, American Joint Committee on Cancer. AJCC cancer staging manual. 7th ed. New York: Springer; 2010.

80. Taliano RJ, LeGolvan M, Resnick MB. Immunohistochemistry of colorectal carcinoma: current practice and evolving applications. Hum Pathol 2013;44:151-163.

81. Shin JH, Bae JH, Lee A, et al. CK7, CK20, CDX2 and MUC2 Immunohistochemical staining used to distinguish metastatic colorectal carcinoma involving ovary from primary ovarian mucinous adenocarcinoma. Jpn J Clin Oncol 2010;40:208-213.

82. Dalerba P, Sahoo D, Paik S, et al. CDX2 as a prognostic biomarker in stage II and stage III Colon cancer. N Engl J Med 2016;374:211-222.

83. Dalerba P, Sahoo D, Clarke MF. CDX2 as a Prognostic Biomarker in Colon Cancer. N Engl J Med 2016;374:2184.

84. Hong KD, Lee D, Lee Y, Lee SI, Moon HY. Reduced CDX2 expression predicts poor overall survival in patients with colorectal cancer. Am Surg. 2013;79(4):353-360.

85. Kim JH, Rhee YY, Bae JM, Cho NY, Kang GH. Loss of CDX2/CK20 expression is associated with poorly differentiated carcinoma, the CpG island methylator phenotype, and adverse prognosis in microsatellite-unstable colorectal cancer. Am J Surg Pathol 2013;37:1532-1541.

86. Terada T. An immunohistochemical study of primary signet-ring cell carcinoma of the stomach and colorectum: I. Cytokeratin profile in 42 cases. Int J Clin Exp Pathol 2013;6:703-710.

87. Abdulkader M, Abdulla K, Rakha E, Kaye P. Routine elastic staining assists detection of vascular invasion in colorectal cancer. Histopathology 2006;49:487-492.

88. Baumhoer D, Thiesler T, Maurer CA, Huber A, Cathomas G. Impact of using elastic stains for detection of venous invasion in the prognosis of patients with lymph node negative colorectal cancer. Int J Colorectal Dis 2010;25:741-746.

89. Howlett CJ, Tweedie EJ, Driman DK. Use of an elastic stain to show venous invasion in colorectal carcinoma: a simple technique for detection of an important prognostic factor. J Clin Pathol 2009;62:1021-1025.

90. Suzuki A, Togashi K, Nokubi M, et al. Evaluation of venous invasion by Elastica van Gieson stain and tumor budding predicts local and distant metastases in patients with T1 stage colorectal cancer. Am J Surg Pathol 2009;33:1601-1607.

91. Sato T, Ueno H, Mochizuki H, et al. Objective criteria for the grading of venous invasion in colorectal cancer. Am J Surg Pathol 2010;34:454-462.

92. Liang P, Nakada I, Hong JW, et al. Prognostic significance of immunohistochemically detected blood and lymphatic vessel invasion in colorectal carcinoma: its impact on prognosis. Ann Surg Oncol 2007;14:470-477.

93. Kai K, Aishima S, Aoki S, et al. Cytokeratin immunohistochemistry improves interobserver variability between unskilled pathologists in the evaluation of tumor budding in T1 colorectal cancer. Pathol Int 2016;66:75-82.

94. Okamura T, Shimada Y, Nogami H, et al. Tumor budding detection by immunohistochemical staining is not superior to hematoxylin and eosin staining for predicting lymph Node metastasis in pt1 colorectal cancer. Dis Colon Rectum 2016;59:396-402.

95. Puppa G, Senore C, Sheahan K, et al. Diagnostic reproducibility of tumour budding in colorectal cancer: a multicentre, multinational study using virtual microscopy. Histopathology 2012;61:562-575.

96. Weixler B, Warschkow R, Guller U, et al. Isolated tumor cells in stage I & II colon cancer patients are associated with significantly worse disease-free and overall survival. BMC Cancer 2016;16D:106.

97. Oh SY, Kim DY, Kim YB, Suh KW. Clinical application of sentinel lymph node mapping in colon cancer: in vivo vs. ex vivo techniques. Ann Surg Treat Res 2014;87:118-122.

98. Braat AE, Pol RA, Oosterhuis JW, de Vries JE, Mesker WE, Tollenaar RA. Excellent prognosis of node negative patients after sentinel node procedure in colon carcinoma: a 5-year follow-up study. Eur J Surg Oncol 2014;40:747-755.

99. Bilchik AJ, Hoon DS, Saha S, et al. Prognostic impact of micrometastases in colon cancer: interim results of a prospective multicenter trial. Ann Surg 2007;246:568-575; discussion 575-567.

100. Redston M, Compton CC, Miedema BW, et al. Analysis of micrometastatic disease in sentinel lymph nodes from resectable colon cancer: results of Cancer and Leukemia Group B Trial 80001. J Clin Oncol 2006;24:878-883.

101. Bartley AN, Hamilton SR. Select biomarkers for tumors of the gastrointestinal tract: present and future. Arch Pathol Lab Med 2015;139:457-468.

102. Washington MK, Berlin J, Branton P, et al. Protocol for the examination of specimens from patients with primary carcinoma of the colon and rectum. Arch Pathol Lab Med 2009;133:1539-1551.

103. Amin M, Edge S, Greene F, et al. AJCC Cancer Staging Manual, 8th ed. Switzerland: Springer International Publishing; 2017.

104. Adam IJ, Mohamdee MO, Martin IG, et al. Role of circumferential margin involvement in the local recurrence of rectal cancer. Lancet 1994;344:707-711.

105. Birbeck KF, Macklin CP, Tiffin NJ, et al. Rates of circumferential resection margin involvement vary between surgeons and predict outcomes in rectal cancer surgery. Ann Surg 2002;235:449-457.

106. Bosch SL, Nagtegaal ID. The Importance of the pathologist's role in assessment of the quality of the mesorectum. Curr Colorectal Cancer Rep 2012;8:90-98.

107. Nagtegaal ID, van de Velde CJ, van der Worp E, et al. Macroscopic evaluation of rectal cancer resection specimen: clinical significance of the pathologist in quality control. J Clin Oncol 2002;20:1729-1734.

108. Sehgal R, Coffey JC. Historical development of mesenteric anatomy provides a universally applicable anatomic paradigm for complete/total mesocolic excision. Gastroenterol Rep (Oxf) 2014;2:245-250.

109. Storli KE, Sondenaa K, Furnes B, et al. Short term results of complete (D3) vs. standard (D2) mesenteric excision in colon cancer shows improved outcome of complete mesenteric excision in patients with TNM stages I-II. Tech Coloproctol 2014;18:557-564.

110. West NP, Morris EJ, Rotimi O, Cairns A, Finan PJ, Quirke P. Pathology grading of colon cancer surgical resection and its association with survival: a retrospective observational study. Lancet Oncol 2008;9:857-865.

111. Kenney BC, Jain D. Identification of lymphatics within the colonic lamina propria in inflammation and neoplasia using the monoclonal antibody D2-40. Yale J Biol Med 2008;81:103-113.

112. Shepherd NA, Baxter KJ, Love SB. The prognostic importance of peritoneal involvement in colonic cancer: a prospective evaluation. Gastroenterology 1997;112:1096-1102.

113. Compton CC. Updated protocol for the examination of specimens from patients with carcinomas of the colon and rectum, excluding carcinoid tumors, lymphomas, sarcomas, and tumors of the vermiform appendix: a basis for checklists. Cancer Committee. Arch Pathol Lab Med 2000;124:1016-1025.

114. Panarelli NC, Schreiner AM, Brandt SM, Shepherd NA, Yantiss RK. Histologic features and cytologic techniques that aid pathologic stage assessment of colonic adenocarcinoma. Am J Surg Pathol 2013;37:1252-1258.

115. Frankel WL, Jin M. Serosal surfaces, mucin pools, and deposits, oh my: challenges in staging colorectal carcinoma. Mod Pathol 2015;28(Suppl 1):S95-108.

116. Gunderson LL, Jessup JM, Sargent DJ, Greene FL, Stewart AK. Revised TN categorization for colon cancer based on national survival outcomes data. J Clin Oncol 2010;28:264-271.

117. Kim B, Giardiello FM. Chemoprevention in familial adenomatous polyposis. Best Pract Res Clin Gastroenterol 2011;25:607-622.

118. Park JS, Choi GS, Hasegawa S, et al. Validation of the seventh edition of the American Joint Committee on cancer tumor node-staging system in patients with colorectal carcinoma in comparison with sixth classification. J Surg Oncol 2012;106:674-679.

119. Petersen VC, Baxter KJ, Love SB, Shepherd NA. Identification of objective pathological prognostic determinants and models of prognosis in Dukes' B colon cancer. Gut 2002;51:65-69.

120. Kim KH, Yang SS, Yoon YS, Lim SB, Yu CS, Kim JC. Validation of the seventh edition of the American Joint Committee on Cancer tumor-node-metastasis (AJCC TNM) staging in patients with stage II and stage III colorectal carcinoma: analysis of 2511 cases from a medical centre in Korea. Colorectal Dis 2011;13:e220-226.

121. Markl B. Stage migration vs immunology: the lymph node count story in colon cancer. World J Gastroenterol 2015;21:12218-12233.

122. McDonald JR, Renehan AG, O'Dwyer ST, Haboubi NY. Lymph node harvest in colon and rectal cancer: Current considerations. World J Gastrointest Surg 2012;4:9-19.

123. Kobayashi H, Mochizuki H, Kato T, et al. Lymph node ratio is a powerful prognostic index in patients with stage III distal rectal cancer: a Japanese multicenter study. Int J Colorectal Dis 2011;26:891-896.

124. Baxter NN, Ricciardi R, Simunovic M, Urbach DR, Virnig BA. An evaluation of the relationship between lymph node number and staging in pT3 colon cancer using population-based data. Dis Colon Rectum 2010;53:65-70.

125. Markl B, Rossle J, Arnholdt HM, et al. The clinical significance of lymph node size in colon cancer. Mod Pathol 2012;25:1413-1422.

126. Budde CN, Tsikitis VL, Deveney KE, Diggs BS, Lu KC, Herzig DO. Increasing the number of lymph nodes examined after colectomy does not improve colon cancer staging. J Am Coll Surg 2014;218:1004-1011.

127. Bui L, Rempel E, Reeson D, Simunovic M. Lymph node counts, rates of positive lymph nodes, and patient survival for colon cancer surgery in Ontario, Canada: a population-based study. J Surg Oncol 2006;93:439-445.

128. Wang H, Safar B, Wexner SD, Denoya P, Berho M. The clinical significance of fat clearance lymph node harvest for invasive rectal adenocarcinoma following neoadjuvant therapy. Dis Colon Rectum 2009;52:1767-1773.

129. Lee MR, Hong CW, Yoon SN, et al. Isolated tumor cells in lymph nodes are not a prognostic marker for patients with stage I and stage II colorectal cancer. J Surg Oncol 2006;93:13-18; discussion 18-19.

130. Mescoli C, Albertoni L, Pucciarelli S, et al. Isolated tumor cells in regional lymph nodes as relapse predictors in stage I and II colorectal cancer. J Clin Oncol 2012;30:965-971.

131. Rock JB, Washington MK, Adsay NV, et al. Debating deposits: an interobserver variability study of lymph nodes and pericolonic tumor deposits in colonic adenocarcinoma. Arch Pathol Lab Med 2014;138:636-642.

132. Song YX, Gao P, Wang ZN, et al. Can the tumor deposits be counted as metastatic lymph nodes in the UICC TNM staging system for colorectal cancer? PLoS One 2012;7:e34087.

133. Ueno H, Hashiguchi Y, Shimazaki H, et al. Peritumoral deposits as an adverse prognostic indicator of colorectal cancer. Am J Surg. 2014;207(1):70-77.

134. Ueno H, Mochizuki H, Hashiguchi Y, et al. Extramural cancer deposits without nodal structure in colorectal cancer: optimal categorization for prognostic staging. Am J Clin Pathol 2007;127:287-294.

135. Yamano T, Semba S, Noda M, et al. Prognostic significance of classified extramural tumor deposits and extracapsular lymph node invasion in T3-4 colorectal cancer: a retrospective single-center study. BMC Cancer 2015;15:859.

136. Goldstein NS, Turner JR. Pericolonic tumor deposits in patients with T3N+MO colon adenocarcinomas: markers of reduced disease free survival and intra-abdominal metastases and their implications for TNM classification. Cancer 2000;88:2228-2238.

137. Wunsch K, Muller J, Jahnig H, Herrmann RA, Arnholdt HM, Markl B. Shape is not associated with the origin of pericolonic tumor deposits. Am J Clin Pathol 2010;133:388-394.

138. Greenson JK, Huang SC, Herron C, et al. Pathologic predictors of microsatellite instability in colorectal cancer. Am J Surg Pathol 2009;33:126-133.

139. Rozek LS, Schmit SL, Greenson JK, et al. Tumor-infiltrating lymphocytes, Crohn's-like lymphoid reaction, and survival from colorectal cancer. J Natl Cancer Inst 2016;108.

140. Rosenbaum MW, Bledsoe JR, Morales-Oyarvide V, Huynh TG, Mino-Kenudson M. PD-L1 expression in colorectal cancer is associated with microsatellite instability, BRAF mutation, medullary morphology and cytotoxic tumor-infiltrating lymphocytes. Mod Pathol 2016;29:1104-1112.

141. Ishii M, Ota M, Saito S, Kinugasa Y, Akamoto S, Ito I. Lymphatic vessel invasion detected by monoclonal antibody D2-40 as a predictor of lymph node metastasis in T1 colorectal cancer. Int J Colorectal Dis 2009;24:1069-1074.

142. Muller S, Chesner IM, Egan MJ, et al. Significance of venous and lymphatic invasion in malignant polyps of the colon and rectum. Gut 1989;30:1385-1391.

143. Wada H, Shiozawa M, Sugano N, et al. Lymphatic invasion identified with D2-40 immunostaining as a risk factor of nodal metastasis in T1 colorectal cancer. Int J Clin Oncol 2013;18:1025-1031.

144. Betge J, Schneider NI, Pollheimer MJ, et al. Is there a rationale to record lymphatic invasion in node-positive colorectal cancer? J Clin Pathol 2012;65:847-850.

145. Betge J, Pollheimer MJ, Lindtner RA, et al. Intramural and extramural vascular invasion in colorectal cancer: prognostic significance and quality of pathology reporting. Cancer 2012;118:628-638.

146. Lai JH, Zhou YJ, Bin D, Qiangchen, Wang SY. Clinical significance of detecting lymphatic and blood vessel invasion in stage II colon cancer using markers D2-40 and CD34 in combination. Asian Pac J Cancer Prev 2014;15:1363-1367.

147. Walgenbach-Bruenagel G, Tolba RH, Varnai AD, Bollmann M, Hirner A, Walgenbach KJ. Detection of lymphatic invasion in early stage primary colorectal cancer with the monoclonal antibody D2-40. Eur Surg Res 2006;38:438-444.

148. Akagi Y, Kinugasa T, Adachi Y, Shirouzu K. Prognostic significance of isolated tumor cells in patients with colorectal cancer in recent 10-year studies. Mol Clin Oncol 2013;1:582-592.

149. Akagi Y, Adachi Y, Ohchi T, Kinugasa T, Shirouzu K. Prognostic impact of lymphatic invasion of colorectal cancer: a single-center analysis of 1,616 patients over 24 years. Anticancer Res 2013;33:2965-2970.

150. Kingston EF, Goulding H, Bateman AC. Vascular invasion is underrecognized in colorectal cancer using conventional hematoxylin and eosin staining. Dis Colon Rectum 2007;50:1867-1872.

151. Inoue T, Mori M, Shimono R, Kuwano H, Sugimachi K. Vascular invasion of colorectal carcinoma readily visible with certain stains. Dis Colon Rectum 1992;35:34-39.

152. Courtney ED, West NJ, Kaur C, et al. Extramural vascular invasion is an adverse prognostic indicator of survival in patients with colorectal cancer. Colorectal Dis 2009;11:150-156.

153. Talbot IC, Ritchie S, Leighton M, Hughes AO, Bussey HJ, Morson BC. Invasion of veins by carcinoma of rectum: method of detection, histological features and significance. Histopathology 1981;5:141-163.

154. Mitrovic B, Schaeffer DF, Riddell RH, Kirsch R. Tumor budding in colorectal carcinoma: time to take notice. Mod Pathol 2012;25:1315-1325.

155. Koelzer VH, Zlobec I, Berger MD, et al. Tumor budding in colorectal cancer revisited: results of a multicenter interobserver study. Virchows Arch 2015;466:485-493.

156. Ogawa T, Yoshida T, Tsuruta T, et al. Tumor budding is predictive of lymphatic involvement and lymph node metastases in submucosal invasive colorectal adenocarcinomas and in non-polypoid compared with polypoid growths. Scand J Gastroenterol 2009;44:605-614.

157. Ueno H, Murphy J, Jass JR, Mochizuki H, Talbot IC. Tumour 'budding' as an index to estimate the potential of aggressiveness in rectal cancer. Histopathology 2002;40:127-132.

158. Zlobec I, Bihl MP, Foerster A, Rufle A, Lugli A. The impact of CpG island methylator phenotype and microsatellite instability on tumour budding in colorectal cancer. Histopathology 2012;61:777-787.

159. Knijn N, Mogk SC, Teerenstra S, Simmer F, Nagtegaal ID. Perineural Invasion is a strong prognostic factor in colorectal cancer: a systematic review. Am J Surg Pathol 2016;40:103-112.

160. Pourmand K, Itzkowitz SH. Small bowel neoplasms and polyps. Curr Gastroenterol Rep 2016;18:23.

161. Choi EH, Mergener K, Semrad C, et al. A multicenter, prospective, randomized comparison of a novel signal transmission capsule endoscope to an existing capsule endoscope. Gastrointest Endosc 2013;78:325-332.

162. Haanstra JF, Al-Toma A, Dekker E, et al. Prevalence of small-bowel neoplasia in Lynch syndrome assessed by video capsule endoscopy. Gut 2015;64:1578-1583.

163. Aparicio T, Svrcek M, Zaanan A, et al. Small bowel adenocarcinoma phenotyping, a clinicobiological prognostic study. Br J Cancer 2013;109:3057-3066.

164. Durno CA, Sherman PM, Aronson M, et al. Phenotypic and genotypic characterisation of biallelic mismatch repair deficiency (BMMR-D) syndrome. Eur J Cancer 2015;51:977-983.

165. Genta RM, Feagins LA. Advanced precancerous lesions in the small bowel mucosa. Best Pract Res Clin Gastroenterol 2013;27:225-233.

166. Genta RM, Hurrell JM, Sonnenberg A. Duodenal adenomas coincide with colorectal neoplasia. Dig Dis Sci 2014;59:2249-2254.

167. Torlakovic EE, Gomez JD, Driman DK, et al. Sessile serrated adenoma (SSA) vs. traditional serrated adenoma (TSA). Am J Surg Pathol 2008;32:21-29.

168. Salaria SN, Abu Alfa AK, Alsaigh NY, Montgomery E, Arnold CA. Composite intestinal adenoma-microcarcinoid clues to diagnosing an under-recognised mimic of invasive adenocarcinoma. J Clin Pathol 2013;66:302-306.

169. Chen ZM, Wang HL. Alteration of cytokeratin 7 and cytokeratin 20 expression profile is uniquely associated with tumorigenesis of primary adenocarcinoma of the small intestine. Am J Surg Pathol 2004;28:1352-1359.

170. Shih IM, Wang TL, Traverso G, et al. Top-down morphogenesis of colorectal tumors. Proc Natl Acad Sci U S A 2001;98:2640-2645.

171. Cameron JL, He J. Two thousand consecutive pancreaticoduodenectomies. J Am Coll Surg 2015;220:530-536.

172. Offerhaus GJ, Entius MM, Giardiello FM. Upper gastrointestinal polyps in familial adenomatous polyposis. Hepatogastroenterology 1999;46:667-669.

173. Offerhaus GJ, Giardiello FM, Krush AJ, et al. The risk of upper gastrointestinal cancer in familial adenomatous polyposis. Gastroenterology 1992;102:1980-1982.

174. Wood LD, Salaria SN, Cruise MW, Giardiello FM, Montgomery EA. Upper GI tract lesions in familial adenomatous polyposis (FAP): enrichment of pyloric gland adenomas and other gastric and duodenal neoplasms. Am J Surg Pathol 2014;38:389-393.

175. Chen ZM, Scudiere JR, Abraham SC, Montgomery E. Pyloric gland adenoma: an entity distinct from gastric foveolar type adenoma. Am J Surg Pathol 2009;33:186-193.

176. Vieth M, Kushima R, Borchard F, Stolte M. Pyloric gland adenoma: a clinico-pathological analysis of 90 cases. Virchows Arch 2003;442:317-321.

177. Vieth M, Montgomery EA. Some observations on pyloric gland adenoma: an uncommon and long ignored entity! J Clin Pathol 2014;67:883-890.

178. Elster K. Histologic classification of gastric polyps. In: Morson B, ed. Pathology of the gastro-intestinal tract. Berlin: Springer; 1976:78-92.

179. Watanabe H GJ, Sobin LH. Histological typing of oesophageal and gastric tumours. WHO classification of gastrointestinal tumours. Berlin: Springer; 1990.

180. Borchard F GA, Kodovsky U, Hengels KJ, Brückmann FW. Gastrale Differenzierung in Adenomen der Magenschleimhaut. Immunhistochemische und elektronenmikroskopische Untersuchungen. Verh Dtsch Ges Pathol 1990;74:528.

181. Park JY, Cornish TC, Lam-Himlin D, Shi C, Montgomery E. Gastric lesions in patients with autoimmune metaplastic atrophic gastritis (AMAG) in a tertiary care setting. Am J Surg Pathol 2010;34:1591-1598.

182. Vieth M, Kushima R, Mukaisho K, Sakai R, Kasami T, Hattori T. Immunohistochemical analysis of pyloric gland adenomas using a series of mucin 2, mucin 5AC, mucin 6, CD10, Ki67 and p53. Virchows Arch 2010;457:529-536.

183. Matsubara A, Sekine S, Kushima R, et al. Frequent GNAS and KRAS mutations in pyloric gland adenoma of the stomach and duodenum. J Pathol 2013;229:579-587.

184. Lee SE, Kang SY, Cho J, et al. Pyloric gland adenoma in Lynch syndrome. Am J Surg Pathol 2014;38:784-792.

185. Park YK, Jeong WJ, Cheon GJ. Slow-growing early adenocarcinoma arising from traditional serrated adenoma in the duodenum. Case Rep Gastroenterol 2016;10:257-263.

186. Rosty C, Campbell C, Clendenning M, Bettington M, Buchanan DD, Brown IS. Do serrated neoplasms of the small intestine represent a distinct entity? Pathological findings and molecular alterations in a series of 13 cases. Histopathology 2015;66:333-342.

187. Aparicio T, Zaanan A, Svrcek M, et al. Small bowel adenocarcinoma: epidemiology, risk factors, diagnosis and treatment. Dig Liver Dis 2014;46:97-104.

188. Estrella JS, Wu TT, Rashid A, Abraham SC. Mucosal colonization by metastatic carcinoma in the gastrointestinal tract: a potential mimic of primary neoplasia. Am J Surg Pathol 2011;35:563-572.

189. Wilentz RE, Su GH, Dai JL, et al. Immunohistochemical labeling for dpc4 mirrors genetic status in pancreatic adenocarcinomas: a new marker of DPC4 inactivation. Am J Pathol 2000;156:37-43.

190. Le DT, Uram JN, Wang H, et al. PD-1 blockade in tumors with mismatch-repair deficiency. N Engl J Med 2015;372:2509-2520.

191. Axelrad JE, Lichtiger S, Yajnik V. Inflammatory bowel disease and cancer: The role of inflammation, immunosuppression, and cancer treatment. World J Gastroenterol 2016;22:4794-4801.

192. Eaden JA, Abrams KR, Mayberry JF. The risk of colorectal cancer in ulcerative colitis: a meta-analysis. Gut 2001;48:526-535.

193. Friedman S, Rubin PH, Bodian C, Goldstein E, Harpaz N, Present DH. Screening and surveillance colonoscopy in chronic Crohn's colitis. Gastroenterology 2001;120:820-826.

194. Jess T, Simonsen J, Jorgensen KT, Pedersen BV, Nielsen NM, Frisch M. Decreasing risk of colorectal cancer in patients with inflammatory bowel disease over 30 years. Gastroenterology 2012;143:375-381 e371; quiz e313-374.

195. Beaugerie L, Svrcek M, Seksik P, et al. Risk of colorectal high-grade dysplasia and cancer in a prospective observational cohort of patients with inflammatory bowel disease. Gastroenterology 2013;145:166-175 e168.

196. Wang R, Leong RW. Primary sclerosing cholangitis as an independent risk factor for colorectal cancer in the context of inflammatory bowel disease: a review of the literature. World J Gastroenterol 2014;20:8783-8789.

197. Dyson JK, Rutter MD. Colorectal cancer in inflammatory bowel disease: what is the real magnitude of the risk? World J Gastroenterol 2012;18:3839-3848.

198. Laine L, Kaltenbach T, Barkun A, et al. SCENIC international consensus statement on surveillance and management of dysplasia in inflammatory bowel disease. Gastroenterology 2015;148:639-651.

199. Rubin DT, Rothe JA, Hetzel JT, Cohen RD, Hanauer SB. Are dysplasia and colorectal cancer endoscopically visible in patients with ulcerative colitis? Gastrointest Endosc 2007;65:998-1004.

200. Ullman T, Croog V, Harpaz N, Sachar D, Itzkowitz S. Progression of flat low-grade dysplasia to advanced neoplasia in patients with ulcerative colitis. Gastroenterology 2003;125:1311-1319.

201. Shergill AK, Farraye FA. Toward a consensus on endoscopic surveillance of patients with colonic inflammatory bowel disease. Gastrointest Endosc Clin N Am 2014;24:469-481.

202. Kisiel JB, Loftus EV Jr, Harmsen WS, Zinsmeister AR, Sandborn WJ. Outcome of sporadic adenomas and adenoma-like dysplasia in patients with ulcerative colitis undergoing polypectomy. Inflamm Bowel Dis 2012;18:226-235.

203. Srivastava A, Redston M, Farraye FA, Yantiss RK, Odze RD. Hyperplastic/serrated polyposis in inflammatory bowel disease: a case series of a previously undescribed entity. Am J Surg Pathol 2008;32:296-303.

204. Vogelstein B, Papadopoulos N, Velculescu VE, Zhou S, Diaz LA Jr, Kinzler KW. Cancer genome landscapes. Science 2013;339:1546-1558.

205. Aust DE, Terdiman JP, Willenbucher RF, et al. The APC/beta-catenin pathway in ulcerative colitis-related colorectal carcinomas: a mutational analysis. Cancer 2002;94:1421-1427.

206. Hussain SP, Amstad P, Raja K, et al. Increased p53 mutation load in noncancerous colon tissue from ulcerative colitis: a cancer-prone chronic inflammatory disease. Cancer Res 2000;60:3333-3337.

207. Walsh SV, Loda M, Torres CM, Antonioli D, Odze RD. P53 and beta catenin expression in chronic ulcerative colitis—associated polypoid dysplasia and sporadic adenomas: an immunohistochemical study. Am J Surg Pathol 1999;23:963-969.

208. Fleisher AS, Esteller M, Harpaz N, et al. Microsatellite instability in inflammatory bowel disease-associated neoplastic lesions is associated with hypermethylation and diminished expression of the DNA mismatch repair gene, hMLH1. Cancer Res 2000;60:4864-4868.

209. Dorer R, Odze RD. AMACR immunostaining is useful in detecting dysplastic epithelium in Barrett's esophagus, ulcerative colitis, and Crohn's disease. Am J Surg Pathol 2006;30:871-877.

210. Wong NA, Mayer NJ, MacKell S, Gilmour HM, Harrison DJ. Immunohistochemical assessment of Ki67 and p53 expression assists the diagnosis and grading of ulcerative colitis-related dysplasia. Histopathology 2000;37:108-114.

211. Odze RD, Farraye FA, Hecht JL, Hornick JL. Long-term follow-up after polypectomy treatment for adenoma-like dysplastic lesions in ulcerative colitis. Clin Gastroenterol Hepatol 2004;2:534-541.

212. Cannon-Albright LA, Skolnick MH, Bishop DT, Lee RG, Burt RW. Common inheritance of susceptibility to colonic adenomatous polyps and associated colorectal cancers. N Engl J Med 1988;319:533-537.

213. Lichtenstein P, Holm NV, Verkasalo PK, et al. Environmental and heritable factors in the causation of cancer—analyses of cohorts of twins from Sweden, Denmark, and Finland. N Engl J Med 2000;343:78-85.

214. Brosens LA, Offerhaus GJ, Giardiello FM. Hereditary colorectal cancer: genetics and screening. Surg Clin North Am 2015;95:1067-1080.

215. Ma C, Giardiello FM, Montgomery EA. Upper tract juvenile polyps in juvenile polyposis patients: dysplasia and malignancy are associated with foveolar, intestinal, and pyloric differentiation. Am J Surg Pathol 2014;38:1618-1626.

216. Ma X, Zhang B, Zheng W. Genetic variants associated with colorectal cancer risk: comprehensive research synopsis, meta-analysis, and epidemiological evidence. Gut 2014;63:326-336.

217. Lynch HT, Lynch JF, Lynch PM, Attard T. Hereditary colorectal cancer syndromes: molecular genetics, genetic counseling, diagnosis and management. Fam Cancer 2008;7:27-39.

218. Gala M, Chung DC. Hereditary colon cancer syndromes. Semin Oncol 2011;38:490-499.

219. Hamilton SR, Liu B, Parsons RE, et al. The molecular basis of Turcot's syndrome. N Engl J Med 1995;332:839-847.

220. Park JG, Vasen HF, Park YJ, et al. Suspected HNPCC and Amsterdam criteria II: evaluation of mutation detection rate, an international collaborative study. Int J Colorectal Dis 2002;17:109-114.

221. Umar A, Boland CR, Terdiman JP, et al. Revised Bethesda Guidelines for hereditary nonpolyposis colorectal cancer (Lynch syndrome) and microsatellite instability. J Natl Cancer Inst 2004;96:261-268.

222. Aronson M, Gallinger S, Cohen Z, et al. Gastrointestinal findings in the largest series of patients with hereditary biallelic mismatch repair deficiency syndrome: report from the International Consortium. Am J Gastroenterol 2016;111:275-284.

223. Durno CA, Holter S, Sherman PM, Gallinger S. The gastrointestinal phenotype of germline biallelic mismatch repair gene mutations. Am J Gastroenterol 2010;105:2449-2456.

224. Bandipalliam P. Syndrome of early onset colon cancers, hematologic malignancies & features of neurofibromatosis in HNPCC families with homozygous mismatch repair gene mutations. Fam Cancer 2005;4:323-333.

225. Kakar S, Smyrk TC. Signet ring cell carcinoma of the colorectum: correlations between microsatellite instability, clinicopathologic features and survival. Mod Pathol 2005;18:244-249.

226. Kakar S, Aksoy S, Burgart LJ, Smyrk TC. Mucinous carcinoma of the colon: correlation of loss of mismatch repair enzymes with clinicopathologic features and survival. Mod Pathol 2004;17:696-700.

227. Smyrk TC, Watson P, Kaul K, Lynch HT. Tumor-infiltrating lymphocytes are a marker for microsatellite instability in colorectal carcinoma. Cancer 2001;91:2417-2422.

228. Sinicrope F, Foster NR, Sargent DJ, et al. Model-based prediction of defective DNA mismatch repair using clinicopathological variables in sporadic colon cancer patients. Cancer 2010; 116:1691-1698.

229. Hitchins M, Williams R, Cheong K, et al. MLH1 germline epimutations as a factor in hereditary nonpolyposis colorectal cancer. Gastroenterology 2005;129:1392-1399.

230. Peltomaki P. Epigenetic mechanisms in the pathogenesis of Lynch syndrome. Clin Genet 2014;85:403-412.

231. Kovacs ME, Papp J, Szentirmay Z, Otto S, Olah E. Deletions removing the last exon of TACSTD1 constitute a distinct class of mutations predisposing to Lynch syndrome. Hum Mutat 2009;30:197-203.

232. Rumilla K, Schowalter KV, Lindor NM, et al. Frequency of deletions of EPCAM (TACSTD1) in MSH2-associated Lynch syndrome cases. J Mol Diagn 2011;13:93-99.

233. Ligtenberg MJ, Kuiper RP, Geurts van Kessel A, Hoogerbrugge N. EPCAM deletion carriers constitute a unique subgroup of Lynch syndrome patients. Fam Cancer 2013;12:169-174.

234. Ligtenberg MJ, Kuiper RP, Chan TL, et al. Heritable somatic methylation and inactivation of MSH2 in families with Lynch syndrome due to deletion of the 3' exons of TACSTD1. Nat Genet 2009;41:112-117.

235. Boland CR, Goel A. Microsatellite instability in colorectal cancer. Gastroenterology 2010;138:2073-2087.

236. Suraweera N, Duval A, Reperant M, et al. Evaluation of tumor microsatellite instability using five quasimonomorphic mononucleotide repeats and pentaplex PCR. Gastroenterology 2002;123:1804-1811.

237. Goel A, Nagasaka T, Hamelin R, Boland CR. An optimized pentaplex PCR for detecting DNA mismatch repair-deficient colorectal cancers. PLoS One 2010;5:e9393.

238. Syngal S, Brand RE, Church JM, et al. ACG clinical guideline: Genetic testing and management of hereditary gastrointestinal cancer syndromes. Am J Gastroenterol 2015;110:223-262; quiz 263.

239. Giardiello FM, Allen JI, Axilbund JE, et al. Guidelines on genetic evaluation and management of Lynch syndrome: a consensus statement by the US Multi-Society Task Force on colorectal cancer. Gastroenterology 2014;147:502-526.

240. Balmana J, Balaguer F, Cervantes A, Arnold D, ESMO Guidelines Working Group. Familial risk-colorectal cancer: ESMO Clinical Practice Guidelines. Ann Oncol 2013;24(Suppl 6):vi73-80.

241. Stoffel EM, Mangu PB, Gruber SB, et al. Hereditary colorectal cancer syndromes: American Society of Clinical Oncology Clinical Practice Guideline endorsement of the familial risk-colorectal cancer: European Society for Medical Oncology Clinical Practice Guidelines. J Clin Oncol 2015;33:209-217.

242. Moreira L, Balaguer F, Lindor N, et al. Identification of Lynch syndrome among patients with colorectal cancer. JAMA 2012;308):1555-1565.

243. Haraldsdottir S, Hampel H, Tomsic J, et al. Colon and endometrial cancers with mismatch repair deficiency can arise from somatic, rather than germline, mutations. Gastroenterology 2014;147:1308-1316.

244. German HNPCC Consortium, Muller A, Beckmann C, et al. Prevalence of the mismatch-repair-deficient phenotype in colonic adenomas arising in HNPCC patients: results of a 5-year follow-up study. Int J Colorectal Dis 2006;21:632-641.

245. Panarelli NC, Vaughn CP, Samowitz WS, Yantiss RK. Sporadic microsatellite instability-high colon cancers rarely display immunohistochemical evidence of Wnt signaling activation. Am J Surg Pathol 2015;39:313-317.

246. Affolter K, Samowitz W, Tripp S, Bronner MP. BRAF V600E mutation detection by immunohistochemistry in colorectal carcinoma. Genes Chromosomes Cancer 2013;52:748-752.

247. Sourrouille I, Coulet F, Lefevre JH, et al. Somatic mosaicism and double somatic hits can lead to MSI colorectal tumors. Fam Cancer 2013;12:27-33.

248. Castillejo A, Vargas G, Castillejo MI, et al. Prevalence of germline MUTYH mutations among Lynch-like syndrome patients. Eur J Cancer 2014;50:2241-2250.

249. Rhees J, Arnold M, Boland CR. Inversion of exons 1-7 of the MSH2 gene is a frequent cause of unexplained Lynch syndrome in one local population. Fam Cancer 2014;13:219-225.

250. Mensenkamp AR, Vogelaar IP, van Zelst-Stams WA, et al. Somatic mutations in MLH1 and MSH2 are a frequent cause of mismatch-repair deficiency in Lynch syndrome-like tumors. Gastroenterology 2014;146:643-646 e648.

251. Goodenberger ML, Thomas BC, Riegert-Johnson D, et al. PMS2 monoallelic mutation carriers: the known unknown. Genet Med 2016;18:13-19.

252. Gavin PG, Colangelo LH, Fumagalli D, et al. Mutation profiling and microsatellite instability in stage II and III colon cancer: an assessment of their prognostic and oxaliplatin predictive value. Clin Cancer Res 2012;18:6531-6541.

253. Llosa NJ, Cruise M, Tam A, et al. The vigorous immune microenvironment of microsatellite instable colon cancer is balanced by multiple counter-inhibitory checkpoints. Cancer Discov 2015;5:43-51.

254. Lindor NM, Rabe K, Petersen GM, et al. Lower cancer incidence in Amsterdam-I criteria families without mismatch repair deficiency: familial colorectal cancer type X. JAMA 2005;293:1979-1985.

255. Shiovitz S, Copeland WK, Passarelli MN, et al. Characterisation of familial colorectal cancer Type X, Lynch syndrome, and non-familial colorectal cancer. Br J Cancer 2014;111:598-602.

256. Nieminen TT, O'Donohue MF, Wu Y, et al. Germline mutation of RPS20, encoding a ribosomal protein, causes predisposition to hereditary nonpolyposis colorectal carcinoma without DNA mismatch repair deficiency. Gastroenterology 2014;147:595-598.

257. Zeng C, Matsuda K, Jia WH, et al. Identification of Susceptibility loci and genes for colorectal cancer risk. Gastroenterology 2016;150:1633-1645.

258. Schulz E, Klampfl P, Holzapfel S, et al. Germline variants in the SEMA4A gene predispose to familial colorectal cancer type X. Nat Commun 2014;5:5191.

259. Wei C, Peng B, Han Y, et al. Mutations of HNRNPA0 and WIF1 predispose members of a large family to multiple cancers. Fam Cancer 2015;14:297-306.

260. Spier I, Drichel D, Kerick M, et al. Low-level APC mutational mosaicism is the underlying cause in a substantial fraction of unexplained colorectal adenomatous polyposis cases. J Med Genet 2016;53:172-179.

261. Schulz AC, Bojarski C, Buhr HJ, Kroesen AJ. Occurrence of adenomas in the pouch and small intestine of FAP patients after proctocolectomy with ileoanal pouch construction. Int J Colorectal Dis 2008;23:437-441.

262. Crail HW. Multiple primary malignancies arising in the rectum, brain, and thyroid; report of a case. U S Nav Med Bull 1949;49:123-128.

263. Turcot J, Despres JP, St Pierre F. Malignant tumors of the central nervous system associated with familial polyposis of the colon: report of two cases. Dis Colon Rectum 1959;2:465-468.

264. Wallis YL, Macdonald F, Hulten M, et al. Genotype-phenotype correlation between position of constitutional APC gene mutation and CHRPE expression in familial adenomatous polyposis. Hum Genet 1994;94:543-548.

265. Arnason T, Liang WY, Alfaro E, et al. Morphology and natural history of familial adenomatous polyposis-associated dysplastic fundic gland polyps. Histopathology 2014;65:353-362.

266. Jass JR. Colorectal polyposes: from phenotype to diagnosis. Pathol Res Pract 2008;204:431-447.

267. Borras E, San Lucas FA, Chang K, et al. Genomic landscape of colorectal mucosa and adenomas. Cancer Prev Res (Phila) 2016;9:417-427.

268. Powell SM, Petersen GM, Krush AJ, et al. Molecular diagnosis of familial adenomatous polyposis. N Engl J Med 1993;329:1982-1987.

269. Leppert M, Burt R, Hughes JP, et al. Genetic analysis of an inherited predisposition to colon cancer in a family with a variable number of adenomatous polyps. N Engl J Med 1990;322:904-908.

270. Spirio LN, Samowitz W, Robertson J, et al. Alleles of APC modulate the frequency and classes of mutations that lead to colon polyps. Nat Genet 1998;20:385-388.

271. Pavicic W, Nieminen TT, Gylling A, et al. Promoter-specific alterations of APC are a rare cause for mutation-negative familial adenomatous polyposis. Genes Chromosomes Cancer 2014;53:857-864.

272. Snow AK, Tuohy TM, Sargent NR, Smith LJ, Burt RW, Neklason DW. APC promoter 1B deletion in seven American families with familial adenomatous polyposis. Clin Genet 2015;88:360-365.

273. Li J, Woods SL, Healey S, et al. Point mutations in exon 1B of APC reveal gastric adenocarcinoma and proximal polyposis of the stomach as a familial adenomatous polyposis variant. Am J Hum Genet 2016;98:830-842.

274. White BD, Chien AJ, Dawson DW. Dysregulation of Wnt/β-catenin signaling in gastrointestinal cancers. Gastroenterology 2012;142:219-232.

275. Lamlum H, Ilyas M, Rowan A, et al. The type of somatic mutation at APC in familial adenomatous polyposis is determined by the site of the germ-line mutation: a new facet to Knudson's 'two-hit' hypothesis. Nat Med 1999;5:1071-1075.

276. Albuquerque C, Breukel C, van der Luijt R, et al. The 'just-right' signaling model: APC somatic mutations are selected based on a specific level of activation of the beta-catenin signaling cascade. Hum Mol Genet 2002;11:1549-1560.

277. Kennedy RD, Potter DD, Moir CR, El-Youssef M. The natural history of familial adenomatous polyposis syndrome: a 24 year review of a single center experience in screening, diagnosis, and outcomes. J Pediatr Surg 2014;49:82-86.

278. Septer S, Lawson CE, Anant S, Attard T. Familial adenomatous polyposis in pediatrics: natural history, emerging surveillance and management protocols, chemopreventive strategies, and areas of ongoing debate. Fam Cancer 2016;15:477-485.

279. Baron TH, Smyrk TC, Rex DK. Recommended intervals between screening and surveillance colonoscopies. Mayo Clin Proc 2013;88:854-858.

280. Samadder NJ, Neklason DW, Boucher KM, et al. Effect of Sulindac and Erlotinib vs placebo on duodenal neoplasia in familial adenomatous polyposis: a randomized clinical trial. JAMA 2016;315:1266-1275.

281. Ricciardiello L, Ahnen DJ, Lynch PM. Chemoprevention of hereditary colon cancers: time for new strategies. Nat Rev Gastroenterol Hepatol 2016;13:352-361.

282. Landon M, Ceulemans S, Saraiya DS, et al. Analysis of current testing practices for biallelic MUTYH mutations in MUTYH-associated polyposis. Clin Genet 2015;87:368-372.

283. Rashid M, Fischer A, Wilson CH, et al. Adenoma development in familial adenomatous polyposis and MUTYH-associated polyposis: somatic landscape and driver genes. J Pathol 2016;238:98-108.

284. Grover S, Kastrinos F, Steyerberg EW, et al. Prevalence and phenotypes of APC and MUTYH mutations in patients with multiple colorectal adenomas. JAMA 2012;308:485-492.

285. Win AK, Reece JC, Dowty JG, et al. Risk of extracolonic cancers for people with biallelic and monoallelic mutations in MUTYH. Int J Cancer 2016;139:1557-1563.

286. Aretz S, Uhlhaas S, Goergens H, et al. MUTYH-associated polyposis: 70 of 71 patients with biallelic mutations present with an attenuated or atypical phenotype. Int J Cancer 2006;119:807-814.

287. Walton SJ, Kallenberg FG, Clark SK, Dekker E, Latchford A. Frequency and features of duodenal adenomas in patients with MUTYH-associated polyposis. Clin Gastroenterol Hepatol 2016;14:986-992.

288. Vogt S, Jones N, Christian D, et al. Expanded extracolonic tumor spectrum in MUTYH-associated polyposis. Gastroenterology 2009;137:1976-1985.

289. Knopperts AP, Nielsen M, Niessen RC, et al. Contribution of bi-allelic germline MUTYH mutations to early-onset and familial colorectal cancer and to low number of adenomatous polyps: case-series and literature review. Fam Cancer 2013;12:43-50.

290. Guarinos C, Juarez M, Egoavil C, et al. Prevalence and characteristics of MUTYH-associated polyposis in patients with multiple adenomatous and serrated polyps. Clin Cancer Res 2014;20:1158-1168.

291. Lefevre JH, Colas C, Coulet F, et al. MYH biallelic mutation can inactivate the two genetic pathways of colorectal cancer by APC or MLH1 transversions. Fam Cancer 2010;9:589-594.

292. Giardiello FM, Hamilton SR, Kern SE, et al. Colorectal neoplasia in juvenile polyposis or juvenile polyps. Arch Dis Child 1991;66;971-975.

293. Delnatte C, Sanlaville D, Mougenot JF, Stoppa-Lyonnet D. [Contiguous gene deletion within chromosome arm 10q is associated with juvenile polyposis of infancy, reflecting cooperation between the BMPR1A and PTEN tumor-suppressor genes.] Med Sci (Paris) 2006;22:912-913. [French]

294. Howe JR, Sayed MG, Ahmed AF, et al. The prevalence of MADH4 and BMPR1A mutations in juvenile polyposis and absence of BMPR2, BMPR1B, and ACVR1 mutations. J Med Genet 2004;41:484-491.

295. Hizawa K, Iida M, Matsumoto T, et al. Cancer in Peutz-Jeghers syndrome. Cancer 1993;72:2777-2781.

296. Hizawa K, Iida M, Matsumoto T, et al. Cancer in Peutz-Jeghers syndrome. Cancer 1993;72:2777-2781.

297. Watanabe H, Suda T. [Precancerous lesions of the colon and rectum]. Gan To Kagaku Ryoho 1984;11:1-9.

298. Snover D, Ahnen D, Burt R, Odze RD. Serrated polyps of the colon and rectum and serrated polyposis. In: Bosman F, Carneiro F, Hruban R, Theise N, eds. WHO Classification of Tumours of the Digestive System. Lyon: IARC; 2010:160-165.

299. Bick BL, Ponugoti PL, Rex DK. High yield of synchronous lesions in referred patients with large lateral spreading colorectal tumors. Gastrointest Endosc 2016. [Epub ahead of print]

300. Chow E, Lipton L, Lynch E, et al. Hyperplastic polyposis syndrome: phenotypic presentations and the role of MBD4 and MYH. Gastroenterology 2006;131:30-39.

301. Jass JR. Gastrointestinal polyposes: clinical, pathological and molecular features. Gastroenterol Clin North Am 2007;36:927-946, viii.

302. Boparai KS, Reitsma JB, Lemmens V, et al. Increased colorectal cancer risk in first-degree relatives of patients with hyperplastic polyposis syndrome. Gut 2010;59:1222-1225.

303. Boparai KS, Mathus-Vliegen EM, Koornstra JJ, et al. Increased colorectal cancer risk during follow-up in patients with hyperplastic polyposis syndrome: a multicentre cohort study. Gut 2010;59:1094-1100.

304. Holme O, Bretthauer M, Eide TJ, et al. Long-term risk of colorectal cancer in individuals with serrated polyps. Gut 2015;64:929-936.

305. Lage P, Cravo M, Sousa R, et al. Management of Portuguese patients with hyperplastic polyposis and screening of at-risk first-degree relatives: a contribution for future guidelines based on a clinical study. Am J Gastroenterol 2004;99:1779-1784.

5 TUMORS AND TUMOR-LIKE LESIONS OF THE VERMIFORM APPENDIX

Primary malignant neoplasms of the appendix are rare, with an age-adjusted incidence of 0.12 cases per 1,000,000 person-years. They are diagnosed unexpectedly in approximately 1 percent of all appendectomy specimens (1,2). About two thirds of cases can be further classified into three major histologic subtypes: *mucinous neoplasms, nonmucinous* (or *colonic-type*) *neoplasms*, and *goblet cell carcinoid tumor* and the associated adenocarcinoma (*adenocarcinoma ex goblet cell carcinoid tumor*) with a predominant signet ring cell morphology. Well-differentiated neuroendocrine (carcinoid) tumor of the appendix is covered in chapter 7.

BENIGN AND DYSPLASTIC HYPERPLASTIC/ SERRATED AND NONINVASIVE LESIONS

General Features. Serrated lesions of colorectum are discussed in chapters 3 and 4. *Serrated appendiceal lesions* have been classified using current diagnostic terminology for the colorectum as described by the World Health Organization (WHO): *hyperplastic polyp (HP), sessile serrated adenoma/polyp (SSA/P), SSA/P with cytologic dysplasia*, and *traditional serrated adenoma (TSA)* (3–6). While these appendiceal lesions are reported to occur in older patients than those of the colorectum (6), most are identified incidentally in appendectomy specimens and their epidemiology is poorly understood.

Microscopic Findings. Most serrated lesions in the appendix circumferentially involve the mucosa (5,6). Given their location in the smallest organ of the gastrointestinal tract, with a very narrow lumen, and the fact that they are almost always cross-sectioned perpendicularly to the length of the appendix for histologic examination, their configuration in the appendix may not be entirely comparable with that of their colorectal counterparts.

HPs are morphologically similar to those in the colorectum, which have tall columnar cells and goblet cells with ample eosinophilic cytoplasm and apical microvesicular mucin. Serration is usually present on the superficial aspect of the lesion, without full length extension to the base of the crypts. Typical SSA/Ps contain both non-goblet columnar cells and goblet cells, which demonstrate prominent crypt serration and dilation that extends the entire length of the crypts to their bases, either with or without branching in the deep mucosa (fig. 5-1A). Both HP and SSA/P lack significant surface cytologic atypia but may show mild nuclear enlargement and hyperchromasia in the deep crypts (fig. 5-1B). While the degree of serration and extent of lumen dilation separate HPs from SSA/Ps, these morphologic criteria are subjective, and in many circumstances, distinction between an appendiceal HP and SSA/P is challenging, particular in suboptimally oriented specimens; sometimes features of both lesions are present in one specimen (fig. 1C).

The morphologic features of dysplasia in serrated lesions of the appendix (SSA/P with cytologic dysplasia) and lesions classified as TSA are comparable with those of their colorectal counterparts (see chapter 3). Neoplastic cells have enlarged but not fully stratified hyperchromatic nuclei and abundant eosinophilic cytoplasm; crypt necrosis may be present (fig. 5-2A,B). Appendiceal adenocarcinomas that arise in association with serrated dysplasia exhibit a nonmucinous and intestinal phenotype, with or without apparent luminal serrations, similar to colorectal adenocarcinomas (discussed in chapter 4) (fig. 5-2C).

Molecular Genetic Findings. A number of molecular genetic investigations have been carried out to characterize various phenotypes and molecular pathways of appendiceal serrated lesions. In contrast to the distinct serrated neoplastic pathway in the colon and rectum characterized by mutations in *BRAF,* progressive DNA methylation, and microsatellite instability

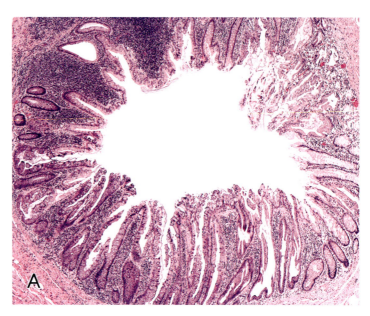

Figure 5-1

NONDYSPLASTIC SERRATED LESIONS

A: Low-power view of a sessile serrated adenoma/polyp (SSA/P), with full length serration, with or without base crypt branching.

B,C: High-power view shows subtle differences between SSA/P (B) and hyperplastic polyp (C), with varying degrees of serration and crypt dilatation.

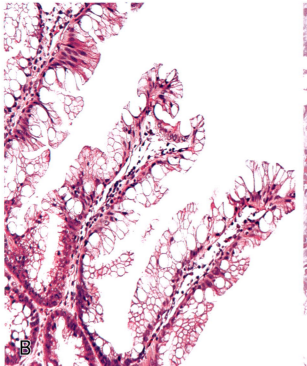

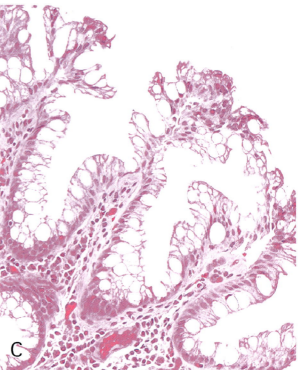

(7,8), appendiceal serrated lesions, either in sporadic cases or in polyposis syndromes, have instead demonstrated a high frequency of *KRAS* mutations (34 to 52 percent) but *BRAF* mutations are infrequent (7 to 29 percent), and high-level CpG island methylator phenotype (CIMP) is not typically identified (5,6,9). Thus the limited molecular studies, with the primary

focus on *KRAS* mutations, *BRAF* mutations, and microsatellite stability, have failed to establish the relationship between appendiceal serrated lesions and appendiceal adenocarcinomas. Next-generation sequencing may result in the discovery of pathways governing the relationship between serrated polyps and appendiceal adenocarcinoma (10), however, the current data

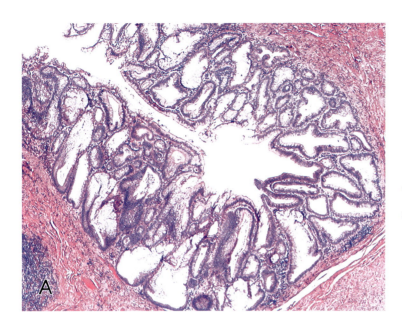

Figure 5-2

DYSPLASTIC SERRATED LESIONS AND ASSOCIATED ADENOCARCINOMA

A: SSA/P with apparent dysplasia.

B: High-power view of a serrated lesion with low- and high-grade dysplasia.

C: Adenocarcinoma arising in a serrated dysplastic lesion.

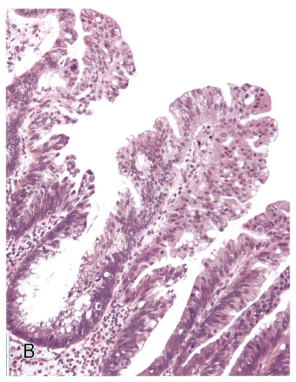

suggest that the appendiceal serrated pathway differs from that in the colorectum.

Treatment and Prognosis. Simple HP and typical SSA/P, although difficult to differentiate from each other, do not progress to invasive or disseminated adenocarcinoma once the appendix is removed; as such, the distinction between the subtypes is of no clinical consequence. SSA/P with cytologic dysplasia and TSA have a risk for the development of invasive appendiceal adenocarcinoma but resection of these precursors is also curative. Given the equivocal morphologic criteria for the subclassification of serrated lesions in the appendix, some observers have suggested classifying them simply as nondysplastic serrated lesions and dysplastic serrated lesions (5,6).

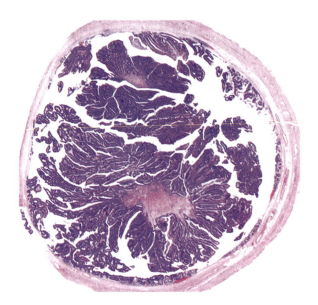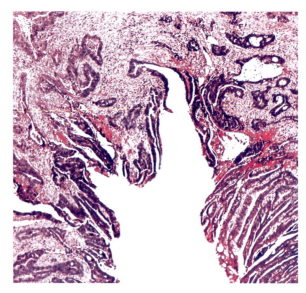

Figure 5-3

CONVENTIONAL TUBULAR ADENOMA AND ASSOCIATED ADENOCARCINOMA

Left: Circumferential involvement of a tubulovillous adenoma.
Right: Adenocarcinoma of colorectal type arising in a conventional adenoma.

CONVENTIONAL TUBULAR/TUBULOVILLOUS ADENOMA OF NONMUCINOUS AND NONSERRATED SUBTYPE AND ASSOCIATED ADENOCARCINOMA

General Features. *Appendiceal colorectal-type adenomas without prominent mucinous features* are rare and the associated adenocarcinomas account for less than 30 percent of all appendiceal malignancies and approximately 40 percent of all appendiceal adenocarcinomas (11). While their genetic alterations are similar to those of adenocarcinomas arising in association with appendiceal mucinous neoplasms (6), given their distinct clinical and pathologic features, the latter are discussed separately below. Appendiceal conventional adenomas may present as sporadic polyps with coexisting colorectal adenomas, or within the spectrum of familial adenomatous polyposis syndrome (discussed in chapter 4) (12,13).

Clinical Features. In contrast to appendiceal mucinous adenocarcinomas, which often present with pseudomyxoma peritonei, nonmucinous adenocarcinomas more commonly present with appendicitis and acute abdomen (14). The pattern of disease progression of appendiceal nonmucinous adenocarcinoma is comparable to that of its colorectal counterpart, with frequent distant solid organ (liver and lung) metastases, and the prognosis of stage IV disease is worse than that of mucinous adenocarcinoma (11,14).

Microscopic Findings. Similar to conventional adenomas of the colorectum, appendiceal nonmucinous adenoma exhibits a predominant tubular or tubulovillous configuration and the epithelium has complete or incomplete mucin depletion with nuclear elongation and stratification (fig. 5-3, left). Increased cellular crowding, nuclear pleomorphism, and loss of cellular polarity are evident as the lesions progress from low- to high-grade dysplasia. Appendiceal adenocarcinomas that develop in association with adenomas exhibit a typical intestinal phenotype (fig. 5-3, right) (4). Other histologic subtypes, as classified by the WHO (15), such as high-grade neuroendocrine carcinoma of small or large cell type and mixed adeno-neuroendocrine carcinoma, are rare.

Molecular Genetic Findings. Appendiceal adenocarcinomas arising in association with adenomatous polyps demonstrate morphologic and genetic progression in the classic colorectal adenoma–adenocarcinoma sequence, although p53 abnormalities are less frequently reported (10,14). This genotype, however, may reflect the inclusion of heterogeneous phenotypes of appendiceal adenocarcinoma, including adenocarcinoma ex goblet cell carcinoid tumor. Appendiceal adenocarcinomas generally have a microsatellite stable phenotype (10,14).

MUCINOUS NEOPLASM

Appendiceal mucinous neoplasm is the most common epithelial neoplasm of the appendix; it comprises approximately 33 percent of all appendiceal neoplasms. The associated adenocarcinomas account for about half of appendiceal adenocarcinomas, compared to 10 percent of colorectal adenocarcinomas that show a mucinous phenotype (16). Mucinous neoplasms are identified incidentally in appendectomy specimens performed for acute appendicitis (11) or present with peritoneal dissemination, i.e., PMP.

Mucinous adenocarcinomas comprise a heterogeneous group of tumors with a prognosis that reflects the histologic subtype, tumor grade, and pathologic stage (11,17–20). There have been many proffered classification and staging schemes for primary appendiceal mucinous neoplasms and their associated PMP, using both the histopathologic and clinical characteristics of the tumor with controversial designations and terminology (Table 5-1) (20–25). The dilemma of tumor classification and nomenclature will likely remain the subject of debate (20,26), and there is considerable confusion in both routine pathology practice and in clinical management of the disease (18,19).

Nomenclature. *Mucocele* denotes gross dilation of the epithelial lumen with mucin accumulation; it is not a histologic diagnosis. It usually develops in the presence of luminal obstruction secondary to a neoplasm, inspissated mucin, or a non-neoplastic process such as fecalith, postinflammatory scar, or endometriosis (27). The epithelial lining of a mucocele may or may not be dysplastic/neoplastic, although most cases are due to neoplasms rather than non-neoplastic etiologies. The term "mucocele" should be eliminated from pathology reports to avoid the confusion regarding the etiology of this group of lesions.

This section intends to acknowledge and consolidate a spectrum of pathologic characteristics of the appendiceal mucinous neoplasm using nomenclatures and classifications that harmonize with those in the American Joint Committee on Cancer (AJCC) and WHO system, in which the staging and classification are generally synchronized throughout the entire gastrointestinal tract. However, under some circumstances, a definitive distinction between an appendiceal mucinous adenoma and a low-grade mucinous adenocarcinoma can be challenging on pathologic assessment alone. Many factors can contribute this uncertainty which include the paucicellular nature of the low-grade neoplasm, mishandling of the gross specimen, and suboptimal orientation of the histologic sections. Thus, for practical purposes, pathology of the following categories associated with appendiceal mucinous neoplasms will be discussed: 1) *mucinous adenoma (including cystadenoma)*; 2) *mucinous adenocarcinoma*; 3) *mucinous neoplasms that are not readily classified as either adenoma or adenocarcinoma;* and 4) *disseminated mucinous adenocarcinoma (PMP)*.

Appendiceal Mucinous Adenoma. *Appendiceal mucinous adenoma* can be defined as a mucinous neoplasm confined to the appendiceal mucosa with intact normal histologic landmarks; it is unassociated with lamina propria fibrosis, obliteration of the muscularis mucosae, or alterations in the appendiceal wall (28). Thus, in the presence of PMP, identification of dysplastic epithelia in appendiceal mucosa supports an appendiceal primary. In contrast to conventional/nonmucinous tubular adenomas in other sites of the gastrointestinal tract, which often present as discrete polyps, appendiceal mucinous adenoma commonly shows circumferential luminal involvement (19), with villous or papillary architecture (fig. 5-4A). It usually contains cytologically bland columnar epithelial cells with basally oriented nuclei. Abundant intracellular mucin can render nuclear stratification less apparent, particularly at the surface, and nuclear atypia is better appreciated towards the crypt base (fig. 5-4B). High-grade dysplasia is uncommon, but appears as nuclear stratification, nucleomegaly, and loss of cellular polarity accompanied by decreased cytoplasmic mucin (fig. 5-4C). Architectural complexity may appear as crypt crowding, cribriform growth, and apical budding from the tips of papillae (fig. 5-4D).

Table 5-1

TERMINOLOGY FOR MUCINOUS APPENDICEAL LESIONS

System	Terminology for Lesions Confined to the Appendix	Terminology for Lesions that have Spread to the Peritoneum	
		Low Grade	High Grade
World Health Organization (WHO)	**Adenoma** (dysplastic epithelium is confined within lamina propria) **Low-grade appendiceal mucinous neoplasm (LAMN)** (neoplastic epithelium is present in atrophic submucosa and/or muscularis propria; lamina propria and muscularis mucosae are lost; neoplastic cells have bland cytology and are arranged in single layer)	**Low-grade mucinous carcinoma peritonei/pseudomyxoma peritonei** (usually associated with LAMN; neoplastic cells form strips or small islands; cells may be very scanty; the mucin may appear acellular)	**High-grade mucinous carcinoma peritonei/pseudomyxoma peritonei** (neoplastic cells form strips, small islands, or cribriform structure with hypercellularity and extensive invasion of underlying organisms
Carr (20)[a]	**Low-grade appendiceal mucinous neoplasm (LAMN)** (mucinous neoplasm with low-grade cytologic atypia and any of: loss of muscularis mucosae; fibrosis of submucosa; "pushing invasion" (expansile or diverticulum-like growth); dissection of acellular mucin in wall; undulating or flattened epithelial growth; rupture of appendix; and mucin and/or cells outside appendix **High-grade appendiceal mucinous neoplasm (HAMN)** *(mucinous neoplasm with the architectural features of LAMN and no infiltrative invasion, but with high-grade cytologic atypia*	**Mucinous adenocarcinoma, well-differentiated** (low-grade mucinous neoplasm with infiltrative invasion within a a desmoplastic stroma)	Mucinous adenocarcinoma, moderately or poorly differentiated (features of infiltrative invasion with tumor budding and/or small, irregular glands within a desmoplastic stroma) **Poorly differentiated (mucinous) adenocarcinoma with signet ring cells** (neoplasm with signet ring cells [≤50% of cells]) **Carcinoma** (neoplasm with signet ring cells [>50% of cells])
Ronnett (21)	Not applicable	Disseminated peritoneal adenomucinosis (PDAM)	Peritoneal mucinous carcinomatosis (PMCA)
Pai (31)	Mucinous Adenoma Mucinous neoplasm of uncertain malignant potential	Mucinous neoplasm of low malignant potential	Mucinous adenocarcinoma
Misdraji (23)	Low-grade appendiceal mucinous neoplasm (LAMN)	Low-grade appendiceal mucinous neoplasm (LAMN)	Mucinous adenocarcinoma

[a]Numbers in parentheses indicate references.

The term *mucinous cystadenoma*, not endorsed by the WHO, has been applied to lesions with prominent appendiceal dilation from mucin produced by the neoplasm. The gross appearance of the appendix varies from localized and diffuse luminal dilatation to a substantial cystic mass (fig. 5-5A,5B). In these cases, the epithelium may be compressed, atrophic, or variably denuded, leaving large portions of the cystic wall devoid of epithelial lining (fig. 5-6A). Progressive distention culminates in attenuation of the appendiceal wall and alteration of normal histologic landmarks with fibrous obliteration of the muscularis mucosae and submucosa, or replacement of the muscularis propria by hyalinized fibrosis (fig. 5-6B). In this situation, distinction between an adenoma and a well differentiated/low- grade mucinous adenocarcinoma with pushing invasion may become challenging, resulting in classification

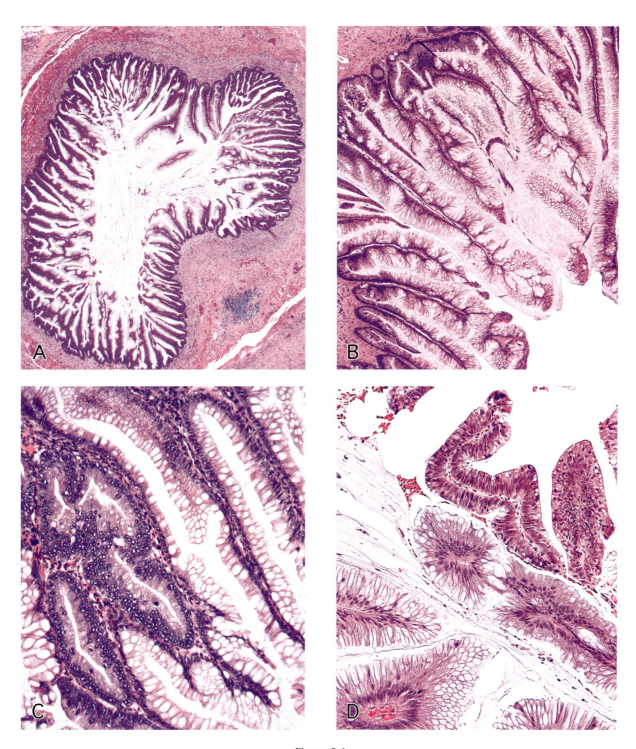

Figure 5-4

MUCINOUS ADENOMA

A: Circumferential involvement by a mucinous adenoma.

B: High-power view of mucinous adenoma with abundant intracellular apical mucin and minimal nuclear stratification on the superficial aspect.

C: Mucinous adenoma with increased dysplasia (from top to bottom).

D: Mucinous adenoma with low-grade (bottom) and high-grade (top) dysplasia.

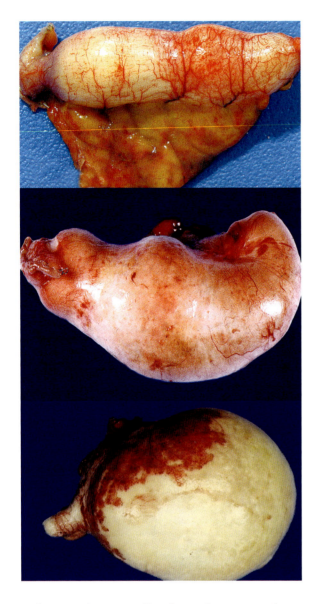

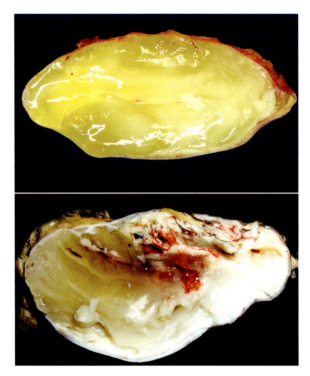

Figure 5-5

MUCINOUS NEOPLASM

Left: Intact appendix with cystic dilation.
Below: Gelatinous (upper) and calcified mucin accumulation (lower) in the lumen.

as low-grade appendiceal mucinous neoplasm (LAMN), as described below (fig. 5-6C) (29). There are no data to suggest that adenomas or low-grade mucinous neoplasms confined to the appendix carry significant risk of recurrence or disseminated peritoneal disease, so the distinction is somewhat arbitrary (20).

Another common and practical issue that may complicate the diagnosis of a non-invasive mucinous adenoma is the presence of an appendiceal diverticulum that results from excessive mucin production by the adenoma. Increased appendiceal luminal pressure may culminate in herniation of mucosal elements through the muscularis propria with associated mucin pools

lying deep in the appendiceal wall, including misplacement of neoplastic epithelium. This is particularly challenging because mucinous adenocarcinomas of the appendix are often well differentiated and display minimal cytological atypia, and they are often indistinguishable from the epithelium of the non-invasive counterpart even at the site of metastasis. Copious lamina propria around misplaced epithelium suggests a benign diverticulum, but it can be essentially impossible to distinguish between herniated neoplastic epithelium and well-differentiated low-grade mucinous adenocarcinoma (fig. 5-7B) (30). If a connection to the luminal surface cannot be established, alternative

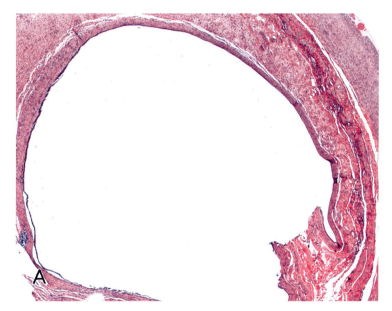

Figure 5-6

MUCINOUS "CYSTADENOMA"

A: Mucinous cystadenoma with a markedly dilated lumen, partially lined by attenuated dysplastic epithelium.

B: Mucinous cystadenoma with loss of muscularis mucosae and submucosal fibrosis.

C: Noninvasive mucinous adenoma with epithelium present in the superficial and hyalinized appendiceal wall simulating invasive adenocarcinoma.

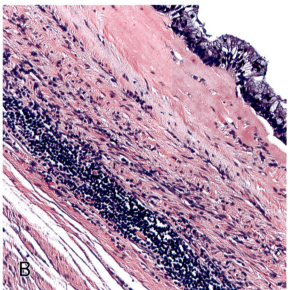

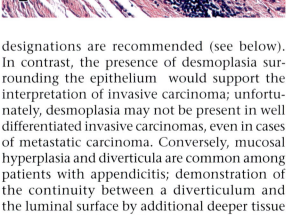

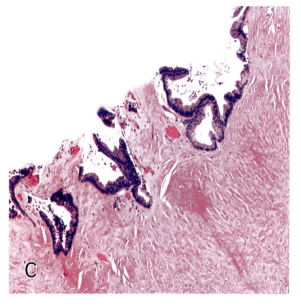

designations are recommended (see below). In contrast, the presence of desmoplasia surrounding the epithelium would support the interpretation of invasive carcinoma; unfortunately, desmoplasia may not be present in well differentiated invasive carcinomas, even in cases of metastatic carcinoma. Conversely, mucosal hyperplasia and diverticula are common among patients with appendicitis; demonstration of the continuity between a diverticulum and the luminal surface by additional deeper tissue sections can help confirm the non-neoplastic nature of the lesion.

The diagnosis of mucinous adenoma should be reserved for adenomatous lesions unequivocally confined to the appendiceal lumen without intra- or extramural neoplastic epithelium. This necessitates diligent handling of appendectomy specimens by both surgeon and pathologist. Particular care must be taken when manipulating the cyst to prevent extramural contamination by cyst contents, which may complicate the microscopic evaluation and assessment of margin status (fig. 5-8) (18). The final diagnosis of a mucinous adenoma can only be established after microscopic examination

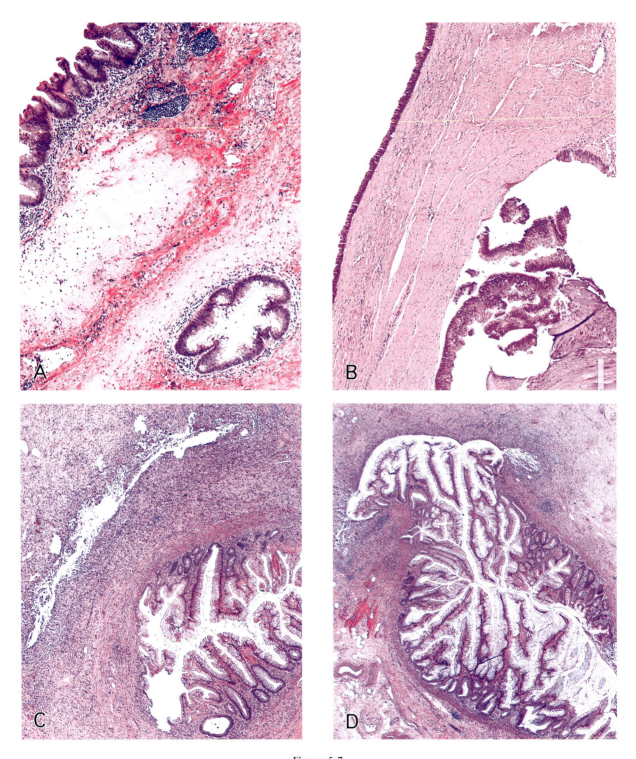

Figure 5-7

MUCINOUS ADENOMA WITH DIVERTICULUM/MUCOSAL HERNIATION

A: Herniated dysplastic epithelium is rimmed by lamina propria, indicating the noninvasive nature.

B: Herniated dysplastic epithelium and mucin simulating invasive adenocarcinoma.

C,D: An appendiceal mucinous adenoma with a diverticulum presents as a mucin pool without epithelium (C) and is better recognized in a deeper section (D).

of the entirely submitted appendectomy specimen. When mucin is found outside the appendix without unequivocal evidence of mural invasive carcinoma, alternative terminology is suggested depending upon whether neoplastic cells are detected within the mucin, as discussed below.

Mucinous Adenocarcinoma. *Mucinous adenocarcinoma* of the appendix shows variable morphologic features. It is important to acknowledge that numerous previous investigations have contributed to the understanding of the natural progression of mucinous neoplasm of the appendix, and it is well established that clinical outcomes are strongly associated with specific histologic characteristics and pathologic stage (21–23,30,31,37). Nevertheless, some of the clinical and pathologic terminology has not been universally accepted. It would now be prudent to consolidate some of the confusing nomenclatures with a standardized classification to facilitate the communication among pathologists and clinicians. Therefore, the diagnostic criteria for invasive mucinous adenocarcinoma of the appendix should be harmonized, as closely as possible, with those for adenocarcinomas in the rest of the gastrointestinal tract. Histologic features that are clinically pertinent and unique to the appendiceal mucinous adenocarcinoma can be used to provide additional prognostic grouping of the carcinoma (Table 5-1).

At one end of the spectrum, extremely low-grade carcinomas consist of paucicellular mucin pools that contain scant, cytologically bland mucinous epithelium. This subtype of mucinous adenocarcinoma possesses the potential for peritoneal dissemination, i.e., PMP with infrequent metastasis to solid organs (e.g., liver, lung), and an indolent but progressive clinical course. The unusual disease distribution, biologic behavior, and deceptively bland appearance of peritoneal disease have led some pathologists and clinicians to question a diagnosis of malignancy for this subtype even when low-grade neoplastic epithelium is present at the metastatic site of peritoneum. Consequently, low-grade mucinous carcinomas of the appendix have been variably designated as *low-grade appendiceal mucinous neoplasm* (LAMN) (20,23), *mucinous neoplasm of low-grade malignant potential* (31),

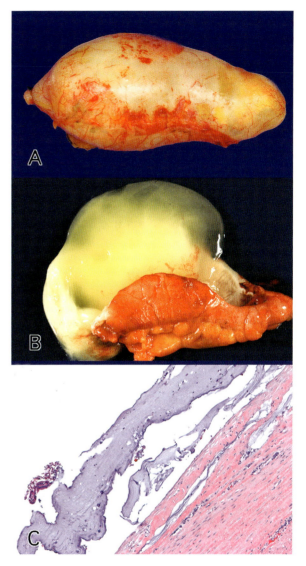

Figure 5-8

MUCINOUS ADENOMA WITH MUCIN CONTAMINATION FROM PROSECTION

A confined mucinous cystadenoma (A) with high luminal pressure and mucin contamination of the outside surface of the appendix (B) culminating in the presence of extramural mucin and detached epithelium (C).

and *mucinous tumor of uncertain malignant potential* (Table 5-1) (28,31).

Low-grade/well-differentiated mucinous carcinoma is often associated with bland neoplastic mucinous epithelium that may be indistinguishable from the non-invasive adenomatous epithelium confined to the mucosa. The pattern of invasion consists of a pushing front with associated hyalinizing stromal fibrosis and mucin dissection (either accompanied by or unassociated with scant epithelial cells) into the surrounding stroma. Desmoplasia is not a typical feature at either the primary site or in metastases (fig. 5-9A). Rather, tumors consist of mucin pools that contain floating strips of bland mucinous epithelium, or epithelium attached to the stroma at the edges of mucin pools (fig. 5-9B). The nuclei of the neoplastic cells are mildly to moderately atypical, and cellular polarization is preserved. Most mucin pools are entirely devoid of malignant epithelium and the likely explanation is that the mural invasive carcinoma is not represented in the sections submitted for evaluation (fig. 5-9C).

It is not uncommon to encounter mucinous neoplasms seemingly confined to the mucosa that are accompanied by paucicellular or acellular mucin dissecting into the appendiceal wall (fig. 5-9D). Diligent pathologic assessment, including a meticulous gross description of the specimen, evaluation of the entirely submitted appendix, and deeper sections of tissue blocks to search for malignant epithelium are necessary to exclude the possibility of extra-appendiceal mucinous epithelium (i.e., mucinous adenocarcinoma).

Some morphologic features may provide clues as to whether extra-appendiceal mucin pools represent part of an invasive carcinoma or spillage secondary to a ruptured cystadenoma (32). Passive mucin spillage induced by high luminal pressure is often associated with an intense inflammatory response that includes lymphocytes, neutrophils, and histiocytes. In contrast, mucin dissection secondary to invasive carcinoma lacks the inflammatory response, which gives rise to a "clean" appearance (fig. 5-10A,B).

When neoplastic epithelium is identified outside the appendiceal wall, a diagnosis of mucinous adenocarcinoma should be established even in the absence of high-grade luminal epithelial dysplasia, and all sites of mural or extramural mucin should be regarded as evidence of carcinoma. If all efforts fail to determine the nature of focal mural mucin pools without epithelial cells, however, a designation of low-grade appendiceal mucinous neoplasm (LAMN) with uncertain malignant potential may be rendered, as discussed below.

At the other end of the spectrum, some appendiceal mucinous adenocarcinomas resemble conventional colorectal type adenocarcinoma with a destructive and infiltrative pattern of invasion and prominent desmoplasia. These tumors may spread to the peritoneal cavity, where they form solid tumor nodules and have potential for lymph node and solid organ metastasis with poor clinical outcome. Most of these tumors show features of moderately to poorly differentiated carcinoma with a high degree of cellularity, complex architecture with irregular gland formation and a cribriform growth, and overtly malignant cytologic abnormalities such as more apparent nuclear atypia and loss of cellular polarity (fig. 5-11A). Poorly differentiated adenocarcinomas may contain solid nests and sheets of malignant cells, or singly infiltrating signet ring cells, accompanied by mucin. Stromal mucin pools may be present, but they are seldom without abundant malignant epithelial cells in contrast to the situation with low grade lesions (fig. 5-11B). There is unanimous agreement that this subtype should be designated and staged as conventional adenocarcinoma (11,20).

Low-Grade Appendiceal Mucinous Neoplasm (LAMN). The definition of *low-grade appendiceal mucinous neoplasm* (LAMN) is not entirely consistent throughout the literature (Table 5-1) (15,20). It includes non-invasive and invasive mucinous neoplasms as well as lesions with uncertain malignant potential. Therefore, a diagnosis of LAMN without further specification with regard to its non-invasive versus invasive nature and localized versus disseminated disease does not provide adequate information for clinical management of the disease, unless these features cannot be defined with the given clinical and pathologic information. Appendiceal mucinous tumors that are not readily classified as either adenoma or adenocarcinoma due to the presence of mural hyalinization or diverticular-like herniation of neoplastic epithelium into the appendiceal wall (fig. 5-12A), mural acellular mucin dissection, and rupture of the appendix of uncertain etiology, may fall under the designation of low-grade appendiceal mucinous neoplasm.

A diagnosis of LAMN should be applied in scenarios where there is no clear evidence to diagnose a completely benign neoplasm (i.e., mucinous adenoma) and to reflect the fact

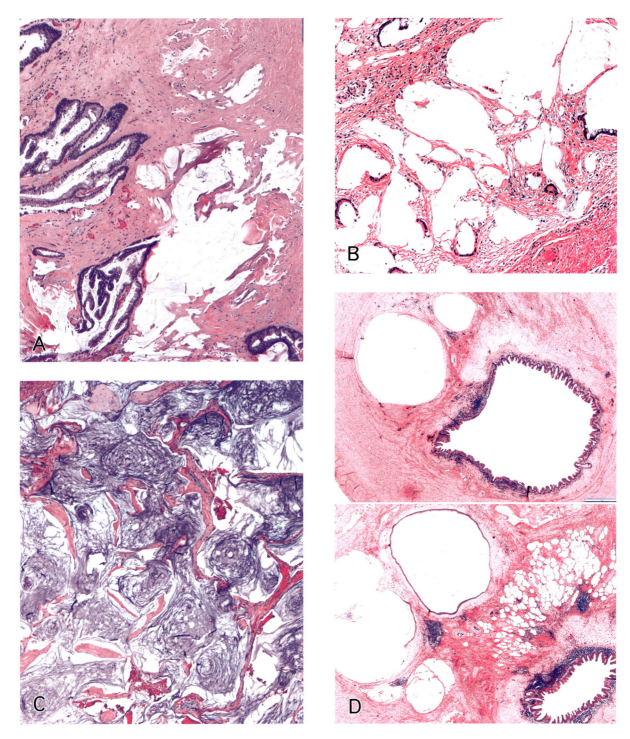

Figure 5-9

**WELL-DIFFERENTIATED MUCINOUS ADENOCARCINOMA WITH
EXPANSILE PATTERN OF INVASION AND WITHOUT STROMAL DESMOPLASIA**

A: Pushing front pattern of invasion with hyalinizing stromal fibrosis.
B: The carcinoma is paucicellular, with scanty and low-grade neoplastic epithelium.
C: Mucin pools associated with invasive carcinoma may be entirely devoid of epithelium.
D: An apparent mucinous adenoma with well-differentiated invasive carcinoma that was not represented on all histologic sections.

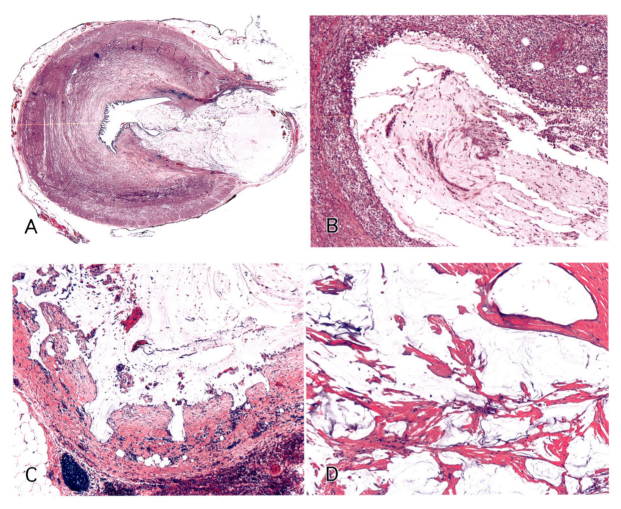

Figure 5-10

**ACELLULAR MUCIN POOLS IN PASSIVE MUCIN SPILLAGE AND
WELL-DIFFERENTIATED INVASIVE MUCINOUS ADENOCARCINOMA**

A,B: Mucin spillage secondary to high luminal pressure is associated with an intense inflammatory response around mural mucin pools.

C,D: Mucin with a pushing front (C) or dissection (D) in association with invasive carcinoma lacks an inflammatory response and has a "clean" appearance.

that it is difficult to completely exclude the possibility of occult invasive carcinoma. Indications for designation of a LAMN often include certain situations in which it is impossible to confidently assure that the patient will not have subsequent PMP. These features can be regarded in some respects as situations in which there is uncertain malignant potential as used by some authors. In addition to the WHO definition of LAMN (Table 5-1), some additional concerning situations include: 1) detection of limited and unexplained mural mucin without associated epithelial cells (spilled mucin from a mucinous adenoma versus an invasive low-grade mucinous carcinoma with paucicellular epithelium not represented in the mucin pool) (fig. 5-12B); 2) limited extramural acellular mucin of undetermined etiology (iatrogenic mucin contamination intraoperatively or during pathology prosection versus perforated appendix from mucinous adenoma with abundant mucin, or an invasive adenocarcinoma with extramural extension) (fig. 5-12C); and 3) extramural scant and isolated mucinous epithelium with

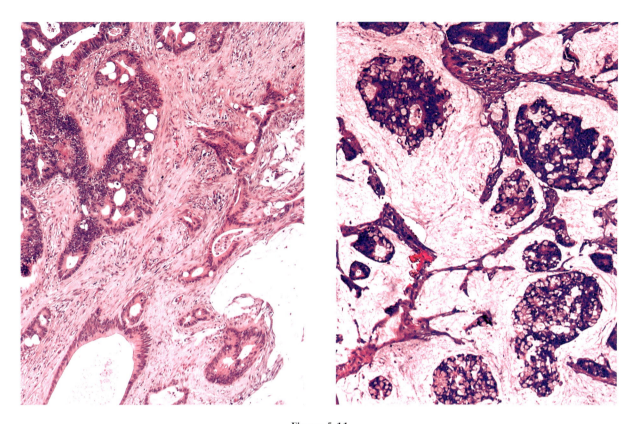

Figure 5-11

HIGH-GRADE MUCINOUS ADENOCARCINOMA WITH INFILTRATIVE PATTERN OF INVASION

Left: Moderately differentiated adenocarcinoma with prominent stomal desmoplasia.
Right: Poorly differentiated adenocarcinoma consists of mucin pools that harbor confluent aggregates of signet ring cells.

otherwise no evidence of invasive carcinoma (displacement of dysplastic mucinous epithelium versus an adenocarcinoma extending to the extra-appendiceal tissue) (fig. 5-12D).

Uncertainty regarding the biologic risk of an appendiceal mucinous neoplasm may result from mishandling or inadequate sampling of appendectomy specimens, poor orientation of the histologic sections, unclear gross descriptions, and lack of clinical information regarding surgical findings and distribution of disease (fig. 5-8). In the absence of malignant epithelium beyond the appendiceal mucosa, one cannot definitively render a diagnosis of carcinoma. The most concerning and difficult situation concerns determining whether the disease has spread beyond the appendix, since it has implications on clinical decisions for further intervention (33,34). It has been suggested that organizing acellular mucin on the serosa, with neovascularization and mesothelial hyperplasia,

likely represents extramural tumor extension rather than benign mucinous extrusion secondary to rupture or manipulation of the specimen (fig. 5-13) (25). Serosal neovascularization and mesothelial hyperplasia, however, may also be observed when there is co-existing acute appendicitis in a non-invasive mucinous cystadenoma. Available data suggest that limited extra-appendiceal mucin without neoplastic epithelial cells is associated with an excellent prognosis when confined to the periappendiceal region; the risk of disease progression after appendectomy is extremely low (35).

Given the extreme hypocellularity of well-differentiated mucinous adenocarcinoma, one can never entirely exclude the possibility of extra-appendiceal epithelium in such cases, especially if the specimen has not been completely submitted for histologic examination.

The revised 8th edition AJCC tumor staging system designates LAMN as in situ neoplasia

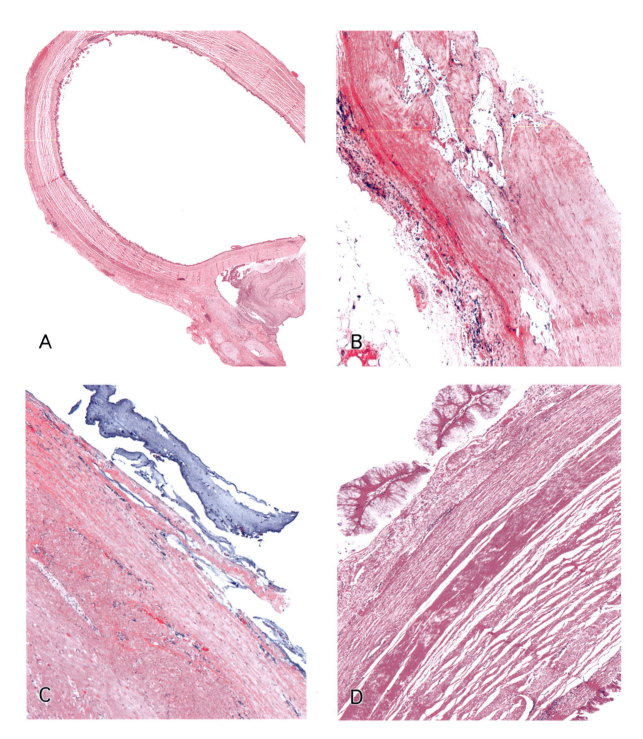

Figure 5-12

MUCINOUS NEOPLASM OF UNCERTAIN MALIGNANT POTENTIAL

A: The presence of mural/extramural mucin and dysplastic epithelium of unknown etiology in a mucinous cystadenoma creates uncertainty in a diagnosis of invasive adenocarcinoma.

B: A mucinous cystadenoma with denuded luminal epithelium and the presence of focal mural mucin without malignant epithelium.

C: A mucinous cystadenoma with focal extramural acellular mucin of uncertain etiology.

D: A mucinous cystadenoma with extramural scant and detached dysplastic epithelium of uncertain etiology.

and introduces the term Tis(LAMN) to specifically describe LAMN with a pushing front and confinement to the muscularis propria (36). Pathologic T1 and T2 stages are not applicable, whereas those with invasion into the subserosa and serosa are staged as T3 and T4, respectively (Table 5-2).

High-Grade Appendiceal Mucinous Neoplasm (HAMN). Some appendiceal mucinous neoplasms display architectural features of LAMN such as cystic appearance, diverticulum-like growth, or pushing invasion and without infiltration, but high-grade cytologic atypia. These *high-grade appendiceal mucinous neoplasms* (HAMN) are believed to represent an aggressive form of mucinous neoplasia more likely to be associated with high-grade disease in the peritoneum. The 8th edition of the AJCC staging manual considers these tumors to represent adenocarcinomas for staging purposes (36).

Pseudomyxoma Peritonei. *Pseudomyxoma peritonei* (PMP) is a condition characterized by mucinous/gelatinous ascites or diffuse mucin deposits within the peritoneal cavity. In the context of a primary appendiceal mucinous neoplasm, the condition is the clinical manifestation of either low- or high-grade disseminated mucinous adenocarcinoma (37–41), although it may rarely be associated with mucinous carcinomas of the ovary, urachus, colon, and pancreas (42–44). Non-neoplastic conditions, such as ruptured diverticula of the appendix or colon, can also result in spillage of mucin into the peritoneal cavity, although it usually remains locally confined and is not associated with mucinous ascites or diffuse mucin deposits (19). Given that the clinical impression of PMP can result from various etiologies, this term should also be avoided as a "first-line" diagnosis. Once there is apparent diffuse mucin accumulation, or neoplastic peritoneal implants, beyond the right lower quadrant, the carcinoma is classified as metastatic disease and staged as M1.

While the classification system and the nomenclature for these tumors will remain the subject of debate, most investigators recognize that disseminated peritoneal mucinous adenocarcinoma is comprised fundamentally of two prognostic groups based on tumor grade (Table 5-1) (25,26). The quality and quantity of PMP is closely associated with the pathologic features

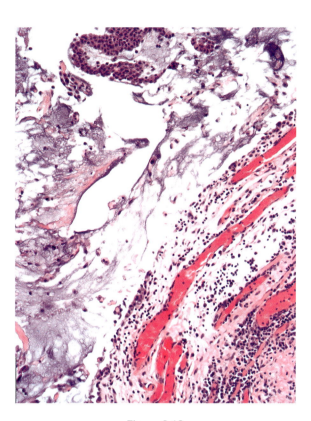

Figure 5-13

MUCINOUS ADENOCARCINOMA

There is serosal mucin and associated mesothelial hyperplasia and neovascularization.

of the mucinous peritoneal adenocarcinoma. Well-differentiated/low-grade mucinous adenocarcinoma usually lacks a destructive invasive pattern and is capable of producing massive gelatinous ascites with very scant malignant epithelium, typically with less than 10 percent cellularity (figs. 5-14, left; 5-9C). Lymph node and distant solid organ metastases are uncommon, although ovarian metastases are frequently present at clinical presentation. In contrast, the high-grade mucinous adenocarcinoma/moderately to poorly differentiated counterpart tends to generate mucinous ascites with solid areas, including omental caking (figs. 5-11A, 5-14, right). Tumors contain more abundant epithelium that may show signet ring cell differentiation (fig. 5-11B), as well as destructive invasion of viscera and desmoplastic stroma. This subtype has a poor outcome that is similar to that of nonmucinous appendiceal adenocarcinoma (14,16,45,46). Therefore, determination of histologic grade

Table 5-2

REVISED TNM STAGING FOR APPENDICEAL ADENOCARCINOMA IN AJCC 8TH EDITION

	Well-Differentiated Mucinous Adenocarcinoma/Low-Grade Appendiceal Mucinous Neoplasm (LAMN)	Moderately and Poorly Differentiated Mucinous Adenocarcinoma/ High-Grade Appendiceal Mucinous Neoplasm (HAMN)
TX	Primary tumor cannot be assessed	
T0	No evidence of primary tumor	
Tis	LAMN confined by the muscularis propria; acellular mucin and mucinous epithelium many invade into muscularis propria	Carcinoma in situ (intramucosal carcinoma; invasion of the lamina propria or extension into, but not through, the muscularis mucosae)
T1	No applicable	Tumor invades the submucosa
T2	No applicable	Tumor invades the muscularis propria
T3	Tumor invades through the muscularis propria into the subserosa or the mesoappendix	
T4a	Tumor invades the visceral peritoneum, including the acellular mucin or mucinous epithelium involving the serosa of the appendix or serosa of the mesoappendix	
T4b	Tumor directly invades or adherent to adjacent organs or structures	
NX	Regional lymph nodes cannot be assessed	
N0	No regional lymph node metastasis	
N1	One to three (1-3) regional lymph nodes are positive (measuring $\leq$0.2 mm) OR any number of tumor deposits is present, and all identifiable lymph nodes are negative	
N1a	One (1) regional lymph node is positive	
N1b	Two (2) or three (3) regional lymph nodes are positive	
	No (0) regional lymph nodes are positive, but there are tumor deposits in the subserosa or mesentery	
N2	Four (4) or more regional lymph nodes are positive	
M0	No distant metastases	
M1	Distant metastasis	
M1a	Intraperitoneal acellular mucin, without identifiable tumor cells in the disseminated peritoneal mucinous deposits	
M1b	Intraperitoneal metastasis only, including peritoneal mucinous deposits containing tumor cells	
M1c	Metastasis to sites other than peritoneum	

Note: For specimens containing mucin without identifiable tumor cells, efforts should be made to obtain additional tissue for thorough histologic examination to evaluate cellularity.

has considerable prognostic significance, even in stage IV disease (11,20).

Stratification of Prognostic Groups and Management of Appendiceal Mucinous Adenocarcinoma

The prognosis of patients with mucinous tumors of the appendix is dictated by multiple clinical and pathologic features. Data from numerous investigations have demonstrated that outcome is driven by the histologic grade and stage of the neoplasm while the pathologic classification of appendiceal mucinous adenocarcinomas has primarily been the basis for stratification of the prognostic groups.

The clinical management of appendiceal mucinous adenocarcinoma differs somewhat from that of conventional colorectal adenocarcinoma (11,17). The treatment decisions regarding right hemicolectomy following appendectomy, cytoreductive surgery, and perioperative or adjuvant chemotherapy are dependent not only on tumor stage, but also tumor grade and classification (11,16,17,47–51). It is, therefore, important to establish a good line of communication between pathologists and clinicians in order to facilitate the mutual understanding of implications for the diagnosis and management of the disease.

Mucinous tumors with dysplastic epithelium confined to the mucosa (mucinous adenoma

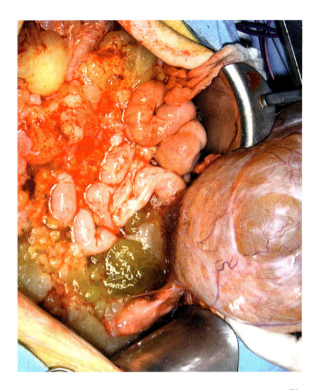 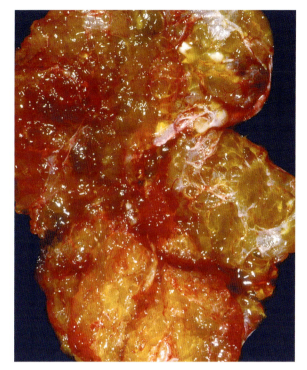

Figure 5-14

MUCINOUS ADENOCARCINOMA WITH PSEUDOMYXOMA PERITONEI

Left: Well-differentiated adenocarcinoma presented as a large cystic mass and mucin ascites.
Right: Poorly differentiated mucinous adenocarcinoma with omental cake.

or cystadenoma) have no potential to spread, regardless of the degree of dysplasia. To diagnose these lesions requires complete removal of the lesion and thorough examination as described above. Low-grade mucinous tumors with a broad front pushing into the muscularis propria, without unequivocal evidence of invasion, do not recur when completely removed and thoroughly examined to exclude more aggressive features. Low-grade mucinous tumors with limited mural mucin, without epithelial cells (undetermined etiology) confined within appendiceal wall, do not carry notable risk for recurrence when completely removed and thoroughly examined to exclude more aggressive features.

Low-grade mucinous tumors with invasion beyond muscularis propria possess the potential for peritoneal dissemination or distant metastasis, and should be graded and staged accordingly.

High-grade appendiceal mucinous tumor and tumors with destructive invasion are graded and staged as adenocarcinomas. Additional right hemicolectomy may be necessary depending on the tumor grade and stage (33,34,51).

Low-grade mucinous neoplasms with limited extramural mucin and without epithelial cells have an uncertain clinical risk that is largely dependent on meticulous pathologic assessment of the initial appendectomy specimen. Such lesions are associated with a risk of disease recurrence ranging from 4 to 8 percent depending on adequacy of sampling (25,35). Even though the recurrent risk is very low, the probability of disease-free survival is not 100 percent, even when the entire appendix has been submitted for histologic evaluation. The clinical management of appendiceal mucinous neoplasms with uncertain malignant potential is controversial. There are no compelling data to indicate right colectomy or intraperitoneal chemotherapy following appendectomy to improve recurrence-free survival. Many may choose close observation of patients with localized disease, particularly with pathology support to ascertain that the adverse features for recurrence are not present.

The likelihood of disease recurrence among patients with extra-appendiceal neoplastic epithelium confined to the right lower quadrant ranges from 33 to 75 percent (25,35). Additional surgical intervention and perioperative chemotherapy may be considered in this situation (11).

Patients with low-grade/well-differentiated mucinous adenocarcinoma in the peritoneal cavity may benefit from cytoreductive surgery as an initial treatment modality. Five-year survival rates range up to 63 percent for patients undergoing complete cytoreductive surgery with perioperative intraperitoneal chemotherapy (11,16,42,51). Patients with high-grade/moderately to poorly differentiated mucinous adenocarcinoma in the peritoneal cavity often have some degree of solid growth in the omentum, lymph node, and distant metastases. Outcomes are poorer with a 5-year survival rate of 23 percent; these patients may benefit from systemic chemotherapy (11,17,42).

Appendiceal mucinous neoplasms are a heterogeneous group of tumors that behave in a grade- and stage-dependent fashion. Unfortunately, a number of terminology and classification systems exist and, while familiar to a small group of specialists, they are confusing to most practicing physicians. Decisions regarding clinical management require clear designation of tumor stage and histologic subtype, which should be delineated in a uniform reporting system harmonized with the rest of the gastrointestinal tract. Secondary histologic features that are specific to appendiceal mucinous neoplasms and their clinical relevance, such as tumor grade, tumor differentiation, pattern of invasion, and nature of disseminated disease, should be reported accordingly. Until there is global harmonization of terminology, terms that the treating physicians understand should be offered as well as terminology in line with the WHO criteria (15).

Molecular and Genetic Features of Appendiceal Mucinous Adenocarcinoma

The combined targeted sequencing of specific genes, next-generation sequencing of cancer-related genes, and immunohistochemistry for selected proteins as surrogate markers of gene alterations have delineated molecular signatures of appendiceal mucinous adenocarcinoma (10,52–56). The highest frequency of somatic mutations occurs in *KRAS* (53 to 100 percent), although *KRAS* mutations do not seem to differentiate between high-grade and low-grade mucinous adenocarcinomas. *KRAS* mutations at codon 12 are more frequent than those at codon 13. Notably, *KRAS* codon 12 mutations have been associated with a mucinous phenotype of colorectal cancers (57).

The second most commonly mutated gene is *GNAS* at codon 201, in 40 to 77 percent of mucinous carcinomas, but is not associated with tumor grade or clinical outcome. Alterations in *GNAS* are associated with a mucinous epithelial phenotype (52,54,55).

Other less common mutations include those of *SMAD4, AKT1, ATM, PIK3CA, APC, p53,* and *RB1* (52). Of all the molecular aberrations, either by gene mutation or abnormal protein expression, *TP53/p53* has a demonstrated association with tumor grade and prognosis (52). *BRAF* mutations are either not detected in most studies or found in rare cases. DNA mismatch repair deficiency is not detected in most appendiceal mucinous adenocarcinomas.

GOBLET CELL CARCINOID AND ASSOCIATED ADENOCARCINOMA

Goblet cell carcinoid (GCC) is a malignant epithelial neoplasm that comprises less than 5 percent of all appendiceal malignancies and about 10 percent of appendiceal carcinomas. In contrast to typical carcinoid tumors of the appendix (see chapter 7), GCCs of the appendix have a mixed phenotype, with partial neuroendocrine differentiation together with intestinal-type goblet cell morphology (58–63). In many respects, however, it can be regarded as a low-grade form of adenocarcinoma with unique morphology.

Throughout the gastrointestinal tract there are many neoplasms that exhibit both glandular and neuroendocrine differentiation (64,65). True hybrid tumors with significant bidirectional differentiation, however, are rare, and in most anatomic locations these neoplasms are designated with a variety of descriptive terms (e.g., adenocarcinoid tumor, mixed carcinoid-adenocarcinoma, amphicrine carcinoma) that do not necessarily reflect a consistent morphology or biologic behavior. GCC, if not unique to the appendix, has only been well characterized in this organ (58,64,66–69).

While GCC and the associated higher-grade adenocarcinomas are rare neoplasms of the appendix, their frequent association with appendicitis raises concerns about adequate initial clinical evaluation and subsequent oncologic management (1,58,64,66–68,70–72). Their adenocarcinoma-like morphology and frequent high-stage tumor presentation have caused confusion as to whether such tumors should be regarded as carcinoid tumors or as adenocarcinomas (58,68). These issues have considerable impact on the management of the disease. Despite a number of hypotheses, the histogenesis of the GCC is not clear (72–74). Morphologically, GCCs arise in the deep mucosa (69) without conventional surface dysplasia as seen in other precursors of adenocarcinoma. Both the clinical and pathologic features of GCCs are sufficiently distinctive that they are best regarded as a separate unique entity, distinct from both classic carcinoid tumors and de novo appendiceal adenocarcinomas (1,68,75). Many GCCs behave aggressively, although a significant number appear to have an indolent clinical course despite presenting at an advanced clinical stage (61,62).

Clinical and Pathologic Features

There are a number of clinical and pathologic features of GCCs that are distinct from either adenocarcinoma or classic carcinoid tumor of the appendix. The median patient age is 50 years, with a range of 29 to 80 years (60–62), which is younger than the reported age for patients with appendiceal adenocarcinoma of conventional/nonmucinous type (median age, 62 years) and well-differentiated mucinous adenocarcinoma (median age, 58 years) (11,61,64); it is older than that of patients with classic carcinoid tumor of the appendix (mean age, 42 years) (76). The disease, particularly when stage IV, exhibits a female predominance (female/male ratio: 3 to 1); metastases are frequently to the ovaries and adnexae (60–62,77).

In contrast to mucinous neoplasms, GCCs do not produce excessive extracellular mucin and thus the appendiceal lumen lacks mucin accumulation and is usually not dilated. Early stage GCC typically causes diffuse thickening of the wall of the entire length of the appendix with a compressed or collapsed lumen (fig. 5-15, left). At an advanced stage, GCC presents as a right lower quadrant mass, with the appendix embedded within the mass. The tumor is commonly mistaken for a cecal or right colon primary (fig. 5-15, right).

The fundamental morphologic features common to all GCCs are: 1) the presence of mucin-containing goblet-shaped epithelial cells arranged in round or oval clusters and 2) neoplastic cells demonstrating (usually focal) positive immunoreactivity for neuroendocrine markers (chromogranin or synaptophysin). Despite its signet ring cell-like morphology, which is reminiscent of a poorly differentiated adenocarcinoma, GCC does not have an apparent association with the adenoma-carcinoma sequence as seen in most conventional-type adenocarcinomas of the gastrointestinal tract. No surface epithelial dysplasia or other preinvasive neoplasia has been identified in any GCCs (61), although in rare situations, a mucinous cystadenoma or classic carcinoid tumor (78,79) may coincide with detection of a GCC.

GCCs can also contain elements that are poorly differentiated, growing either as a signet ring cell adenocarcinoma without the typical histologic features of GCC or even as an undifferentiated carcinoma (62,61). These frankly carcinomatous elements appear to represent transformation of the low-grade GCC into a more histologically aggressive neoplasm (adenocarcinoma ex GCC). GCCs are thus separated into two histologic groups: typical GCC and adenocarcinoma ex GCC; the latter may manifest predominant signet ring cell morphology or a poorly/undifferentiated phenotype. The criteria for this classification, along with other morphologic features, are detailed below (Table 5-3) (61). The classification of the two histologic subtypes is based upon tumor characteristics present in the appendiceal primary since the histologic features at metastatic sites are often heterogeneous and cannot be reliably used to predict the outcome (61,62).

Classification of GCC

Typical GCC. Typical GCCs are initially characterized by an exuberant proliferation of cytologically bland epithelial cells arranged either in tight clusters or ill-defined clusters, at the base of the crypts and in the lamina propria

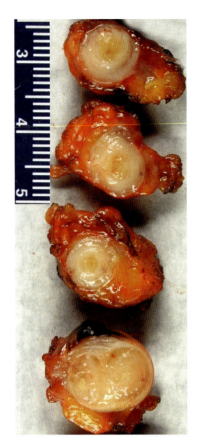
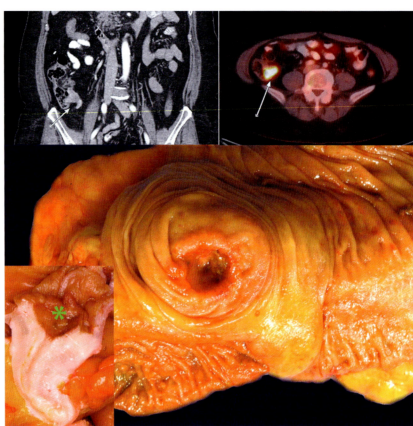

Figure 5-15

GOBLET CELL CARCINOID AND ASSOCIATED ADENOCARCINOMA

Left: The tumor involves the entire length of the appendix, with wall thickening and lumen obliteration.

Right: The tumor presents on radiographic images as a cecal mass (upper panels); on gross examination, the tumor protrudes from the appendiceal orifice to the cecum without a discrete mass (*) in the appendix other than mural thickening (insert).

Table 5-3

MORPHOLOGIC CRITERIA FOR PATHOLOGIC CLASSIFICATION OF GOBLET CELL CARCINOID[a,b]

Morphologic Criteria	
Typical goblet cell carcinoid	Well defined goblet cells arranged in clusters, acinar, or linear pattern Minimal cytologic atypia Minimal to no desmoplasia Minimal architectural distortion of the appendiceal wall Degenerative change with extracellular mucin is acceptable Cytologic atypia associated with acute inflammation is acceptable
Adenocarcinoma ex goblet cell carcinoid	Goblet cells or signet ring cells arranged in irregular clusters and sheets, fused or cribriform glands/tables Single cell infiltrating pattern Component of otherwise indistinguishable from a poorly differentiated/ undifferentiated or high-grade neuroendocrine adenocarcinoma Significant cytologic atypia Marked desmoplasia Destruction of appendiceal wall

[a]Adapted from a table in reference 61.
[b]Based upon morphologic features at the primary site: appendix only.

(fig. 5-16A); the surface epithelium lacks dysplasia. As the tumor invades into the muscularis propria and subserosal adipose tissues, it usually contain well-formed oval or round tumor cells arranged in an acinar configuration, resembling normal appendiceal crypts, with well-preserved and uniform goblet cells and small nuclei that do not show significant cytologic atypia (fig. 5-16B). As the tumor cells infiltrate through the muscularis propria, the clusters often exhibit a compressed linear configuration oriented parallel to the muscle cells, giving rise to a single file pattern reminiscent of that of a poorly differentiated signet ring cell adenocarcinoma (fig. 5-16C). The tumor cells still remain in groups and appear cohesive. Mitotic figures are rarely identifiable. Prominent perineural invasion by tumor cells is a common feature.

Since many GCCs are incidentally identified in appendectomy specimens removed for acute appendicitis, the diagnostic dilemma is that the tumor may display concerning morphologic alterations when present within an acutely inflamed appendix. Common findings in this setting include: 1) a degenerative change that is associated with signet ring cells present in extracellular mucin; the tumor cells demonstrate cytoplasmic ballooning and complete or incomplete loss of cell membrane, but the nuclei do not have high-grade cytologic features (fig. 5-17A); 2) loss of intracellular mucin produces irregularly shaped clusters of the tumor cells or even gives rise to a tubular appearance (fig. 5-17B); 3) similar to the situation of active inflammation occurring in mucosa at any site, the epithelial atypia of GCC can be significant, particularly when neutrophils are present within the epithelium (fig. 5-17B,C). These features may make separating typical GCC from adenocarcinoma ex GCC difficult.

Adenocarcinoma ex GCC. In addition to having residual areas of typical GCC, this subgroup of tumors also demonstrates regions with either a partial or a nearly complete loss of goblet cell clusters, with neoplastic cells instead arranged individually and infiltrating in a discohesive pattern throughout the appendix. In some cases, focally preserved goblet cell architecture is the only evidence of the diagnosis of GCC.

The morphologic features of adenocarcinoma ex GCC include a disorganized arrangement of the tumor cells with prominent signet ring cell features and an associated desmoplastic stromal reaction (fig. 5-18A). The signet ring cells infiltrate singly or are arranged in irregular clusters or confluent sheets (fig. 5-18B). Compared with tumor cells in typical GCC, the signet ring cells in this group of tumors demonstrate significant cytologic atypia with pleomorphic and hyperchromatic nuclei (fig. 5-18C).

Rarely, adenocarcinoma ex GCC presents with poorly differentiated/undifferentiated features, either as a gland/tubule-forming adenocarcinoma, as confluent sheets of malignant epithelial cells with or without signet ring cell features, or with the morphologic features of a high-grade neuroendocrine carcinoma (fig. 5-18D) (61,62). This poorly differentiated histologic subtype was previously designated separately from the more common signet ring cell subtype (61). However, since most cases of adenocarcinoma ex GCC are of advanced stage (62) and managed similarly, the simplified classification of typical GCC or adenocarcinoma ex GCC is adequate, with the latter designated as a signet ring cell or poorly differentiated subtype, respectively, to indicate their different clinical outcomes.

Immunoprofile

Evidence of neuroendocrine differentiation is provided by immunoreactivity for chromogranin and synaptophysin in these tumors, although the staining is often focal, and is almost always much less extensive than that in classic carcinoid tumors (fig. 5-19, left). These findings are supported by studies that have demonstrated genetic alterations in GCCs compatible with a neuroendocrine origin and different from appendiceal adenocarcinomas (73,80,81). The scant immunoreactivity for neuroendocrine markers could be explained by the presence of large intracellular mucin globules in tumor cells that inflate the cytoplasmic space and dilute the concentration of neuroendocrine secretory granules for detection. When an adenocarcinoma ex GCC has predominantly tubular/glandular and diffuse signet ring cell morphology, with minimal or no foci of typical GCC at the metastatic site, a primary conventional adenocarcinoma should be considered in the differential diagnosis. Previous studies have suggested that typical GCC and adenocarcinoma

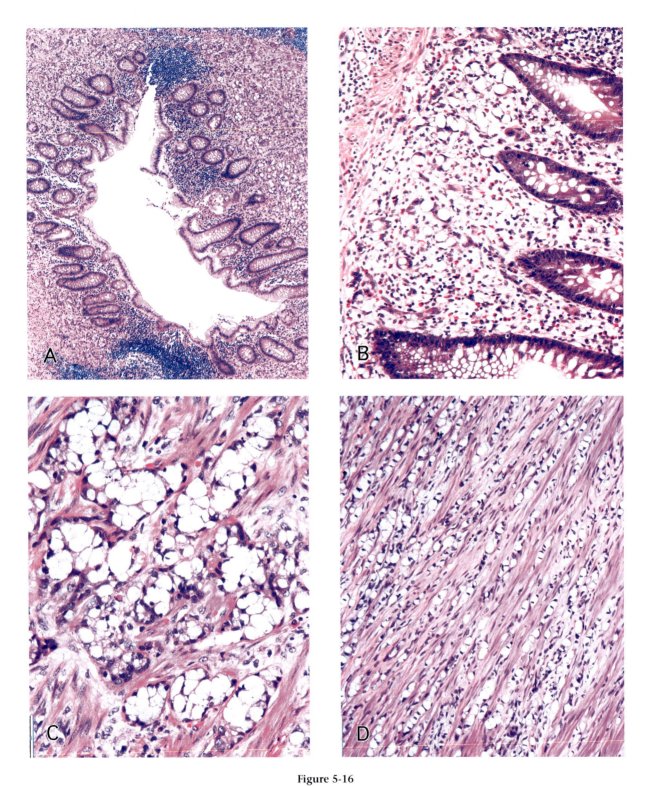

Figure 5-16

TYPICAL GOBLET CELL CARCINOID TUMOR

A,B: The tumor originates from base crypts and lamina propria without epithelial dysplasia on the mucosal surface.
C: The tumor cells are arranged in an acinar configuration with minimal nuclear atypia.
D: The tumor cells exhibit a linear configuration when infiltrating between muscle fibers.

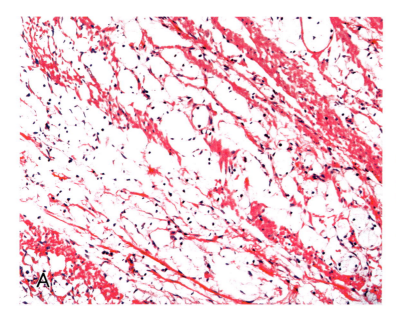

Figure 5-17

GOBLET CELL CARCINOID WITH CHANGES ASSOCIATED WITH ACUTE APPENDICITIS

A: Degenerative tumor cells with cytoplasmic ballooning and extracelluar mucin.

B: Tumor cells in acute inflammation with loss of intracellular mucin, tubule formation, presence of intraepithelial neutrophils, and extracellular mucin.

C: Cytologic atypia is accentuated when the tumor cells are infiltrated by neutrophils.

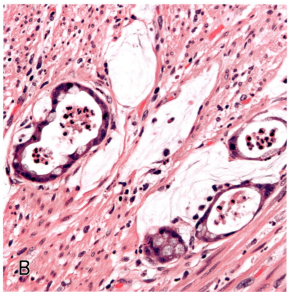

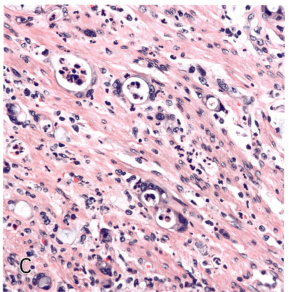

ex GCC of signet ring cell type do not demonstrate the characteristic immunophenotype of conventional adenocarcinomas (61).

Many adenocarcinomas of the colon and the appendix are associated with *CTNNB1* (the gene that encodes for β-catenin, 70 to 80 percent) and *TP53* (50 percent) mutations (82,83). However, there is no specific immunoprofile that can definitively distinguish a conventional lower gastrointestinal tract adenocarcinoma from an adenocarcinoma ex GCC.

Previous investigations have demonstrated an alternate profile of mucin glycoproteins (MUCs)

in adenocarcinoma of colonic type (84,85). Normal colorectal epithelial cells (including the glands of the appendix) only express MUC2. In most conventional colonic adenocarcinomas, MUC1 is overexpressed and MUC2 is lost. Conversely, MUC1 is not expressed and MUC2 is preserved in typical GCCs (fig. 5-19, right), but MUC2 is lost and MUC1 is expressed in poorly differentiated adenocarcinoma ex GCC (61). These findings suggest that the morphologic transformation from typical GCC to adenocarcinoma ex GCC may be correlated with a molecular phenotype and genotype transformation.

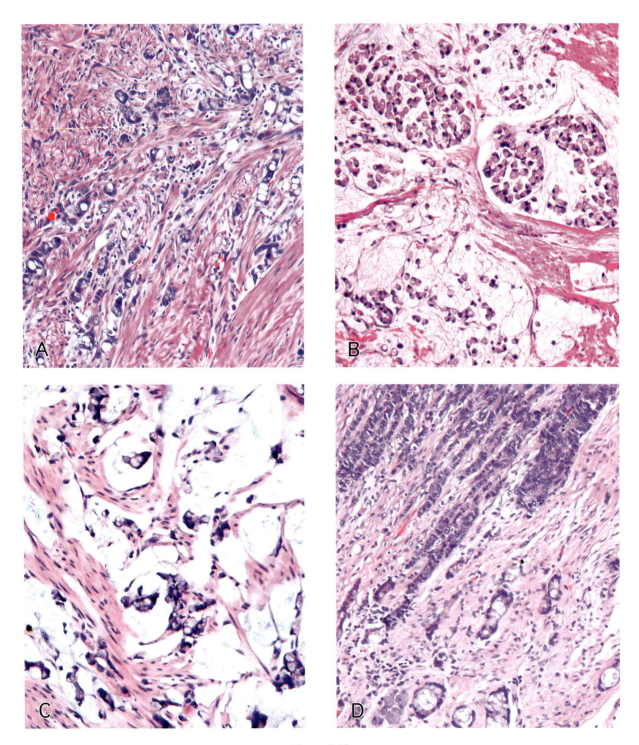

Figure 5-18

ADENOCARCINOMA EX GOBLET CELL CARCINOID

A: The carcinoma has a disorganized architecture, with signet ring cell features and stromal desmoplasia.

B: The signet ring carcinoma cells grow in confluent sheets.

C: The tumor cells are arranged in irregular clusters with hyperchromatic nuclei and marked cytologic atypia.

D: The tumor presents as a poorly differentiated/undifferentiated carcinoma with minimal evidence of residual better differentiated goblet cell tumor morphology (right).

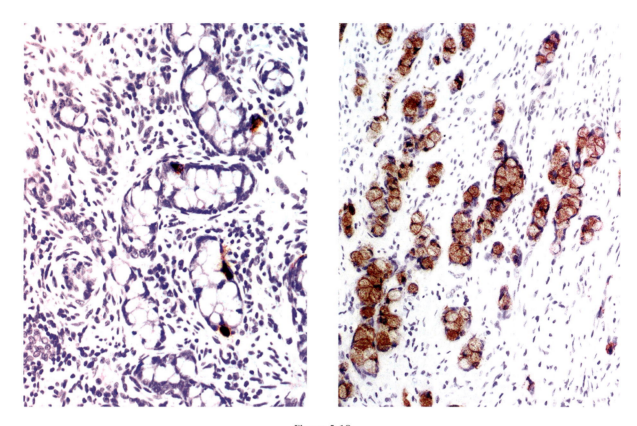

Figure 5-19

IMMUNOPROFILE OF GOBLET CELL CARCINOID

Left: The tumor cells typically show focal immunoreactivity for neuroendocrine markers (chromogranin or synaptophysin). Right: Typical goblet cell carcinoid tumor cells usually exhibit positive immunoreactivity with MUC2.

Stratification of Prognostic Groups and Recommended Management

Despite the pathologic differences from conventional appendiceal adenocarcinomas, the family of GCCs, particularly adenocarcinoma ex GCC, appears to be associated with a clinical behavior closer to that of adenocarcinoma than that of classic appendiceal carcinoid. The high pathologic stage at presentation is in contrast to classic carcinoid tumors of the appendix, in which the majority present with localized disease (75). Lymph node metastases are rare in classical appendiceal carcinoid tumors (1.4 to 8.8 percent) (75). In contrast, they are detected in 34 to 73 percent of all patients with GCCs depending on the subtype (60–62); appendiceal adenocarcinoma (other than the well-differentiated mucinous type) has a lymph node positivity rate of about 31 percent (colonic type) to about 64 percent (signet ring cell type).

GCC of the appendix appears to spread selectively to the pelvic organs, peritoneum, and omentum, similar to well-differentiated appendiceal mucinous adenocarcinoma, although mucinous ascites is uncommon. Rare liver metastasis of GCC has been reported (62,64,68). Over 85 percent women with clinical stage IV GCC have initially consulted gynecologic oncologists for ovarian masses; identifying a primary site for the ovarian metastasis can be challenging since the histologic pattern of adenocarcinoma ex GCC in the ovary is extremely heterogeneous and does not resemble that of most gastrointestinal tract primaries (62,77).

Some of the morphologic features of GCC may correlate with clinical outcome (58,61,62,66). The subclassification of GCCs demonstrates clear prognostic significance, with a progressively worse prognosis between those with typical GCC and those whose tumor has transformed to adenocarcinoma. Patients with typical GCCs have a fairly favorable long-term survival rate, despite the fact that 33 percent present with stage IV disease (61,62). It is not clear to what extent the favorable outcome is attributable to the use of adjuvant chemotherapy, rather than the inherent biology of the neoplasm, but it is evident that this outcome is better than might be predicted for tose with similarly staged de novo appendiceal adenocarcinomas. In contrast, the adenocarcinoma ex GCC subtype has an outcome similar to that of stage-matched conventional-type colorectal or appendiceal adenocarcinoma. These data further support the recognition of GCCs as a separate and distinct clinicopathologic entity (61).

Due to the inconsistency in terminology in diagnostic criteria, the malignant potential of some GCCs may have been underestimated, since the term "appendiceal carcinoid" implies an indolent lesion. Conversely, low-grade and low-stage typical GCCs of the appendix may be overtreated if they carry a diagnosis of "poorly differentiated or signet ring cell adenocarcinoma."

Historically, the malignant potential of low-grade GCC tumors was generally considered comparable to that of classic carcinoid tumors of the appendix, and management recommendations were based on the guidelines generally applicable to conventional carcinoid tumors (64,86); thus, right hemicolectomy was performed for locally advanced disease or if the tumor size exceeded 2 cm, given the potential for lymph node metastases. This management strategy is based upon the fact that the classic carcinoid tumor of the appendix does not exhibit morphologically defined grades; thus, the size of the tumor has been the only means to assess malignant potential.

This size criterion may not be equally applicable in the management of GCCs. First, the size of a GCC may be difficult to measure accurately due to the diffuse pattern of infiltration, lack of a discrete grossly identifiable mass (see fig. 5-16), and more importantly, the histologic grade rather than the size of the tumor is more indicative of the behavior of subtypes of GCC. This is particularly relevant in typical GCC since most adenocarcinomas ex GCC are larger than 2 cm. Thus, appendectomy alone with close follow-up may be adequate management for patients with a localized (pT1 or pT2) low-grade GCC with

negative resection margins without perforation. This surgical decision is also supported by a previously conducted meta-analysis of 13 studies, which recommended appendectomy alone in localized cases in which the lesion is confined to the muscularis propria of the appendix and the tumor histology is low grade (87). Available data suggest that 1) typical GCCs that present with perforation or positive appendectomy resection margin, 2) tumors that have extended beyond muscularis propria, or 3) tumors that have any features of adenocarcinoma ex GCCs should all be treated as conventional adenocarcinoma using right hemicolectomy with adequate lymph node staging (61,87,88).

Regardless of the grade and differentiation, it may be appropriate for all patients with stage IV GCC to be treated with chemotherapy because of the tendency for peritoneal spread and because some of the favorable long-term survival statistics in the group with typical GCCs may be attributable to the efficacy of the chemotherapy that was given. Nevertheless, there are no data that rigorously support the efficacy of a specific chemotherapeutic regimen for this tumor type (88,89). Given the pattern of spread, with a predominant peritoneal predilection, intraperitoneal chemotherapy combined with or without systemic chemotherapy has been recommended (90). Management of GCCs should be based on both the grade and the stage of the tumor as they are considered as variants of adenocarcinoma and should be staged as such. Female patients with locally advanced disease or adenocarcinoma ex GCC have a high propensity for ovarian metastases, and therefore bilateral oophorectomy in selected postmenopausal patients, at the time of right hemicolectomy, should be considered (91).

Molecular Genetic Features

Given its rarity, few molecular investigations have specifically focused on subtypes of GCC and the associated adenocarcinomas. The available data analysis is further complicated since many studies of de novo appendiceal mucinous adenocarcinomas have included "signet ring cell carcinoma," many of which could represent adenocarcinoma ex GCC without a recognizable typical GCC counterpart (10,52). Nevertheless, lesions reported as appendiceal signet ring cell carcinoma and adenocarcinoma, with goblet cell features, appear to harbor fewer *KRAS* and *GNAS* mutations than conventional adenocarcinoma but instead have frequent *TP53* and *SMAD4* mutations (10,70).

OTHER TUMOR AND TUMOR-LIKE LESIONS OF THE APPENDIX

There are a number of incidental and accidental lesions that are identified in the appendix. Some of them are of no clinical significance and others necessitate further clinical evaluation to exclude possible systemic involvement or metastatic diseases.

Intussusception and Inversion of the Appendix

While this is not a neoplastic condition, *intussusception* and *inversion of the appendix* can present as an intraluminal polypoid mass at the base of the cecum on CT scans. The etiology is either non-neoplastic or neoplastic (92). Intussusception of the appendix more commonly affects young boys (93). Predisposing factors include thin mesoappendix, conical shaped appendix, and the presence of mass lesions such as follicular lymphoid hyperplasia, endometriosis, appendiceal polyps (hyperplastic polyp, adenoma), well-differentiated neuroendocrine tumor (carcinoid), primary adenocarcinoma, and metastatic tumors (94). Occasionally, the appendix may auto-amputate following repeated intussusception and volvulus.

Appendiceal mucosal inflammation, erosion, and ischemia are evident on microscopic examination. Appendiceal wall thickening with hyperplasia of the mucosa and muscular layers may be present in recurrent intussusception. The intussuscepted appendix should be carefully examined for possible neoplasms.

Neurofibroma and Ganglioneuroma

As a rare component of gastrointestinal tract involvement by von Recklinghausen disease (neurofibromatosis type-1, NF1), the appendix may contain various neural proliferations. Grossly, there is wall thickening and a nodule or mass extending into the mesentery (fig. 5-20) (95–97). Histologic evaluation of these lesions typically reveals plexiform *neurofibromas* with proliferations of ganglion cells. *Ganglioneuromas* may also be present in association with NF1.

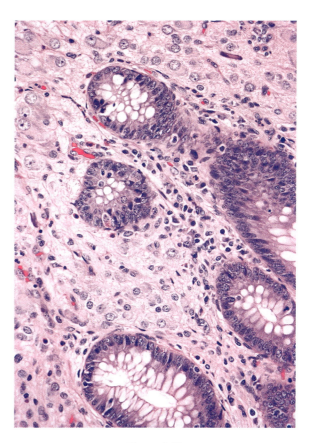

Figure 5-20

GANGLIONEUROMA

The lamina propria is involved by a ganglioneuroma.

Fibrous Obliteration (Appendiceal Neuroma)

Neither the designation *fibrous obliteration* nor *neuroma* is ideal terminology to define this lesion, perhaps because the true pathologic etiology of the lesion is not clear. Appendiceal neuroma is a benign condition, which may cause symptoms similar to those of appendicitis, but many neuromas are incidental findings in asymptomatic patients (97). Appendiceal neuroma exhibits nerve tissue proliferation involving the mucosa in the early stage, which continues to the mural appendiceal wall and consists of spindle cells reflecting unmyelinated nerves and Schwann cells (98). The process is thought to progress through a series of stages of mucosal atrophy to fibrous obliteration of the appendiceal lumen (80). Perhaps the condition is better explained by a response to trauma and chronic inflammation such as fecalith, which could be

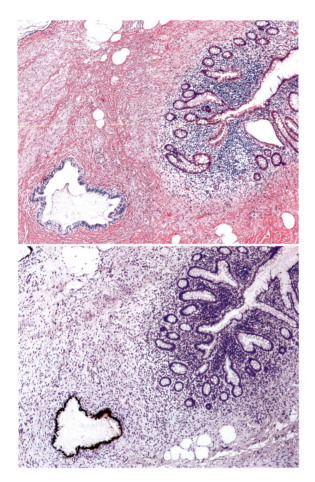

Figure 5-21

ENDOMETRIOSIS

Mural involvement by endometriosis, which is confirmed by an immunostain for estrogen receptor (lower).

comparable with traumatic neuroma occurring elsewhere in the body. Pseudoneuroma is probably a better term to describe the lesion.

Endometriosis and Endosalpingiosis

Endometriosis is present in up to 2.6 percent of appendectomy specimens as a component of gastrointestinal tract involvement by the condition (99–101). Although some patients are asymptomatic, most present with symptoms of acute appendicitis with associated abdominal pain that is often localized to the right lower quadrant. In uncommon cases, appendical endometriosis can cause intussusception of the appendix into the cecum, retention mucocele, intestinal hemorrhage, and appendiceal perforation.

On gross examination, dark brown and blue cysts or nodules may be present on the serosal surface of the appendix. Distortion of the appendix can be seen in cases of diffuse involvement by endometriosis. Microscopically, endometrial-type glands, surrounded by a variable amount of endometrial stroma, are present in appendiceal mucosa, muscularis propria, and serosa (fig. 5-21). As discussed in chapter 10, intestinal metaplasia in endometriosis can mimic LAMN.

The presence of mural glandular epithelium can raise concern for metastatic carcinoma of either a colorectal or mullerian primary. The presence of endometrial stroma and hemosiderin deposition provide clues for the diagnosis of endometriosis. The distinct immunoprofile of colorectum (positive for CK20 and CDX2; negative for CK7) and endometrium (positive for CK7, PAX8, and estrogen receptor; negative for CK20 and CDX2) can facilitate the differential diagnosis (fig. 5-22).

Appendiceal *endosalpingiosis* is usually an incidental finding in appendectomy specimens resected for other reasons. Patients are asymptomatic and there are no significant clinical implications associated with this condition. Histologically, appendiceal endosalpingiosis can elicit a differential diagnosis of metastatic adenocarcinoma. However, the glandular epithelium of endosalpingiosis comprises bland and ciliated cuboidal cells without adjoining endometrial stroma. The mullerian immunophenotype (positive for CK7, PAX8, and estrogen receptors) confirms the nature of the lesion.

Atypical Mesothelial Proliferation and Mesothelioma

The solo presentation of *mesothelial lesions* at the appendix is uncommon, although there have been case reports of localized benign cystic mesothelioma and diffuse malignant mesothelioma (102–104). When these lesions are present in appendectomy specimens performed for other conditions, they merit further clinical evaluation to exclude the possibility of potentially diffuse malignant tumors present in the peritoneum (97).

Mesenchymal Tumors

Mesenchymal neoplasms of almost all lineages have been reported in the appendix (97), all of which are extremely rare. Most are identified incidentally during appendectomy surgery or at time of autopsy; some present with symptoms related to obstruction and associated inflammation, torsion, bleeding, and rupture of the appendix.

Leiomyoma is reportedly the most frequent appendiceal mesenchymal tumor (1.7 percent) (105). About a dozen *gastrointestinal stromal tumors* (GIST) have been reported in the literature (106,107). Other reported mesenchymal tumors include *leiomyosarcoma, Kaposi sarcoma* as a concomitant presentation of multifocal gastrointestinal involvement in immune compromised individuals (108), *granular cell tumor* (fig. 5-22) (109), *gangliocytic paraganglioma* (47), *schwannoma, lipoma*, and *hemangioma* (97). The histologic features of these mesenchymal tumors are similar to those of their counterpart in the intestinal tract (see chapter 8).

Lymphoma

While the gastrointestinal tract is the frequent site of involvement for extranodal lymphoma, isolated *primary appendiceal lymphoma* accounts for less than 1 percent of cases (105,110); all have been non-Hodgkin lymphomas. Patients present with symptoms of acute appendicitis, palpable masses, intussusception, bleeding, or perforation. *Burkitt lymphoma* presents almost exclusively in children and young adults (111) and *diffuse large B-cell lymphoma* is the most common type appendiceal lymphoma in adults (112). Extranodal marginal zone B-cell lymphoma of mucosa-associated lymphoid tissue (MALT) type, mantle cell lymphoma, follicular lymphoma (113), small lymphocytic lymphoma/chronic lymphocytic leukemia (CLL), anaplastic large T-cell lymphoma, and peripheral

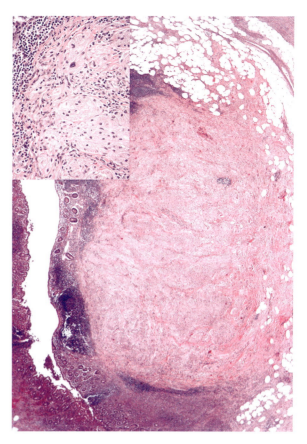

Figure 5-22

GRANULAR CELL TUMOR

A large granular cell tumor presents as a mural mass with abundant granular cytoplasm and bland cytologic features.

T-cell lymphoma, have been reported in the appendix (113–116). The histologic features of lymphomas are similar throughout the intestinal tract as discussed in chapter 9.

REFERENCES

1. McCusker ME, Cote TR, Clegg LX, Sobin LH. Primary malignant neoplasms of the appendix: a population-based study from the surveillance, epidemiology and end-results program, 1973-1998. Cancer 2002;94:3307-3312.

2. Connor SJ, Hanna GB, Frizelle FA. Appendiceal tumors: retrospective clinicopathologic analysis of appendiceal tumors from 7,970 appendectomies. Dis Colon Rectum 1998;41:75-80.

3. Snover DC, Ahnen D, Burt R, Odze RD. Serrated polyps of the colon and rectum and serrated polyposis. In: Bosman FT, Carneiro F, Hruban RH, Theise ND. Lyon: IARC Press; 2010.

4. Bellizzi AM, Rock J, Marsh WL, Frankel WL. Serrated lesions of the appendix: a morphologic and immunohistochemical appraisal. Am J Clin Pathol 2010;133:623-632.

5. Yantiss RK, Panczykowski A, Misdraji J, et al. A comprehensive study of nondysplastic and dysplastic serrated polyps of the vermiform appendix. Am J Surg Pathol 2007;31:1742-1753.

6. Pai RK, Hartman DJ, Gonzalo DH, et al. Serrated lesions of the appendix frequently harbor KRAS mutations and not BRAF mutations indicating a distinctly different serrated neoplastic pathway in the appendix. Hum Pathol 2014;45:227-235.

7. Snover DC, Jass JR, Fenoglio-Preiser C, Batts KP. Serrated polyps of the large intestine: a morphologic and molecular review of an evolving concept. Am J Clin Pathol 2005;124:380-391.

8. Weisenberger DJ, Siegmund KD, Campan M, et al. CpG island methylator phenotype underlies sporadic microsatellite instability and is tightly associated with BRAF mutation in colorectal cancer. Nat Genet 2006;38:787-793.

9. Bettington M, Brown IS, Rosty C. Serrated lesions of the appendix in serrated polyposis patients. Pathology 2016;48:30-34.

10. Liu X, Mody K, de Abreu FB, et al. Molecular profiling of appendiceal epithelial tumors using massively parallel sequencing to identify somatic mutations. Clin Chem 2014;60:1004-1011.

11. Asare EA, Compton CC, Hanna NN, et al. The impact of stage, grade, and mucinous histology on the efficacy of systemic chemotherapy in adenocarcinomas of the appendix: Analysis of the National Cancer Data Base. Cancer 2016;122:213-221.

12. Parker GM, Stollman NH, Rogers A. Adenomatous polyposis coli presenting as adenocarcinoma of the appendix. Am J Gastroenterol 1996;91:801-802.

13. Koorey D, Basha NJ, Tomaras C, Freiman J, Robson L, Smith A. Appendiceal carcinoma complicating adenomatous polyposis in a young woman with a de novo constitutional reciprocal translocation t(5;8)(q22;p23.1). J Med Genet 2000;37:71-75.

14. Kabbani W, Houlihan PS, Luthra R, Hamilton SR, Rashid A. Mucinous and nonmucinous appendiceal adenocarcinomas: different clinicopathological features but similar genetic alterations. Mod Pathol 2002;15:599-605.

15. Bosman FT, Carneiro F, Hruban RH, Theise ND. WHO Classification of tumours of the digestive system. World Health Organization. 2010.

16. Overman MJ, Fournier K, Hu CY, et al. Improving the AJCC/TNM staging for adenocarcinomas of the appendix: the prognostic impact of histological grade. Ann Surg 2013;257:1072-1078.

17. Tejani MA, ter Veer A, Milne D, et al. Systemic therapy for advanced appendiceal adenocarcinoma: an analysis from the NCCN Oncology Outcomes Database for colorectal cancer. J Natl Compr Canc Netw 2014;12:1123-1130.

18. Tang LH. Epithelial neoplasms of the appendix. Arch Pathol Lab Med 2010;134:1612-1620.

19. Panarelli NC, Yantiss RK. Mucinous neoplasms of the appendix and peritoneum. Arch Pathol Lab Med 2011;135:1261-1268.

20. Carr NJ, Cecil TD, Mohamed F, et al. A consensus for classification and pathologic reporting of pseudomyxoma peritonei and associated appendiceal neoplasia: the results of the Peritoneal Surface Oncology Group International (PSOGI) Modified Delphi Process. Am J Surg Pathol 2016;40:14-26.

21. Ronnett BM, Yan H, Kurman RJ, Shmookler BM, Wu L, Sugarbaker PH. Patients with pseudomyxoma peritonei associated with disseminated peritoneal adenomucinosis have a significantly more favorable prognosis than patients with peritoneal mucinous carcinomatosis. Cancer 2001;92:85-91.

22. Bradley RF, Stewart JH 4th, Russell GB, Levine EA, Geisinger KR. Pseudomyxoma peritonei of appendiceal origin: a clinicopathologic analysis of 101 patients uniformly treated at a single institution, with literature review. Am J Surg Pathol 2006;30:551-559.

23. Misdraji J, Yantiss RK, Graeme-Cook FM, Balis UJ, Young RH. Appendiceal mucinous neoplasms: a clinicopathologic analysis of 107 cases. Am J Surg Pathol 2003;27:1089-1103.

24. Turaga KK, Pappas SG, Gamblin T. Importance of histologic subtype in the staging of appendiceal tumors. Ann Surg Oncol 2012;19:1379-1385.

25. Pai RK, Beck AH, Norton JA, Longacre TA. Appendiceal mucinous neoplasms: clinicopathologic study of 116 cases with analysis of factors predicting recurrence. Am J Surg Pathol 2009;33:1425-1439.

26. Ronnett BM. Pseudomyxoma peritonei: a rose by any other name. Am J Surg Pathol 2006;30:1483-1484; author reply 1484-1485.

27. Aho AJ, Heinonen R, Lauren P. Benign and malignant mucocele of the appendix. Histological types and prognosis. Acta Chir Scand 1973;139:392-400.

28. Carr NJ, Sobin LH. Adenocarcinoma of the Appendix. In: Bosman FT, Carneiro, F., Hruban, R.H., Theise, N.D., ed. WHO Classification of Tumors of the Digestive System Vol 3. Lyon, France: IARC Press; 2010:120-125.

29. Edge S, Byrd D, Compton C, Fritz A, Greene FL, Trotti A. AJCC Cancer Staging Manual. 7th ed. New York, NY: Springer. 2010:133-141.

30. Lamps LW, Gray GF Jr, Dilday BR, Washington MK. The coexistence of low-grade mucinous neoplasms of the appendix and appendiceal diverticula: a possible role in the pathogenesis of pseudomyxoma peritonei. Mod Pathol 2000;13:495-501.

31. Pai RK, Longacre TA. Appendiceal mucinous tumors and pseudomyxoma peritonei: histologic features, diagnostic problems, and proposed classification. Adv Anat Pathol 2005;12:291-311.

32. Molavi D, Argani P. Distinguishing benign dissecting mucin (stromal mucin pools) from invasive mucinous carcinoma. Adv Anat Pathol 2008;15:1-17.

33. Nitecki SS, Wolff BG, Schlinkert R, Sarr MG. The natural history of surgically treated primary adenocarcinoma of the appendix. Ann Surg 1994;219:51-57.

34. Nash GM, Smith JD, Tang L, et al. Lymph node metastasis predicts disease recurrence in a single-center experience of 70 stages 1-3 appendix cancers: a retrospective review. Ann Surg Oncol 2015;22:3613-3617.

35. Yantiss RK, Shia J, Klimstra DS, Hahn HP, Odze RD, Misdraji J. Prognostic significance of localized extra-appendiceal mucin deposition in appendiceal mucinous neoplasms. Am J Surg Pathol 2009;33:248-255.

36. Amin MB, Greene FL, Edge SB, et al. The eighth edition AJCC cancer staging manual: continuing to build a bridge from a population-based to a more "personalized" approach to cancer staging. CA Cancer J Clin 2017;67:93-99.

37. Prayson RA, Hart WR, Petras RE. Pseudomyxoma peritonei. A clinicopathologic study of 19 cases with emphasis on site of origin and nature of associated ovarian tumors. Am J Surg Pathol 1994;18:591-603.

38. Seidman JD, Elsayed AM, Sobin LH, Tavassoli FA. Association of mucinous tumors of the ovary and appendix. A clinicopathologic study of 25 cases. Am J Surg Pathol 1993;17:22-34.

39. Young RH. Pseudomyxoma peritonei and selected other aspects of the spread of appendiceal neoplasms. Semin Diagn Pathol 2004;21:134-150.

40. Szych C, Staebler A, Connolly DC, Wu R, Cho KR, Ronnett BM. Molecular genetic evidence supporting the clonality and appendiceal origin of Pseudomyxoma peritonei in women. Am J Pathol 1999;154:1849-1855.

41. Cuatrecasas M, Matias-Guiu X, Prat J. Synchronous mucinous tumors of the appendix and the ovary associated with pseudomyxoma peritonei. A clinicopathologic study of six cases with comparative analysis of c-Ki-ras mutations. Am J Surg Pathol 1996;20:739-746.

42. Carr NJ, Finch J, Ilesley IC, et al. Pathology and prognosis in pseudomyxoma peritonei: a review of 274 cases. J Clin Pathol 2012;65:919-923.

43. Rosenberger LH, Stein LH, Witkiewicz AK, Kennedy EP, Yeo CJ. Intraductal papillary mucinous neoplasm (IPMN) with extra-pancreatic mucin: a case series and review of the literature. J Gastrointest Surg 2012;16:762-770.

44. Agrawal AK, Bobinski P, Grzebieniak Z, et al. Pseudomyxoma peritonei originating from urachus-case report and review of the literature. Curr Oncol 2014;21:e155-165.

45. Lieu CH, Lambert LA, Wolff RA, et al. Systemic chemotherapy and surgical cytoreduction for poorly differentiated and signet ring cell adenocarcinomas of the appendix. Ann Oncol 2012;23:652-658.

46. Shapiro JF, Chase JL, Wolff RA, et al. Modern systemic chemotherapy in surgically unresectable neoplasms of appendiceal origin: a single-institution experience. Cancer 2010;116:316-322.

47. Abdelbaqi MQ, Tahmasbi M, Ghayouri M. Gangliocytic paraganglioma of the appendix with features suggestive of malignancy, a rare case report and review of the literature. Int J Clin Exp Pathol 2013;6:1948-1952.

48. Gough DB, Donohue JH, Schutt AJ, et al. Pseudomyxoma peritonei. Long-term patient survival with an aggressive regional approach. Ann Surg 1994;219:112-119.

49. Loungnarath R, Causeret S, Bossard N, et al. Cytoreductive surgery with intraperitoneal chemohyperthermia for the treatment of pseudomyxoma peritonei: a prospective study. Dis Colon Rectum 2005;48:1372-1379.

50. Sugarbaker PH. The natural history, gross pathology, and histopathology of appendiceal epithelial neoplasms. Eur J Surg Oncol. Aug 2006;32:644-647.

51. Sugarbaker PH, Alderman R, Edwards G, et al. Prospective morbidity and mortality assessment of cytoreductive surgery plus perioperative intraperitoneal chemotherapy to treat peritoneal dissemination of appendiceal mucinous malignancy. Ann Surg Oncol 2006;13:635-644.

52. Nummela P, Saarinen L, Thiel A, et al. Genomic profile of pseudomyxoma peritonei analyzed using next-generation sequencing and immunohistochemistry. Int J Cancer 2015;136:E282-289.

53. Hara K, Saito T, Hayashi T, et al. A mutation spectrum that includes GNAS, KRAS and TP53 may be shared by mucinous neoplasms of the appendix. Pathol Res Pract 2015;211:657-664.

54. Singhi AD, Davison JM, Choudry HA, et al. GNAS is frequently mutated in both low-grade and high-grade disseminated appendiceal mucinous neoplasms but does not affect survival. Hum Pathol 2014;45:1737-1743.

55. Nishikawa G, Sekine S, Ogawa R, et al. Frequent GNAS mutations in low-grade appendiceal mucinous neoplasms. Br J Cancer 2013;108:951-958.

56. Shetty S, Thomas P, Ramanan B, Sharma P, Govindarajan V, Loggie B. Kras mutations and p53 overexpression in pseudomyxoma peritonei: association with phenotype and prognosis. J Surg Res 2013;180:97-103.

57. Bazan V, Migliavacca M, Zanna I, et al. Specific codon 13 K-ras mutations are predictive of clinical outcome in colorectal cancer patients, whereas codon 12 K-ras mutations are associated with mucinous histotype. Ann Oncol 2002;13:1438-1446.

58. Burke AP, Sobin LH, Federspiel BH, Shekitka KM, Helwig EB. Goblet cell carcinoids and related tumors of the vermiform appendix. Am J Clin Pathol 1990;94:27-35.

59. van Eeden S, Offerhaus GJ, Hart AA, et al. Goblet cell carcinoid of the appendix: a specific type of carcinoma. Histopathology 2007;51:763-773.

60. Taggart MW, Abraham SC, Overman MJ, Mansfield PF, Rashid A. Goblet cell carcinoid tumor, mixed goblet cell carcinoid-adenocarcinoma, and adenocarcinoma of the appendix: comparison of clinicopathologic features and prognosis. Arch Pathol Lab Med 2015;139:782-790.

61. Tang LH, Shia J, Soslow RA, et al. Pathologic classification and clinical behavior of the spectrum of goblet cell carcinoid tumors of the appendix. Am J Surg Pathol 2008;32:1429-1443.

62. Reid MD, Basturk O, Shaib WL, et al. Adenocarcinoma ex-goblet cell carcinoid (appendiceal-type crypt cell adenocarcinoma) is a morphologically distinct entity with highly aggressive behavior and frequent association with peritoneal/intra-abdominal dissemination: an analysis of 77 cases. Mod Pathol 2016;29:1243-1253.

63. Hofler H, Kloppel G, Heitz PU. Combined production of mucus, amines and peptides by goblet-cell carcinoids of the appendix and ileum. Pathol Res Pract 1984;178:555-561.

64. Bak M, Asschenfeldt P. Adenocarcinoid of the vermiform appendix. A clinicopathologic study of 20 cases. Dis Colon Rectum 1988;31:605-612.

65. Capella C, Solcia E, Sobin L. R.A. Pathology & Genetics. Tumours of the Digestive System. IARC Press; 2000:53-57.

66. Warkel RL, Cooper PH, Helwig EB. Adenocarcinoid, a mucin-producing carcinoid tumor of the appendix: a study of 39 cases. Cancer 1978;42:2781-2793.

67. Chen V, Qizilbash AH. Goblet cell carcinoid tumor of the appendix. Report of five cases and review of the literature. Arch Pathol Lab Med 1979;103:180-182.

68. Watson PH, Alguacil-Garcia A. Mixed crypt cell carcinoma. A clinicopathological study of the so-called 'goblet cell carcinoid'. Virchows Arch A Pathol Anat Histopathol 1987;412:175-182.

69. Isaacson P. Crypt cell carcinoma of the appendix (so-called adenocarcinoid tumor). Am J Surg Pathol 1981;5:213-224.

70. Ramnani DM, Wistuba II, Behrens C, Gazdar AF, Sobin LH, Albores-Saavedra J. K-ras and p53 mutations in the pathogenesis of classical and goblet cell carcinoids of the appendix. Cancer 1999;86:14-21.

71. Lin BT, Gown AM. Mixed carcinoid and adenocarcinoma of the appendix: report of 4 cases with immunohistochemical studies and a review of the literature. Appl Immunohistochem Mol Morphol 2004;12:271-276.

72. Goede AC, Caplin ME, Winslet MC. Carcinoid tumour of the appendix. Br J Surg 2003;90:1317-1322.

73. Anderson NH, Somerville JE, Johnston CF, Hayes DM, Buchanan KD, Sloan JM. Appendiceal goblet cell carcinoids: a clinicopathological and immunohistochemical study. Histopathology 1991;18:61-65.

74. Burke A, Sobin L. The histogenesis of appendiceal carcinoid tumours. Histopathology 1992;21:600-601.

75. Riddell R, Petras RE, Williams G, Sobin L. Tumors of the intestines. AFIP Atlas of Tumor Pathology, 3rd Series, Fascicle 32. Washington, DC. American Registry of Pathology; 2003;32:303-304.

76. Sandor A, Modlin IM. A retrospective analysis of 1570 appendiceal carcinoids. Am J Gastroenterol 1998;93:422-428.

77. Hristov AC, Young RH, Vang R, Yemelyanova AV, Seidman JD, Ronnett BM. Ovarian metastases of appendiceal tumors with goblet cell carcinoidlike and signet ring cell patterns: a report of 30 cases. Am J Surg Pathol 2007;31:1502-1511.

78. Carr NJ, Remotti H, Sobin LH. Dual carcinoid/epithelial neoplasia of the appendix. Histopathology 1995;27:557-562.

79. Chetty R, Klimstra DS, Henson DE, Albores-Saavedra J. Combined classical carcinoid and goblet cell carcinoid tumor: a new morphologic variant of carcinoid tumor of the appendix. Am J Surg Pathol 2010;34:1163-1167.

80. Masson P. Carcinoids (Argentaffin-Cell Tumors) and Nerve Hyperplasia of the Appendicular Mucosa. Am J Pathol 1928;4:181-212

81. Shaw PA. Carcinoid tumours of the appendix are different. J Pathol 1990;162:189-190.

82. Kinzler KW, Vogelstein B. Lessons from hereditary colorectal cancer. Cell 1996;87159-170.

83. Neibergs HL, Hein DW, Spratt JS. Genetic profiling of colon cancer. J Surg Oncol 2002;80:204-213.

84. Ajioka Y, Xing PX, Hinoda Y, Jass JR. Correlative histochemical study providing evidence for the dual nature of human colorectal cancer mucin. Histochem J 1997;29:143-152.

85. Matsuda K, Masaki T, Watanabe T, et al. Clinical significance of MUC1 and MUC2 mucin and p53 protein expression in colorectal carcinoma. Jpn J Clin Oncol 2000;30:89-94.

86. Bucher P, Gervaz P, Ris F, Oulhaci W, Egger JF, Morel P. Surgical treatment of appendiceal adenocarcinoid (goblet cell carcinoid). World J Surg 2005;29:1436-1439.

87. Varisco B, McAlvin B, Dias J, Franga D. Adenocarcinoid of the appendix: is right hemicolectomy necessary? A meta-analysis of retrospective chart reviews. Am Surg 2004;70:593-599.

88. Pham TH, Wolff B, Abraham SC, Drelichman E. Surgical and chemotherapy treatment outcomes of goblet cell carcinoid: a tertiary cancer center experience. Ann Surg Oncol 2006;13:370-376.

89. Mahteme H, Sugarbaker PH. Treatment of peritoneal carcinomatosis from adenocarcinoid of appendiceal origin. Br J Surg 2004;91:1168-1173.

90. Shaib WL, Martin LK, Choi M, et al. Hyperthermic Intraperitoneal chemotherapy following cytoreductive surgery improves outcome in patients with primary appendiceal mucinous adenocarcinoma: a pooled analysis from three tertiary care centers. Oncologist 2015;20:907-914.

91. Butler JA, Houshiar A, Lin F, Wilson SE. Goblet cell carcinoid of the appendix. Am J Surg 1994;168:685-687.

92. Jevon GP, Daya D, Qizilbash AH. Intussusception of the appendix. A report of four cases and review of the literature. Arch Pathol Lab Med 1992;116:960-964.

93. Forshall I. Intussusception of the vermiform appendix with a report of seven cases in children. Br J Surg 1953;40:305-312.

94. Langsam LB, Raj PK, Galang CF. Intussusception of the appendix. Dis Colon Rectum 1984;27:387-392.

95. Lie KA, Lindboe CF, Kolmannskog SK, Haugen SE, Grammeltvedt AT. Giant appendix with diffuse ganglioneuromatosis. An unusual presentation of von Recklinghausen's disease. Eur J Surg 1992;158:127-128.

96. Merck C, Kindblom LG. Neurofibromatosis of the appendix in von Recklinghausen's disease. A report of a case. Acta Pathol Microbiol Scand A 1975;83:623-627.

97. Misdraji J, Graeme-Cook FM. Miscellaneous conditions of the appendix. Semin Diagn Pathol 2004;21:151-163.

98. Olsen BS. Giant appendicular neurofibroma. A light and immunohistochemical study. Histopathology 1987;11:851-855.

99. Pittaway DE. Appendectomy in the surgical treatment of endometriosis. Obstet Gynecol 1983;61:421-424.

100. Saleem A, Navarro P, Munson JL, Hall J. Endometriosis of the appendix: Report of three cases. Int J Surg Case Rep 2011;2:16-19.

101. Yantiss RK, Clement PB, Young RH. Endometriosis of the intestinal tract: a study of 44 cases of a disease that may cause diverse challenges in clinical and pathologic evaluation. Am J Surg Pathol 2001;25:445-454.

102. Bansal A, Zakhour HD. Benign mesothelioma of the appendix: an incidental finding in a case of sigmoid diverticular disease. J Clin Pathol 2006;59:108-110.

103. O'Connor DB, Beddy D, Aremu MA. Benign cystic mesothelioma of the appendix presenting in a woman: a case report. J Med Case Rep 2010;4:394.

104. Hayashi K, Takamura M, Sato Y, et al. Primary malignant mesothelioma of the appendix. Intern Med 2012;51:1027-1030.

105. Collins DC. 71,000 human appendix specimens. A final report, summarizing forty years' study. Am J Proctol 1963;14:265-281.

106. Agaimy A, Pelz AF, Wieacker P, Roessner A, Wunsch PH, Schneider-Stock R. Gastrointestinal stromal tumors of the vermiform appendix: clinicopathologic, immunohistochemical, and molecular study of 2 cases with literature review. Hum Pathol 2008;39:1252-1257.

107. Vassos N, Agaimy A, Gunther K, Hohenberger W, Schneider-Stock R, Croner RS. A novel complex KIT mutation in a gastrointestinal stromal tumor of the vermiform appendix. Hum Pathol 2013;44:651-655.

108. Chetty R, Arendse MP. Gastro-intestinal Kaposi's sarcoma, with special reference to the appendix. S Afr J Surg 1999;37:9-11.

109. Gavelli A, Clement N, Marmorale A, et al. [Granular cell tumor involving the appendix]. Gastroenterol Clin Biol 2005;29:211-212. [French]

110. Lewin KJ, Ranchod M, Dorfman RF. Lymphomas of the gastrointestinal tract: a study of 117 cases presenting with gastrointestinal disease. Cancer 1978;42:693-707.

111. Sin IC, Ling ET, Prentice RS. Burkitt's lymphoma of the appendix: report of two cases. Hum Pathol 1980;11:465-470.

112. Stewart RJ, Mirakhur M. Primary malignant lymphoma of the appendix. Ulster Med J 1986;55:187-189.

113. Furuse M, Aoyagi K, Esaki M, et al. Endoscopic appearance of primary appendiceal lymphoma. Gastrointest Endosc 1998;48:86-87.

114. Muller G, Dargent JL, Duwel V, et al. Leukaemia and lymphoma of the appendix presenting as acute appendicitis or acute abdomen. Four case reports with a review of the literature. J Cancer Res Clin Oncol 1997;123:560-564.

115. Kitamura Y, Ohta T, Terada T. Primary T-cell non-Hodgkin's malignant lymphoma of the appendix. Pathol Int 2000;50:313-317.

116. Pasquale MD, Shabahang M, Bitterman P, Lack EE, Evans SR. Primary lymphoma of the appendix. Case report and review of the literature. Surg Oncol 1994;3:243-248.

CONDYLOMAS AND ANAL INTRAEPITHELIAL NEOPLASIA/BOWEN DISEASE

General Features. Most anal squamous lesions, whether they are *condylomas, flat squamous dysplasia/anal intraepithelial neoplasia* (AIN), or *invasive squamous cell carcinoma,* are related to human papillomavirus (HPV). HPV is a double-stranded DNA virus that is transmitted by skin-to-skin contact or mucosa-to-mucosa contact. There are over 150 types and it is estimated that over half are associated with the formation of warty lesions of the hands and feet, genital area, anus, and oropharynx. It is estimated that up to 20 million persons in the United States are infected annually and the total number of infected persons is 80 to 110 million (see http://www.cdc.gov/std/hpv/). Most individuals who are infected are able to clear the virus without intervention but some infections progress to neoplasia. Affected sites include uterine cervix, oropharynx, anus, vulva, vagina, and penis.

The most common HPV types that cause neoplasia are HPV16 and 18 but men who have sex with men and are HPV16 positive often have co-infections with types 11, 51, 52, 6, 68, 74, 45, 26, 44, 70, 53, 54, 82, 31, 33, 56, 58, and 59 (1). The HPV types considered "at least possibly carcinogenic to humans" include 16, 18, 31, 33, 35, 39, 51, 52, 56, 58, 59, and 68 (2). A vaccine to prevent HPV16 and 18 as well as types 6 and 11 (which produce warts) was introduced in 2006 and some long-term efficacy data are available as of this writing (3). In the population of human immunodeficiency virus (HIV)-infected men who have sex with men (MSM), and who have nearly 40-fold the risk for anal squamous carcinoma than the general population, vaccination has been shown to be cost effective (4). Furthermore, the Centers for Disease Control (CDC) published a formal endorsement of HPV vaccination in both young men and young women as of 2013 (5).

The incidence of anogenital warts (condylomas) has been estimated at about 100 to 170 persons per 100,000 in Canada and Europe (3) and at 205 cases per 100,000 per year in the United States (6). For men, risk factors for acquiring HPV infection include a high number of female sexual partners; the number of male anal-sexual partners and clearance of virus seems to increase with age (7). In HIV-positive women (8) the prevalence of anal high-risk (HR)-HPV is 16 to 85 percent. The reported prevalence of anal HR-HPV infection in HIV-negative women ranges from 4 to 86 percent, similar to that of HIV-infected women, evidence that most women clear the infection. The prevalence of anal HR-HPV in HIV-negative women with HPV-related pathology of the female genital tract varies from 23 to 86 percent compared with 5 to 22 percent in women with no known HPV-related genital pathology. Histologic anal high-grade squamous intraepithelial lesions (AIN 2 or greater) has been reported in 3 to 26 percent of HIV-positive women, 0 to 9 percent of HIV-negative women with lower genital tract pathology, and 0 to 3 percent of women who are HIV negative and lack known lower genital tract pathology.

Most cases of AIN do not progress to cancer: it has been estimated that the rate of progression of high-grade AIN to squamous cell carcinoma is 1 to 3 percent at 5 years in the MSM population (9) and it is probably far lower in fully immunocompetent persons. In HIV-infected MSM without high-grade AIN at baseline, the cumulative incidence of biopsy-confirmed high-grade AIN has been estimated at about 7 percent at 1 year, 16 percent at 2 years, and about 25 percent at 3 years (10). Those taking antiretroviral treatment and in stable relationships were protected from progression (10).

Clinical Features and Gross Findings. Condylomas are polypoid cauliflower-like warty anogenital papules (fig. 6-1), typically diagnosed

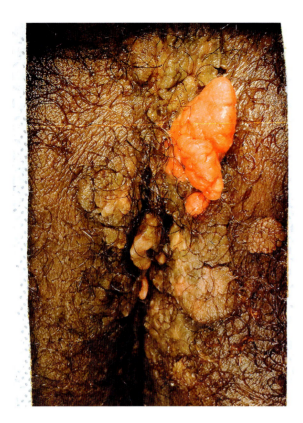

Figure 6-1

CONDYLOMA

This is an extensive lesion exhibiting multiple polypoid excrescences.

by gynecologists in women and dermatologists in men. As above, most are associated with HPV types 6 and 11, and they only exceptionally progress to squamous cell carcinomas.

Bowen disease is a high-grade squamous intraepithelial lesion/squamous cell carcinoma in situ in the hair-bearing perianal skin or on the penis/vulva. It presents as an erythematous scaly patch or plaque ranging from 1 to 3 cm. A subset of lesions is pruritic. Some examples in the anogenital region, termed *bowenoid papulosis*, consist of crops of papules resembling small condylomas. The term *erythroplasia of Queyrat* has been applied to histologically identical lesions of the prepuce or glans penis and vulva. Such lesions, like condylomas and AIN, are HPV associated, usually with HPV16 rather than with HPV6 or 11 (typically the types associated with classic condylomas). The likelihood that any of them will progress to carcinoma is 1 to 3 percent.

AIN refers to lesions that usually arise at the junction of the columnar colonic-type mucosa and the squamous mucosa. On high-resolution anoscopy, the findings are similar to those encountered at the junction of the uterine cervix and endocervix at colposcopy (11), namely, flat leukoplakia, hyperkeratotic leukoplakia, zones that are either acetowhite or lugol negative, and areas of abnormal vascularity (10).

Microscopic Findings. Like the uterine cervix, the anal canal has a transformation zone but it cannot be visualized without the use of anoscopy, so a procedure is required even for cytologic screening. In biopsies obtained from this area (anoscopically at the dentate/pectinate line), there are typically fragments of rectal-type mucosa adjoining, or separate from, the lesion. The histology of anal squamous intraepithelial lesions is essentially like that found in the uterine cervix. Such lesions have been classified as AIN1, AIN2, and AIN3, but now, as for the cervix, most observers prefer to separate low- and high-grade lesions, with the AIN2 subsumed under high grade. In AIN1, immature mitotically active basaloid cells extend into the lower third of the squamous epithelium, in AIN2 they extend between one third and two thirds of the thickness of the epithelium, and in AIN3 atypical cells extend for more than two thirds of the epithelial thickness (figs. 6-2–6-13). Findings sought on biopsy are loss of nuclear stratification and polarity, nuclear pleomorphism and hyperchromatism (with or without keratinization or HPV viral cytopathic changes), and increased mitoses high in the epithelium. HPV viral cytopathic changes (koilocytes) are seen in exophytic (condyloma acuminata) or flat lesions. Dysplasia may extend into colonic glands and should not be mistaken for invasive tumor.

Bowen disease, as above, is the eponymous term used for squamous carcinoma in situ at the anal margin (in contrast to lesions seen at the transition zone, inside the canal, and at the dentate line). In other words, Bowen disease is essentially an AIN lesion that arises in perianal skin (12). Biopsies display full thickness dysplasia with disorganized nuclei, disorderly maturation, mitoses at all levels, and dyskeratosis, sometimes extending into skin appendages (pilosebaceous units).

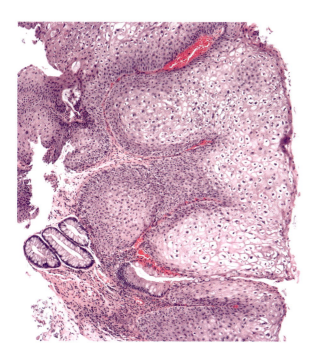

Figure 6-2

LOW-GRADE ANAL INTRAEPITHELIAL NEOPLASIA (AIN)

This lesion shows features of a flat condyloma and has developed at the transition between the anal squamous and colonic-type mucosa. Colorectal glands are seen in the lower part of the field. The lesion displays numerous koilocytes.

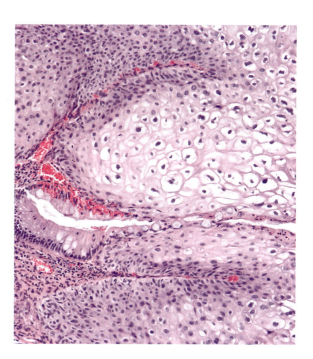

Figure 6-3

KOILOCYTES

These cells are infected with human papillomavirus (HPV) and display enlarged hyperchromatic nuclei suspended in a large perinuclear cavity.

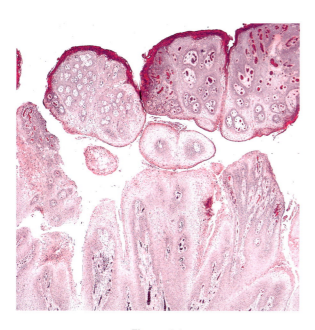

Figure 6-4

CONDYLOMA

This lesion of perianal skin shows multiple papillary fronds, each with a fibrovascular core and a hyperkeratotic surface.

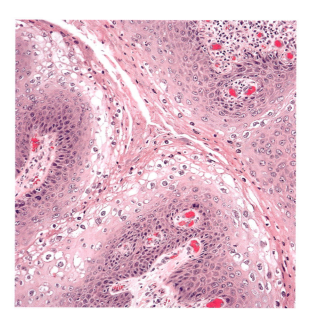

Figure 6-5

CONDYLOMA

The fibrovascular cores are readily identified and numerous koilocytes are present in the center of the field.

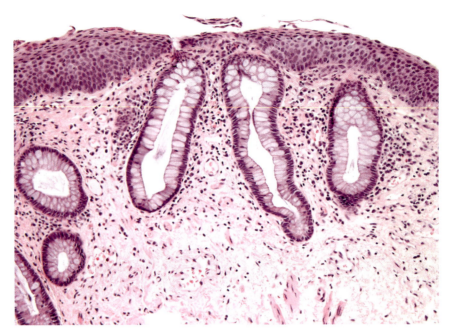

Figure 6-6

HIGH-GRADE ANAL INTRAEPITHELIAL NEOPLASIA

The squamous lesion has large nuclei that extend to more than half of the thickness of the epithelium.

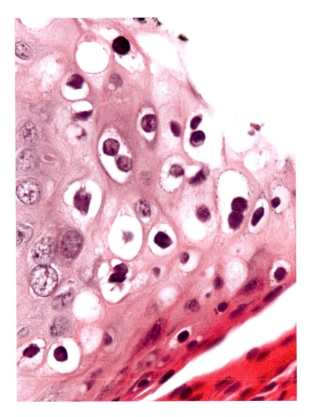

Figure 6-7

CONDYLOMA

Several binucleated cells are present, a common feature in condylomas.

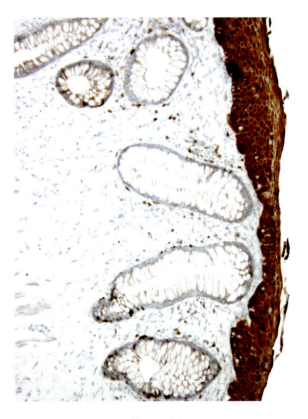

Figure 6-8

HIGH-GRADE ANAL INTRAEPITHELIAL NEOPLASIA

Note the strong p16 labeling.

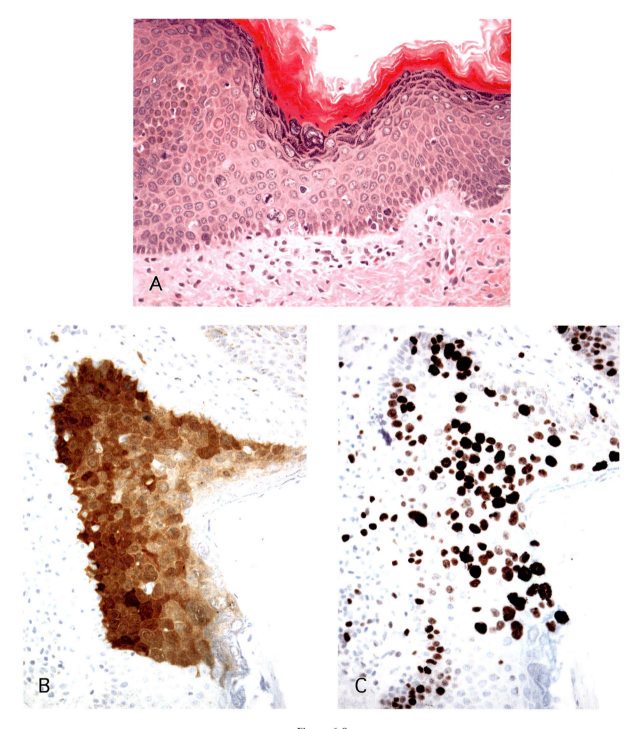

Figure 6-9

HIGH-GRADE ANAL INTRAEPITHELIAL NEOPLASIA

A: This lesion is very subtle on hematoxylin and eosin (H&E) stain but several atypical mitoses suggest that this is a high-grade lesion. However, this case would be controversial.

B: This p16 preparation is from the area depicted in A. Strong p16 immunolabeling is good evidence of high-grade AIN.

C: There is Ki-67 labeling throughout the thickness of the squamous epithelium in the case depicted in A. A positive result is defined as the presence of a cluster of at least two strongly stained epithelial nuclei in the upper two thirds of the epithelial thickness. This labeling pattern is not useful for separating low- and high-grade AIN.

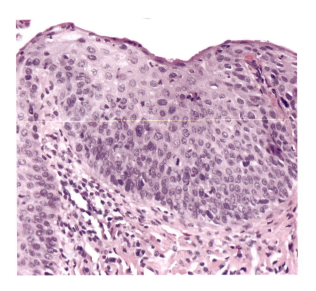

Figure 6-10

HIGH-GRADE ANAL INTRAEPITHELIAL NEOPLASIA

This lesion has a more classic appearance than that seen in figure 6-9, with hyperchromatic basaloid nuclei extending almost to the surface.

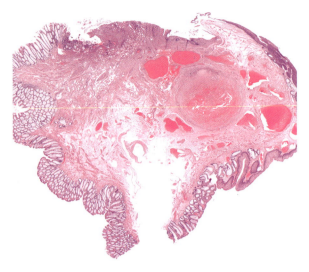

Figure 6-12

HIGH-GRADE ANAL INTRAEPITHELIAL NEOPLASIA IN A HEMORRHOIDECTOMY SAMPLE

It is important to always scan such samples for squamous lesions, which are sometimes detected incidentally. The lesion is at the upper right of the field.

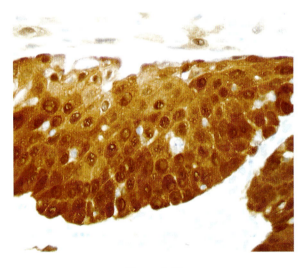

Figure 6-11

HIGH-GRADE ANAL INTRAEPITHELIAL NEOPLASIA: P16 IMMUNOLABELING

There is strong diffuse immunolabeling.

Immunohistochemical Findings. Since interpretation of AIN samples is somewhat hampered by observer variation, the use of immunolabeling helps confirm a diagnosis (figs. 6-9B,C; 6-11; 6-13A,B). Ki-67 (MIB-1) labeling as well as p16 immunolabeling are useful for assessing dysplasia in biopsies and are well studied (13,14).

Ki-67, used according to guidelines, is a sensitive and specific marker for dysplasia in mature squamous epithelium and is therefore helpful for the confirmation of AIN1 and condyloma. A Ki-67-positive result is defined as the presence of a cluster of at least two strongly stained epithelial nuclei in the upper two thirds of the epithelial thickness. The key point of this labeling pattern is that is it not for separating low- and high-grade intraepithelial neoplasia. Additionally, it does not separate low-risk from high-risk HPV type lesions. Reactive lymphocytes express Ki-67 and should not be interpreted as epithelial cells. Lastly, it does not distinguish reparative changes from intraepithelial neoplasia.

Based on the limitations of Ki-67 labeling, it is useful to combine it with p16 immunolabeling, which is evaluated using a two-tier system: an absent or discontinuous, patchy nuclear and cytoplasmic staining pattern is considered a negative result; a positive result consists of diffuse and strong staining of cells of the basal and parabasal layers of the squamous epithelium, with or without superficial staining. P16 is a regulatory protein that inhibits the cell cycle by interfering with retinoblastoma tumor suppressor protein (pRB) phosphorylation. Cells

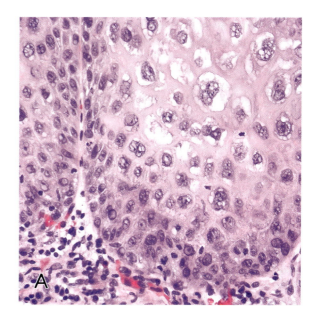

Figure 6-13

LOW-GRADE ANAL INTRAEPITHELIAL NEOPLASIA

A: Large hyperchromatic basal cells extend less than half the thickness of the epithelium.

B: With Ki-67 immunolabeling there are clusters of positive nuclei in the sample shown in A. This pattern does not separate low- and high-dysplasia but can confirm that dysplasia is present.

C: This example is nonreactive for p16, which, together with the morphology (A) and Ki-67 labeling pattern, is supportive of an interpretation of low-grade AIN.

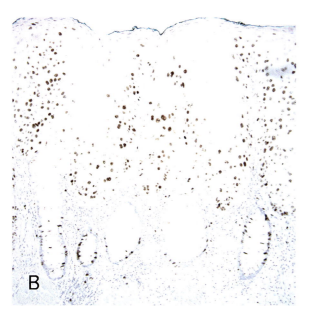

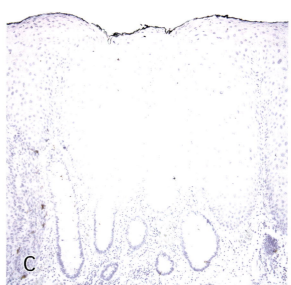

that are infected with oncogenic HPVs have functional overexpression of p16 because pRB proliferation is abrogated by E7 HPV oncoprotein. P16 labeling is an excellent marker of high-grade AIN but has limited value in confirming a diagnosis of low-grade AIN.

Other studied antibodies include stathmin-1, ProEx C, phosphorylated S6, SOX2, p53, and capsid protein L1 (13,14).

Molecular Genetic Findings. The viral molecular underpinnings of these lesions mirror those of invasive squamous cell carcinoma and

are further discussed below. For daily diagnostic work, HPV DNA in situ hybridization is less sensitive than immunolabeling for both low- and high-grade AIN. Newer HPV RNA probes for E6/E7 mRNA appear promising as of this writing (15).

Treatment and Prognosis. Current treatment options for AIN include electrofulguration, infrared coagulation, immunomodulation therapy with imiquimod 5 percent cream, and surgical excision. Most lesions do not progress to cancer.

SQUAMOUS CELL CARCINOMA

General Features and Risk Factors. The number of cases of anal carcinoma in the United States is low: for 2016, the estimated number of anal cancers is about 8,100, with a female to male ratio of 1.7 to 1.0 (16). About 1,100 deaths are estimated (16). This contrasts with an expected number of about 135,000 new colorectal cancers (16). Based on the National Cancer Institute's (NCI) Surveillance, Epidemiology, and End Results (SEER) data, however, the number of anal cancers and in situ carcinomas is steadily increasing, an increase attributed to increasing HPV infections (17).

Most anal cancers in the United States are squamous carcinomas. The precursors noted above are the major risk factors, even condylomas (18), as are lifetime number of sexual partners, receptive anal intercourse, and HIV infection, but these factors are all intertwined with HPV as the common denominator. There is also some association with smoking. Incidence estimates range from 0.2 to 4.4 cases per 100,000 people per year with a female predominance, but these increase to about 35 per 100,000 for MSM and to 750-135 per 100,000 for HIV infected persons (19).

There is little, if any, risk associated with the presence of hemorrhoids, fissures, or fistulae. Furthermore, a history of inflammatory bowel disease has now been shown not to predispose patients to anal cancer, in contrast to prior anecdotal views. Frisch et al. (20) linked the hospital records of 68,549 patients with the Danish Cancer Registry and found no anal cancers in any of the 651 patients with Crohn disease or the 509 patients with ulcerative colitis.

Clinical Features. Rectal bleeding is the most common initial symptom of squamous cell carcinoma of the anus, occurring in about half of patients and sometimes attributed to hemorrhoids (21). A history of anorectal condylomas can be elicited in about half of MSM with anal cancer, but in only 20 percent of women and men who have sex with women with anal cancer (21).

Gross Findings. In the past, the pathologist often encountered a firm, indurated or ulcerated tumor in the anal canal but typically anal carcinomas are biopsied and treated with chemoradiation so such samples are seldom

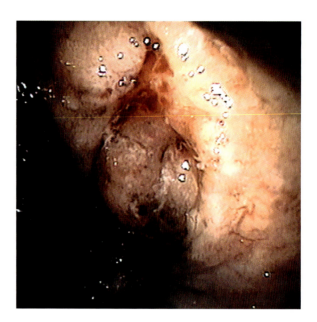

Figure 6-14

ANAL SQUAMOUS CELL CARCINOMA

Endoscopic image shows a polypoid and ulcerated lesion.

encountered. Many lesions present as polyps or anal tags (fig. 6-14).

Microscopic Findings. Tumors arising within the anal canal distal to the dentate line are often keratinizing squamous cell carcinomas, whereas those appearing in the transitional mucosa above the dentate line are frequently nonkeratinizing squamous cell carcinomas. The nonkeratinizing subtypes were once referred to as transitional cell and cloacogenic; they are now, however, recognized as variants of squamous cell carcinoma that lack classic terminal differentiation. One type is composed of large cells and the other is characterized by small cells (figs. 6-15–6-19). Many tumors show more than one morphologic subtype but most are diagnosed on small biopsies, which likely do not represent the entire tumor morphology.

The bladder and anus share a common embryologic origin, thus giving rise to the similar (i.e., transitional or cloacogenic) morphology. The biology and prognosis of keratinizing and nonkeratinizing tumors of the anal canal are essentially the same, so prior concern about subclassification of anal tumors is probably not warranted. Furthermore, pathologists do not always reproducibly separate the categories, further

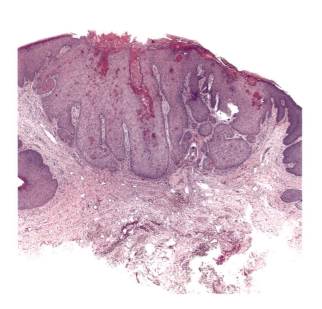 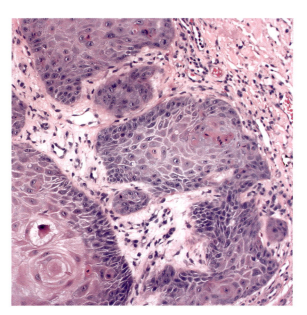

Figure 6-15

ANAL SQUAMOUS CELL CARCINOMA

Left: This is a highly differentiated carcinoma arising in perianal skin. Skin appendages are seen at the right side of the image. The tumor has a verrucous appearance but an infiltrative deep border.

Right: At higher magnification, the deep portion of the lesion is shown.

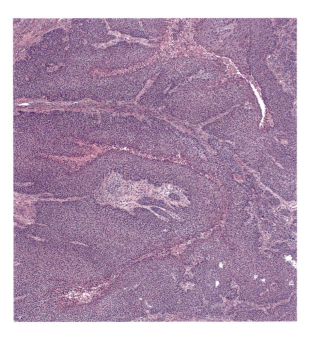

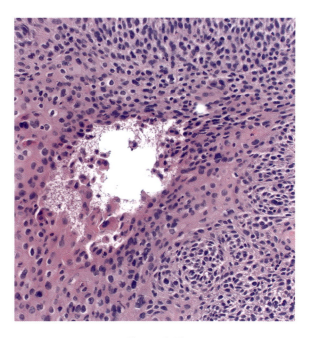

Figure 6-16

ANAL SQUAMOUS CELL CARCINOMA

This is a basaloid squamous cell carcinoma. Such tumors were referred to as "cloacogenic" carcinomas in the past. The tumor consists of small hyperchromatic basal-type cells. In this field, the lesion looks in situ, but it was from the center of a bulky mass.

Figure 6-17

ANAL SQUAMOUS CELL CARCINOMA

At times it can be difficult to separate basaloid squamous cell carcinomas from other neoplasms. Often a careful search yields zones with brightly eosinophilic keratinized cells, a clue to the diagnosis.

237

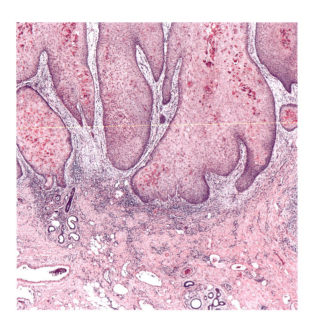 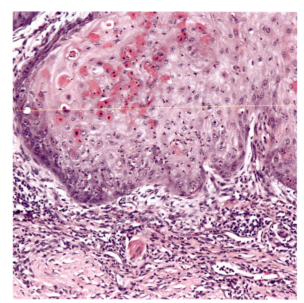

Figure 6-18

ANAL SQUAMOUS CELL CARCINOMA

Left: This lesion, like the one in figure 6-15, has verrucous features. This one arose within the anal canal and has overall pushing borders. Such tumors have a favorable outcome.

Right: Higher magnification shows pushing borders.

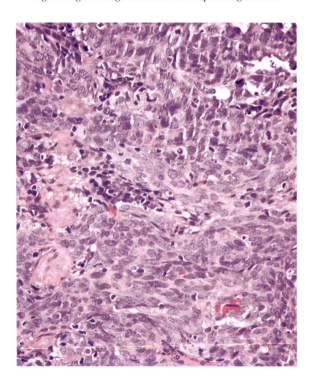 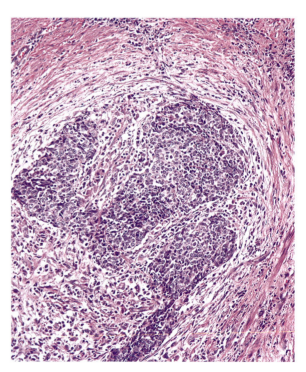

Figure 6-19

ANAL SQUAMOUS CELL CARCINOMA

Left: This basaloid squamous cell carcinoma has a spindled appearance, along with streaming hyperchromatic nuclei.

Right: In another field, tumor infiltrating lymphocytes are seen.

limiting their utility (22). Tumor differentiation, however, should be included in the report, since poorly differentiated neoplasms are associated with a higher risk of death than well to moderately differentiated examples (23).

Squamous carcinomas of the anorectum have essentially the same morphology as those in other anatomic sites other than their proclivity to have a basaloid appearance. An exception to the usual striking epithelial changes is the rare *verrucous carcinoma* (fig. 6-18), which displays broad-based squamous papillae that are sheet-like in a sclerotic background. They are often accompanied by many neutrophils and a peculiar pattern of abnormal keratinization at all levels of the markedly thickened epithelial proliferation. Verrucous carcinoma has been termed the *giant condyloma of Buschke-Löwenstein* and may involve the external genitalia and perianal skin. It resembles a condyloma, but is, if anything, cytologically blander, with less striking viral cytopathic changes. Koilocytes with nuclear cavities are not seen. Verrucous carcinoma lacks the true papillary configuration with fibrovascular cores seen in large condylomas. Metastases from verrucous carcinomas are rare and, when present, should prompt a diagnosis of squamous cell carcinoma.

Staging. Anal canal tumors are staged by size rather than depth of invasion. As such, a T1 tumor is 2 cm or less, a T2 lesion is greater than 2 cm but less than 5 cm, a T3 tumor is 5 cm or larger, and a T4 tumor invades other structures. Lymphatic drainage of anal cancer depends on the location of the tumor. Above the dentate line, drainage flows to perirectal and paravertebral nodes (like rectal adenocarcinoma); below the dentate line, drainage is through the inguinal and femoral nodes.

Immunohistochemical Findings. Anal squamous cell carcinomas express the same markers as squamous carcinomas elsewhere, including CK5/6, pankeratins, p63, and p40. An important pitfall is their ability to label with CD117, which can result in an interpretation as gastrointestinal stromal tumor (fig. 6-20).

Molecular Genetic Findings. The genes that are active in anal squamous cell carcinogenesis include *TP53*, *p21*, *EGFR*, and the PI3K/AKT pathway but HPV DNA integration is a key element (19). The HPV genome encodes for several early structural genes (*E1*, *E2*, *E4*, *E5*, *E6*, and *E7*) believed to be responsible for viral replication, and late structural genes (*L1–L2*). It is the L1 capsid protein that has been used to develop vaccines.

As above, there are over 150 HPV types, with HPV16 associated with the highest carcinoma risk. This potential for carcinogenesis has been attributed to the expression of the *E6* and *E7* oncogenes and their protein products. These have been shown to be necessary to immortalize cells. These proteins can target the products of the tumor suppressor genes *TP53* and *pRb*. The E6 oncoprotein binds to and promotes degradation of the p53 protein such that the *TP53* gene product is unable to induce growth arrest, similar to having a *TP53* mutation. The E7 oncoprotein serves as a cell-cycle deregulator. In its quiescent state, pRb is hypophosphorylated and associated with E2F transcription factor molecules that inhibit their transcriptional activity. The phosphorylation of pRb releases the E2F heterodimer, allowing cell proliferation. When the E7 oncoprotein forms complexes with pRb, pRb is degraded, ultimately mimicking phosphorylation of pRb and allowing cellular proliferation.

Treatment and Prognosis. Standard treatment for anal squamous carcinoma is chemoradiotherapy with fluorouracil and mitomycin C, which allows sphincter preservation, and considerably preferable to abdomino-perineal resection. Newer radiation techniques target radiation better to the tumor and some protocols include cisplatin (19).

Tumor size, nodal status, and the presence of distal metastases are the most important prognostic factors for patients with cancer of the anal canal (23). Mobile lesions that are less than 2 cm in diameter can be cured in approximately 80 percent of cases, whereas those 5 cm or larger are cured in less than half the cases. The probability of nodal involvement is also directly related to the size of the tumor.

Rare Carcinomas. Rare *high-grade neuroendocrine (small and large cell) carcinomas* (figs. 6-21–6-23) can be encountered in the anal canal, some of which can reflect spread from prostatic (or other) or female genital tract primary lesions. Unfortunately, these can be difficult to separate. For example, most prostatic small cell carcinomas lack prostate markers (24) (although some

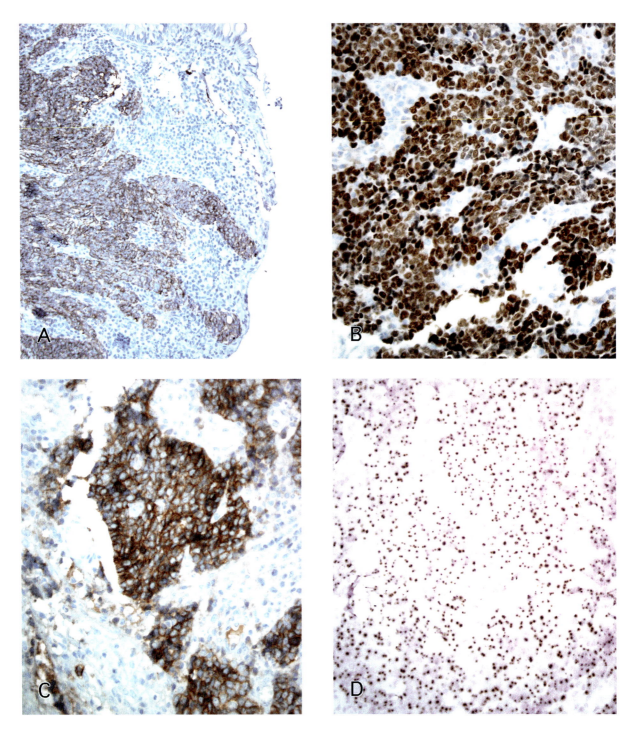

Figure 6-20

ANAL SQUAMOUS CELL CARCINOMA

A: In the same field as seen in figure 6-19, CK5/6 immunostain was used. The tumor arose at the junction of the squamous and colorectal type mucosa. Colorectal type glands are present at the upper right.

B: p63 immunostain.

C: This neoplasm (shown in fig. 6-19) had been interpreted as a gastrointestinal stromal tumor based on this nonspecific immunolabeling (CD117 stain).

D: There is nuclear hybridization in most cells (HPV16 DNA in situ hybridization).

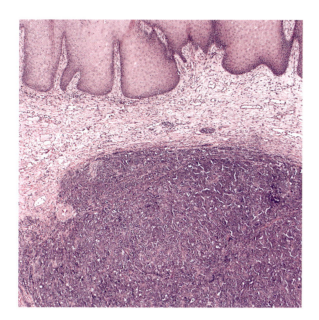

Figure 6-21

**ANAL NEUROENDOCRINE
CARCINOMA, LARGE CELL TYPE**

Even at low magnification, this tumor has the appearances of a high-grade malignant neoplasm. The vascular space between the main tumor mass and the anal squamous epithelium is invaded.

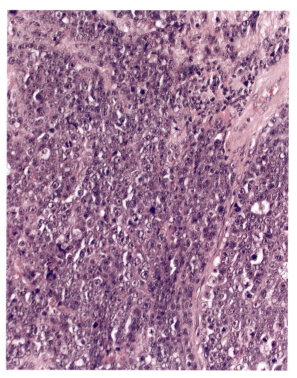

Figure 6-22

**ANAL NEUROENDOCRINE
CARCINOMA, LARGE CELL TYPE**

Many of the malignant cells have prominent nucleoli.

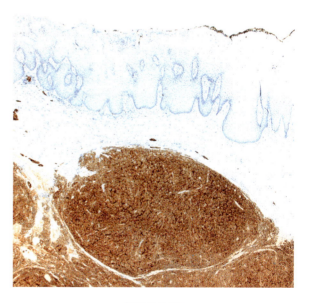

Figure 6-23

**ANAL NEUROENDOCRINE CARCINOMA,
LARGE CELL TYPE: SYNAPTOPHYSIN STAIN**

Note the strong labeling of this subepithelial malignant neoplasm

lesions do express such markers) and about 45 percent have *ERG* gene rearrangements (25). Imaging studies are sometimes the best tool to determine the primary site when a neuroendocrine carcinoma is biopsied from the anus. Anal small cell carcinoma can be associated with squamous cell carcinoma. Well-differentiated neuroendocrine (carcinoid) tumors are extremely rare in the anal canal, although they can create a diagnostic pitfall by occasionally mimicking AIN (fig. 6-24).

Rare *adenosquamous carcinomas* of the anus appear similar to adenosquamous carcinomas elsewhere in the body with areas of both squamous and glandular differentiation (figs. 6-25–6-27). When in doubt, a mucin stain helps identify intracellular mucin. Most of these cases are encountered in the sigmoid colon, rectum, and anus. Patients with localized disease have an overall survival rate similar to those with colorectal adenocarcinoma but survival in the setting of regional and distant disease is significantly lower. Individuals with distal disease (sigmoid, rectum, and anus) have a better prognosis than patients with proximal tumors (26).

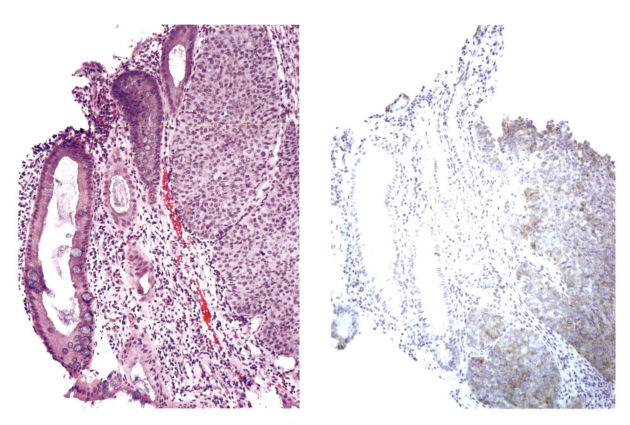

Figure 6-24

WELL-DIFFERENTIATED NEUROENDOCRINE (CARCINOID) TUMOR MIMICKING ANAL INTRAEPITHELIAL NEOPLASIA

Left: Reactive changes are seen in the adjoining colorectal epithelium at the lower right portion of the field.
Right: This synaptophysin stain highlights the neoplasm at the right.

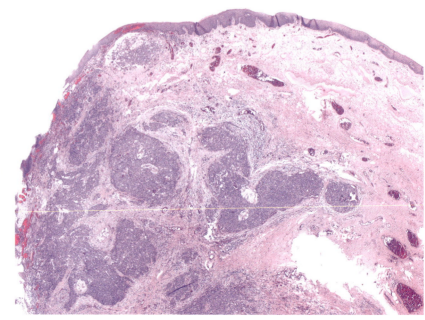

Figure 6-25

ANAL ADENOSQUAMOUS CARCINOMA

Tumor proliferates in solid nests.

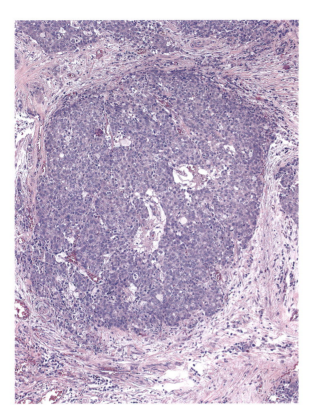 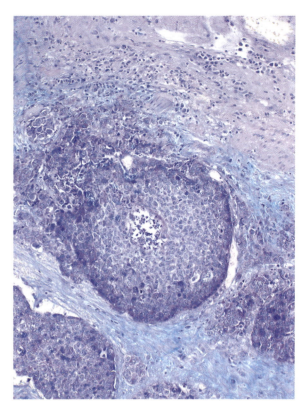

Figure 6-26

ANAL ADENOSQUAMOUS CARCINOMA

Left: Foci of mucin production are apparent.
Right: Alcianophilic mucin is present (periodic acid–Schiff [PAS]/alcian blue stain).

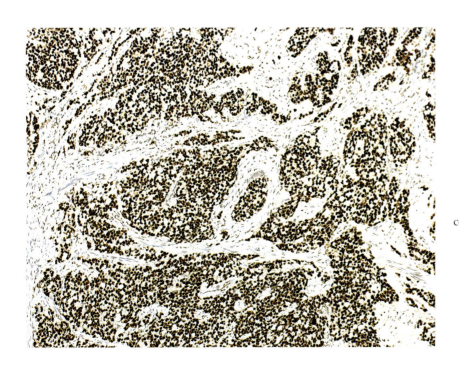

Figure 6-27

ANAL ADENOSQUAMOUS CARCINOMA: p63 NUCLEAR LABELING

Labeling is seen in the squamous component.

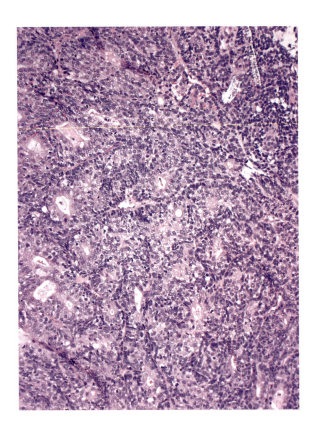 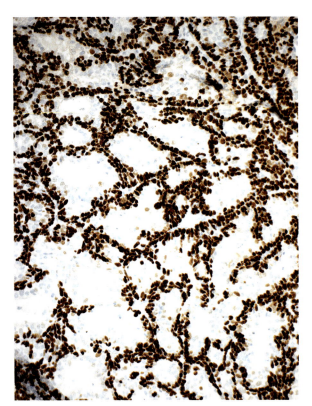

Figure 6-28

ANAL ADENOSQUAMOUS CARCINOMA

Left: Glands are surrounded by basaloid malignant squamous cells.
Right: The nuclei of the squamous component label with p63 but the intermingled glands do not.

ANAL PAGET DISEASE

General Features. Extramammary *Paget disease* typically affects apocrine gland-rich sites, namely, the perianal zone. Pure examples are believed to be an intraepithelial skin appendage-type tumor; some, however, are instead a reflection of intraepithelial spread of separate carcinomas of the colon or female genital tract. A subset is associated with an invasive skin appendage-type tumor.

Clinical Features. Perianal Paget disease is rare and is believed to account for about 6 percent of all cases of Paget disease and about 20 percent of cases of extramammary Paget disease (27). Lesions usually present in the sixth to seventh decades of life (mean age, about 63 years). The prototype patient is a postmenopausal Caucasian woman. The affected areas include the vulva, perineum, perianal skin, scrotum, penis, and pubic area. Lesions tend to recur many times and those associated with anorectal carcinomas can metastasize. Involved lymph nodes include inguinal, perirectal, retroperitoneal, and even periaortic nodes. Curiously, even intraepithelial Paget disease can metastasize, although rarely (28).

Gross Findings. Paget disease presents as a slowly growing, erythematous, eczematoid plaque that may extend internally to the dentate line (fig. 6-29).

Microscopic Findings. On biopsies, part or all of the squamous epithelial thickness is infiltrated by large pale cells, some of which may have signet cell features, and some of which may be large and eosinophilic (figs. 6-30–6-33). In some cases, a mucus droplet is readily identified in the intraepithelial neoplastic cells. If the epithelium is crushed or altered in any way, it can be difficult to separate the Paget cells from atypical keratinocytes, or from melanoma. For this reason, Paget disease is readily mistaken for squamous intraepithelial neoplasia/dysplasia.

Immunohistochemical Findings. True Paget disease, defined as an intraepithelial carcinoma with skin appendage differentiation, shows apocrine cell differentiation. The malignant cells express CK8/18 (using CAM 5.2), carcinoembryonic antigen (CEA), gross cystic disease fluid protein (GCDFP), and CK7, and they contain mucin (29). Both Merkel cells and Toker cells also express CK7, a feature the pathologist must consider when evaluating these stains (30,31).

About half of cases described using the term perianal Paget disease reflect pagetoid extension of an underlying typical colorectal cancer into squamous epithelium (figs. 6-32, 6-33). Such lesions lack GCDFP labeling and are often CK20(+), CK7(-), and CDX2(+). However, the occasional microsatellite unstable colorectal carcinoma may not express CK20 (32), although most such tumors are found in the right colon rather than the rectum. The best way to determine whether any given case of anal Paget disease is associated with an invasive cancer is by a careful clinical examination. About 5 percent of cutaneous squamous cell carcinomas in situ have a nested pattern, referred to as *pagetoid cutaneous squamous cell carcinomas in situ,*

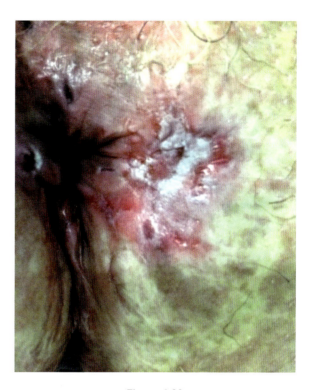

Figure 6-29

ANAL PAGET DISEASE

The lesion is a yellowish plaque with areas of ulceration.

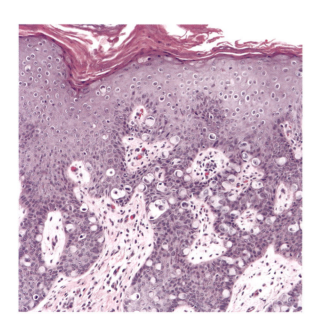
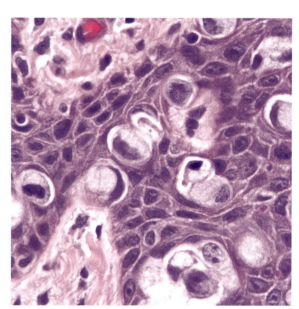

Figure 6-30

ANAL PAGET DISEASE

Left: Paget cells are seen within the squamous epithelium. This example is essentially an intraepithelial carcinoma composed of sweat duct type cells.

Right: At high magnification, mucin-producing cells are seen scattered within the squamous epithelium.

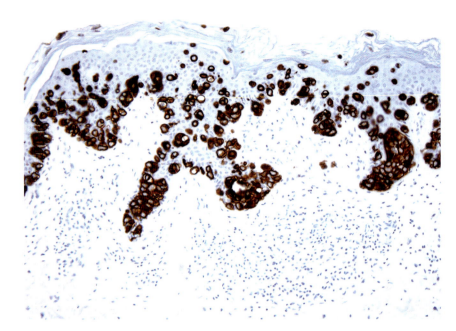

Figure 6-31

**ANAL PAGET DISEASE:
CK7 IMMUNOSTAIN**

CK7 expression is strong.

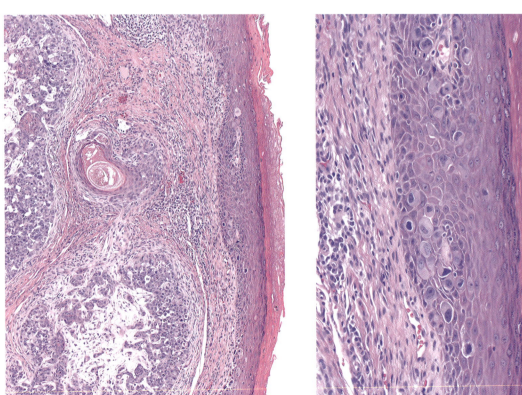

Figure 6-32

ANAL PAGET DISEASE, EXTENSION FROM A COLORECTAL-TYPE ADENOCARCINOMA

Left: This field shows striking pseudoepitheliomatous squamous hyperplasia peppered with single malignant cells. Note the malignant cells in the surface epithelium.

Right: Malignant cells are in the squamous epithelium. Such cells can be impossible to distinguish from a primary lesion.

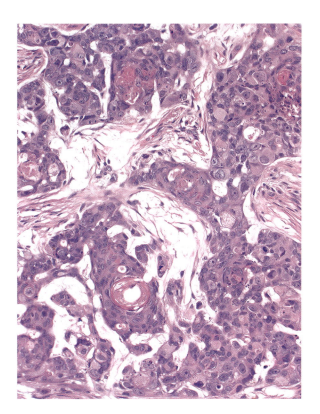
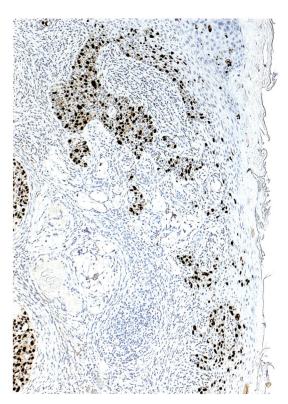

Figure 6-33

ANAL PAGET DISEASE, EXTENSION FROM A COLORECTAL-TYPE ADENOCARCINOMA

Left: Numerous malignant cells are proliferating within pseudoepitheliomatous hyperplasia.

Right: CDX2 stain shows that much of the lesion is pseudoepitheliomatous squamous hyperplasia; the tumor cells are CDX2 reactive.

or *pagetoid Bowen disease*. This growth pattern may simulate extramammary Paget disease and, more importantly, display CK7 expression (33). Thus, a panel approach is warranted. Occasionally reactive squamous cells in areas adjoining Paget cells can mimic AIN lesions. These cells lack nuclear p16 expression.

Molecular Genetic Findings. There are few data on the molecular profile of extramammary Paget disease but one tested case was found to have an *ERBB2/HER2* mutation and treated with targeted therapy (34).

Treatment and Prognosis. True Paget disease cases that are epidermotrophic apocrine neoplasms have a high local recurrence rate and can eventually become invasive. Those that reflect the epidermotropism of "ordinary" adenocarcinomas behave as the associated cancers, and are managed as such; stage is the primary prognostic marker.

Treatment revolves around the stage at presentation. Stage I (Paget cells in perianal epidermis) and IIA (cutaneous lesions associated with adnexal carcinoma) lesions are treated with wide local excision whereas IIB (cutaneous Paget disease with associated anorectal adenocarcinoma) tumors are managed by abdominoperineal resection. Stage III tumors (Paget disease with associated carcinoma present in regional nodes) is managed by as per stage IIB, with the addition of inguinal lymph node dissection. Stage IV (with distant metastases) is managed by chemotherapy, radiotherapy, and local palliation (27).

ANAL ADENOCARCINOMA, INCLUDING ANAL DUCT CARCINOMAS

Most *adenocarcinomas* arising in the anus are of the rectal type, arising in the upper zone of the anus, but rare anal adenocarcinomas are distal (fig. 6-34). These are identical to true rectal carcinomas and are managed as such. On biopsies, they appear identical to rectal adenocarcinomas, and their immunohistochemical profile is similarly identical: CK20 positive, CK7 (usually) negative. These tumors are characterized by elongated nuclei, abundant necrosis, and the usual overall pattern of colorectal carcinoma, with frequent association with an adenoma. Like rectal cancers, some are mucinous and some can be poorly differentiated.

Anal adenocarcinomas seldom pose diagnostic problems, although the differential diagnosis includes mucosal prolapse polyps (inflammatory cloacogenic polyps) with prominent colitis cystic profunda, which are distinguished by their diamond-shaped glands, fibromuscular mucosal stranding, and bland cytology. Anal adenocarcinomas with a poorly differentiated morphology confer a worse prognosis than well-differentiated ones (35).

A subset of anal carcinomas arises in association with chronic anal fistulas. Most of these fistula-associated carcinomas are clinically unsuspected, arising from longstanding tracts (10 to 26 years). Some of these patients have a history of Crohn disease and previous anorectal surgery.

An interesting group of anal adenocarcinomas is believed to arise in association with, or at least display, differentiation toward anal ducts. They are sufficiently unusual that the former Armed Forces Institute of Pathology (AFIP) was only able to amass seven bona fide cases (36). These tumors consist of tubules proliferating in association with the ducts that open onto the mucosal surface (fig. 6-35). They are intramural, lacking a luminal in situ component, although they may show pagetoid spread into the overlying squamous epithelium. There is variable overlying surface ulceration. On immunohistochemical staining, anal duct carcinomas are typically CK7 positive and CK20 negative, as per anal glands and ducts. Unlike normal anal glands, however, anal gland carcinoma lacks immunoreactivity with CK5/6 and p63. Both benign and malignant anal glands are negative for CDX2 (37,38). When these tumors are found, they need to be separated from prostate cancer (which is often negative for CK7 and CK20) and gynecologic carcinomas. Tested anal duct/gland carcinomas lack prostate-specific antigen (PSA) and prostatic acid phosphatase (39), hormone receptor

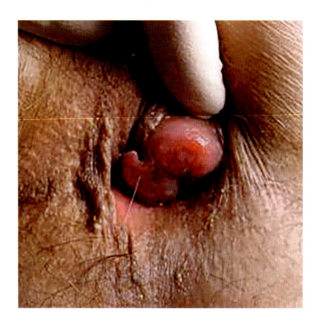

Figure 6-34

ANAL ADENOCARCINOMA

Like other anal neoplasms, this lesion is readily mistaken for a hemorrhoid.

expression, and HPV by in situ hybridization (40). Many behave aggressively (40).

ANAL MELANOMA

General Features. *Anal melanomas*, like other mucosal melanomas, are rare. Mucosal melanomas account for 1.3 to 1.4 percent of all melanomas (41); anal melanomas account for 0.2 to 0.3 percent of all melanomas and about 4 percent of anal neoplasms (41). The overwhelming majority of melanomas arise in the skin, but the mucosal sites that can be affected are those that contain melanocytes. These include uvea, leptomeninges, and mucosa of the eye, gastrointestinal tract (especially mouth and anus), respiratory tract, and genitourinary tract, i.e., neuroectodermal sites (reviewed by Seetharamu et al. [42]).

Clinical Features. Anal melanomas present in older persons than those of skin (about 67 years compared to 55 years) and they tend to present at a late stage since they are not visible. There seems to be no racial predilection for mucosal melanomas, although mucosal melanomas account for about 1 percent of melanomas in whites and about 12 percent of

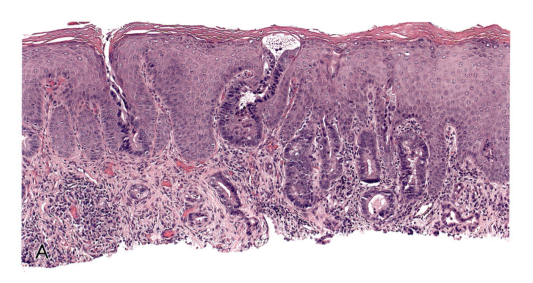

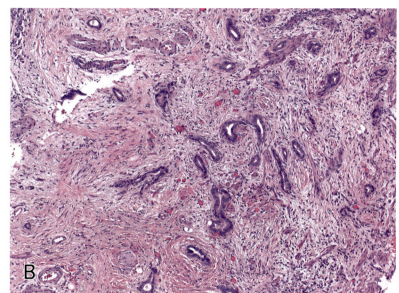

Figure 6-35

ANAL DUCT/ANAL GLAND CARCINOMA

A: The tubules display pagetoid extension onto the surface.

B: The tumor consists of subepithelial tubules composed of cells with atypical nuclei. There is a desmoplastic stroma.

C: Carcinomas of this type express CK7 in the manner of anal ducts.

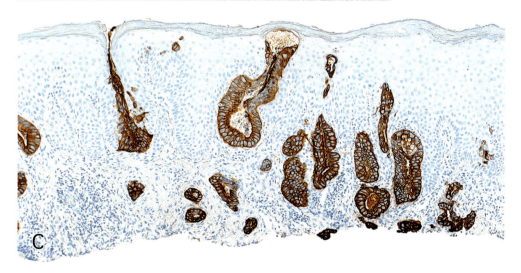

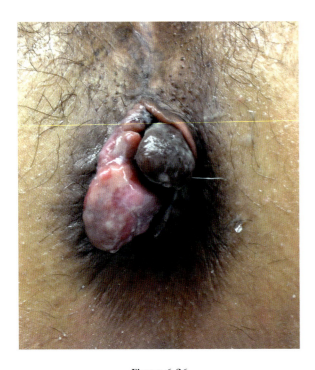

Figure 6-36

ANAL MELANOMA

Much of the lesion is amelanotic but the portion to the right shows pigmentation that is similar to that of the perianal skin.

melanomas in African Americans (41). Mucosal melanomas are more likely to lack pigmentation than cutaneous neoplasms. Patients present with rectal bleeding, which is often attributed to hemorrhoids, and small nodules are dismissed as anal tags or rectal polyps (see below).

Gross Findings. Lesions appear grossly flat or polypoid (fig. 6-36). Many appear black on cut surface, but about 25 percent of anorectal melanomas lack pigment. They resemble sarcomas grossly, with a fish-flesh type appearance.

Microscopic Findings. Like all melanomas, anorectal melanomas display a wide range of appearances (figs. 6-37, 6-38) and thus may be difficult to diagnose if an in situ component is not seen. An immunolabeling panel is often required for diagnosis. They can be pleomorphic and sarcomatoid as well as epithelioid. Some examples consist of uniform monotonous cells that suggest benign lesions.

Immunohistochemical Findings. Like melanomas in other sites, anorectal ones nearly always label with S-100 protein and SOX10 and variably with so-called "melanoma markers" such as tyrosinase, HMB45, MART1, and MELAN-A. An important pitfall is that spindle cell melanomas

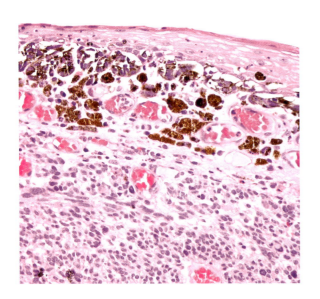 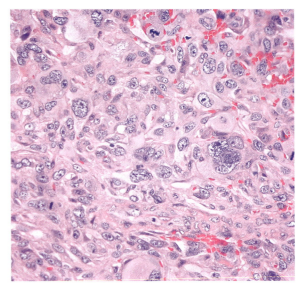

Figure 6-37

ANAL MELANOMA

Left: These tumors are readily diagnosed if an in situ component is present, as in this case. The spindled appearance can result in misinterpretation as a gastrointestinal stromal tumor.

Right: This example is epithelioid and pleomorphic and was unassociated with a recognizable in situ component. In such cases, immunolabeling is often required for diagnosis.

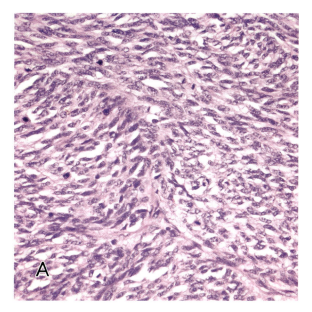

Figure 6-38

ANAL MELANOMA

A: The monotonous nuclei resulted in a misinterpretation as gastrointestinal stromal tumor.

B: The S-100 protein stain shows both nuclear and cytoplasmic labeling, which is important in interpreting the stain as reactive.

C: This strong membranous and cytoplasmic CD117 expression is common in melanomas and resulted in an incorrect diagnosis in this case. This finding sometimes correlates with *KIT* mutations in mucosal melanomas.

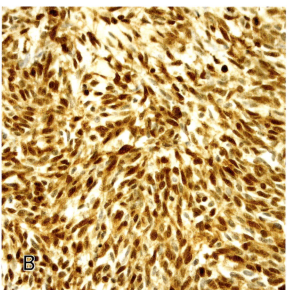

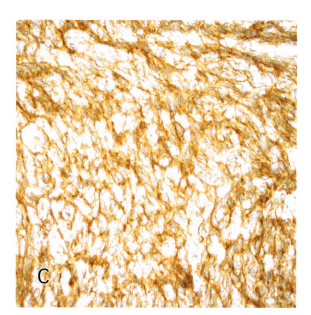

often lack labeling with melanoma markers, only showing S-100 protein and SOX10 positivity. Furthermore, melanomas (including spindle cell examples) often show CD117/KIT immunostaining, even in the absence of *KIT* mutations, which can result in misinterpretation as gastrointestinal stromal tumor (fig. 6-38B,C).

Molecular Genetic Findings. Mucosal melanomas have *KIT* mutations in up to a third of cases (about 20 percent in most studies) in contrast to cutaneous ones that only rarely have *KIT* mutations. *BRAF* mutations are rare in mucosal melanomas but common in cutaneous ones (see below).

Treatment and Prognosis. Overall, anal melanomas are highly aggressive malignancies associated with overall survival in the range of 3 years (43); the 5-year survival rate is about 7 to 15 percent (44,45). Up to about 60 percent of patients present with distant metastatic disease. Patients with early lesions, however, often have a favorable 5-year survival rate (80 to 90 percent) (43,46). Staging has been problematic for mucosal melanomas since lesions tend to be advanced at presentation and thus an equivalent to Breslow levels is not relevant. Simply using the American Joint Committee on Cancer (AJCC) system already in place for rectum and anus results in good correlation with outcome based on stage (46).

There are no randomized treatment trials since anorectal melanoma is rare. Surgery is still the mainstay of treatment and can result in clinical cure. There are no advantages in performing abdominoperineal resection over local excision (42). Adjuvant radiation is often offered, although it is typically not a component of the treatment plan for skin melanomas. Since many patients have micrometastases at presentation, adjuvant therapy is often suggested.

As of this writing there are no data on response to PD1-related (programmed death 1) targeted immunotherapy (47) specifically in anal melanoma, which might improve outcome. Since many anal mucosal melanomas harbor *KIT* mutations (20 to 30 percent), there has been some success with targeted therapy with tyrosine kinase inhibitors (imatinib and sorafenib) (43,48–51). *KIT* mutations are typically absent in sun-exposed skin with the exception of skin in acral sites (52,53). About 70 percent of melanomas in sun-exposed sites have *BRAF* mutations, but most anal melanomas lack *BRAF* mutations, and thus cannot be treated using vemurafenib, but rare cases harboring such mutations have been reported (54).

MISCELLANEOUS ANAL LESIONS

Many processes, both reactive and neoplastic, can produce anal tumefaction. These include, but are not limited to, fibroepithelial polyps, skin appendage tumors, mucosal prolapse polyps, granular cells tumors, inflammatory fibroid polyps (discussed elsewhere), and even rare lesions such as Langerhans cell histiocytosis (fig. 6-39) (55). While melanomas are rare, benign melanocytic lesions are rarer still, although nevi are occasionally encountered, including blue nevi (fig. 6-40).

Fibroepithelial Polyps

Fibroepithelial polyps are also called *anal tags*. Removal may be extremely painful and, in the case of those associated with Crohn disease, may result in additional morbidity due to incomplete healing. Fibroepithelial polyps are projections of anal mucosa and submucosa. When they arise at the edge of an anal ulcer or fissure, the term "sentinel tag" has been used. They are often submitted to the pathologist as hemorrhoids, but fibroepithelial polyps lack prominent vessels.

Fibroepithelial polyps consist of myxoid or collagenous stroma covered by squamous epithelium. Stromal cells, including multinucleated cells, are usually found, and large fibroepithelial polyps can contain atypical stromal cells. Mast cells are frequent. The stromal cells express vimentin, CD34, and sometimes desmin. As in cases of uterine prolapse, surface changes can superficially resemble viral cytopathic effect and should not be diagnosed as such (figs. 6-41, 6-42). When fibroepithelial polyps are examined, the overlying mucosa should be evaluated for AIN.

Skin Appendage Tumors

Theoretically, any skin appendage tumor can be found in the anal area but the one that is likely to result in diagnostic problems is *hidradenoma papilliferum*. This is a cystic and papillary benign apocrine neoplasm that arises in the perianal skin and vulva. The prototype patient is a white woman over the age of 30 years. The key affected sites are the labia majora, perineum, and perianal skin (56–58), although extragenital tumors do occur.

The lesion forms an epithelial-lined cyst in the mid-dermis, displaying elaborate papillary infoldings with fibrovascular cores. The epithelium contains two layers of cuboidal epithelium with foci of bridging and tuft formation (fig. 6-43). Inflammation is usually absent, and the superficial portions of the cyst are often lined by a flattened squamous layer. If the pathologist is concerned that this lesion is a metastasis, CK5/6 staining, which has a limited expression profile and is fairly specific for mesothelium and other "pavement"-type epithelia (such as squamous epithelium), is useful. Immunoreactivity with CK5/6 is seen in these tumors, and excludes an adenocarcinoma. Hidradenoma papilliferum also expresses estrogen receptor, a potential problem if the pathologist is concerned about a metastasis from the breast or female genital tract.

Some anal skin appendage tumors are difficult to classify precisely as hidradenoma papilliferum or syringocystadenoma papilliferum, but they can usually be classified as "skin appendage tumors" rather than adenocarcinomas. Rare anal tumors have the appearances of mammary-like gland adenomas (59) and others have

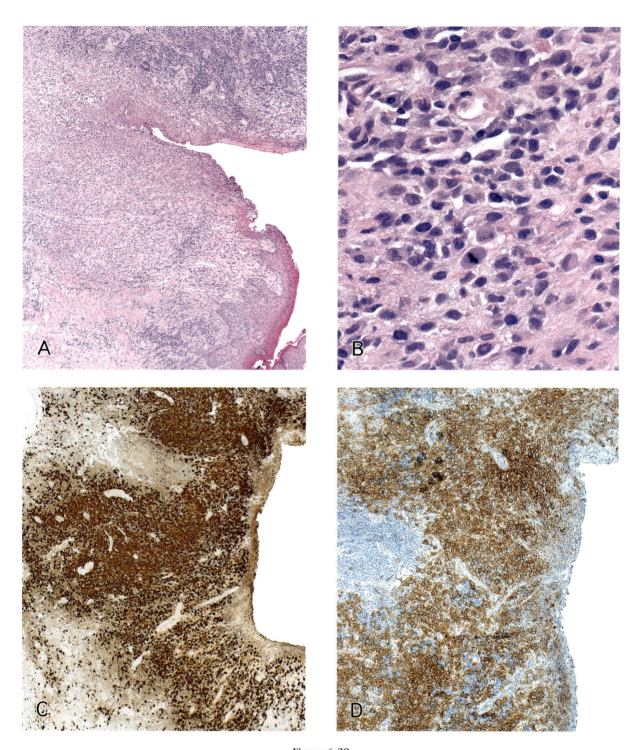

Figure 6-39

ANAL LANGERHANS CELL HISTIOCYTOSIS

A: This lesion presented as a chronic ulcer. There is a nonspecific lymphoid infiltrate on the left but the central lesion is more eosinophilic.

B: At high magnification, there are atypical nuclei, some with nuclear grooves.

C: There is strong nuclear and cytoplasmic S-100 protein expression.

D: There is cytoplasmic and membranous CD1a expression.

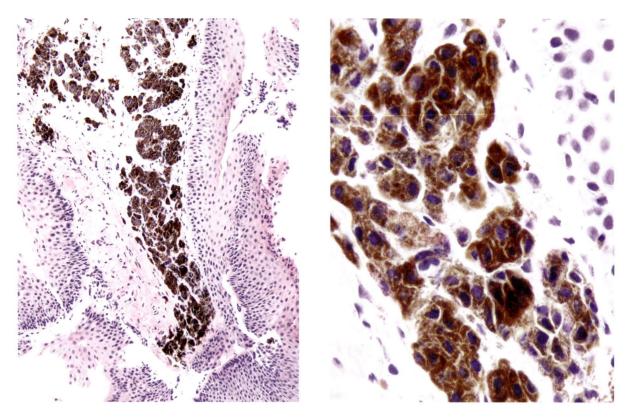

Figure 6-40

ANAL NEVUS

Left: Anal nevi are rare but an example is seen in this mucosal biopsy.
Right: The cytologic features are bland.

Figure 6-41

ANAL FIBROEPITHELIAL POLYP/ANAL TAG

These are analogous to acrochordons/skin tags and are prone to surface damage and peculiar epithelial changes, as seen in the surface of this lesion.

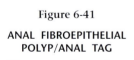

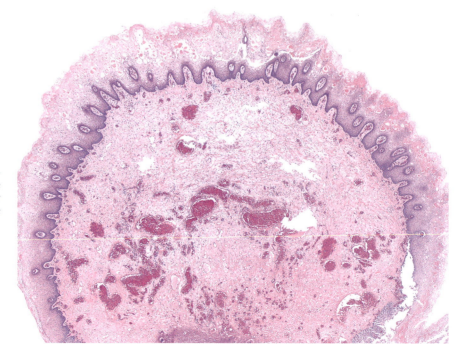

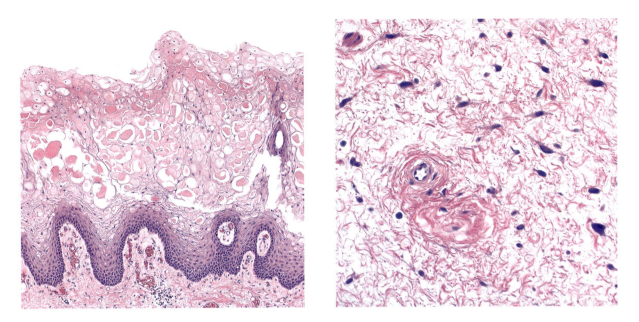

Figure 6-42

ANAL FIBROEPITHELIAL POLYP/ANAL TAG

Left: These reactive surface changes are sometimes mistaken for either koilocytotic atypia or Paget disease. Some observers have used the term "pagetoid dyskeratosis," however, the nuclei in the cells are small, in contrast to those in koilocytes or in Paget cells.

Right: These lesions often contain reactive stromal fibroblasts.

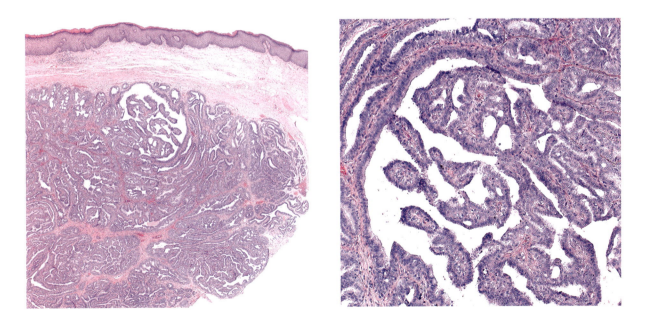

Figure 6-43

HIDRADENOMA PAPILLIFERUM

Left: These tumors typically arise in the perineum of middle-aged women. Complex glands are present, however, the process is well-marginated and has not resulted in a desmoplastic stroma.

Right: The two cell layers are seen at high magnification.

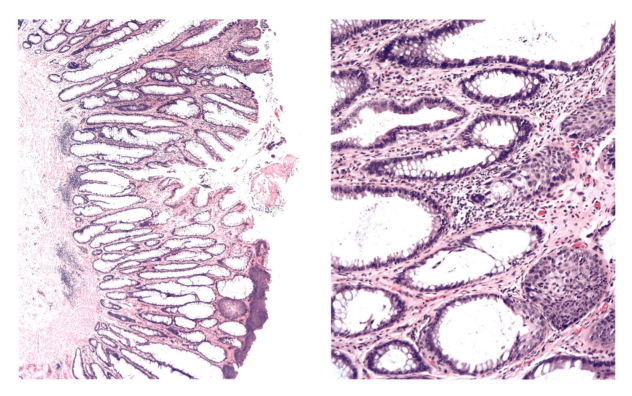

Figure 6-44

INFLAMMATORY CLOACOGENIC POLYP

Left: This is essentially a mucosal prolapse polyp at the anorectal transition zone. As such, each crypt becomes invested in smooth muscle and some of the crypts are angulated and have been termed "diamond-shaped crypts." In this example, there is high-grade AIN in the squamous epithelium at the upper right.

Right: Strands of smooth muscle surround each crypt. High-grade AIN is present in the adjoining squamous epithelium.

hybrid features (60). Such tumors also display pagetoid spread into the overlying epithelium. In contrast to anal gland carcinomas (above), they usually have a myoepithelial component (and thus areas with two cell layers).

Cysts of the lower female genital tract also present as anal lesions, although they generally appear benign. Most contain squamous epithelium, although *müllerian cysts* are lined by varying components of columnar, mucinous, endocervical-type, or ciliated epithelium. *Mesonephric* (*Gartner duct cysts*) and *urothelial cysts* are also occasionally encountered in the anus.

Anal Mucosal Prolapse Polyps

Inflammatory cloacogenic polyp is a mucosal prolapse polyp arising at the anorectal transition, such that these lesions are coated by both squamous and columnar mucosa (fig. 6-44)

(61,62). Patients present with hematochezia, and the polyps typically arise on the anterior or wall of the anal canal. These polyps have a tubulovillous growth pattern, with surface ulceration, displaced clusters of crypts into the submucosa, and abundant fibromuscular stroma that extends into the mucosa. They are essentially the anal form of solitary rectal ulcer. Occasionally, AIN is encountered in the overlying squamous epithelium (fig. 6-44).

Inflammatory Conditions

Various inflammatory conditions can also produce a mass. The ability of sexually transmitted *infectious proctitis* to produce a mass has been recently highlighted (fig. 6-45) (63–65) and *anal inflammatory polyps* can be encountered in the setting of inflammatory bowel disease, especially Crohn disease.

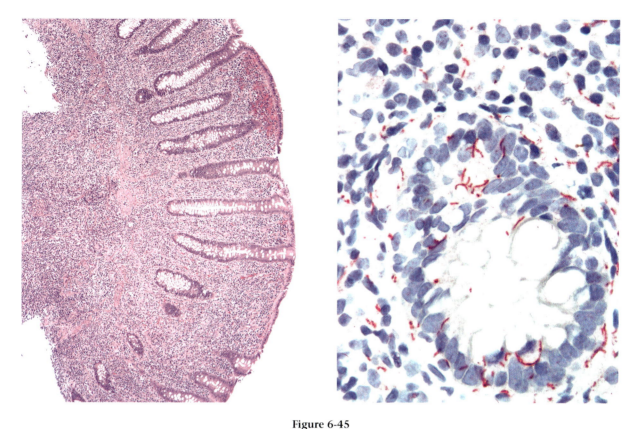

Figure 6-45

SYPHILIS PROCTITIS

Left: This lesion produced a polyp in a man with human immunodeficiency virus (HIV) who had sex with men (MSM). There is an expanded lamina propria and prominent submucosal chronic inflammation. There is essentially no crypt distortion. Lymphogranuloma venereum proctitis produces essentially the same findings so patients with these findings need to be tested for both of these processes.

Right: This is a *Treponema pallidum* immunostain, which highlights numerous organisms. It should be noted, however, that a negative immunostain does not exclude syphilis proctitis.

REFERENCES

1. Mendez-Martinez R, Rivera-Martinez NE, Crabtree-Ramirez B, et al. Multiple human papillomavirus infections are highly prevalent in the anal canal of human immunodeficiency virus-positive men who have sex with men. BMC Infect Dis 2014;14:671.

2. Bouvard V, Baan R, Straif K, et al. A review of human carcinogens—Part B: biological agents. Lancet Oncol 2009;10:321-322.

3. Handler NS, Handler MZ, Majewski S, Schwartz RA. Human papillomavirus vaccine trials and tribulations: vaccine efficacy. J Am Acad Dermatol 2015;73:759-767; quiz 767-758.

4. Deshmukh AA, Chhatwal J, Chiao EY, Nyitray AG, Das P, Cantor SB. Long-term outcomes of adding HPV vaccine to the anal intraepithelial neoplasia treatment regimen in HIV-positive men who have sex with men. Clin Infect Dis 2015;61:1527-1535.

5. Advisory Committee on Immunization P. Recommended adult immunization schedule: United States, 2013. Ann Intern Med 2013;158:191-199.

6. Koshiol JE, Laurent SA, Pimenta JM. Rate and predictors of new genital warts claims and genital warts-related healthcare utilization among privately insured patients in the United States. Sex Transm Dis 2004;31:748-752.

7. Giuliano AR, Lee JH, Fulp W, et al. Incidence and clearance of genital human papillomavirus infection in men (HIM): a cohort study. Lancet 2011;377:932-940.

8. Stier EA, Sebring MC, Mendez AE, Ba FS, Trimble DD, Chiao EY. Prevalence of anal human papillomavirus infection and anal HPV-related disorders in women: a systematic review. Am J Obstet Gynecol 2015;213:278-309.

9. Machalek DA, Poynten M, Jin F, et al. Anal human papillomavirus infection and associated neoplastic lesions in men who have sex with men: a systematic review and meta-analysis. Lancet Oncol 2012;13:487-500.

10. Burgos J, Curran A, Tallada N, et al. Risk of progression to high-grade anal intraepithelial neoplasia in HIV-infected MSM. AIDS 2015;29:695-702.

11. Walker P, Dexeus S, De Palo G, et al. International terminology of colposcopy: an updated report from the International Federation for Cervical Pathology and Colposcopy. Obstet Gynecol 2003;101:175-177.

12. Bosman F, Carneiro F, Hruban R, Theise N. WHO Classification of tumours of the digestive system. In: Bosman F, Jaffee E, Lakhani S, Ohgaki H, eds. World Health Organization Classification of Tumours. Lyon: IARC; 2010.

13. Patil DT, Yang B. Utility of human papillomavirus capsid protein L1 and p16 in the assessment and accurate classification of anal squamous intraepithelial lesions. Am J Clin Pathol 2015;144:113-121.

14. Pirog EC. Immunohistochemistry and in situ hybridization for the diagnosis and classification of squamous lesions of the anogenital region. Semin Diagn Pathol 2015;32:409-418.

15. Ukpo OC, Flanagan JJ, Ma XJ, Luo Y, Thorstad WL, Lewis JS Jr. High-risk human papillomavirus E6/E7 mRNA detection by a novel in situ hybridization assay strongly correlates with p16 expression and patient outcomes in oropharyngeal squamous cell carcinoma. Am J Surg Pathol 2011;35:1343-1350.

16. Siegel RL, Miller KD, Jemal A. Cancer statistics, 2016. CA Cancer J Clin 2016;66:7-30.

17. Shiels MS, Kreimer AR, Coghill AE, Darragh TM, Devesa SS. Anal cancer incidence in the United States, 1977-2011: distinct patterns by histology and behavior. Cancer Epidemiol Biomarkers Prev 2015;24:1548-1556.

18. Blomberg M, Friis S, Munk C, Bautz A, Kjaer SK. Genital warts and risk of cancer: a Danish study of nearly 50,000 patients with genital warts. J Infect Dis 2012;205:1544-1553.

19. Bernardi MP, Ngan SY, Michael M, et al. Molecular biology of anal squamous cell carcinoma: implications for future research and clinical intervention. Lancet Oncol 2015;16:e611-621.

20. Frisch M, Johansen C. Anal carcinoma in inflammatory bowel disease. Br J Cancer 2000;83:89-90.

21. Ryan DP, Compton CC, Mayer RJ. Carcinoma of the anal canal. N Engl J Med 2000;342:792-800.

22. Fenger C, Frisch M, Jass JJ, Williams GT, Hilden J. Anal cancer subtype reproducibility study. Virchows Arch 2000;436:229-233.

23. Bilimoria KY, Bentrem DJ, Rock CE, Stewart AK, Ko CY, Halverson A. Outcomes and prognostic factors for squamous-cell carcinoma of the anal canal: analysis of patients from the National Cancer Data Base. Dis Colon Rectum 2009;52:624-631.

24. Wang W, Epstein JI. Small cell carcinoma of the prostate. A morphologic and immunohistochemical study of 95 cases. Am J Surg Pathol 2008;32:65-71.

25. Lotan TL, Gupta NS, Wang W, et al. ERG gene rearrangements are common in prostatic small cell carcinomas. Mod Pathol 2011;24:820-828.

26. Cagir B, Nagy MW, Topham A, Rakinic J, Fry RD. Adenosquamous carcinoma of the colon, rectum, and anus: epidemiology, distribution, and survival characteristics. Dis Colon Rectum 1999;42:258-263.

27. Kyriazanos ID, Stamos NP, Miliadis L, Noussis G, Stoidis CN. Extra-mammary Paget's disease of the perianal region: a review of the literature emphasizing the operative management technique. Surg Oncol 2011;20:e61-71.

28. Khoubehi B, Schofield A, Leslie M, Slevin ML, Talbot IC, Northover JM. Metastatic in-situ perianal Paget's disease. J R Soc Med 2001;94:137-138.

29. Goldblum JR, Hart WR. Perianal Paget's disease: a histologic and immunohistochemical study of 11 cases with and without associated rectal adenocarcinoma. Am J Surg Pathol 1998;22:170-179.

30. Lundquist K, Kohler S, Rouse RV. Intraepidermal cytokeratin 7 expression is not restricted to Paget cells but is also seen in Toker cells and Merkel cells. Am J Surg Pathol 1999;23:212-219.

31. van der Putte SC. Clear cells of Toker in the developing anogenital region of male and female fetuses. Am J Dermatopathol 2011;33:811-818.

32. McGregor DK, Wu TT, Rashid A, Luthra R, Hamilton SR. Reduced expression of cytokeratin 20 in colorectal carcinomas with high levels of microsatellite instability. Am J Surg Pathol 2004;28:712-718.

33. Raju RR, Goldblum JR, Hart WR. Pagetoid squamous cell carcinoma in situ (pagetoid Bowen's disease) of the external genitalia. Int J Gynecol Pathol 2003;22:127-135.

34. Vornicova O, Hershkovitz D, Yablonski-Peretz T, Ben-Itzhak O, Keidar Z, Bar-Sela G. Treatment of metastatic extramammary Paget's disease associated with adnexal adenocarcinoma, with anti-HER2 drugs based on genomic alteration ERBB2 S310F. Oncologist 2014;19:1006-1007.

35. Chang GJ, Gonzalez RJ, Skibber JM, Eng C, Das P, Rodriguez-Bigas MA. A twenty-year experience with adenocarcinoma of the anal canal. Dis Colon Rectum 2009;52:1375-1380.

36. Hobbs CM, Lowry MA, Owen D, Sobin LH. Anal gland carcinoma. Cancer 2001;92:2045-2049.

37. Lisovsky M, Patel K, Cymes K, Chase D, Bhuiya T, Morgenstern N. Immunophenotypic characterization of anal gland carcinoma: loss of p63 and cytokeratin 5/6. Arch Pathol Lab Med 2007;131:1304-1311.

38. Carpenter JB, Rennels MA. Immunophenotypic characteristics of anal gland carcinoma. Arch Pathol Lab Med 2008;132:1547-1548.

39. Ballo MT, Gershenwald JE, Zagars GK, et al. Sphincter-sparing local excision and adjuvant radiation for anal-rectal melanoma. J Clin Oncol 2002;20:4555-4558.

40. Meriden Z, Montgomery EA. Anal duct carcinoma: a report of 5 cases. Hum Pathol 2011;43:216-220.

41. Chang AE, Karnell LH, Menck HR. The National Cancer Data Base report on cutaneous and non-cutaneous melanoma: a summary of 84,836 cases from the past decade. The American College of Surgeons Commission on Cancer and the American Cancer Society. Cancer 1998;83:1664-1678.

42. Seetharamu N, Ott PA, Pavlick AC. Mucosal melanomas: a case-based review of the literature. Oncologist 2010;15:772-781.

43. Knowles J, Lynch AC, Warrier SK, Henderson M, Heriot AG. A case series of anal melanoma including the results of treatment with Imatinib in selected patients. Colorectal Dis 2016;18:877-882.

44. Brady MS, Kavolius JP, Quan SH. Anorectal melanoma. A 64-year experience at Memorial Sloan-Kettering Cancer Center. Dis Colon Rectum 1995;38:146-151.

45. Cooper PH, Mills SE, Allen MS Jr. Malignant melanoma of the anus: report of 12 patients and analysis of 255 additional cases. Dis Colon Rectum 1982;25:693-703.

46. Chae WY, Lee JL, Cho DH, Yu CS, Roh J, Kim JC. Preliminary suggestion about staging of anorectal malignant melanoma may be used to predict prognosis. Cancer Res Treat 2016;48:240-249.

47. Topalian SL, Hodi FS, Brahmer JR, et al. Safety, activity, and immune correlates of anti-PD-1 antibody in cancer. N Engl J Med 2012;366:2443-2454.

48. Antonescu CR, Busam KJ, Francone TD, et al. L576P KIT mutation in anal melanomas correlates with KIT protein expression and is sensitive to specific kinase inhibition. Int J Cancer 2007;121:257-264.

49. Carvajal RD, Antonescu CR, Wolchok JD, et al. KIT as a therapeutic target in metastatic melanoma. JAMA 2011;305:2327-2334.

50. Quintas-Cardama A, Lazar AJ, Woodman SE, Kim K, Ross M, Hwu P. Complete response of stage IV anal mucosal melanoma expressing KIT Val560Asp to the multikinase inhibitor sorafenib. Nat Clin Pract Oncol 2008;5:737-740.

51. Satzger I, Schaefer T, Kuettler U, et al. Analysis of c-KIT expression and KIT gene mutation in human mucosal melanomas. Br J Cancer 2008;99:2065-2069.

52. Curtin JA, Busam K, Pinkel D, Bastian BC. Somatic activation of KIT in distinct subtypes of melanoma. J Clin Oncol 2006;24:4340-4346.

53. Curtin JA, Fridlyand J, Kageshita T, et al. Distinct sets of genetic alterations in melanoma. N Engl J Med 2005;353:2135-2147.

54. Martinez-Cadenas C, Bosch N, Penas L, et al. Malignant melanoma arising from a perianal fistula and harbouring a BRAF gene mutation: a case report. BMC Cancer 2011;11:343.

55. Singhi AD, Montgomery EA. Gastrointestinal tract langerhans cell histiocytosis: A clinicopathologic study of 12 patients. Am J Surg Pathol 2011;35:305-310.

56. Goette DK. Hidradenoma papilliferum. J Am Acad Dermatol 1988;19(Pt 1):133-135.

57. Handa Y, Yamanaka N, Inagaki H, Tomita Y. Large ulcerated perianal hidradenoma papilliferum in a young female. Dermatol Surg 2003;29:790-792.

58. Loane J, Kealy WF, Mulcahy G. Perianal hidradenoma papilliferum occurring in a male: a case report. Ir J Med Sci 1998;167:26-27.

59. Scurry J, van der Putte SC, Pyman J, Chetty N, Szabo R. Mammary-like gland adenoma of the vulva: review of 46 cases. Pathology 2009;41:372-378.

60. Nishie W, Sawamura D, Mayuzumi M, Takahashi S, Shimizu H. Hidradenoma papilliferum with mixed histopathologic features of syringocystadenoma papilliferum and anogenital mammary-like glands. J Cutan Pathol 2004;31:561-564.

61. Lobert PF, Appelman HD. Inflammatory cloacogenic polyp. A unique inflammatory lesion of the anal transitional zone. Am J Surg Pathol 1981;5:761-766.

62. Saul SH. Inflammatory cloacogenic polyp: relationship to solitary rectal ulcer syndrome/mucosal prolapse and other bowel disorders. Hum Pathol 1987;18:1120-1125.

63. Arnold CA, Limketkai BN, Illei PB, Montgomery E, Voltaggio L. Syphilitic and lymphogranuloma venereum (LGV) proctocolitis: clues to a frequently missed diagnosis. Am J Surg Pathol 2013;37:38-46.

64. Arnold CA, Montgomery EA, Voltaggio L. From the pathologist: review of sexual behaviors should be a routine component of clinical histories. Gastrointest Endosc 2013;78:385-386.

65. Arnold CA, Roth R, Arsenescu R, et al. Sexually transmitted infectious colitis vs inflammatory bowel disease: distinguishing features from a case-controlled study. Am J Clin Pathol 2015;144:771-781.

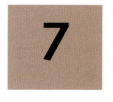

7   WELL-DIFFERENTIATED NEUROENDOCRINE TUMORS OF THE INTESTINES

Intestinal neuroendocrine tumors (NETs) are distinct from conventional adenocarcinomas with neuroendocrine differentiation and poorly differentiated neuroendocrine carcinoma of either small cell or large cell type (discussed in chapter 4). In contrast to neuroendocrine carcinomas (NEC), which usually develop from a crypt/glandular epithelial precursor and are closely related to conventional adenocarcinoma, well-differentiated NETs differentiate along the lines of the normal counterpart neuroendocrine cell lineage, i.e., the diffuse neuroendocrine cell system.

Recognition of these distinct entities (NET versus NEC) is of clinical significance. They not only exhibit marked differences in clinical presentation and prognosis, their clinical management is remarkably different. In addition, whereas for other chapters, the history of classification of the neoplasms is of little interest for daily practice, the historical context is relevant with neuroendocrine neoplasms and, in addition to diagnostic criteria, is outlined in this chapter.

DIFFUSE NEUROENDOCRINE CELL SYSTEM OF THE GASTROINTESTINAL TRACT

First recognized by German physiologist Heiderhain in 1870 (1) and followed by the Russian anatomist Kultchitzky in 1897 (2), gastrointestinal (GI) neuroendocrine cells spread as single cells or clusters of cells between crypt and glandular epithelial cells throughout the mucosa, to comprise a grossly invisible diffuse neuroendocrine cell system (fig. 7-1). Similar to the classic endocrine system with discernible endocrine organs, the diffuse neuroendocrine cell system plays an important role in the regulation of body homeostasis. At the cellular and ultrastructural levels, these cells possess long dendritic processes and contain secretory granules of various size, shape, and electron density.

The origins of the concept of a GI neuroendocrine system reflect the interrelationship between nerves, endocrine cells, and intestinal motility and secretory activity as regulated by amines, peptides, and hormones. These chemical messengers are delivered via multiple pathways, including direct cell-cell interactions and endocrine and paracrine mechanisms. The distinction between neuroectoderm-derived enteric neurons and endoderm-derived neuroendocrine cells must be recognized. While the anatomic proximity between the two elements may suggest a spectrum ranging from GI neurons to open-type (connected to crypt lumen) and close-type enteroendocrine cells, the distinct developmental origins of enteric neurons and intestinal diffuse neuroendocrine cells have been acknowledged (3–5).

In 1938, the Austrian pathologist Feyrter (6) proposed that NETs were derived from the diffuse endocrine system, based on his observation of "clear cells" (helle Zellen) sparsely intermingled with crypts and ducts throughout the tubular GI tract and pancreas, and displayed characteristic light microscopic and histochemical features in their reactions with silver salts (i.e., argentaffinity and argyrophilia) (7,8). In 1966, Pearse (9), a histochemist from London, recognized the common biochemical characteristics of intestinal neuroendocrine cells and provided a classification system that unified the variety of diffusely scattered neuroendocrine cells by introducing the term APUD (amine precursor uptake and decarboxylation).

The first intestinal neuroendocrine cell was designated by Carmèlo Ciaccio (10,11) in 1906 as "enterochromaffin" to depict the staining of the helle Zellen with chromium salts. Depending on their location in the GI tract, numerous subtypes of neuroendocrine cells have been recognized based upon their histochemical

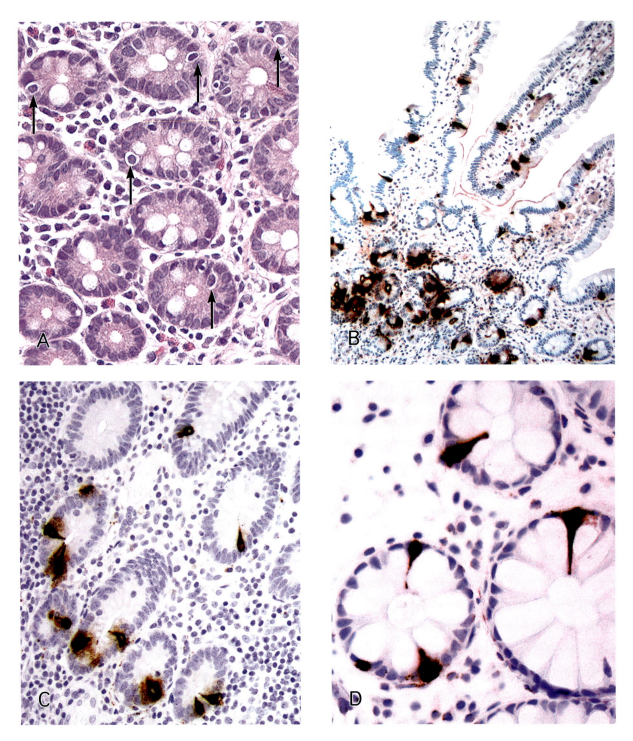

Figure 7-1

NEUROENDOCRINE TUMOR (NET): DIFFUSE NEUROENDOCRINE CELLS OF THE INTESTINE

A: Diffuse neuroendocrine cells (arrows) are difficult to appreciate on hematoxylin and eosin (H&E)- stained sections. They have round to ovoid nuclei encircled by pale halos; they are better appreciated with chromogranin A immunostaining.

B,C: Diffuse neuroendocrine cells are abundant in the deep crypts in the small intestine (B) and colon (C).

D: These cells are located in the base of the crypts, with long dendritic processes that reach to the lumen and adjacent epithelial cells.

Table 7-1

GASTROINTESTINAL NEUROENDOCRINE CELLS: SUBTYPE, LOCATION, AND SECRETORY PRODUCTS[a]

Cell Type	Location	Secretory Products
G	Antrum, duodenum	Gastrin
ECL	Stomach	Histamine
D	Antrum, SI,[b] LI	Somatostatin
D1	Stomach, SI	Ghrelin
EC	Stomach, SI, LI, APP	Serotonin, substance P
I (CCK)	Duodenum, jejunum	CCK
K (GIP)	Duodenum, jejunum	GIP
M	Duodenum, jejunum	Motilin
S	Duodenum, jejunum	Secretin
PP	Pancreas, duodenum	Pancreatic polypeptide
L	SI, LI	Enteroglucagon, peptide YY
N	SI	Neurotensin

[a]Data from reference 20.

[b]SI = small intestine; LI = large intestine; APP = appendix; GRP = gastrin-releasing peptide; CCK = cholecystokinin; GIP = gastric-inhibitory peptide.

properties, cellular and ultrastructural characteristics by electron microscopy, and their secretory products (Table 7-1) (12–19).

In current practice, the normal neuroendocrine cells of the gut and the corresponding tumors derived from them are identified by generic neuroendocrine markers such as chromogranin and synaptophysin (fig. 7-1B); less specific neuroendocrine markers such as neuron-specific enolase (NSE) and CD56 are not recommended for the confirmation of the diagnosis of NET. While the morphologic identification of these neuroendocrine cells preceded the characterization of their secretory products and physiologic functions, most known neuroendocrine cell types have corresponding amine/peptide hormones and regulatory functions (Table 7-1) (20).

NEUROENDOCRINE TUMORS OF THE INTESTINE

The term "carcinoid" was proposed in 1907 by Siegfried Oberndorfer (21). He also regarded NETs as "tumorlets" when they were detected in the small intestine (fig. 7-2). The name carcinoid was intended to express the distinctions and similarities in morphologic and clinical characteristics between these relatively indolent lesions compared to more overtly malignant carcinomas. Obendorfer (22) initially described these tumors as small and often multiple, with minimal or no indications of gland formation, without a tendency to penetrate into the surrounding tissues in an infiltrative pattern, with exceptionally slow growth and a seemingly harmless nature. Obendorfer later recognized that some carcinoid tumors were malignant and had associated metastases. It is now evident that this tumor entity exhibits considerable heterogeneity in pathobiology, clinical presentation, and molecular characteristics.

Classification

In 1963, Williams and Sandler (23) proposed classifying well-differentiated NETs according to their embryologic origin, i.e., foregut (lung, thymus, stomach, duodenum, proximal jejunum, and pancreas), midgut (distal jejunum, ileum, appendix, and cecum), or hindgut (colon and rectum) lesions. This stratification was developed prior to the elucidation of the various neuroendocrine cell subtypes and the recognition that an embryologic classification did not reflect the pathobiology of the disease. Upon the establishment of the APUD concept by Pearse (9), particularly the uptake of

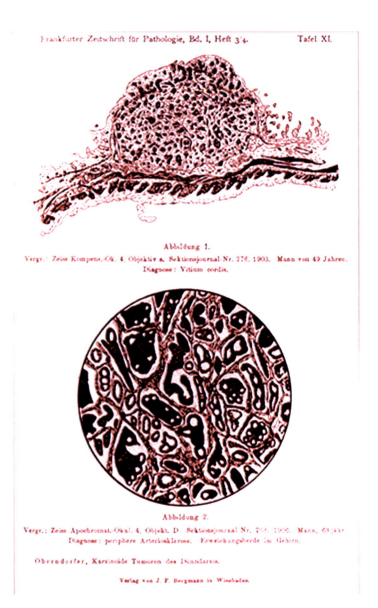

Figure 7-2

NEUROENDOCRINE TUMOR

This image shows the histopathologic features of a small intestine NET (carcinoid) depicted by Oberdorfer in 1907.

5-hydroxytryptophan (5-HT) and its conversion to 5-HT in the neuroendocrine cells of the GI tract, the term "apudoma" appeared, describing a patient with an adrenocorticotropic hormone (ACTH)-producing neuroendocrine tumor (24).

In the 1980 World Health Organization (WHO) classification for neuroendocrine neoplasms, the term carcinoid tumor applied to all tumors derived from the diffuse neuroendocrine system excluding pancreatic endocrine tumors. The carcinoids were then subclassified on the basis of various silver and other staining characteristics of their secretory granules: 1) enterochromaffin (EC) cell carcinoids, 2) gastrin (G) cell carcinoids, and 3) other carcinoids. With the wide application of progressively refined techniques in pathology, including biochemistry, histochemistry, immunocytochemistry, and molecular biology, NETs have revealed substantial heterogeneity. The clinically characterized carcinoid syndrome only relates to the EC-cell carcinoid, which produces active serotonin and substance P while non-EC-cell carcinoids are associated either with other hypersecreting hormonal syndromes or are functionally silent. While carcinoid is a historic-honored term, it may carry a deceptively benevolent connotation; the preferred terminology is well-differentiated neuroendocrine tumor for both the primary and metastatic lesions (25).

A classification proposed in 1995 eliminated the term carcinoid and was subsequently adopted by WHO in 2000 (26). The revised classification system separated NETs by their anatomic sites and emphasized the prognostic groups of the tumors by introducing several pathologic elements, such as tumor differentiation and size, extent of invasion, and lymphovascular invasion. However, the lack of understanding of the pathobiology and the molecular distinctions between well-differentiated NET and poorly differentiated NEC at the time culminated in confusing terminology. In the 2000 WHO classification system, well-differentiated NET was without metastasis, well-differentiated NEC had metastasis, and poorly differentiated NEC was a high-grade carcinoma. While useful for clinical outcome projections, dividing NETs into "benign," "low-grade malignant," and "high-grade malignant" categories mixed pathologic staging parameters (size, extent of invasion, and metastasis) with other prognostic factors (tumor differentiation, grade, and lymphovascular invasion).

The 2010 WHO classification (27) for GI neuroendocrine neoplasms, the most current at this writing, recognizes the pathologic distinction between well-differentiated NET and poorly differentiated NEC. These two entities are defined by the combined morphologic features and proliferative activities of the tumor, i.e., mitotic count and Ki-67 (MIB-1) proliferative index (Table 7-2). Given its close association with conventional carcinomas by clinical, pathologic, and molecular characteristics, poorly differentiated NEC is classified and staged as carcinomas at other sites of the GI tract and discussed in chapter 4. In contrast to NECs, which are inevitably high grade, well-differentiated NETs exhibit a spectrum of grades, i.e., low grade (WHO G1), intermediate grade (WHO G2), and even breach the Ki-67 index threshold for a high-grade (WHO G3) NET although a homogeneous high-grade component is uncommon in well-

Table 7-2

2010 WORLD HEALTH ORGANIZATION (WHO) CLASSIFICATION OF NEUROENDOCRINE TUMORS[a]

	Mitoses	Ki-67 Index
Well-differentiated NET[b] - G1	<2/10 HPF	<3%
Well-differentiated NET - G2	2-20/10 HPF	3-20%
Poorly differentiated NEC - G3	>20/10 HPF	>20%

[a]Modified from reference 27.
[b]NET = neuroendocrine tumor; HPF = high-power fields; NEC = neuroendocrine carcinoma.

differentiated NETs of the intestine (28). Thus, proliferative activity alone cannot adequately distinguish between NET and NEC. Given the significant difference in treatment and survival, the combined assessment of clinical characteristics and pathologic features of the tumor are necessary for an accurate diagnosis (28,29).

Depending on their anatomic location and their specific subtype, well-differentiated intestinal NETs produce a variety of amines and polypeptides/hormones. Most intestinal NETs are clinically silent (nonfunctioning) even though immunolabeling and serum studies demonstrate the presence of various hormones produced by the tumor cells. The term "functioning" NET is restricted to those NETs that cause a clinical syndrome secondary to inappropriate hormone hyperfunction.

Clinical and Biochemical Diagnosis of Well-Differentiated Neuroendocrine Tumors

Chromogranin A is the most widely used generic biomarker for NETs, with a sensitivity of 60 to 90 percent, although its specificity (50 percent) is hindered by numerous metabolites in the food, proton pump inhibitors, and hepatic, renal, and cardiac functions (30). Recent studies have suggested that pancreastatin, a post-translational fragment of chromogranin A, is a reliable biomarker for NETs that is not influenced by acid inhibitory medications (31). Depending on the neuroendocrine cell types that comprise the specific NET, the amines and polypeptide/hormones, and their corresponding byproducts, may be detected in the plasma or urine. Urine 24-hour 5-HIAA exhibits high specificity for the detection of small intestinal NETs that are derived from EC cells (32).

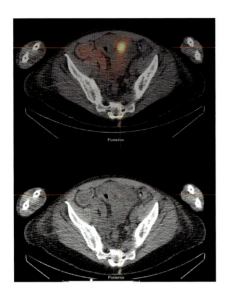
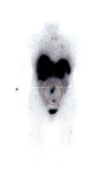
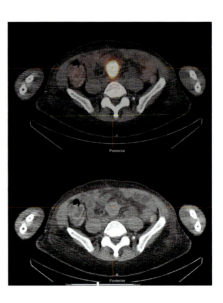

Figure 7-3

NEUROENDOCRINE TUMOR

This Octreotidescan™ highlights an occult primary NET and is useful for determining the stage of the disease. The patient initially presented with extensive liver metastases. Additional abdominal/pelvic lesions were identified on Octreoscan™ (middle panel in red circle), which corresponded to a minute NET of the small intestine (left upper panel) that was difficult to classify on computerized tomography (CT) scan (left lower panel), and a large mesenteric mass on CT (right lower panel) that was intensely avid on Octreoscan™ (right upper panel).

In addition to standard imaging evaluations by computerized tomography (CT) or magnetic resonance imaging (MRI), somatostatin-receptor scintigraphy (SRS; OctreoScan™ or 68Ga-DOTATATE scan) is useful for either the initial diagnosis and staging of NETs or for the assessment of disease recurrence after treatment since over 85 percent of intestinal NETs express somatostatin type 2 receptors (fig. 7-3) (33). Endoscopic ultrasound is frequently used to evaluate the depth of tumor invasion and regional lymph node metastasis for duodenal and rectal NETs, with an estimated accuracy of 80 to 100 percent (34,35).

Tumor Staging

There are a number of staging systems for NETs of the intestine, including those developed by the European Neuroendocrine Tumor Society (ENETS) in 2006 (36,37) accompanied by a grading system, and the Union for International Cancer Control (UICC)/American Joint Commission for Cancer (AJCC 7th edition) in 2009 and revised AJCC 8th edition in 2016 (38). There are some discrepancies in these systems and it should be stated in the pathology report

which staging system is used for intestinal NETs (Table 7-3).

Molecular Genetic Features

NETs of the GI tract generally occur as sporadic tumors with rare somatic gene mutations/alterations, although they may present as part of complex familial endocrine syndromes with germline mutations. About 20 percent of NETs of the GI tract and the pancreas occur in the context of a genetic syndrome, with at least 10 recognized NET syndromes (39,40). However, *multiple endocrine neoplasia type 1* (MEN1) and *neurofibromatosis type 1* (NF1) are the only conditions that manifest intestinal NETs, primarily in the duodenum. Additional rare susceptibility genes associated with a smaller fraction of intestinal NETs have also been identified (39,40).

The MEN1 syndrome is an autosomal dominant disorder which results from an inactivating mutation of the *MEN1* gene. MEN1 can be diagnosed clinically if a patient has two of three tumors: duodenopancreatic NETs, anterior pituitary tumors, and parathyroid tumors. Other endocrinopathies may be present, including NETs of the thymus and lung, adrenal gland tumors,

Table 7-3

COMPARISON OF AMERICAN JOINT COMMITTEE ON CANCER (AJCC) AND EUROPEAN NEUROENDOCRINE TUMOR SOCIETY (ENETS) TNM STAGING FOR NEUROENDOCRINE TUMORS OF THE INTESTINE[a]

A. TNM Staging for Neuroendocrine Tumors of the Duodenum and Ampulla of Vater

	AJCC TNM (8th Edition)	ENETS TNM
TX	Primary tumor cannot be assessed	Primary tumor cannot be assessed
T0		No evidence of primary tumor
T1	Duodenum: tumor invades mucosa/lamina propria or submucosa and size ≤1 cm	Duodenum: tumor invades mucosa/lamina propria or submucosa and size ≤1 cm
	Ampulla: tumor ≤1 cm and confined within the sphincter of Oddi	Tumor limited to ampulla of Vater for ampullary ganglioctyic paraganglioma
T2	Duodenum: tumor invades the muscularis propria or is >1 cm	Duodenum: tumor invades the muscularis propria or is >1 cm
	Ampulla: tumor invades through sphincter into duodenal submucosa or muscularis propria, or is >1 cm	
T3	Tumor invades the pancreas or peripancreatic adipose tissue	Tumor invades the pancreas or peripancreatic adipose tissue
T4	Tumor invades peritoneum (serosa) or other organs	Tumor invades peritoneum (serosa) or other organs
	For any T, add (m) for multiple tumors [TX(#) or TX(m)] # = number of primary tumors	*For any T add (m) for multiple tumors*
NX	Regional lymph nodes cannot be assessed	Regional lymph nodes cannot be assessed
N0	No regional lymph node metastasis	No regional lymph node metastasis
N1	Regional lymph node metastasis	Regional lymph node metastasis
MX		Distant metastasis cannot be assessed
M0	No distant metastases	No distant metastases
M1	Distant metastasis	Distant metastasis (specify sites)
M1a	Metastasis confined to the liver	
M1b	Metastases in at least one extrahepatic site (e.g., lung, ovary, nonregional lymph node, peritoneum, bone)	
M1c	Both hepatic and extrahepatic metastases	

B. TNM Staging for Neuroendocrine Tumors of the Jejunum and Ileum

	AJCC TNM (8th Edition)	ENETS TNM
TX	Primary tumor cannot be assessed	Primary tumor cannot be assessed
T0	No evidence of primary tumor	No evidence of primary tumor
T1	Tumor invades mucosa/lamina propria or submucosa and size ≤1 cm	Tumor invades mucosa/lamina propria or submucosa and size ≤1 cm
T2	Tumor invades muscularis propria or size >1 cm	Tumor invades muscularis propria or size >1 cm
T3	Tumor invades subserosa without penetrating overlying serosa	Tumor invades subserosa without penetrating overlying serosa
T4	Tumor invades visceral peritoneum (serosal) or other organs or adjacent structures	Tumor invades peritoneum/other organs
	For any T, add (m) for multiple tumors [TX(#) or TX(m)] # = number of primary tumors	*For any T add (m) for multiple tumors*
NX	Regional lymph nodes cannot be assessed	Regional lymph nodes cannot be assessed
N0	No regional lymph node metastasis	No regional lymph node metastasis
N1	Regional lymph node metastasis less than 12 nodes	Regional lymph node metastasis
N2	Large mesenteric masses (>2 cm) and/or extensive nodal deposits (12 or greater), especially those that encase the superior mesenteric vessels	
M	Distant metastasis	Distant metastasis
MX	Distant metastasis cannot be assessed	Distant metastasis cannot be assessed
M0	No distant metastases	

Table 7-3, continued

B. TNM Staging for Neuroendocrine Tumors of the Jejunum and Ileum, continued

AJCC TNM (8th Edition)	ENETS TNM
M1 Distant metastasis	Distant metastasis (specify sites)
M1a Metastasis confided to the liver	
M1b Metastases in at least one extrahepatic site (e.g., lung, ovary, nonregional lymph node, peritoneum, bone)	
M1c Both hepatic and extrahepatic metastases	

C. TNM Staging for Neuroendocrine Tumors of the Appendix

AJCC TNM (8th Edition)	ENETS TNM
TX	Primary tumor cannot be assessed
T0	No evidence of primary tumor
T1 Tumor 2 cm or less in greatest dimension	Tumor ≤1 cm invading submucosa and muscularis propria
T2 Tumor more than 2 cm but less than or equal to 4 cm	Tumor ≤2 cm invading submucosa, muscularis propria and/or minimally (up to 3 mm) invading subserosa/mesoappendix
T3 Tumor more than 4 cm or with subserosal invasion or involvement of the mesoappendix	Tumor >2 cm and/or extensive (more than 3 mm) invasion of subserosa/mesoappendix
T4 Tumor perforates the peritoneum or directly invades other adjacent organs or structures, e.g., abdominal wall and skeletal muscle *(excluding direct mural extension to adjacent subserosa of adjacent bowel)*	Tumor invades peritoneum/other organs
NX	Regional lymph nodes cannot be assessed
N0	No regional lymph node metastasis
N1	Regional lymph node metastasis
M	Distant metastasis
MX	Distant metastasis cannot be assessed
M0	No distant metastases
M1 Distant metastasis	Distant metastasis (specify sites)
M1a Metastasis confined to the liver	
M1b Metastases in at least one extrahepatic site (e.g., lung, ovary, nonregional lymph node, peritoneum, bone)	
M1c Both hepatic and extrahepatic metastases	

lipomas, and multiple skin lesions. More than 1,300 different *MEN1* mutations have been identified in MEN1 patients; the majority of the MEN1-related NETs develop after somatic loss of heterozygosity (LOH) on chromosome 11q13. The prevalence of duodenopancreatic NETs in MEN1 is about 50 percent (41). The majority of MEN1-related gastrinomas are located in the submucosa of the duodenum. Duodenal NETs in MEN1 are usually multiple and associated with multifocal hyperplasia of gastrin-producing G cells (42).

NF1 (von Recklinghausen disease) is an autosomal dominant syndrome caused by loss of function mutations in *NF1* that have been linked to deregulation of both rat sarcoma viral oncogene homolog (RAS) proteins and the ERK/MAPK signaling pathway (40). The condition is characterized by multiple endocrinopathies and nervous system manifestations. The most common features are fibromatous skin tumors, Lisch eye nodules, optic gliomas, and cafe´-au-lait spots. Endocrinopathies are less common and include pheochromocytoma and duodenal

Table 7-3, continued

D. TNM Staging for Neuroendocrine Tumors of the Colorectum

	AJCC TNM (8th Edition)	ENETS TNM
TX	Primary tumor cannot be assessed	
T0	No evidence of primary tumor	
T1	Tumor invades mucosa/lamina propria or submucosa $\leq$2 cm	
	T1a size <1 cm	
	T1b size 1–2 cm	
T2	Tumor invades muscularis propria or size >2 cm	
T3	Tumor invades subserosa/pericolic/perirectal fat without penetration of overlying serosa	
T4	Tumor invades the visceral peritoneum (serosa) or other organs or adjacent structures	
NX	Regional lymph nodes cannot be assessed	
N0	No regional lymph node metastasis	
N1	Regional lymph node metastasis	
M	Distant metastasis	
MX		Distant metastasis cannot be assessed
M0	No distant metastases	
M1	Distant metastasis	Distant metastasis (specify sites)
M1a	Metastasis confined to the liver	
M1b	Metastases in at least one extrahepatic site (e.g., lung, ovary, nonregional lymph node, peritoneum, bone)	
M1c	Both hepatic and extrahepatic metastases	

[a]Data from references 36 through 38.

NETs, i.e., somatostatinoma/glandular NET (43,44).

Familial jejunoileal NETs have also been described in a small fraction of patients (45,46). Despite substantial efforts, no definitive genetic basis for this phenomenon has been elucidated. The genomic landscape of these NETs has been investigated by next-generation sequencing and recurrent mutations are only identified in the *CDKN1B* gene in about 9 percent tumors (47–49). Instead, the most frequent genomic alteration is hemizygous deletions affecting chromosome 18q, which have been identified in both familial and sporadic jejunoileal NETs (45,47,48). Other investigations have demonstrated several altered cancer-related pathways, including the PI3K/Akt/mTOR signaling pathway, the TGF-β pathway (through mutations in *SMAD* genes), and the *SRC* oncogene (48,50).

No hereditary syndromes have been associated with colorectal and appendiceal well-differentiated NETs. There are limited data on their molecular characteristics.

Treatment and Prognosis

Treatment strategies for intestinal NETs are highly individualized based on the diverse range of tumor burden and symptoms. The best therapeutic options for individual patients depend on whether the aim of treatment is to slow tumor growth or ameliorate symptoms by inhibition of the secretion of bioactive agents. One of the difficulties in treating these patients is that there are no clearly defined measures to predict which tumors will respond to a particular modality or to rigorously assess therapeutic efficacy (51–54).

Surgery is essential in many phases of intestinal NET management and remains the primary chance for cure in patients with localized disease. For patients with advanced disease, cytoreductive surgery is recommended for palliation, symptom amelioration, and prolonged survival.

The liver is the primary site of metastasis for intestinal NETs. The reduction of hepatic tumor burden by means of surgical intervention is associated with a 5-year survival rate of 60 percent compared to 30 percent without surgical intervention in highly selected patients (55,56). Resection of hepatic metastases can be done by enucleation, segmental resection, or lobar resection. Cytoreduction procedures depend on arterial embolization, ablation by radiofrequency, other modalities (57,58).

Somatostatin analog therapy is recommended as first-line medical treatment for functioning tumors. It provides symptomatic improvement in 70 to 80 percent of patients and stabilizes tumor growth in up to half for varying durations (59–63). Additionally, an oral serotonin inhibitor (telotristat epitrate) has been developed for the management of refractory diarrhea in patients with carcinoid syndrome (64).

Conventional cytotoxic chemotherapy is ineffective in WHO G1/G2 NETs. Newer agents, including antiangiogenic medications (bevacizumab), tyrosine kinase inhibitors (sunitinib, sorafenib, vatalanib), and mTOR inhibitors (everolimus), are optional medical treatment for patients with intestinal NETs but clinical responses are marginal (30,65,66). Targeting somatostatin receptor with radiolabeled analogs, i.e., peptide receptor radiotherapy (PRRT), is safe and effective for patients whose tumors express adequate densities of somatostatin receptors as evaluated on diagnostic somatostatin receptor scintigraphy. PRRT is recommended in selected patients with unresectable metastatic disease and large tumor burden (67).

NEUROENDOCRINE TUMORS OF THE DUODENUM

Epidemiology and Clinical Presentation

While *duodenal NETs* are rare among intestinal NETs (2 to 3 percent), with an age-adjusted annual incidence of 0.19/100,000 to the 2000 US standard population (68), they are the most diverse group of neoplasms. They have unusual clinical presentations, involve several subtypes of neuroendocrine cells, have unique pathologic characteristics, and are often syndromic (69). The median age of onset is 67 years for sporadic lesions and one decade younger for syndromic tumors.

NETs with G-cell differentiation are the most common subtype, accounting for approximately 50 percent of all duodenal NETs (70). About 50 percent of these tumors are functional, i.e., gastrinomas. Patients present with markedly elevated serum gastrin levels and associated clinical symptoms of acid hypersecretion, peptic ulcer disease, gastroesophageal reflux disease, and diarrhea (Zollinger-Ellison syndrome) (71). Gastrinomas may be present in the pancreas, duodenum, and first jejunal loop. In addition to G-cell neoplasia, secondary enterochromaffin-like (ECL) cell hyperplasia and neoplasia can occur in the stomach (type II gastric NET) due to hypergastrin stimulation of ECL cells. While gastrin was discovered as early as 1905 by British physiologist Edkins (72), it was not initially linked to Zollinger-Ellison syndrome until 1967 when British physiologist Gregory et al. (73) extracted gastrin from a pancreatic NET. The clinical presentation of multiple pancreatic gastrinomas indicates MEN1 whereas 40 percent of sporadic gastrinomas with associated Zollinger-Ellison syndrome arise in the duodenum (74).

Duodenal gastrinoma is known for its disproportional systemic manifestations in the face of occult primaries on endoscopic and imaging evaluations, and its frequent locoregional lymph node and distant metastases (70). If noted on endoscopy, duodenal NETs are readily mistaken for Brunner gland adenoma/hamartoma or gastric heterotopia. When nonfunctioning, gastrin-expressing NET is designated as a G-cell tumor; these are usually solitary and located in the first portion of the duodenum (D1).

The ampullary portion of the duodenum is the primary location of somatostatin-expressing D-cell NETs (somatostatinoma/glandular NETs) and gangliocytic paragangliomas, which constitute about 30 percent of all duodenal NETs. Both entities have known associations with NF1 and MEN1, although the hereditary association is much less common for gangliocytic paraganglioma (75). In contrast to pancreatic lesions, which often manifest as somatostatinoma and present with somatostatin hypersecretion-related symptoms of diarrhea, cholelithiasis, dyspepsia, and diabetes, somatostatin-expressing duodenal tumors are almost never functional. Given their exclusive location at or around the major or minor ampulla, somatostatinomas frequently cause obstructive symptoms, i.e., acute pancreatitis, jaundice, and intestinal bleeding. Somatostatinomas and gangliocytic

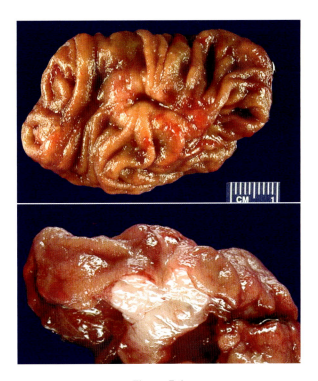

Figure 7-4

DUODENAL NEUROENDOCRINE TUMOR

The tumor is a polypoid mass with mucosal erosion (top); on cut surface the tumor is fleshy, yellow-tan, and centered in the submucosa (bottom).

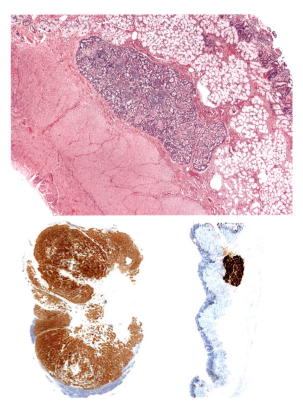

Figure 7-5

DUODENAL GASTRINOMA

Top: An occult gastrinoma was identified in the entirely submitted duodenal submucosa.

Bottom: An immunostain for gastrin highlights an occult gastrinoma (3 mm) that gave rise to an enlarged periportal lymph node (25 mm).

paragangliomas are also discussed in Tumors of the Gallbladder, Extrahepatic Bile Ducts, and Vaterian System (75a).

Asymptomatic serotonin-expressing EC-cell NETs of the duodenum are usually identified incidentally at an early stage, which can be accredited to frequent GI surveillance by endoscopy. Larger tumors may cause mucosal erosion and intestinal bleeding, and patients with liver metastasis may present with carcinoid syndrome as seen in their jejunoileal NET counterpart (see below). Other rare duodenal NETs have a nonspecific neuroendocrine cell lineage and express a variety of intestinal and pancreatic peptide hormones on immunohistochemistry (76,77).

Pathologic Features

Macroscopically, duodenal NETs present as soft submucosal polyps or masses, with or without surface erosion. The tumors are tan-yellow with a fleshy consistency on cut surface (fig. 7-4). The initial presentation of gastrinoma is

frequently the identification of enlarged lymph nodes in the periduodenal/peripancreatic/portal region, associated with diminutive occult primary duodenal NETs that are millimeters in size and may only be evident by endoscopic ultrasound or after extensive microscopic examination of the entirely submitted duodenum (fig. 7-5). When the duodenal mucosa is inadequately sampled these occult microgastrinomas are the likely origin of the reported and supposed "primary" lymph node gastrinomas (78–80). Nonfunctioning G-cell NETs are usually incidentally identified in the segment of duodenum proximal to the bulb. Somatostatinomas are exclusively located at the ampulla. Gangliocytic paragangliomas are frequently indented at the shoulder of the ampulla/periampulla, thus the clinical presentation of jaundice is less common.

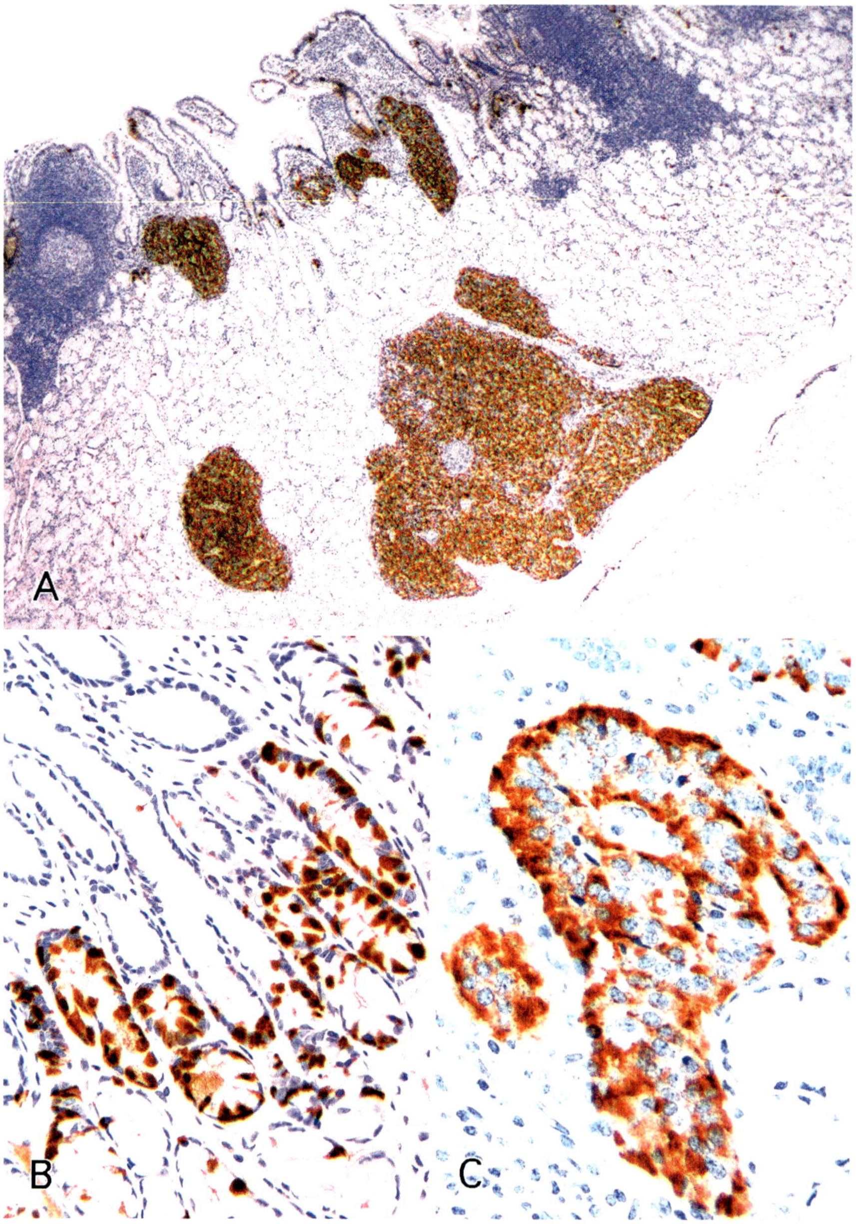

Figure 7-6

**G-CELL HYPERPLASIA
IN MULTIPLE ENDOCRINE
NEOPLASIA (MEN)
1-ASSOCIATED DUODENAL
GASTRINOMA**

A: Multifocal duodenal gastrinomas are highlighted by immunostaining for gastrin.

B: Diffuse G-cell hyperplasia in a circumferential and linear pattern.

C: Micronodular and macronodular G-cell neoplasia.

Precursor lesions exist in patients with MEN1-associated duodenal gastrinomas. This is documented as progressive hyperplasia-neoplasia: from diffusely increased numbers of individual G cells, to linear arrangement of G cells, to micronodule and macronodule formation, and eventually to invasive G-cell tumors (fig. 7-6) (74). Microscopically, small gastrinomas are typically identified in the submucosa, with interanastomosing trabeculae or acini arranged in loosely cohesive nests that may have a gyriform pattern (fig. 7-7). The tumor is richly vascularized and may have capillaries filled with erythrocytes. Delicate to moderate fibrous septa may be present between large tumor nests.

Somatostatin-expressing D-cell NETs commonly exhibit a glandular growth pattern with psammomatous calcifications in the gland lumens; they are also known as glandular carcinoid and psammomatous somatostatinomas (fig. 7-8). These calcifications are highly characteristic of NF1-associated tumors (seen in virtually every case) and they are present in about 60 percent of sporadic somatostatin-expressing neoplasms

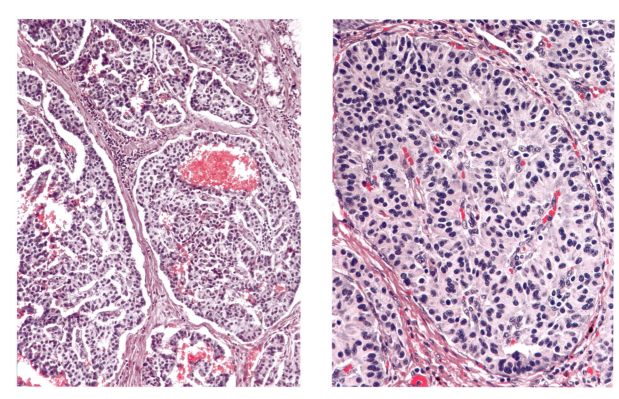

Figure 7-7

DUODENAL GASTRINOMA

The tumor is composed of anastomosing trabeculae that form loosely cohesive and richly vascularized nests with a gyriform pattern at both low (left) and high (right) magnification.

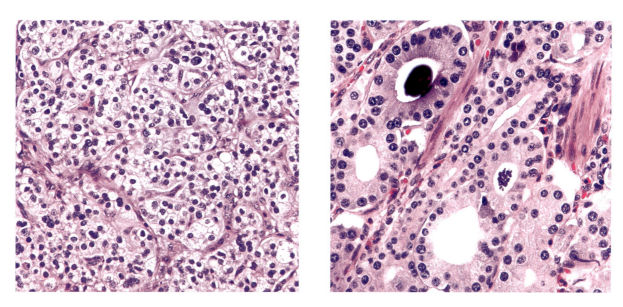

Figure 7-8

DUODENAL SOMATOSTATIN-EXPRESSING D-CELL NET

Left: The tumor cells are arranged in small acini with clear/vacuolated or foamy cytoplasm.
Right: The tumor cells also form glands with psammomatous luminal calcifications.

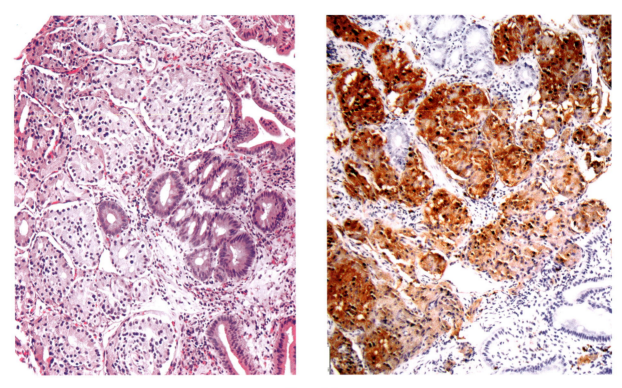

Figure 7-9

DUODENAL SOMATOSTATIN-EXPRESSING D-CELL NET

Left: The tumor is composed of cells with pale cytoplasm, small and basally located nuclei, and an acinar arrangement that may mimic the appearance of benign duodenal Brunner glands.

Right: Immunostain for somatostatin confirms the diagnosis of somatostatin-expressing D-cell NET.

(75). In addition to the glandular pattern, the tumor cells may be arranged in an acinar configuration, with pale or vacuolated cytoplasm (fig. 7-8). As a result, a submucosal somatostatin-expressing D-cell NET can mimic benign Brunner glands (fig. 7-9). These tumors often lack a well-circumscribed border and infiltrate deeply into the smooth muscle of the sphincter of Oddi, abutting or invading the pancreas without eliciting a desmoplastic reaction. As a result, negative deep resection margins are difficult to achieve from local excisions via either endoscopic intervention or ampullectomy (fig. 7-10). Given the combined clinical presentation of jaundice and the gland-forming histology, somatostatinomas are prone to misinterpretation as ampullary adenocarcinoma in mucosal biopsy specimens (fig. 7-11).

The pathologic features of serotonin-expressing EC-cell NETs are similar to those of their jejunoileal counterparts (see below). Other miscellaneous subtypes of duodenal NETs do not have characteristic histologic phenotypes; they may present with any of the common patterns of well-differentiated NETs observed in the GI tract and pancreas, including insular, trabecular, acinar, tubular/glandular, and loosely cohesive architecture. Focal mucin production can be observed in well-differentiated NETs.

All subtypes of duodenal NET exhibit homogeneous and round to ovoid nuclei with stippled chromatin and moderate amounts of granular cytoplasm. Tumor necrosis is almost never present in small tumors and mitotic activity is generally in the range of 0 to 2 mitoses per 10 high-power fields (WHO G1 grade), although Ki-67 proliferative indices of over 2 percent may place them in the WHO G2 grade.

Gangliocytic paraganglioma is a unique type of neuroendocrine tumor with trilineage differentiation, including neuroendocrine-type epithelium, schwannian/nerve sheath spindle cells, and ganglion components (fig. 7-12). Immunohistochemically, the tumor cells are generally reactive for chromogranin and

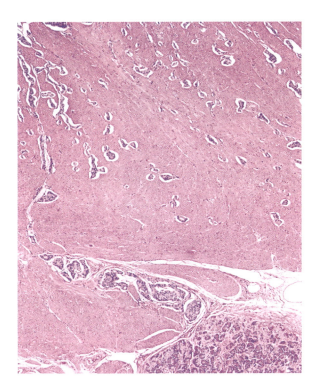

Figure 7-10

DUODENAL SOMATOSTATIN-EXPRESSING D-CELL NET

The tumor lacks a circumscribed border and infiltrates the muscularis propria without eliciting reactive desmoplasia. It abuts the pancreatic parenchyma (bottom right).

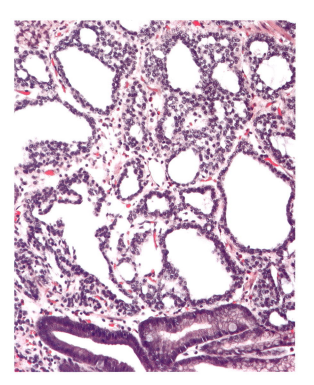

Figure 7-11

SOMATOSTATIN-EXPRESSING D-CELL NET

In the absence of abundant granular cytoplasm, the glandular epithelium of the tumor may appear atypical and could be misinterpreted as adenocarcinoma, particularly in small biopsies.

synaptophysin. The epithelial component may not be immunoreactive to cytokeratin in up to 50 percent cases, but the tumor cells usually express pancreatic polypeptide (PP), somatostatin, or vasoactive intestinal peptide (VIP). The schwannian competent of the tumor is immunoreactive for S-100 protein (fig. 7-12). This tumor entity is also discussed in chapter 8.

Treatment and Prognosis

The majority (81 percent) of duodenal NETs present with localized disease, 10 percent with locally advanced disease, and 9 percent with distant metastasis; the median survival period is 99 months (68). There are, however, significant differences in outcome for patients with different subtypes of NET. The rates of lymph node and liver metastases between functioning gastrinomas and nonfunctioning G-cell NETs are 75 versus 6 percent and 20 versus 0 percent, respectively (70). Thus patients with Zollinger-Ellison syndrome-associated gastrinomas who

do not have MEN1 should be offered surgical intervention for possible cure (81). In most cases of MEN1-associated gastrinoma, patients are not surgical candidates due to the multifocality of small and occult lesions and the wide distribution of lesions in the pancreas and duodenum (82). Small (less than 1 cm), superficial, and incidentally identified duodenal NETs (including G-cell tumors, EC-cell tumors, and NETs not otherwise specified) without clinical evidence of locoregional and distant metastases can be safely managed by endoscopic removal and are associated with an excellent prognosis (35,83).

While lymph node (about 30 percent) and liver (about 5 percent) metastases occur in somatostatinoma and gangliocytic paraganglioma, most patients have favorable outcomes after complete removal of the disease. A Whipple procedure may be required because of the ampullary location of the tumor. The 10-year survival rate is over 70 percent (75).

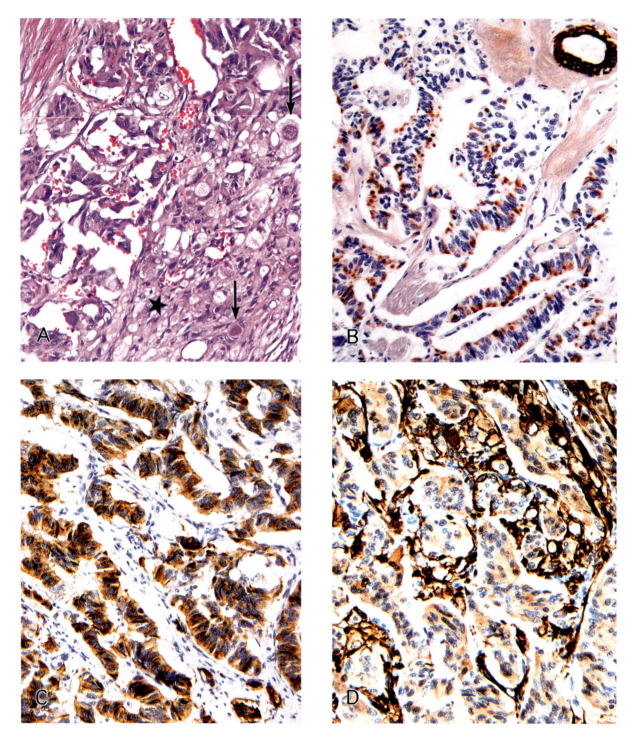

Figure 7-12

DUODENAL GANGLIOCYTIC PARAGANGLIOMA

A: This neoplasm displays trilineage differentiation of endocrine epithelial-type (left), ganglionic (arrows), and schwannian (star) components.

B: Immunostain for cytokeratin may be negative in the epithelial component or have a focal and dot-like pattern.

C: The epithelial component is immunoreactive for pancreatic polypeptide (PP).

D: The schwannian element is immunoreactive for S-100 protein.

NEUROENDOCRINE TUMORS OF THE JEJUNUM AND ILEUM

Jejunoileal NETs are the "classic carcinoids" initially described by Obendorfer in 1907 (21) and "midgut carcinoids" classified by Williams and Sandler (see fig. 7-1) (23). Over 95 percent differentiate along the lines of serotonin- and substance P-producing EC cells with argentaffinity; the rest are argyrophilic tumors with G-cell, enteroglucagon, or pancreatic polypeptide (L-cell) differentiation.

Epidemiology and Clinical Presentation

The incidence of neuroendocrine tumors of the small intestine, particularly the distal jejunum and ileum, is the second highest among GI NETs after rectal primary NETs. The age-adjusted annual incidence is 0.67/100,000 to the 2000 US standard population; they account for approximately 27 percent of GI NETs (68,84). The median age at initial diagnosis is 66 years, with similar prevalence in men and women. The African-American to Caucasian patient ratio is 1.32 and the incidence in Asian-Pacific Islanders and American Indian/Alaskan natives is much lower (one third compared with Caucasians and African-Americans). Up to 75 percent of patients present with liver metastasis and in many cases the primary intestinal NET has not been identified at the time of initial diagnosis.

Individuals with undetected (from autopsy series) and incidentally detected jejunoileal NETs are usually asymptomatic despite the fact that they may have elevated serum neuroendocrine markers (chromogranin A) and urine 5-HIAA, and even liver metastases. Due to small primary size and limitations of endoscopic assessment, in the event of liver metastasis, the identification of the primary tumor site in the jejunoileum can be challenging. When present, symptoms include abdominal pain, bowel obstruction, intussusception, and ischemia, all of which are unrelated to hormone hypersecretion.

Less than 10 percent of jejunoileal NETs are clinically functional with associated carcinoid syndrome, a consequence of liver metastasis leading to the release of tumor derived serotonin and other vasoactive substances directly into the systemic circulation via the hepatic vein. Nevertheless, less than 20 percent of patients with liver metastases present with carcinoid syndrome (85). Carcinoid syndrome does not occur in localized or locally advanced NETs involving mesentery lymph nodes since the secretory products from the tumor are inactivated in the liver when drained into the portal venous system. The carcinoid syndrome is manifested by episodes of cutaneous flushing of the neck and face, with associated sweating, diarrhea, wheezing, and heart disease (Hedinger syndrome) secondary to fibrosis of the tricuspid valve, pulmonic valve, and subendocardium of the right side of the heart (86). Carcinoid crisis is a severe, potentially fatal exacerbation of hormonal symptoms often provoked by anesthesia or invasive surgical procedures. Patients present with classic carcinoid syndrome, with either hypotension or hypertension, severe bronchospasm, and cardiac arrest (87).

Pathologic Features

The terminal ileum is the classic site for jejunoileal NETs (fig. 7-13), although this may be related to its accessible location by colonoscopy during routine surveillance. About a third of jejunoileal NETs are multifocal (88,89), although it is not clear whether some of these tumors are intramucosal/intramural metastases from a solitary primary tumor (fig. 7-14). The primary tumor is usually small, and most range in size from less than 1 to 2 cm, but can present with bowel obstruction, ischemia, or insuccation (figs. 7-15, 7-16). The gross appearance of tumors in the small bowel lumen is that of firm nodules or polypoid lesions under the intact mucosal surface (figs. 7-13–7-16). Intestinal hemorrhage may occur when tumor erodes the mucosa, potentially culminating in a medical emergency.

On cut surface, the tumors are usually white-yellow and centered in the submucosa, with infiltration into the deep muscularis propria (fig. 7-13). Mesenteric involvement by small intestinal NET is common and results in a mass that is usually much larger than its counterpart mural primary tumor (fig. 7-15). A mesenteric mass is caused by either matted metastatic lymph nodes or extensive peritoneal fibrosis induced by fibroblastic growth factor released from the tumor (85,90). NETs of EC-cell lineage also arise in Meckel diverticula (91) and intestinal duplication cysts (92).

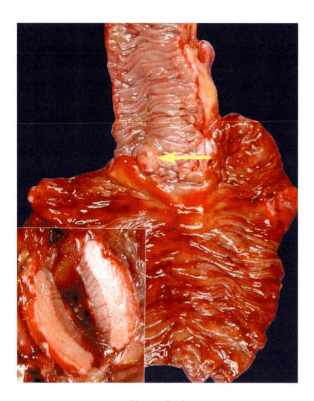

Figure 7-13

NEUROENDOCRINE TUMOR: TERMINAL ILEUM

The terminal ileum is a common location for small intestine NET, particularly at the ileocecal junction (arrow). On cut section (insert), the tumor is present under intact mucosa and infiltrates the muscularis propria.

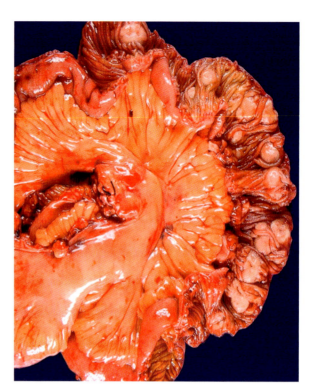

Figure 7-14

NEUROENDOCRINE TUMOR: SMALL INTESTINE

Multiple neuroendocrine tumors present in the small intestine.

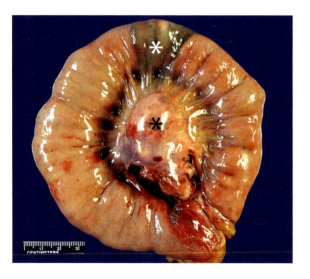

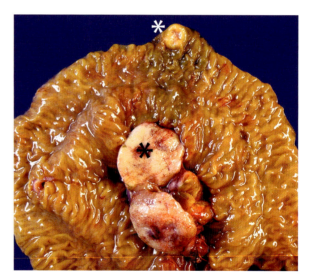

Figure 7-15

NEUROENDOCRINE TUMOR: SMALL INTESTINE

Left: Partial bowel obstruction (white *) and ischemia are associated with a large mesenteric mass (black *).

Right: The primary NET measures less than 1 cm (white *) and the mesenteric mass is formed by matted lymph nodes (black *).

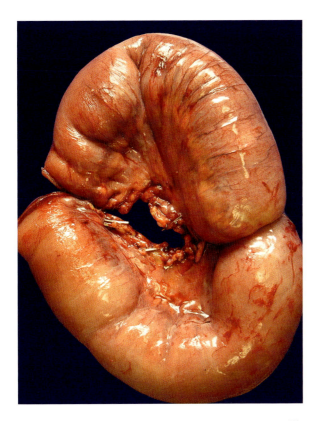 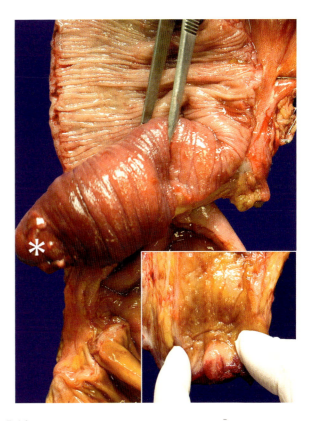

Figure 7-16

NEUROENDOCRINE TUMOR: SMALL INTESTINE

Clinically symptomatic bowel obstruction secondary to intussusception (left) resulted in this resection. A tumor is present at the tip of the intussuscepted bowel (right, white *). On cut section, a small tumor was identified (insert).

Microscopically, the tumor is composed of solid, smooth-bordered, insular or acinar nests with irregular shapes. Eosinophilic cytoplasmic secretory granules are accentuated in the tumor cells located at the periphery of the nests, resulting in the appearance of peripheral palisading (fig. 7-17). In well-fixed specimens, the tumors cells are tightly packed but evenly spaced within the nests, with a moderate amount of granular cytoplasm; the nuclei are round or ovoid in shape with minimal pleomorphism and finely stippled chromatin (fig. 7-18, right). In poorly preserved specimens, the tumor cells may show nuclear crowding, pleomorphism, and coarse/clumped chromatin (fig. 7-18, left). The stroma between the tumor nests consists of either rich vasculature or dense fibrosis; the latter is particularly prominent in the submucosa, subserosa, and mesentery (fig. 7-19). Both perineural invasion and lymphovascular invasion are common. The mitotic activity is nil to low in most small intestinal NETs (0 to 2 per 10 high-power fields), which is classified as WHO G1, but Ki-67 proliferative indices may be higher than 2 percent in some tumors, which places them in the WHO G2 grade (fig. 7-20).

The histologic features of NETs derived from EC cells are fairly specific. Liver metastases (from an unknown primary) can facilitate the identification of a distal small intestine location.

EC-cell tumors are usually diffusely positive for neuroendocrine markers, particularly chromogranin with strong intensity. They are also reactive with serotonin and substance P antibodies.

Treatment and Prognosis

Most low-grade (WHO G1/G2) jejunoileal NETs have a protracted clinical course although there is significant variability in prognosis impacted by patient age, gender, and ethnicity, and tumor grade and stage (68). The overall median survival period of patients with jejunoileal NET

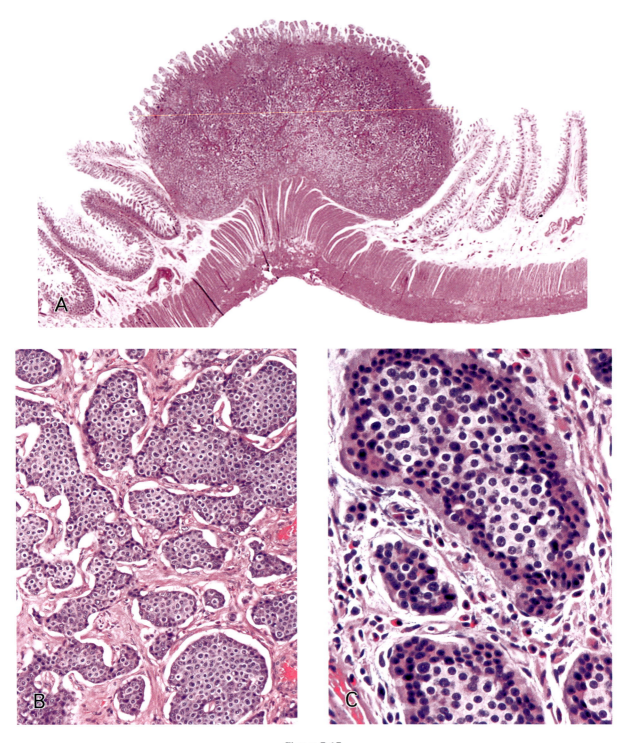

Figure 7-17

JEJUNOILEAL EC-CELL NET

A: Low-power magnification view of an ileal NET located in the mucosa without involvement of surface epithelium.

B: The tumor cells are arranged in solid nests.

C: High-power view shows the tumor nests encircled by cells with eosinophilic granules resulting in an appearance of palisading.

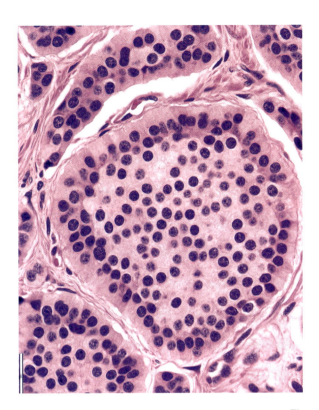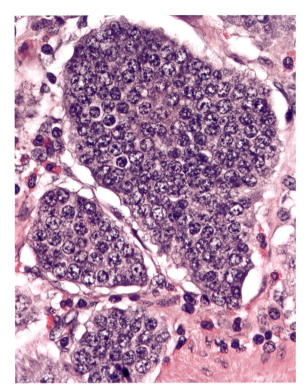

Figure 7-18

JEJUNOILEAL EC-CELL NET

Left: In a well-fixed specimen, the tumor cells are evenly spaced, with round or ovoid nuclei and stippled chromatin.
Right: In a poorly fixed specimen, the tumor cells appear to have nuclear atypia, crowding, and clumped chromatin.

is 88 months, with median survival of 115 months, 107 months, and 65 months among patients with localized, regional, and metastatic disease, respectively (68).

Patients with localized or locally advanced jejunoileal NETs typically undergo surgical resection, consisting of either right hemicolectomy or partial small bowel resection. The majority (72 percent) of resected tumors involve locoregional lymph nodes. The long-term recurrence rate in this group of patients is approximately 50 percent and metastasis can occur many years after surgical resection (93,94).

NEUROENDOCRINE TUMORS OF THE APPENDIX

The first description of what may have been an appendiceal carcinoid was by Glazebrook in 1895 (95). He noted that during an autopsy a primary appendiceal tumor ("the size and shape of a pigeon's egg") was incidentally discovered in the appendiceal wall. A microscopic examination of the tumor, even in view of the unavailability of specific stains, is clearly consistent with features of a well-differentiated NET (carcinoid).

NETs of the appendix constitute approximately 5 percent of GI NETs, and they are the most common appendiceal neoplasm (96). While ubiquitous, these tumors are often overlooked and can present management difficulties because their metastatic potential, although extremely low, is difficult to predict. In particular, problems arise when NETs are diagnosed serendipitously at laparoscopy or unexpectedly identified in appendectomy specimens.

Epidemiology and Clinical Presentation

Surveillance Epidemiology and End Results (SEER) databases in the United States set the incidence of NETs of the appendix in the general population at 0.1 to 0.2/100,000 per year, a figure stable over the last 30 years, with a slight female predominance and a median age of 47

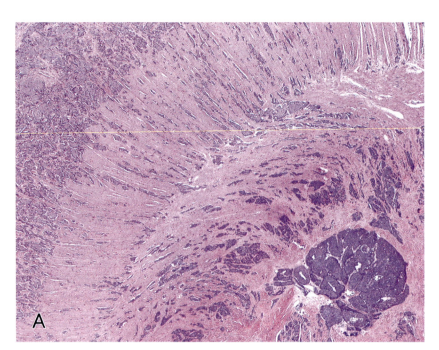

Figure 7-19

JEJUNOILEAL EC-CELL NEUROENDOCRINE TUMOR

A: This ileal NET shows diffuse infiltration into the muscularis propria, with associated subserosal and mesenteric fibrosis.

B,C: The stroma of these tumors can be richly vascularized (B) or densely fibrotic (C).

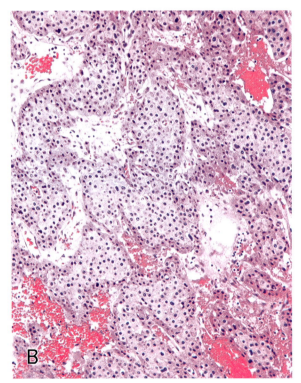

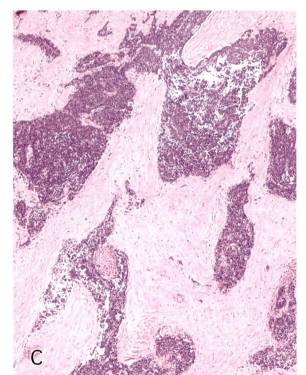

years (68,97). In surgical case series, NETs are encountered in fewer than 0.5 percent of all appendectomy specimens (98,99).

Almost all typical appendiceal NETs are clinically "silent" and are discovered incidentally during surgery performed for symptoms of acute appendicitis or during opportunistic appendectomy in the course of other abdominal surgical procedures. The diagnosis is usually made at laparotomy or laparoscopy, although abdominal ultrasound may occasionally establish a preoperative diagnosis (100).

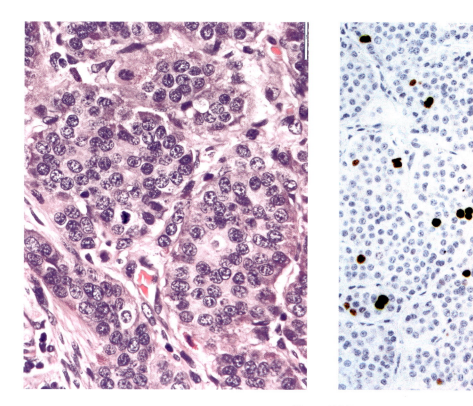

Figure 7-20

JEJUNOILEAL EC-CELL NET

Left: Rare mitotic figures are identified in this tumor and the estimated mitotic count is 1 per10 high-power fields (World Health Organization [WHO] G1/grade 1).

Right: The 4 percent Ki-67 proliferative index, however, places this tumor in WHO G2/grade 2 category.

Pathologic Features

Most typical appendiceal NETs (70 to 80 percent) occur at the tip of the organ (fig. 7-21). They are usually small, measuring less than 1 cm, rarely more than 2 cm, in diameter. Macroscopically, they appear as well-demarcated, firm, gray or yellow intramural nodules that may cause narrowing or complete obliteration of the lumen. They may also exhibit a diffuse growth pattern involving the longitudinal appendiceal wall. Tumors originating in the proximal portion of the appendix (7 to 8 percent) can present as acute appendicitis secondary to obstruction or may rarely be identified at colonoscopy (101).

Typical NETs of the appendix exhibit two to three microscopic patterns that are histogenetically associated with their neuroendocrine cell lineage and peptide amine production (102). The more common type is the serotonin-ex-pressing EC-cell tumor (103), which is generally indistinguishable histologically from the counterpart that occurs in the jejunoileum. There is a classic insular growth pattern with solid nests of uniform polygonal cells and stippled chromatin, situated in the deep lamina propria (fig. 7-22). This corresponds to the location of a population of endocrine cells that are present in the appendiceal lamina propria, separate from the surface epithelium (104). The tumor cells may be arranged in an acinar pattern with a rosette appearance. The cytoplasmic secretory granules of EC tumors, often enriched in the cells lining the periphery of the tumor nests (fig. 7-22, left), are argentaffin reactive and immunoreactive to both serotonin and substance P. Some tumors have no mucosal component and are encountered entirely within the submucosa or muscularis propria. Unique to the appendix, the nests of tumor cells are partly surrounded by S-100 protein-reactive spindle cells, presumably

283

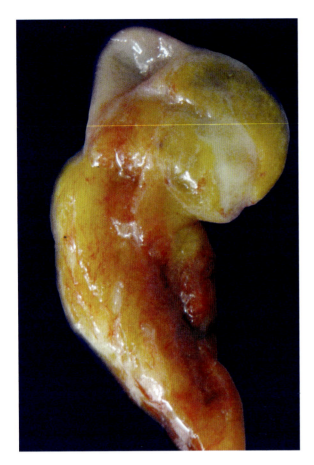
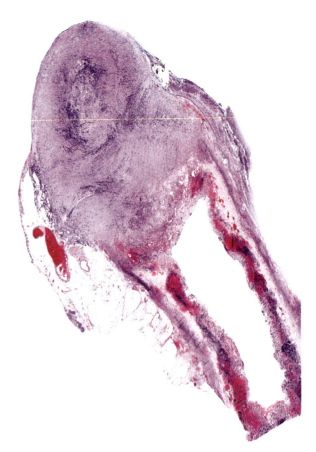

Figure 7-21

APPENDICEAL NET

Left: The NET is located at the tip of the appendix.
Right: The corresponding whole mount photograph shows the histopathologic appearance.

schwannian in nature, a phenomenon described by Masson over 80 years ago (105).

The second type is the less common L-cell NET, which produces glucagon-like peptides (enteroglucagons) and peptide YY. These tumors are even smaller than appendiceal EC-cell tumors. They are argyrophil positive but nonargentaffin reactive (106). Microscopically, these tumors are similar to the L-cell tumors of the rectum, with short trabecular and small ribbon-like architecture. The tumor cells are separated by abundant collagen-rich stroma and located in the muscularis propria of the appendix. When they exhibit a tubular growth pattern (tubular carcinoid), mainly in young women (fig. 7-22, right), they must be distinguished from goblet cell carcinoid tumor (see chapter 5) and adenocarcinoma, since the latter

two pathologic entities require a significantly different intervention from that required for typical carcinoid tumors.

Both types of NETs usually exhibit a low proliferative index; in fact, mitotic figures are not identifiable in many examples, and a count of less than 2 per 10 high-power microscopic fields is common. Necrosis is also almost never present. The concept of an atypical NET with a higher mitotic rate (2 to 20 per 10 high-power fields) and necrosis, as has been proposed for the lung and other sites in the GI tract, is not well accepted in the appendix due to the lack of reliable clinical data (107). Immunohistochemically, NETs of the appendix express general endocrine markers such as chromogranin and synaptophysin, in addition to the peptides and bioamines mentioned above.

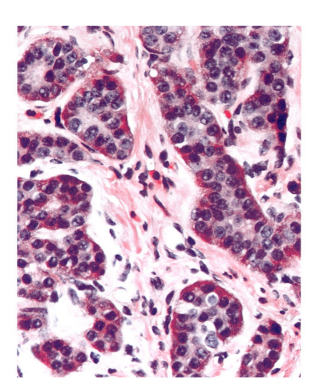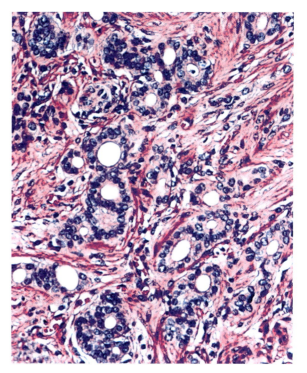

Figure 7-22

APPENDICEAL NET

Left: An EC-cell NET exhibits an insular growth pattern.
Right: Tumor cells with eosinophilic granules are present at the periphery of the tumor nests.

Treatment and Prognosis

Regardless of their histologic pattern, metastases from typical appendiceal NETs are rare. Given their smaller size, tubular carcinoid tumors almost never metastasize. The overall prognosis of patients with typical appendiceal NET is favorable, with a 10-year disease-specific survival rate of nearly 100 percent with localized disease (97). When rare metastases occur (1 to 2 percent of EC-cell tumors), they usually involve regional lymph nodes (108). Distant metastasis is even less common, and individuals with hepatic metastases may present with carcinoid syndrome due to circulation of bioactive serotonin and other peptide-amines produced by the EC-cell tumor (109,110). In addition to the stage of the tumor, adverse prognostic features include onset at an age older than the median of 34 years and mesoappendix involvement (97,111). Tumor grade between WHO G1 and G2 does not impact on survival.

Treatment recommendations subsequent to appendectomy are controversial: collective considerations include tumor size, tumor grade, resection margin status, lymphovascular invasion, depth of tumor invasion, and complications of a perforation in acute appendicitis (112–115). Since the rate of metastasis is less than 1 percent for neoplasms between 1 and 2 cm, appendectomy alone is adequate treatment for most typical appendiceal carcinoid tumors that are under 2 cm, with a negative resection margin and without evidence of perforation or transmural invasion. Conversely, a right hemicolectomy should be considered in patients with tumors over 2 cm in diameter, tumors extending to the mesoappendix, and those with a positive resection margin, associated perforation, or evidence of locoregional lymph node metastasis.

Since most typical appendiceal carcinoid tumors exhibit minimal cytologic atypia and negligible mitotic activity, the mitotic count may vary only marginally in many high-power fields. It is thus not practical to use mitotic activity alone for treatment decisions unless it is brisk, and this occurs rarely. Similarly, a Ki-67 labeling index of 1 to 5 percent is unlikely to separate tumors with metastatic potential from those with a benign clinical course. Thus, typical appendiceal NETs confer the best prognosis among all types of NETs, and this essentially benign course reflects the anatomic site, early detection and removal, and the biology of the tumor itself.

NEUROENDOCRINE TUMORS OF THE COLORECTUM

Neuroendocrine tumors of colorectum are classified by their primary sites: colon and rectum. They differ in histogenesis, ethnic prevalence, and natural clinical history.

Epidemiology and Clinical Presentation

Colonic NETs are rare and the age-adjusted annual incidence is 0.36 per 100,000 to the 2000 US standard population in SEER databases. About half of the lesions are noted in the cecum, which raises the possibility that some cases in these databases may have included NETs from the terminal ileum or the appendix that extended to the cecum (68,116). Thus the true incidence of colonic NETs is likely much less than reported. Many of these tumors have EC-cell differentiation and produce serotonin. Nonappendiceal and nonileal primary colonic NETs predilect to Caucasians. The onset age, pattern of disease spread, and survival rates are comparable with those of jejunoileal primary NETs. The similar clinical and pathologic characteristics of NETs of the distal small intestine and the proximal and mid-colon likely represent their shared embryologic lineage. The EC-cell type will not be further discussed in this section (refer to the section of NETs of jejunoileum above).

Most rectal NETs differentiate along the lines of the L-cell subtype of neuroendocrine cells, which produces enteroglucagon and pancreatic polypeptide-related hormones. The incidence of rectal NETs is the highest among GI NETs, with an age-adjusted annual incidence of 0.86 per 100,000 per year to the 2000 US standard population (68,84). Rectal NETs occur at a markedly higher frequency among Asian-Pacific Island (41 percent), American Indian/Alaskan Native (32 percent), and African-American (26

percent) patients than among white (12 percent) patients. The increasing incidence of rectal NETs is associated with frequent endoscopic surveillance in recent years. The median age of initial diagnosis of rectal NET is 56 years and there is no significant male/female prevalence.

Most rectal NETs are small (under 1 cm) and are identified incidentally on routine colonoscopy, thus these patients are usually asymptomatic. Larger lesions may cause mucosal ulceration, rectal bleeding, and stenosis. Functional NETs derived from L cells are extremely rare, although carcinoid syndrome can occur in patients with colorectal NETs of EC-cell origin.

Pathologic Features

On gross examination, colorectal L-cell NETs are located between 4 and 20 cm above the dentate line on the anterior or lateral rectal wall. Small tumors form firm nodules or polypoid lesions in the submucosa, without involvement of the surface mucosa (fig. 7-23, left). Larger tumors may circumferentially involve the colorectum, mimicking the appearance of conventional colorectal adenocarcinoma (fig. 7-23, right). On cut section, the tumor is centered in the lamina propria and submucosa (fig. 7-24).

Colorectal NETs exhibit typical L-cell tumor features with a trabecular growth pattern, but the tumor cells may be arranged in small acini, tubules, or glands (fig. 7-25). The tumor trabeculae may anastomose with each other, resulting in a gyriform or a cribriform pattern (fig. 7-26A), or they may not have a specific pattern but present as individual columnar or cuboidal trabeculae/cores (fig. 7-26C,D). The tumor stroma is either richly vascularized with erythrocytes within the vascular channels (fig. 7-25) or has prominent hyalinization/fibrosis (fig. 7-26D). The tumor cells have round to ovoid homogeneous nuclei with stippled chromatin and moderate amounts of granular cytoplasm.

Most colorectal NETs are low grade (WHO G1/G2). The presence of tumor necrosis, usually in a punctate pattern, increased mitotic activity and Ki-67 proliferative index, and lymphovascular invasion are associated with unfavorable clinical outcome, and these features should be mentioned in the pathology report.

Unlike in EC-cell NETs, chromogranin A immunoreactivity may vary in L-cell NETs of the

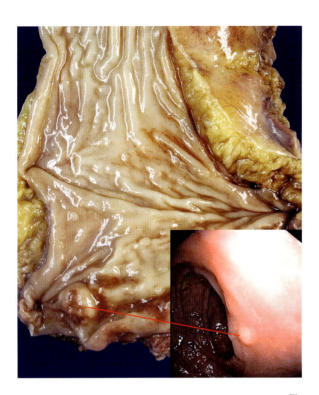
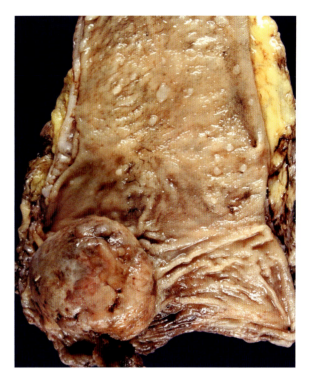

Figure 7-23

RECTAL NET

Left: This rectal NET was identified on colonoscopy as a submucosa nodule without involvement of the surface mucosa; the surgically removed tumor was located in the distal rectum.

Right: A large rectal NET shows surface erosion and exhibits the gross features of an adenocarcinoma.

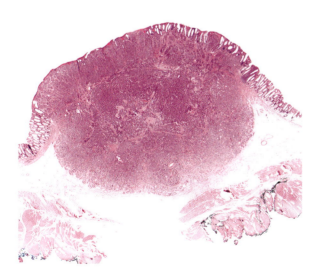

Figure 7-24

RECTAL NET

This small rectal NET undermining rectal mucosa was completely removed by local excision.

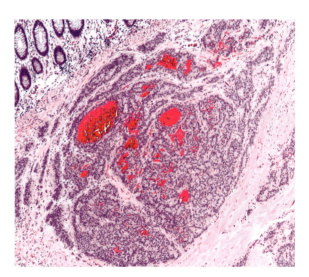

Figure 7-25

RECTAL NET

The tumor is composed of loosely cohesive nests, with tumor cells arranged in anastomosing trabeculae and acini. Rich vascularization is highlighted by congested small vessels stuffed with erythrocytes.

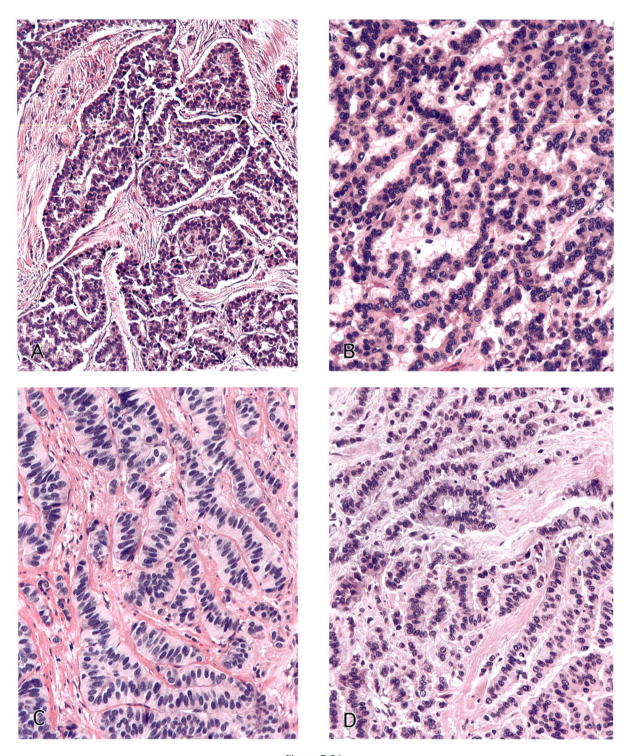

Figure 7-26

RECTAL NET: HISTOLOGIC PATTERNS

A: Tumor trabeculae are arranged within irregular nests with a gyriform appearance.
B: Cuboidal tumor cells are loosely dispersed in a lacy pattern.
C: Tall columnar tumor cells are arranged in a trabecular pattern.
D: Cuboidal tumor trabeculae are separated by fibrotic stroma.

colorectum, and they are usually more immunoreactive to synaptophysin. They also co-express a range of enteroglucagons and glicentin-related hormones including glucagon, pancreatic polypeptide (PP), and peptide YY, although these markers are rarely used as a diagnostic modality in primary tumors. More than 80 percent of colorectal NETs are also immunoreactive for prostatic acid phosphatase; thus in cases with concerning features for prostatic adenocarcinoma, additional more specific prostatic markers (prostatic specific antigen [PSA], prostate-specific membrane antigen [PSMA], and NKX3-1) should be evaluated by immunohistochemistry (see chapter 10).

Treatment and Prognosis

Most patients (92 percent) with rectal NETs present with localized disease, 4 percent have locally advanced disease, and 5 percent have distant metastasis; the corresponding 5-year survival rates are 90 percent, 62 percent, and 24 percent, respectively (68,117). The majority of the tumors are smaller than 1 cm (79 percent) and about 2 percent metastasize. Thus small rectal NETs that are confined within the mucosa and submucosa and without adverse pathologic features can be managed by local endoscopic resection (118,119).

The metastatic potential of rectal NETs increases as the tumors grow, particularly for those larger than 2 cm (117,120). The presence of atypical pathologic features such as tumor invasion into and through the muscularis propria, lymphovascular invasion, necrosis, and increased proliferative activity warrants consideration of anterior resection or abdominal peritoneal excision.

REFERENCES

1. Herderhain R. Untersuchungen uber den Bau der Labdrusen. Arch fur Mikrosk Anat. 1870(6):368-406.
2. Kulchitzky N. Zur Frage uber den Bau des Darmcanals. Arch fur Mikrosk Anat. 1897(49):7-35.
3. Fontaine J, Le Douarin NM. Analysis of endoderm formation in the avian blastoderm by the use of quail-chick chimaeras. The problem of the neurectodermal origin of the cells of the APUD series. J Embryol Exp Morphol 1977;41:209-222.
4. Falkmer S. Phylogeny and ontogeny of the neuroendocrine cells of the gastrointestinal tract. Endocrinol Metab Clin North Am 1993;22:731-752.
5. Molavi D, Argani P. Distinguishing benign dissecting mucin (stromal mucin pools) from invasive mucinous carcinoma. Adv Anat Pathol 2008;15:1-17.
6. Feyrter F. Uber diffuse endokrine epitheliale Organe. Barth Leipzig; 1938.
7. Masson P. La glande endocrine de l'intestin chez l'homme. C R Acad Sci Paris 1914(158):52-61.
8. Gosset AM. Tumeurs endocrines de l'appendice Presse Med 1914(25):237-238.
9. Pearse AG. The diffuse endocrine system and the implications of the APUD concept. Int Surg 1979;64:5-7.
10. Ciaccio C. Ricerche istologiche e citologiche sul timo degli Uccelli. Anat Anz. 1906(29):597-600.
11. Kull H. Die chromaffinen Zellen des Verdauungstraktes. Z Mikrosk Anat Forsch. 1925;2:163-200.
12. Pearse AG, Coulling I, Weavers B, Friesen S. The endocrine polypeptide cells of the human stomach, duodenum, and jejunum. Gut 1970;11:649-658.
13. Polak JM, Bloom SR, Kuzio M, Brown JC, Pearse AG. Cellular localization of gastric inhibitory polypeptide in the duodenum and jejunum. Gut 1973;14:284-288.
14. Bencosme SA, Lechago J. Staining procedures for the endocrine cells of the upper gastrointestinal mucosa: light-electron microscopic correlation for the gastrin-producing cell. J Clin Pathol 1973;26:427-434.
15. Buffa R, Polak JM, Pearse AG, Solcia E, Grimelius L, Capella C. Identification of the intestinal cell storing gastric inhibitory peptide. Histochemistry 1975;43:249-255.

16. Buchan AM, Polak JM, Capella C, Solcia E, Pearse AG. Electronimmunocytochemical evidence for the K cell localization of gastric inhibitory polypeptide (GIP) in man. Histochemistry 1978;56:37-44.

17. Solcia E, Capella C, Buffa R, et al. The diffuse endocrine-paracrine system of the gut in health and disease: ultrastructural features. Scand J Gastroenterol Suppl 1981;70:25-36.

18. Yamada J, Campos VJ, Kitamura N, Pacheco AC, Yamashita T, Yanaihara N. An immunohistochemical study of the endocrine cells in the gastrointestinal mucosa of the Caiman latirostris. Arch Histol Jpn 1987;50:229-241.

19. Rindi G, Necchi V, Savio A, et al. Characterisation of gastric ghrelin cells in man and other mammals: studies in adult and fetal tissues. Histochem Cell Biol 2002;117:511-519.

20. Solcia E, Vanoli A. Histogenesis and natural history of gut neuroendocrine tumors: present status. Endocr Pathol 2014;25:165-170.

21. Obendorfer S. Karzinoide Tumoren des Dunndarms. Frankf Z fur Pathol 1907(1):426-429.

22. Kloppel G, Anlauf M. Gastrinoma—morphological aspects. Wien Klin Wochenschr 2007;119:579-584.

23. Williams ED, Sandler M. The classification of carcinoid tumours. Lancet 1963;1:238-239.

24. Szijj I, Csapo Z, Laszlo FA, Kovacs K. Medullary cancer of the thyroid gland associated with hypercorticism. Cancer 1969;24:167-173.

25. Capella C, Heitz PU, Hofler H, Solcia E, Kloppel G. Revised classification of neuroendocrine tumours of the lung, pancreas and gut. Virchows Arch 1995;425:547-560.

26. Solcia EK, ??G. Sobin LH. Histological typing of endocrine tumours. Berlin, Heidelberg, New York Springer Verlag; 2000.

27. Bosman FT, Carneiro F, Hruban RH, Theise, N.D. WHO Classification of tumours of the digestive system. World Health Organization 2010.

28. Tang LH, Untch BR, Reidy DL, et al. Well-differentiated neuroendocrine tumors with a morphologically apparent high-grade component: a pathway distinct from poorly differentiated neuroendocrine carcinomas. Clin Cancer Res 2016;22:1011-1017.

29. Tang LH, Basturk O, Sue JJ, Klimstra DS. A practical approach to the classification of WHO grade 3 (G3) well-differentiated neuroendocrine tumor (WD-NET) and poorly differentiated neuroendocrine carcinoma (PD-NEC) of the pancreas. Am J Surg Pathol 2016;40:1192-1202.

30. Modlin IM, Moss SF, Oberg K, et al. Gastrointestinal neuroendocrine (carcinoid) tumours: current diagnosis and management. Med J Aust 2010;193:46-52.

31. Sherman SK, Maxwell JE, O'Dorisio MS, O'Dorisio TM, Howe JR. Pancreastatin predicts survival in neuroendocrine tumors. Ann Surg Oncol 2014;21:2971-2980.

32. Oberg K, Modlin IM, De Herder W, et al. Consensus on biomarkers for neuroendocrine tumour disease. Lancet Oncol 2015;16:e435-446.

33. Sadowski SM, Neychev V, Millo C, et al. Prospective study of 68Ga-DOTATATE positron emission tomography/computed tomography for detecting gastro-entero-pancreatic neuroendocrine tumors and unknown primary sites. J Clin Oncol 2016;34:588-596.

34. Yoshikane H, Tsukamoto Y, Niwa Y, et al. Carcinoid tumors of the gastrointestinal tract: evaluation with endoscopic ultrasonography. Gastrointest Endosc 1993;39:375-383.

35. Shroff SR, Kushnir VM, Wani SB, et al. Efficacy of endoscopic mucosal resection for management of small duodenal neuroendocrine tumors. Surg Laparosc Endosc Percutan Tech 2015;25:e134-139.

36. Rindi G, Kloppel G, Alhman H, et al. TNM staging of foregut (neuro)endocrine tumors: a consensus proposal including a grading system. Virchows Arch 2006;449:395-401.

37. Rindi G, Kloppel G, Couvelard A, et al. TNM staging of midgut and hindgut (neuro) endocrine tumors: a consensus proposal including a grading system. Virchows Arch 2007;451:757-762.

38. Kattan MW, Hess KR, Amin MB, et al. American Joint Committee on Cancer acceptance criteria for inclusion of risk models for individualized prognosis in the practice of precision medicine. CA Cancer J Clin 2016;66:370-374.

39. Minnetti M, Grossman A. Somatic and germline mutations in NETs: implications for their diagnosis and management. Best Pract Res Clin Endocrinol Metab 2016;30:115-127.

40. Crona J, Skogseid B. GEP- NETS UPDATE: Genetics of neuroendocrine tumors. Eur J Endocrinol 2016;174:R275-290.

41. Goudet P, Bonithon-Kopp C, Murat A, et al. Gender-related differences in MEN1 lesion occurrence and diagnosis: a cohort study of 734 cases from the Groupe d'etude des Tumeurs Endocrines. Eur J Endocrinol 2011;165:97-105.

42. Anlauf M, Perren A, Meyer CL, et al. Precursor lesions in patients with multiple endocrine neoplasia type 1-associated duodenal gastrinomas. Gastroenterology 2005;128:1187-1198.

43. Griffiths DF, Jasani B, Newman GR, Williams ED, Williams GT. Glandular duodenal carcinoid—a somatostatin rich tumour with neuroendocrine associations. J Clin Pathol 1984;37:163-169.

44. Griffiths DF, Williams GT, Williams ED. Duodenal carcinoid tumours, phaeochromocytoma and neurofibromatosis: islet cell tumour, phaeochro-

mocytoma and the von Hippel-Lindau complex: two distinctive neuroendocrine syndromes. Q J Med 1987;64:769-782.

45. Cunningham JL, Diaz de Stahl T, Sjoblom T, Westin G, Dumanski JP, Janson ET. Common pathogenetic mechanism involving human chromosome 18 in familial and sporadic ileal carcinoid tumors. Genes Chromosomes Cancer 2011;50:82-94.

46. Neklason DW, VanDerslice J, Curtin K, Cannon-Albright LA. Evidence for a heritable contribution to neuroendocrine tumors of the small intestine. Endocr Relat Cancer 2016;23:93-100.

47. Francis JM, Kiezun A, Ramos AH, et al. Somatic mutation of CDKN1B in small intestine neuroendocrine tumors. Nat Genet 2013;45:1483-1486.

48. Banck MS, Kanwar R, Kulkarni AA, et al. The genomic landscape of small intestine neuroendocrine tumors. J Clin Invest 2013;123:2502-2508.

49. Crona J, Gustavsson T, Norlen O, et al. Somatic mutations and genetic heterogeneity at the CDKN1B locus in small intestinal neuroendocrine tumors. Ann Surg Oncol 2015;22(Suppl 3):S1428-1435.

50. Banck MS, Beutler AS. Advances in small bowel neuroendocrine neoplasia. Curr Opin Gastroenterol 2014;30:163-167.

51. Anthony LB, Strosberg JR, Klimstra DS, et al. The NANETS consensus guidelines for the diagnosis and management of gastrointestinal neuroendocrine tumors (nets): well-differentiated nets of the distal colon and rectum. Pancreas 2010;39:767-774.

52. Boudreaux JP, Klimstra DS, Hassan MM, et al. The NANETS consensus guideline for the diagnosis and management of neuroendocrine tumors: well-differentiated neuroendocrine tumors of the jejunum, ileum, appendix, and cecum. Pancreas 2010;39:753-766.

53. Pavel M, Sers C. Women In Cancer Thematic Review: Systemic therapies in neuroendocrine tumors and novel approaches towards personalised medicine. Endocr Relat Cancer 2016;23:T135-T154.

54. O'Toole D, Kianmanesh R, Caplin M. ENETS 2016 consensus guidelines for the management of patients with digestive neuroendocrine tumors: an update. Neuroendocrinology 2016;103:117-118.

55. Eriksson J, Stalberg P, Nilsson A, et al. Surgery and radiofrequency ablation for treatment of liver metastases from midgut and foregut carcinoids and endocrine pancreatic tumors. World J Surg 2008;32:930-938.

56. Frilling A, Modlin IM, Kidd M, et al. Recommendations for management of patients with neuroendocrine liver metastases. Lancet Oncol 2014;15:e8-21.

57. Steinmuller T, Kianmanesh R, Falconi M, et al. Consensus guidelines for the management of patients with liver metastases from digestive (neuro)endocrine tumors: foregut, midgut, hindgut, and unknown primary. Neuroendocrinology 2008;87:47-62.

58. Kennedy A, Bester L, Salem R, Sharma RA, Parks RW, Ruszniewski P. Role of hepatic intra-arterial therapies in metastatic neuroendocrine tumours (NET): guidelines from the NET-Liver-Metastases Consensus Conference. HPB (Oxford) 2015;17:29-37.

59. Kvols LK, Oberg KE, O'Dorisio TM, et al. Pasireotide (SOM230) shows efficacy and tolerability in the treatment of patients with advanced neuroendocrine tumors refractory or resistant to octreotide LAR: results from a phase II study. Endocr Relat Cancer 2012;19:657-666.

60. Rinke A, Wittenberg M, Schade-Brittinger C, et al. Placebo-controlled, double-blind, prospective, randomized study on the effect of octreotide LAR in the control of tumor growth in patients with metastatic neuroendocrine midgut tumors (PROMID): results of long-term survival. Neuroendocrinology 2017;104:26-32.

61. Caplin ME, Pavel M, Cwikla JB, et al. Lanreotide in metastatic enteropancreatic neuroendocrine tumors. N Engl J Med 2014;371:224-233.

62. Laskaratos FM, Walker M, Naik K, et al. Predictive factors of antiproliferative activity of octreotide LAR as first-line therapy for advanced neuroendocrine tumours. Br J Cancer 2016;115:1321-1327.

63. Pokuri VK, Fong MK, Iyer R. Octreotide and Lanreotide in Gastroenteropancreatic Neuroendocrine Tumors. Curr Oncol Rep 2016;18:7.

64. Kulke MH, O'Dorisio T, Phan A, et al. Telotristat etiprate, a novel serotonin synthesis inhibitor, in patients with carcinoid syndrome and diarrhea not adequately controlled by octreotide. Endocr Relat Cancer 2014;21:705-714.

65. Chan J, Kulke M. Targeting the mTOR signaling pathway in neuroendocrine tumors. Curr Treat Options Oncol 2014;15:365-379.

66. Oberg K. Neuroendocrine tumors of the digestive tract: impact of new classifications and new agents on therapeutic approaches. Curr Opin Oncol 2012;24:433-440.

67. Kwekkeboom DJ, Krenning EP, Lebtahi R, et al. ENETS consensus guidelines for the Standards of Care in Neuroendocrine Tumors: peptide receptor radionuclide therapy with radiolabeled somatostatin analogs. Neuroendocrinology 2009;90:220-226.

68. Yao JC, Hassan M, Phan A, et al. One hundred years after "carcinoid": epidemiology of and prognostic factors for neuroendocrine tumors in 35,825 cases in the United States. J Clin Oncol 2008;26:3063-3072.

69. Hoffmann KM, Furukawa M, Jensen RT. Duodenal neuroendocrine tumors: classification, functional syndromes, diagnosis and medical treatment. Best Pract Res Clin Gastroenterol 2005;19:675-697.

70. Rosentraeger MJ, Garbrecht N, Anlauf M, et al. Syndromic versus non-syndromic sporadic gastrin-producing neuroendocrine tumors of the duodenum: comparison of pathological features and biological behavior. Virchows Arch 2016;468:277-287.

71. Zollinger RM, Ellison EH. Primary peptic ulcerations of the jejunum associated with islet cell tumors of the pancreas. Ann Surg 1955;142:709-723; discussion, 724-708.

72. Edkins JS. On the chemical mechanism of gastric secretion. Proc R Soc Lond 1905;76:376.

73. Gregory RA, Grossman MI, Tracy HJ, Bentley PH. Nature of the gastric secretagogue in Zollinger-Ellison tumours. Lancet 1967;2:543-544.

74. Anlauf M, Garbrecht N, Henopp T, et al. Sporadic versus hereditary gastrinomas of the duodenum and pancreas: distinct clinico-pathological and epidemiological features. World J Gastroenterol 2006;12:5440-5446.

75. Garbrecht N, Anlauf M, Schmitt A, et al. Somatostatin-producing neuroendocrine tumors of the duodenum and pancreas: incidence, types, biological behavior, association with inherited syndromes, and functional activity. Endocr Relat Cancer 2008;15:229-241.

75a. Albores-Saavedra J, Henson DE, Klimstra DS. Tumors of the gallbladder, extrahepatic bile ducts, and vaterian system. AFIP Atlas of Tumor Pathology, 4th Series, Fascicle 23. Washington, DC: 2015:441-461.

76. Burke AP, Sobin LH, Federspiel BH, Shekitka KM. Appendiceal carcinoids: correlation of histology and immunohistochemistry. Mod Pathol 1989;2:630-637.

77. Sanchez-Sosa S, Angeles Angeles A, Orozco H, Larriva-Sahd J. Neuroendocrine carcinoma of the ampulla of vater. A case of absence of somatostatin in a vasoactive intestinal polypeptide-, bombesin-, and cholecystokinin-producing tumor. Am J Clin Pathol 1991;95:51-54.

78. Imamura M, Kanda M, Takahashi K, et al. Clinicopathological characteristics of duodenal microgastrinomas. W J Surg 1992;16:703-709; discussion 709-710.

79. Anlauf M, Enosawa T, Henopp T, et al. Primary lymph node gastrinoma or occult duodenal microgastrinoma with lymph node metastases in a MEN1 patient: the need for a systematic search for the primary tumor. Am J Surg Pathol 2008;32:1101-1105.

80. Harper S, Carroll RW, Frilling A, Wickremesekera SK, Bann S. Primary lymph node gastrinoma: 2 cases and a review of the literature. J Gastrointest Surg 2015;19:651-655.

81. Norton JA, Fraker DL, Alexander HR, et al. Surgery to cure the Zollinger-Ellison syndrome. N Engl J Med 1999;341:635-644.

82. Norton JA, Krampitz G, Jensen RT. Multiple endocrine neoplasia: genetics and clinical management. Surg Oncol Clin N Am 2015;24:795-832.

83. Untch BR, Bonner KP, Roggin KK, et al. Pathologic grade and tumor size are associated with recurrence-free survival in patients with duodenal neuroendocrine tumors. J Gastrointest Surg 2014;18:457-462; discussion 462-453.

84. Lawrence B, Gustafsson BI, Chan A, Svejda B, Kidd M, Modlin IM. The epidemiology of gastroenteropancreatic neuroendocrine tumors. Endocrinol Metab Clin North Am 2011;40:1-18, vii.

85. Druce M, Rockall A, Grossman AB. Fibrosis and carcinoid syndrome: from causation to future therapy. Nat Rev Endocrinol 2009;5:276-283.

86. Luis SA, Pellikka PA. Carcinoid heart disease: Diagnosis and management. Best Pract Res Clin Endocrinol Metab 2016;30:149-158.

87. Kvols LK, Martin JK, Marsh HM, Moertel CG. Rapid reversal of carcinoid crisis with a somatostatin analogue. N Engl J Med 1985;313:1229-1230.

88. Burke AP, Thomas RM, Elsayed AM, Sobin LH. Carcinoids of the jejunum and ileum: an immunohistochemical and clinicopathologic study of 167 cases. Cancer 1997;79:1086-1093.

89. Yantiss RK, Odze RD, Farraye FA, Rosenberg AE. Solitary versus multiple carcinoid tumors of the ileum: a clinical and pathologic review of 68 cases. Am J Surg Pathol 2003;27:811-817.

90. Modlin IM, Shapiro MD, Kidd M. Carcinoid tumors and fibrosis: an association with no explanation. Am J Gastroenterol 2004;99:2466-2478.

91. Caracappa D, Gulla N, Lombardo F, et al. Incidental finding of carcinoid tumor on Meckel's diverticulum: case report and literature review, should prophylactic resection be recommended? World J Surg Oncol 2014;12:144.

92. Hata H, Hiraoka N, Ojima H, Shimada K, Kosuge T, Shimoda T. Carcinoid tumor arising in a duplication cyst of the duodenum. Pathol Int 2006;56:272-278.

93. Le Roux C, Lombard-Bohas C, Delmas C, et al. Relapse factors for ileal neuroendocrine tumours after curative surgery: a retrospective French multicentre study. Dig Liver Dis 2011;43:828-833.

94. Dieckhoff P, Runkel H, Daniel H, et al. Well-differentiated neuroendocrine neoplasia: relapse-free survival and predictors of recurrence after curative intended resections. Digestion 2014;90:89-97.

95. L G. Case of endothelial sarcomata of vermiform appendix Virg Med Month. 1895;xxii:211.

96. Modlin IM, Kidd M, Latich I, Zikusoka MN, Shapiro MD. Current status of gastrointestinal carcinoids. Gastroenterology 2005;128:1717-1751.

97. Volante M, Daniele L, Asioli S, et al. Tumor staging but not grading is associated with adverse clinical outcome in neuroendocrine tumors of the appendix: a retrospective clinical pathologic analysis of 138 cases. Am J Surg Pathol 2013;37:606-612.

98. Marudanayagam R, Williams GT, Rees BI. Review of the pathological results of 2660 appendicectomy specimens. J Gastroenterol 2006;41:745-749.

99. Shapiro R, Eldar S, Sadot E, Papa MZ, Zippel DB. Appendiceal carcinoid at a large tertiary center: pathologic findings and long-term follow-up evaluation. Am J Surg 2011;201:805-808.

100. Connor SJ, Hanna GB, Frizelle FA. Appendiceal tumors: retrospective clinicopathologic analysis of appendiceal tumors from 7,970 appendectomies. Dis Colon Rectum 1998;41:75-80.

101. Carr NJ, Sobin LH. Neuroendocrine tumors of the appendix. Semin Diagn Pathol 2004;21:108-119.

102. Shaw PA. Carcinoid tumours of the appendix are different. J Pathol 1990;162:189-190.

103. Rode J, Dhillon AP, Papadaki L. Serotonin-immunoreactive cells in the lamina propria plexus of the appendix. Hum Pathol 1983;14:464-469.

104. Dhillon AP, Williams RA, Rode J. Age, site and distribution of subepithelial neurosecretory cells in the appendix. Pathology 1992;24:56-59.

105. Masson P. Carcinoids (argentaffin-cell tumors) and nerve hyperplasia of the appendicular mucosa. Am J Pathol 1928;4:181-212.119.

106. Iwafuchi M, Watanabe H, Ajioka Y, Shimoda T, Iwashita A, Ito S. Immunohistochemical and ultrastructural studies of twelve argentaffin and six argyrophil carcinoids of the appendix vermiformis. Hum Pathol 1990;21:773-780.

107. Edge S, Byrd D, Compton C, Fritz A, Greene FL, Trotti A. AJCC cancer staging manual, 7th ed. New York: Springer; 2010:133-141.

108. Pape UF, Perren A, Niederle B, et al. ENETS Consensus Guidelines for the management of patients with neuroendocrine neoplasms from the jejuno-ileum and the appendix including goblet cell carcinomas. Neuroendocrinology 2012;95:135-156.

109. Jann H, Roll S, Couvelard A, et al. Neuroendocrine tumors of midgut and hindgut origin: tumor-node-metastasis classification determines clinical outcome. Cancer 2011;117:3332-3341.

110. Alexandraki KI, Griniatsos J, Bramis KI, et al. Clinical value of right hemicolectomy for appendiceal carcinoids using pathologic criteria. J Endocrinol Invest 2011;34:255-259.

111. Syracuse DC, Perzin KH, Price JB, Wiedel PD, Mesa-Tejada R. Carcinoid tumors of the appendix. Mesoappendiceal extension and nodal metastases. Ann Surg 1979;190:58-63.

112. Safioleas MC, Moulakakis KG, Kontzoglou K, et al. Carcinoid tumors of the appendix. Prognostic factors and evaluation of indications for right hemicolectomy. Hepatogastroenterology 2005;52:123-127.

113. Rouanet P, Saingra B, Simony-Lafontaine J, Pujol H. Prognostic factors of carcinoid tumor of the appendix smaller than two centimeters. Surgery 1993;113:595.

114. Rothmund M, Kisker O. Surgical treatment of carcinoid tumors of the small bowel, appendix, colon and rectum. Digestion 1994;55(Suppl 3):86-91.

115. Stinner B, Kisker O, Zielke A, Rothmund M. Surgical management for carcinoid tumors of small bowel, appendix, colon, and rectum. World J Surg 1996;20:183-188.

116. Modlin IM, Lye KD, Kidd M. A 5-decade analysis of 13,715 carcinoid tumors. Cancer 2003;97:934-959.

117. McDermott FD, Heeney A, Courtney D, Mohan H, Winter D. Rectal carcinoids: a systematic review. Surg Endosc 2014;28:2020-2026.

118. Kaneko H, Hirasawa K, Koh R, et al. Treatment outcomes of endoscopic resection for rectal carcinoid tumors: an analysis of the resectability and long-term results from 46 consecutive cases. Scand J Gastroenterol 2016;51:1489-1494.

119. McConnell YJ. Surgical management of rectal carcinoids: trends and outcomes from the Surveillance, Epidemiology, and End Results database (1988 to 2012). Am J Surg 2016;211:877-885.

120. Fahy BN, Tang LH, Klimstra D, et al. Carcinoid of the rectum risk stratification (CaRRS): a strategy for preoperative outcome assessment. Ann Surg Oncol 2007;14:396-404.

8 MESENCHYMAL TUMORS OF THE INTESTINES

Mesenchymal tumors of the intestines can be approached by considering which types of lesions are likely to be encountered and in which layer they are prone to arise. Gastrointestinal stromal tumors (GISTs) are the most likely lesions and pathologists often make efforts to exclude GISTs before considering other entities. Most GISTs, however, arise in the stomach rather than the intestines, so other mesenchymal tumors are often encountered, particularly in the era of extensive screening colonoscopy in some populations. Many small mesenchymal lesions that present as polyps are truly incidental findings. A list of some of the mesenchymal lesions of the gastrointestinal (GI) tract and their most likely sites and depths appears in Table 8-1.

GASTROINTESTINAL STROMAL TUMORS

General Features. *Gastrointestinal stromal tumors* (GISTS) are the most common mesenchymal lesions throughout the GI tract with two exceptions: in both the esophagus and colon, leiomyomas outnumber GISTs (1). GIST differentiate along the lines of interstitial cells

Table 8-1

LOCATION OF MESENCHYMAL LESIONS IN THE GASTROINTESTINAL TRACT BY LAYER AND ANATOMIC SITE[a]

Lesion	Favored Site in Gastrointestinal Tract	Mucosa	Submucosa	Muscularis Propria	Mesentery
Benign epithelioid nerve sheath tumor	colon	x	x		
Sporadic ganglioneuroma	colon	x			
Schwann cell hamartoma	colon	x			
Benign fibroblastic polyp/perineurioma	colon	x			
Leiomyoma	colon	x (associated with muscularis mucosae)			
Inflammatory fibroid polyp	stomach (antrum); terminal ileum		x		
Synovial sarcoma	stomach	x	x	x	
Gangliocytic paraganglioma	small bowel (duodenum)	x	x		
Glomus tumor	stomach			x	
Plexiform fibromyxoma	stomach			x	
Gastrointestinal stromal tumor	stomach			x	
Gastrointestinal schwannoma	stomach			x	
Leiomyoma	esophagus			x	
Gastrointestinal clear cell sarcoma	small intestine (ileum)			x	
Ganglioneuromatosis	colon	x	x	x	x
Mesenteric fibromatosis	small intestine			x	x
Inflammatory myofibroblastic tumor				x	x
Sclerosing mesenteritis					x

[a]Modified from a table in Montgomery E, Voltaggio L. Biopsy interpretation of the gastrointestinal tract, 2nd ed. Philadelphia: Wolters Kluwer/Lippincott Williams & Wilkins; 2012.

of Cajal (2), and most examples have either a *KIT* (CD117, a receptor tyrosine kinase) or a *PDGFRA* (platelet-derived growth factor alpha) mutation. The discussion here will revolve primarily around *KIT*-mutated neoplasms since *PDGFRA*-mutated ones almost always affect the stomach (1). Some GISTs exhibit neither of these mutations, especially those found in children and associated with various genetic syndromes; these GISTs harbor different mutations that affect downstream signaling. With the exception of GISTs found in patients with neurofibromatosis type 1 (NF1), those that lack *KIT* and *PDGFRA* mutations usually affect the stomach.

The histologic appearance of the cells comprising GISTs varies from spindled to epithelioid. Evolving pharmacologic treatments, developed through the growing understanding of molecular pathogenesis (3), have become increasingly effective, underscoring the importance of accurate identification of GISTs.

GISTs (including all sites) usually arise in adults over the age 50 years (median, 55 to 60 years) and are rare in children (less than 1 percent) (4,5). There is no gender predilection, but there is a male predominance for malignant GISTs. The classic presentation is GI bleeding: both acute (melena or hematemesis) and occult (anemia) bleeding (4). Symptoms of obstruction may be the first sign of the tumor.

GISTs are encountered throughout the GI tract: about 60 percent in the stomach, 35 percent in the small intestine, and less than 5 percent in the rectum, esophagus, omentum, and mesentery; most GISTs found in the last site are metastatic rather than primary. About 5 percent of GISTs arise in patients with NF1 (multiple small intestinal tumors [6]) and Carney triad (paraganglioma, GIST, and pulmonary chondroma, usually in young females [7]). Familial GISTs arise in patients with inherited germline *KIT* or *PDGFRA* mutations. Most recently, succinate dehydrogenase-deficient GISTs have been described (8–22), but these are restricted to the stomach (including those described in Carney triad as well as in the Carney-Stratakis syndrome [paraganglioma and gastric stromal tumors] and are not further discussed here).

The types of GISTs with a proclivity for the small bowel include those associated with NF1 and those that have *BRAF* mutations (11). Several kindreds have been reported in which family members have germline mutations in *KIT* or *PDGFRA*. As summarized by Ricci (23), patients with germline *KIT* mutations present at an age about 10 years younger than those with sporadic lesions. This is an autosomal dominant condition with no gender predilection and the GISTs in these patients are found throughout the GI tract (mostly in the stomach and small intestine). Affected patients also have diffuse hyperplasia of interstitial cells of Cajal, skin pigment alterations, and sometimes, mast cell disorders. Patients with germline mutations of *PDGFRA* develop both GISTs and inflammatory fibroid polyps (discussed below) and virtually all their GISTs, as mentioned, arise in the stomach.

Clinical Features. Tumors of the duodenum, jejunum, and ileum present in adults usually in the sixth (24) or seventh (25) decade. There seems to be an overall slight male predominance (24,25). In the largest available series of jejunoileal lesions (25), the most common presentation was GI bleeding, often in the form of anemia rather than melena, followed by acute abdomen needing urgent surgery. Some cases were detected by imaging studies performed to address abdominal pain or even on pelvic exam, but many neoplasms were discovered incidentally. These tumors are detected during evaluation of patients with NF1 as well (25).

Duodenal GISTs are equally represented in males and females (26) and a subset manifests in patients with NF1. Like those in the jejunum and ileum, they peak in adults in the sixth decade and the patients most commonly have evidence of GI bleeding. All small bowel GISTs are rare in children. In the large series of jejunal and ileal GISTs by Miettinen et al. (25), less than 1 percent of patients were under the age of 21 years, and the youngest patient was 13 years old. The youngest patient with a duodenal GIST reported by the same group was age 10 years (26).

Patients with GISTs associated with NF1 are on average about 10 years younger than those with sporadic GISTs (median age, about 50 years), with a female predominance. They tend to have multiple tumors in the jejunum and ileum (6).

Stromal tumors of the colorectum and anus (27,28) are far less common than those of the

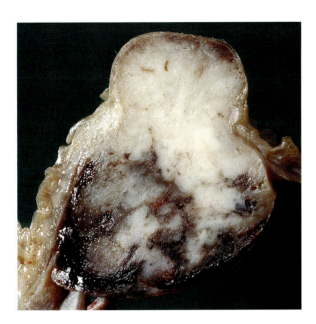

Figure 8-1

GASTROINTESTINAL STROMAL TUMOR (GIST)

This clinically malignant lesion arose in the duodenum and spread to the liver. It is hemorrhagic on the serosal side and centered in the muscularis propria. Note the coating of mucosa overlying the surface.

stomach and small bowel, so there are fewer accumulated data on them and diagnostic algorithms are less evidence based than they are for gastric and small intestinal ones (29). Anal canal tumors are rare: only three were identified in the files of the former Armed Forces Institute of Pathology at the time that their data were published (27). Distal lesions tend to present as prostatic tumors in men (30) and can be a pitfall on needle biopsy samples that are believed to be derived from the prostate gland.

There appears to be a male predominance for anorectal lesions but no gender predominance for lesions of the abdominal colon (26,31). For abdominal colon lesions, the median age is in the seventh decade and for anorectal lesions, the sixth decade. No pediatric examples were seen although a few teens had such tumors.

Appendiceal GISTs are truly rare, with less than 20 cases reported in the English language literature at the time of this writing (5,32–36), including a single lesion reported in a child (35). The mean age of the reported patients is about 65 years, with a male predominance. Patients tend to present with appendicitis over half the

time but many lesions are incidentally detected in opportunistic appendectomy samples.

Gross Findings. Duodenal GISTs most commonly involve the second part of the duodenum (26) and are usually well marginated but occasionally dumbbell shaped, with both luminal and serosal components. Gross ulceration of the mucosal surface is common. Large duodenal GISTs often form a retroperitoneal mass in addition to the duodenal component. Small duodenal GISTs are generally firm, rubbery, and pink tan.

Jejunoileal tumors are described as intraluminal polyps, hourglass-shaped, pedunculated, or solid external masses and some are cavitary (25). Generally they are described as pink-tan (25).

Colonic lesions are transmural and frequently fungating, some with cystic degeneration or an annular shape (31). They are soft and fish flesh-like and tan to pink (31).

Anorectal examples are described as firm, and whitish, tan, or pink-tan (27). They form well-marginated masses with occasional cystic spaces in large lesions (27). Examples of intestinal GISTs are shown in figures 8-1 and 8-2.

Microscopic Findings. Duodenal GISTs display the classic GIST features described in the stomach: either spindle or epithelioid (or mixed) but with the addition of skeinoid fibers (dense wiry collagen fibers) in about half the cases. Most duodenal GISTs are spindled with a minority of mixed lesions and rare purely epithelioid lesions, which tend to be malignant. Other features include calcifications, hemangiopericytoma-like vessels, intersecting fascicles of spindle cells, and palisading similar to that seen in nerve sheath tumors. There is minimal global nuclear pleomorphism in duodenal GISTs overall but it is commonly encountered focally in any given tumor.

GISTs in the jejunum and ileum are also typically spindled, with a subset mixed with an epithelioid component, but completely epithelioid examples are rare. They may also show skeinoid fibers and palisading, or calcifications. Some lack nuclear atypia but some have focal or diffuse nuclear atypia.

Most colorectal GISTs are spindle cell tumors with rare purely epithelioid morphology. They tend to be malignant, with densely packed spindle cells. GISTs found in patients with NF1

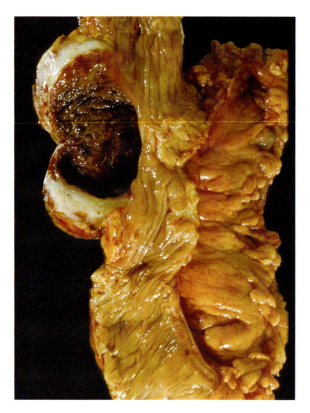

Figure 8-2

GASTROINTESTINAL STROMAL TUMOR

This colon neoplasm shows necrotic cyst formation.

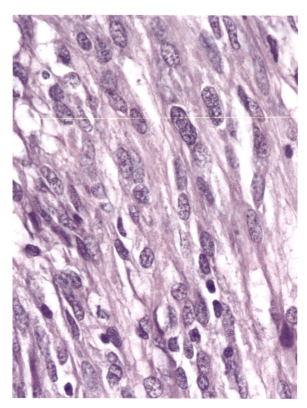

Figure 8-3

GASTROINTESTINAL STROMAL TUMOR

A spindle cell example with monotonous nuclei and fibrillary cytoplasm.

appear similar to other GISTs. Examples of small intestinal and colorectal GISTs are shown in figures 8-3 to 8-10.

Lesions termed "gastrointestinal autonomic tumor" are now regarded as variants of GIST but were first identified as small bowel ("plexosarcomas") lesions (37). The term *gastrointestinal autonomic nerve tumor* (GANT) was introduced because of ultrastructural evidence of axonal differentiation and the presence of dense core granules (fig. 8-11) (38). Since they are GISTs, lesions described as GANTs usually express CD117 but may also express S-100 protein, neuron-specific enolase, synaptophysin, and PGP9.5. CD34 shows variable staining. A subset of GISTs shows either de novo or post-treatment dedifferentiation to high-grade unclassifiable pleomorphic sarcomas. Those reported have mostly arisen in the stomach (39).

Immunohistochemical Findings. Virtually all duodenal GISTs express KIT, about 60 percent express CD34, and about 40 percent express focal smooth muscle actin but lack desmin (26). Keratin expression is occasionally detected as is S-100 protein (GANT) (38).

Almost all jejunoileal GISTs express KIT, sometimes in a dot-like Golgi zone distribution, whereas CD34 is found in only about 40 percent of cases. Smooth muscle actin expression occurs in about a third of cases and desmin expression is exceptional and focal. S-100 protein expression is found in about 15 percent.

KIT expression is seen in about 90 percent of cases in the abdominal colon but in almost all rectal lesions; CD34 expression in about 60 percent of abdominal colon lesions but almost all rectal ones. Desmin and S-100 protein expression are absent.

The addition of DOG1 (discovered on GIST1, also known as anoctamin 1, ANO1, and ORAOV2 [overexpressed in oral carcinoma]) to the diagnostic armamentarium for GISTs has

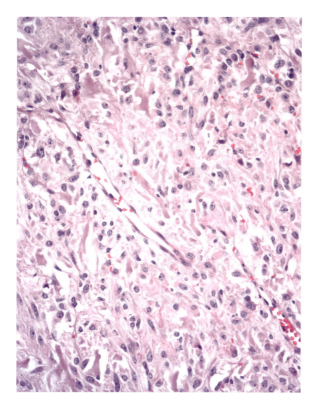

Figure 8-4

GASTROINTESTINAL STROMAL TUMOR

This small bowel tumor has prominent wiry collagen, so called skenoid bodies, named years ago for their ultrastructural appearance reminiscent of skeins of yarn.

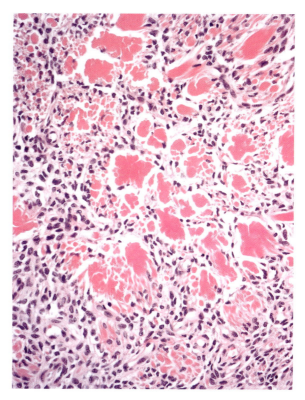

Figure 8-5

GASTROINTESTINAL STROMAL TUMOR

This example shows striking skeinoid bodies. This appearance can also be encountered in endometrial stromal sarcoma, a consideration that can be resolved with immunolabeling.

been useful, but more so for gastric GISTs than intestinal ones (11). DOG1 is a chloride channel protein that was found to be overexpressed in GISTs by gene profiling studies (40–42). It is expressed by about 95 percent of GISTs. Overall DOG1 is expressed in 36 to 92 percent of KIT-negative GISTs (11). Unfortunately, KIT is more sensitive for intestinal GISTs than DOG1; the two markers together (1), however, diagnose nearly all GISTs.

Molecular Genetic Findings. The most common mutations in GISTs are those of exon 11 of the *KIT* gene. These arise in all sites of the GI tract and are highly sensitive to imatinib treatment. About 20 percent of GISTs have mutations in exon 9 instead, and these usually arise in the intestines (small and large) and are less sensitive to imatinib than tumors with exon 11 mutations. Tumors with mutations in exons 13, 17, and 8 also tend to affect the small bowel although there are limited data on the

latter (1,11). Small intestinal GISTs occasionally harbor *BRAF* V600E mutations. So-called dedifferentiated GISTs harbor various *KIT* mutations in both the low- and high-grade components but there are limited data on these rare tumors (39). Table 8-2 outlines these findings.

Prognostication Based on Mitotic Activity, Location, and Size. For years, measuring size and mitotic counts has been the mainstay of prognostication for patients with GISTs at all sites, including the small and large intestines (25–27,31). The primary data are largely based on studies by Miettinen et al. (31) performed on imatinib-naive GISTs. Prior to the availability of extensive outcome data, size and mitotic counts were alone used, but this system failed to take into account the intrinsically worse prognosis of GISTs in sites outside the stomach (43).

Miettinen's data have now been converted into staging schemes, nomograms, and

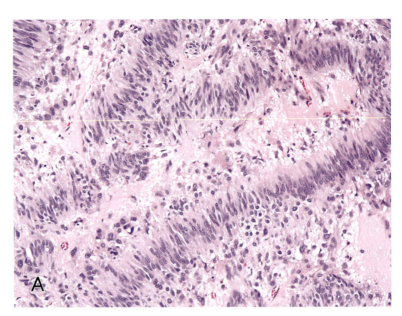

Figure 8-6

GASTROINTESTINAL STROMAL TUMOR

A: This tumor displays more prominent nuclear palisading than most schwannomas.

B: A CD34 immunostain.

C: A KIT/CD117 stain.

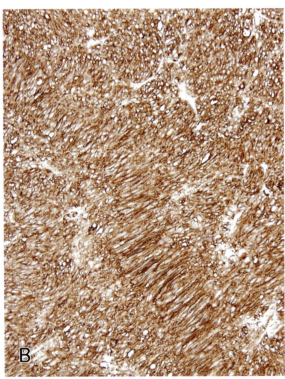

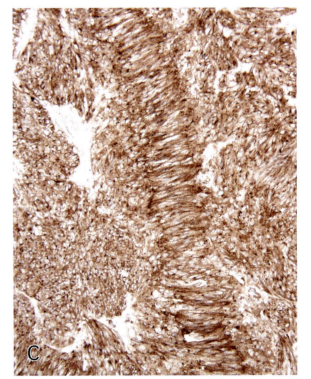

conditional disease-free survival assessments (29, 44–46). These schemes all perform well in prognostication using only site, size, and mitotic counts of the GIST, but the addition of demographic and treatment data can enhance the accuracy of the prediction. Male sex, older age, small bowel and rectal origin, large tumor size, high mitotic rate, and lack of adjuvant tyrosine kinase inhibitor treatment are all poor prognostic factors using a model incorporating various factors in addition to tumor size, mitotic count, and anatomic location (46). Curiously, NF1-associated GISTs are associated with a better outcome than small bowel GISTs in general, even if they are multifocal (6), although 15 to 20 percent are aggressive. A summary of the

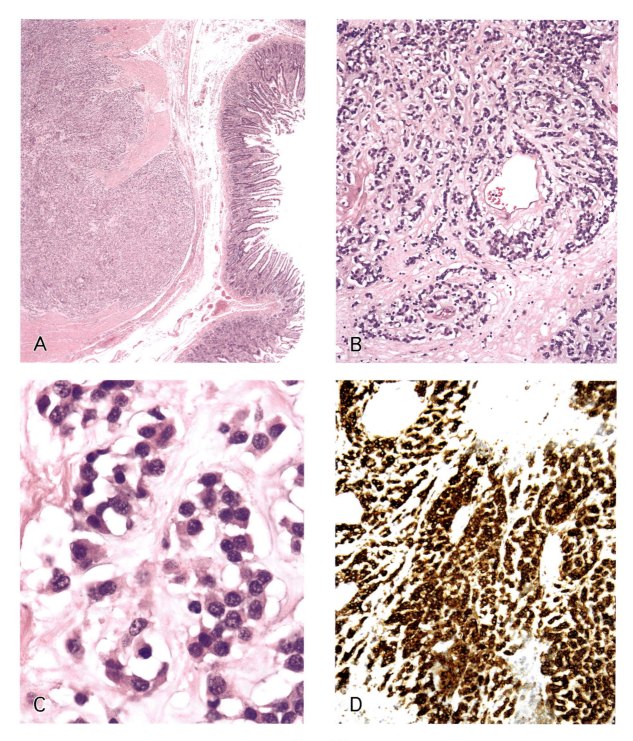

Figure 8-7

GASTROINTESTINAL STROMAL TUMOR

A: This lesion, centered in the muscularis propria, has a distinctly eosinophilic appearance at low magnification. Even at this scanning magnification, the lesion appears epithelioid.

B: At higher magnification, the epithelioid appearance of the cells is clear.

C: The nuclei have a plasmacytoid appearance.

D: A KIT stain.

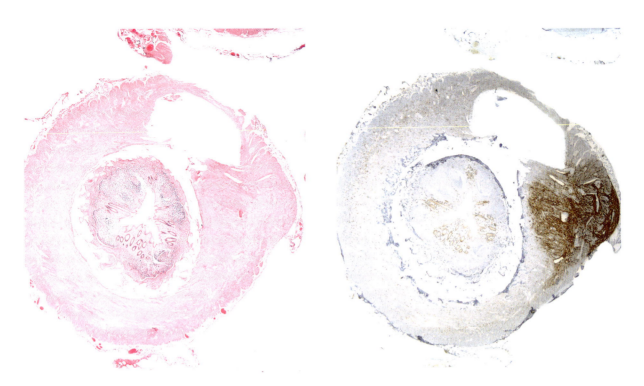

Figure 8-8

GASTROINTESTINAL STROMAL TUMOR: APPENDIX

Left: GISTs are rare in the appendix. The lesion is small and incidental and seen at the right of the field.
Right: A KIT stain.

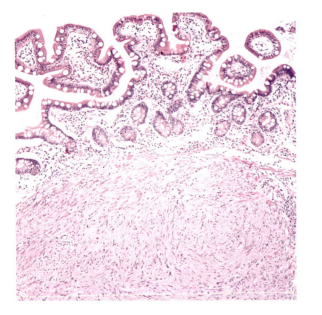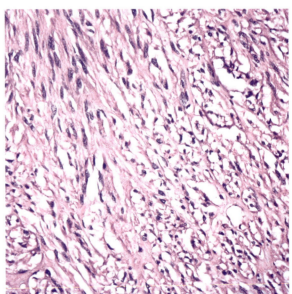

Figure 8-9

GASTROINTESTINAL STROMAL TUMOR

Left: The patient had neurofibromatosis, type 1 (NF1). The tumor was in the muscularis propria but has extended into the muscularis mucosae. The uniform spindled nuclei have a bland appearance.
Right: High magnification view.

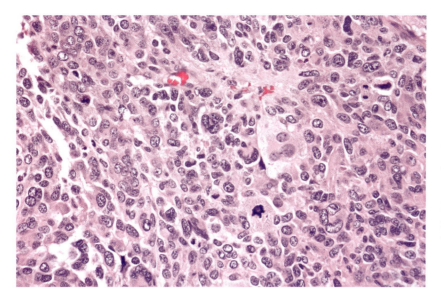

Figure 8-10

GASTROINTESTINAL STROMAL TUMOR

This a dedifferentiated GIST that arose in a patient who had been treated with imatinib for several years for an aggressive but typical-appearing GIST. This finding can be encountered *de novo* as well. It is essentially unrecognizable as a GIST and lacked expression of KIT (but retained *KIT* mutations). Prominent nuclear pleomorphism and dense cellularity are seen.

Figure 8-11

GASTROINTESTINAL STROMAL TUMOR

A: This nested spindled and epithelioid lesion is a "gastro-intestinal autonomic nervous tumor/GANT." It is essentially a GIST with neural differentiation.

B: High magnification shows the delicate fibrillary cytoplasm at the bottom of the field and the uniform nuclei.

C: An S-100 protein stain demonstrates both nuclear and cytoplasmic immunolabeling.

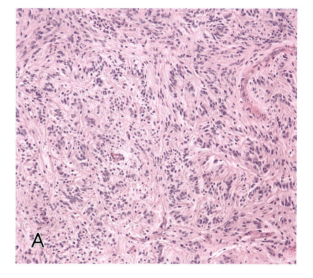

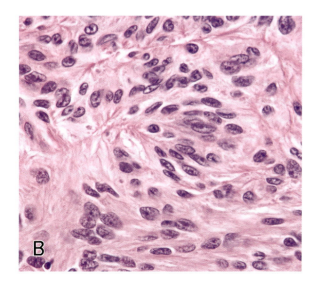

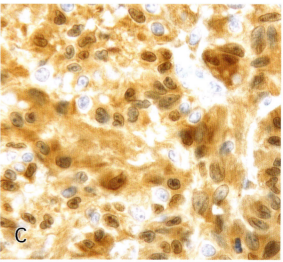

Table 8-2

INTESTINAL STROMAL TUMORS AND KEY MUTATIONS[a]

Mutation	Anatomic Location	Comments
KIT exon 11	All sites	Good response to imatinib, usually spindled or mixed
KIT exon 9	Small intestine and colorectum	Need high-dose tyrosine kinase inhibitor treatment, usually spindled or mixed
KIT exon 13	Small intestine	Modest response to tyrosine kinase inhibitor treatment, spindled
KIT exon 17	Small intestine	Modest response to tyrosine kinase inhibitor treatment, spindled
KIT exon 8	Small intestine	Rare so minimal information available
BRAF mutated (V600E)	Small intestine	Poor response to tyrosine kinase inhibitor treatment, spindled
NF1-associated	Small intestine	Poor response to tyrosine kinase inhibitor treatment, spindled

[a]Modified from reference 11.

Table 8-3

RISK ASSESSMENT IN INTESTINAL GASTROINTESTINAL STROMAL TUMORS[a]

Tumor Characteristic		Risk of Metastasis			AJCC System		
Size	Mitotic rate	Small Bowel	Duodenum	Rectum	T stage	Mitotic rate	AJCC Stage[b]
≤2 cm	<5/50 HPF[c]	Weak data	Weak data	Weak data	T1	≤5/50 HPF	I
>2 to ≤5 cm		Low	Low	Low	T2	(low)	I
>5 to ≤10 cm		Moderate	High	High	T3		II
>10 cm		High	Weak data	Weak data	T4		IIIA
≤2 cm	>5/50 HPF	Weak data	Weak data	High	T1	>5/50 HPF	IIIA
>2 to ≤5 cm		High	High	High	T2	(high)	IIIB
>5 to ≤10 cm		High	High	High	T3		IIIB
>10 cm		High	High	Weak data	T4		IIIB

[a]Table modified from reference 44.
[b]Any metastases (either lymph node or distant) convert the stage to IV.
[c]HPF = high-power field; this can be regarded as per 5mm^2 (closer to 20 hpf using modern microscopes); AJCC 8th edition.

primary data concerning outcomes and the staging for intestinal GISTs appears in Table 8-3.

Treatment. As summarized by Corless (47), treatment with tyrosine kinase inhibitors such as imatinib, sunitinib, and regorafenib is effective in controlling unresectable disease. Unfortunately, drug resistance caused by secondary *KIT* or *PDGFRA* mutations is ultimately detected in over 90 percent of treated individuals. Because of this, many authors suggest adjuvant therapy with imatinib to reduce the likelihood of disease recurrence after primary surgery, and for this reason assessing the prognosis of newly resected tumors is a key issue for pathologists. Routine genotyping has thus been proposed for optimal management of GISTs, as the type and dose of drug used for treatment is dependent on the mutation identified. For example, *BRAF*-mutated tumors may respond to debrafenib (48). NF1-related GISTs do not respond to imatinib (23) and, as above, tumors with exon 11 *KIT* mutations are most amenable to targeted treatment. Overall, the median survival period for patients with advanced disease treated with imatinib is about 5 years, but a third of such patients live nearly 10 years (49).

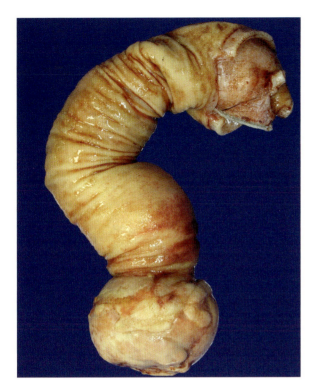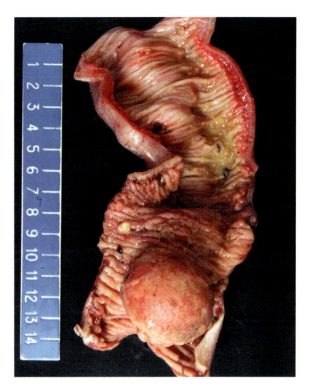

Figure 8-12

INFLAMMATORY FIBROID POLYP

Left: The tumor has resulted in a small bowel intussusception.
Right: The lead point of the intussusception is at the right. The surface of the tumor is eroded. It is based in the submucosa.

INFLAMMATORY FIBROID POLYP OF THE SMALL INTESTINE AND COLON

Inflammatory fibroid polyps were first reported in the stomach as "gastric submucosal granuloma with eosinophilic infiltration" (50). The present term was coined by Helwig and Ranier in 1953 (51). In most series, the majority arise in the stomach and terminal ileum (51,52), but in one series there was a more even distribution in the stomach and colon, which may have reflected consultation bias (53). An interesting family in Devon, England has been reported, in which three generations of women harbor these lesions, predominantly in the small intestine (54). Most arise in adults of a median age of around 60 years, but there are rare pediatric cases reported in the literature and summarized by Righetti et al. (55). Families with known germline mutations in *PDGFRA* are also prone to develop these tumors (23).

Inflammatory fibroid polyps often present clinically as nonspecific polyps, but their surfaces can erode, resulting in hemorrhage. Small bowel examples present as intussusception in about half of cases (fig. 8-12) (53) and gastric antral examples may present with gastric outlet obstruction. Colonic polyps can present in a fashion similar to that of inflammatory bowel disease. The tumors range in size from well under 1 cm to 4 to 5 cm, with a median size of about 2 cm. They are always centered in the submucosa but nearly 90 percent extend into the mucosa and a small number extend into the muscularis propria.

Microscopically, these are submucosal-based lesions composed of uniform spindle cells; in about half of cases, vessels are encircled in an "onion-skin" pattern. Over 90 percent of cases feature a backdrop of numerous eosinophils, although some lack this component and tend to be more sclerotic. Lymphoid aggregates are common (fig. 8-13) and many tumors contain giant cells. Small lesions tend to have an ulcerated surface and thus reactive changes overlie the lesion.

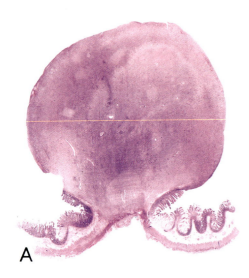

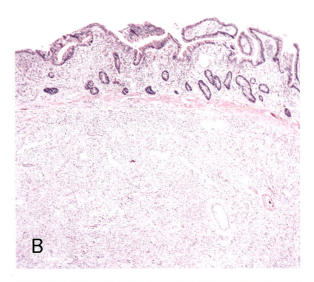

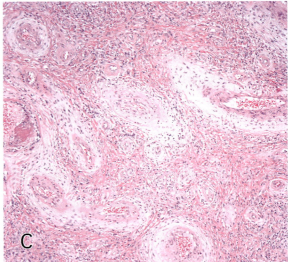

Figure 8-13

INFLAMMATORY FIBROID POLYP

A: The tumor is centered in the submucosa with an eroded surface microscopically.

B: This example has extended into the lamina propria of the small bowel. Prominent edema is seen in the submucosal component. Even at this magnification, the tumor cells have small pale nuclei.

C: There is striking whorling of tumor cells around thickened vessels (onion skin appearance).

D: The eosinophils are prominent.

E: Most cases have many eosinophils. This high-power image highlights the bland appearance of the tumor cell nuclei.

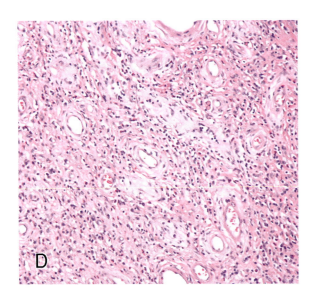

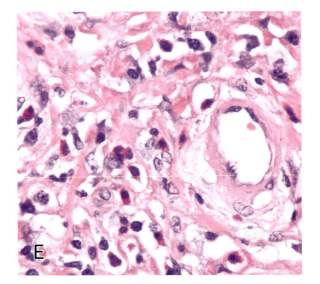

On immunolabeling, 80 to 90 percent express CD34 and most express PDGFRA protein (53,56). They do not express KIT or DOG1, and S-100 protein immunolabeling is always negative. The expression of cyclin D1, fascin, and CD34 has led some observers to suggest that these polyps show differentiation along the lines of dendritic cells (57). These tumors were initially believed to be reactive, but the detection of *PDGFRA* mutations in 70 percent of gastric lesions and 55 percent of small bowel examples supports a benign neoplasm (56,58).

NEURAL TUMORS OF THE INTESTINES

Most *nerve sheath tumors* found in the intestines are benign incidental lesions detected in the course of routine screening colonoscopy. Nevertheless, syndromic intestinal nerve sheath lesions are found in patients with multiple endocrine neoplasia (MEN)2B, neurofibromatosis (von Recklinghausen disease), *PTEN* hamartoma tumor syndrome, which encompasses the eponymous disorders Cowden and Bannayan-Riley-Ruvalcaba diseases. The colon is the typical site for colon nerve sheath lesions whereas gangliocytic paraganglioma (which is not precisely a nerve sheath tumor but has a nerve sheath component) virtually always arises in the duodenum. Nerve sheath tumors of the GI tract are rare, accounting for only about 5 percent of mesenchymal lesions in this area, whereas GISTs account for about 50 percent (59).

Schwannoma

Gastrointestinal lesions that have been termed *schwannomas* most commonly arise in the stomach rather than the colorectum (60). They are unassociated with MEN2B but have occasionally been reported in patients with NF1 (59). Most are reported as isolated cases, but in a series of 15 such tumors, they were lesions of adults, with one exception arising in an adolescent (61). The tumors appear to preferentially involve the right colon but can be found throughout the colon.

Patients present with rectal bleeding, intestinal obstruction, abdominal pain, or intussusceptions. The tumors are macroscopically well marginated but unencapsulated, and are almost always centered in the muscularis propria, although a luminal component may be present. They generally attain a size of 3 cm. They have a homogeneous cut surface lacking zones of necrosis.

Microscopically, schwannomas are characteristically surrounded by a discontinuous cuff showing lymphoid hyperplasia (fig. 8-14). The tumors have moderate to high cellularity and are composed of spindle cells in fascicles, with poorly developed palisading structures but without Verocay bodies. There is a moderate backdrop of lymphoplasmacytic cells scattered throughout the tumor. In contrast to conventional schwannomas of the somatic soft tissues, GI schwannomas generally lack thick-walled vessels, a capsule, and hemosiderin deposition. Scattered mitotic figures can be encountered. A reticular pattern reminiscent of that of reticular perineurioma has been reported (59,62–64), as has a hybrid schwannoma/perineurioma (65) analogous to those reported in soft tissues (66).

On immunolabeling, GI schwannomas strongly express S-100 protein and glial fibrillary acidic protein (GFAP) and a subset displays CD34 expression, but these lesions are negative for CD117, DOG1, neurofilament proteins, keratins, calretinin, and HMB45. In contrast to conventional schwannomas, GI schwannomas lack *NF2* gene alterations (67). Colorectal schwannomas consistently behave in a benign fashion and can sometimes be managed endoscopically but are often resected based on the clinical impression that they are GISTs (68).

Related lesions displaying an epithelioid appearance have been termed *epithelioid schwannomas* or *mucosal benign epithelioid nerve sheath tumors* (69), terminology that underscores their usual site, namely the mucosa, where they are encountered as small colon polyps at screening colonoscopy. Usually seen in the colon, they are rare in the small intestine, occasionally seen as transmural lesions. In contrast to the spindle cell schwannomas above, epithelioid schwannomas are usually less than 1 cm in greatest dimension, with rare exceptions (61), and involve the distal rather than proximal colon.

Histologically, schwannomas have an infiltrative growth pattern and are composed of spindled to predominantly epithelioid cells arranged in nests and whorls. The epicenter of the lesion is in the lamina propria but can extend to the superficial submucosa, or rarely, into the muscularis propria. The proliferating cells have

Figure 8-14

GASTROINTESTINAL TRACT SCHWANNOMA

A: These tumors are uncommon. They are usually found in the stomach followed by the colon. This is a rare small intestinal example. A ring of lymphoid aggregates surrounds the tumor, which has bulged out into the subserosal tissue. Regardless of this locally infiltrative appearance, these tumors are always benign.

B: This image shows the lymphoid cuff to advantage.

C: The degree of nuclear variability is in excess of that expected for a GIST but there is no mitotic activity. These tumors display strong S-100 protein labeling and lack KIT and DOG1 expression.

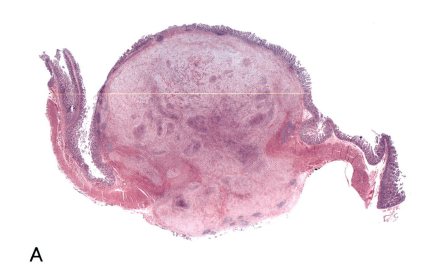

A

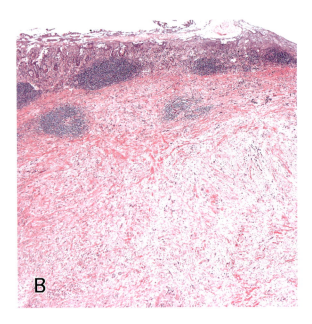

B

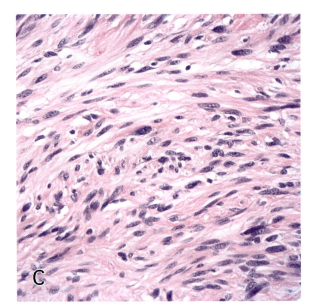

C

uniform round to oval nuclei with frequent intranuclear pseudoinclusions and eosinophilic fibrillary cytoplasm. Some cases display cystic spaces and a pseudoglandular pattern. No mitoses are seen. If Ki-67 is performed, all have a low proliferative index. These tumors express S-100 protein diffusely but lack melanoma markers. They have variable CD34 labeling in supporting cells. Tumors lack CD117 and calretinin, and SMI31 shows no intralesional neuraxons. These are benign lesions treated by excision.

Schwann Cell Hamartoma

Mucosal *Schwann cell hamartoma* is characterized by a diffuse, ill-defined proliferation of spindle cells within the lamina propria, which surrounds colonic crypts (70). While predominantly encountered in the rectosigmoid, these polyps may arise anywhere in the colon. They are usually small (1 to 6 mm) and found incidentally at colonoscopy in adults. The spindle cells show indistinct cell borders and are bland appearing, with elongated or wavy nuclei and ample eosinophilic

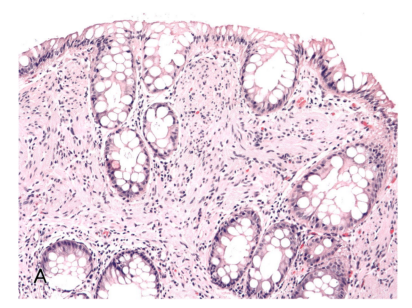

Figure 8-15

SCHWANN CELL HAMARTOMA

A: The nuclei are small and vaguely palisaded, and the cells proliferate in the mucosa between glands. These tumors are unassociated with any known syndromes.

B: The cytoplasm of the tumor cells is fibrillary and very eosinophilic.

C: An S-100 protein stain.

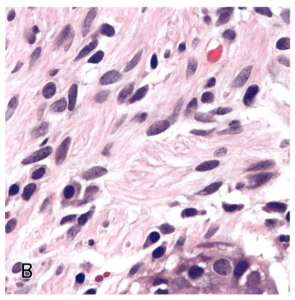

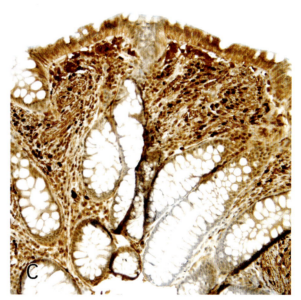

cytoplasm (fig. 8-15). Mucosal ulceration, nuclear atypia, and mitotic activity are absent.

The lesional cells are diffusely immunoreactive with S-100 protein. In some cases, rare associated axons are highlighted with a neurofilament protein immunostain. The spindle cells are negative for CD34, GFAP, epithelial membrane antigen (EMA), smooth muscle actin (SMA), and CD117.

The main differential diagnosis is with colonic neurofibroma, an important distinction given its clinical association with NF1. While histologically very similar, colonic neurofibro-

mas display more cellular heterogeneity, more nuclear variability, and varying amounts of cytoplasm. The spindle cells in neurofibromas are only focally immunoreactive with S-100 protein and all contain associated axons, which are highlighted with a neurofilament protein immunostain. Unlike neurofibromas and ganglioneuromas, mucosal Schwann cell hamartomas are unassociated with syndromic states.

The differential diagnosis also includes lesions that are regarded as epithelioid schwannomas (see above) (fig. 8-16) (69). They consist of epithelioid cells with prominent intranuclear

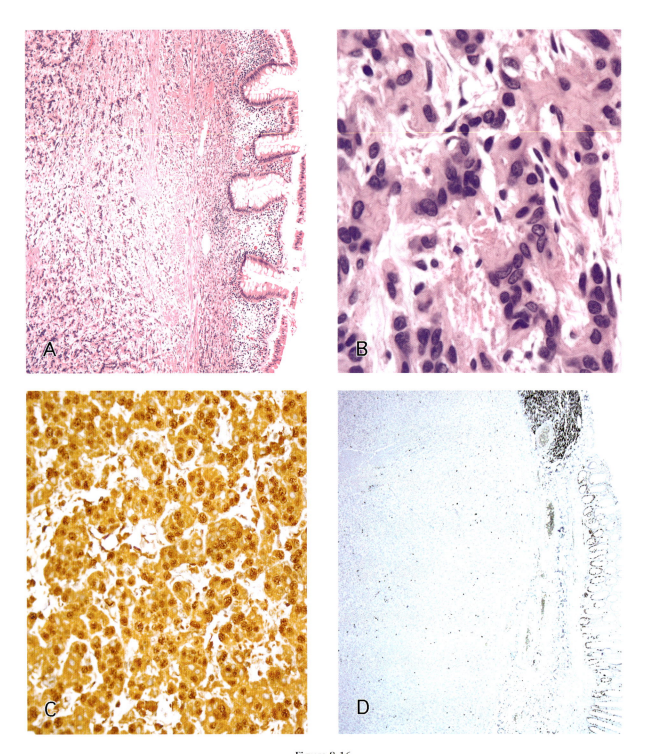

Figure 8-16

EPITHELIOID SCHWANNOMA

A: The tumor is centered in the colonic mucosa and submucosa.

B: Epithelioid pink cytoplasm is seen.

C: This is an S-100 protein stain.

D: A Ki-67/MIB1 stain shows a very low proliferative index. The black pigment at the top left is India ink, which was used to mark the lesion at the time of a mucosal biopsy.

inclusions centered in the lamina propria and superficial submucosa (although we have encountered rare transmural examples). On immunolabeling, they express S-100 protein but no "melanoma markers" and they behave in a benign fashion. They are rare, but of interest since they simulate metastatic melanoma. They differ from it both by the lack of expression of melanoma markers and by their essential lack of mitotic activity.

Rare psammomatous melanotic schwannomas (fig. 8-17) are also seen in the colon, where they have behaved in a benign fashion (59,71). Their importance is that they simulate melanoma.

Schwann cell hamartomas are benign lesions treated by polypectomy. Endoscopic follow-up is not necessary after diagnosis.

Benign Fibroblastic Polyp/Perineurioma

Benign fibroblastic polyps are incidental lesions detected in adult patients undergoing screening colonoscopy. As such, the mean age in reported series ranges from 56 to 64 years (72–76). They present as small, solitary, asymptomatic polyps (size range, 0.2 to 1.5 cm) usually in the rectosigmoid colon (73).

The polyps consist of an expansion of the lamina propria by a bland, monomorphic spindle cell population with abundant pale eosinophilic cytoplasm focally arranged in a concentric fashion around vessels and crypts. There is no mitotic activity or necrosis. Some are intimately admixed with serrated polyps (either sessile serrated adenomas or hyperplastic polyps) (75), which suggests "epithelial stromal interactions" (fig. 8-18) (72).

Traditionally, these polyps were described as usually "vimentin-only" lesions, lacking CD31, S-100 protein, CD117/c-kit, BCL-2, and desmin. However, most express at least one perineurial marker (EMA, claudin-1, and glucose transporter-1), and as such, are also termed *colonic perineuriomas* (74,76); some cases display focal SMA and CD34 (72). The Ki-67 index is low, at approximately 1 percent. In one study of 22 cases associated with serrated polyps, the authors detected *BRAF* and *KRAS* mutations in 63 percent and 4 percent of cases, respectively, presumably in the serrated polyp component (72).

Although most of these lesions are limited to the mucosa, they can, rarely, extend into the superficial submucosa. Benign fibroblastic polyps are managed by simple polypectomy and require no endoscopic follow-up.

Neurofibroma

Neurofibromas of the GI tract are extremely rare as sporadic lesions and even rarer in the setting of NF1. They include plexiform neurofibromas that tend to involve the serosal surfaces or diffuse mucosal lesions (59). Syndromic (NF1) GI neurofibromas display features similar to those encountered in the somatic soft tissues. They are composed of spindled cells embedded in a matrix with myxoid change and wire-like collagen. Zones with a reticular pattern can be encountered at the periphery of the lesion. Infiltrative examples involve the mucosa, where S-100 protein-reactive spindle cells infiltrate between intestinal crypts. These are benign lesions with minimal risk for transformation to malignant peripheral nerve sheath tumor.

Ganglioneuroma and Ganglioneuromatosis

General and Clinical Features. *Ganglioneuromas* occur in two general settings: as solitary isolated lesions and syndromically as multiple lesions that either produce multiple exophytic polyps (*ganglioneuromatous polyposis*) or poorly demarcated transmural proliferations (*ganglioneuromatosis*) (77). In solitary examples, there is no gender predominance and the lesions are detected in adults from 20 to 90 years of age, with a peak incidence between the ages of 40 and 60 (mean age, 48 years). Most are found in the colon, usually on the left side. Most patients are asymptomatic, and the lesions are detected during routine colonoscopy. Solitary lesions are not associated with genetic syndromes.

Ganglioneuromatous polyposis is associated with Cowden syndrome, and diffuse ganglioneuromatosis is associated with MEN2B and NF1. Diffuse ganglioneuromatosis is found in most patients with MEN2B and often antedates the development of the endocrine neoplasms. Patients with MEN-2B and ganglioneuromatosis present with diverse GI symptoms, which may include constipation, diarrhea, difficulty in feeding, projectile vomiting, and crampy abdominal pain. Most syndromic GI tract ganglioneuromas

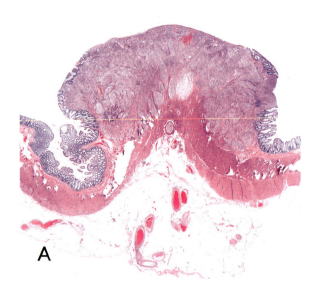

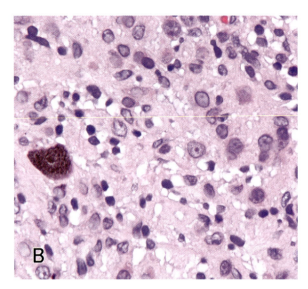

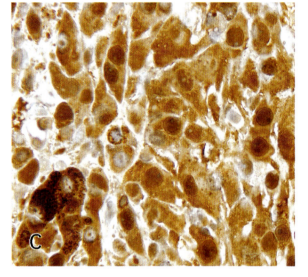

Figure 8-17

PSAMMOMATOUS MELANOTIC SCHWANNOMA

A: These are rare lesions that can be encountered in the colon. This example resulted in a resection. The tumor is centered in the mucosa and submucosa, with a small satellite lesion in the muscularis propria.

B: The nuclei have a bland appearance. A melanocytic cell is present at the left.

C: An S-100 protein immunostain shows both nuclear and cytoplasmic labeling.

D: An HMB45 immunostain.

E: This Ki-67 stain is reassuring in excluding melanoma.

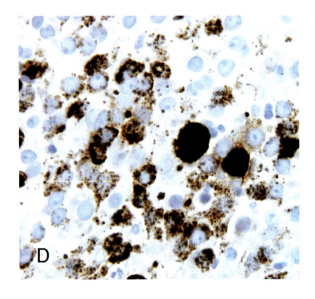

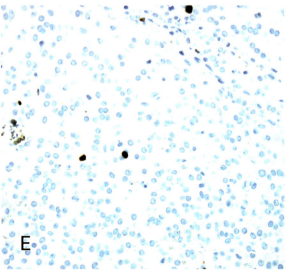

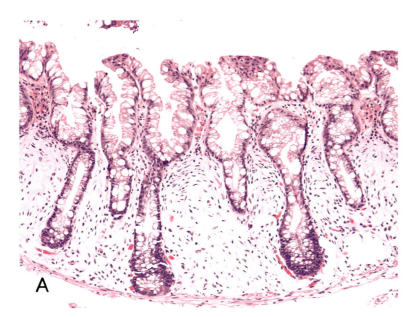

Figure 8-18

**BENIGN FIBROBLASTIC POLYP
OF THE COLON/PERINEURIOMA**

A: The lesion is present between the colon crypts. In this case, the epithelial component is a hyperplastic polyp. These two types of lesions tend to arise in an intermingled fashion.

B: The long cytoplasmic processes are a clue that these lesions have perineurial differentiation.

C: GLUT1 stains both erythrocytes and the lesion itself.

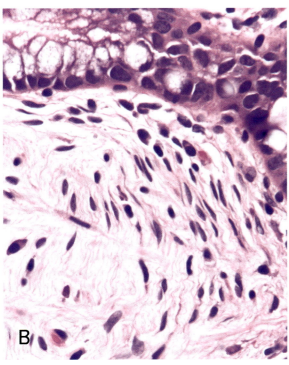

are found in the colorectum and in patients younger (mean age, about 35 years) than those who have sporadic isolated ganglioneuromas.

Polypoid isolated ganglioneuromas are small sessile or pedunculated polyps that grossly resemble juvenile polyp, or adenomas, and are 1 to 2 cm. The polyps in ganglioneuromatous polyposis are multiple (20 to 40) and display greater variability in size than sporadic ones,

ranging from 1 mm to over 2 cm. Some are filiform. Rare pediatric examples of ganglioneuromatous polyposis are associated with the production of vasoactive intestinal polypeptide, which produces the watery diarrhea, hypokalemia, and achlorhydria syndrome (78,79). Diffuse ganglioneuromatosis results in a poorly demarcated, whitish thickening that may be transmural.

Figure 8-19

GANGLIONEUROMA

A: Plump ganglion cells are seen in the lower part of the lamina propria and the more spindled schwannian cells toward the surface.

B: The ganglion cells have unusual appearances in some cases. The Nissl substance in the cell at the right has a clumped distribution.

C: The schwannian component appears similar to a neurofibroma or Schwann cell hamartoma. Ganglioneuromas have the same appearance whether sporadic or syndromic.

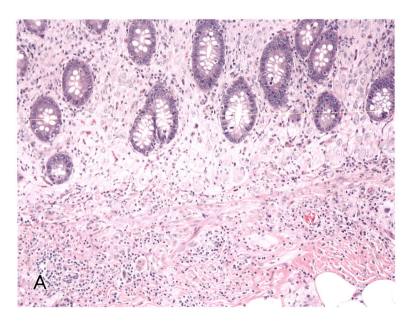

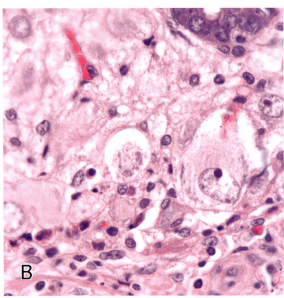

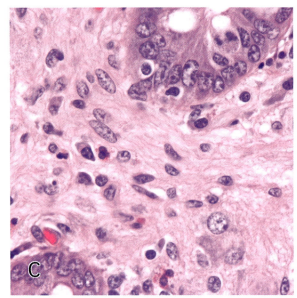

Microscopic Findings. At low magnification, polypoid sporadic ganglioneuromas often resemble juvenile or inflammatory polyps: they have disturbed crypt architecture and expanded lamina propria. At higher magnification, the lamina propria is expanded by collections of spindle cells within a fibrillary matrix, and there are irregular nests and groups of ganglion cells (fig. 8-19). Sporadic examples may also have submucosal extension and a plexiform arrangement involving the submucosal nerve plexus, such that they superficially resemble neurofibromas (differing by the presence of many ganglion cells).

The ganglioneuromas in ganglioneuromatous polyposis show overlapping features with sporadic ganglioneuromas, but tend to be more variable and have more numerous ganglion cells and filiform architecture. In diffuse ganglioneuromatosis, the process is centered around the myenteric plexus, is either diffusely intramural or transmural, and consists of fusiform expansions or confluent transmural ganglioneuromatous proliferations.

These lesions are easily diagnosed without immunohistochemistry, but the spindle cells react with S-100 protein and the ganglion cells mark with neuron-specific enolase (NSE), synaptophysin, and neurofilament protein.

Differential Diagnosis. The primary distinction is from neurofibroma, and is based on the presence of ganglion cells in ganglioneuromas and their lack in neurofibromas. When ganglion cells are sparse, NSE or synaptophysin staining may help detect them. Ganglioneuromas are distinguished from gangliocytic paragangliomas by the presence of epithelioid cells in the latter; these epithelioid cells may be keratin positive. Additionally, gangliocytic paragangliomas arise primarily in the duodenum, rather than the colon.

Treatment and Prognosis. Sporadic ganglioneuromas are treated by polypectomy and seldom recur. Patients with syndromic ganglioneuromas must be carefully followed, based on their specific syndromes. Those with NF1 may develop other neural lesions, including malignant peripheral sheath tumors; those with MEN2B may develop endocrine neoplasms. Polypoid ganglioneuromas may herald Cowden disease, tuberous sclerosis, familial adenomatous polyposis, and juvenile polyposis, whereas the diffuse type is most likely associated with NF1 and MEN2B. This latter type may cause strictures requiring resections, but the ganglioneuromas, themselves, are all benign.

MEN2B-Associated Neuroma

Multiple endocrine neoplasia type 2B (MEN2B) is a rare autosomal dominant disease caused by germline mutations in the *RET* proto-oncogene. It is characterized by medullary thyroid carcinoma, pheochromocytoma, and mucosal neuromas. Whereas the other neoplasms present later in life, the mucosal neuromas generally develop from early childhood and recognizing them is a clue to the disease. Mucosal neuromas generally arise in the lips, tongue, and buccal mucosa, and less commonly in the palate, intestinal mucosa, and conjunctiva, where they form clusters of small nodules. As time goes by, mucosal neuromas can increase in size and number or show no change. Because mucosal neuromas have no specific symptoms and no malignant changes, no further treatment is needed except for cosmetic purposes

In some respects, mucosal neuromas and ganglioneuromas histologically resemble traumatic neuromas (fig. 8-20), consisting of bundles of neural proliferations, often surrounded by a cuff of perineurium. The neural proliferation can appear solid or myxoid, although, in our experience, mucosal neuromas of the GI tract are more likely to appear myxoid whereas oral lesions manifest a more solid appearance. These are benign lesions.

Nerve Sheath Proliferations Found in PTEN Hamartoma Tumor Syndrome (Cowden and Bannayan-Riley-Ruvalcaba Syndromes)

The *PTEN* (phosphatase and tensin homolog) *hamartoma syndrome*, discussed elsewhere, includes Cowden and Bannayan-Riley-Ruvalcaba syndromes, and some examples of Proteus-like syndrome. *Cowden syndrome* features hamartomatous lesions and is transmitted in an autosomal dominant fashion. Tumors that are found in patients with Cowden syndrome include tricholemmomas, oral papillomas, and malignant neoplasms of thyroid gland, breast, and uterus. *Bannayan-Riley-Ruvalcaba syndrome* is typified by lipomas and vascular malformations. Hamartomatous gastrointestinal polyps accompany both disorders.

The skin is the key disease site for patients with the PTEN hamartoma syndrome. Both ganglioneuromas as well as mucocutaneous neuromas are known to arise patients with this syndrome (80). The morphologic features are the same as those in other sites and settings. These tumors are benign.

Granular Cell Tumor

The colon is the second most common GI tract site for *granular cell tumors* (after the esophagus), but they are still rare. They display the features of granular cell tumors elsewhere (including S-100 protein expression) (81), but can be subtle when encountered in the colonic lamina propria. The largest series published to date included only 26 examples (82) and demonstrated an equal gender distribution and a mean age of about 50 years. Unlike their esophageal counterparts, colorectal granular cell tumors appear to be slightly more common in whites than African-Americans. Most examples are incidentally discovered at colonoscopy, are located in the right colon, and are small (mean, 0.6 cm).

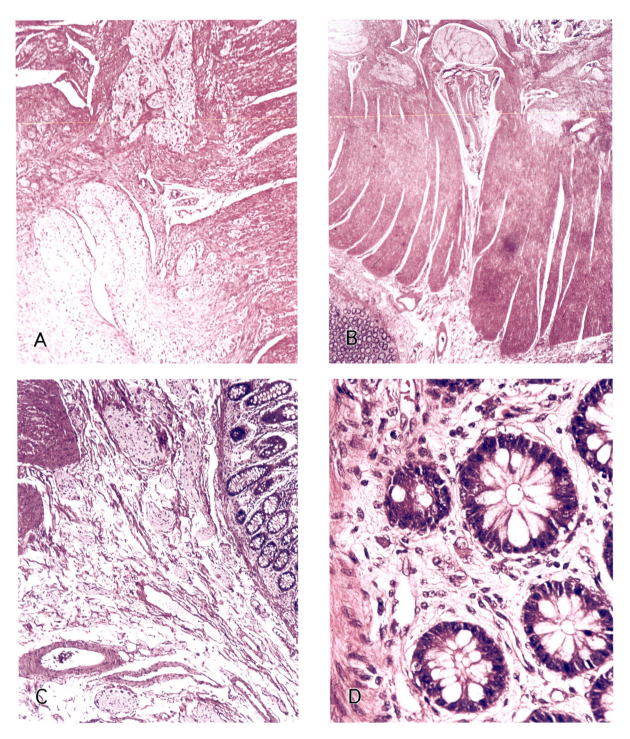

Figure 8-20

NEURAL LESIONS IN PATIENT WITH MULTIPLE ENDOCRINE NEOPLASIA (MEN) 2B

A: The lesion shows transmural extension. Each part of the lesion is surrounded by a rim of perineurium as per a traumatic neuroma but some of the nodules contain ganglion cells as well as Schwann cells (ganglioneuromatosis).

B: This is an extensive process, affecting all bowel layers.

C: Well-delineated neuromatous lesions are seen in the submucosa.

D: This area has the appearance of a sporadic ganglioneuroma, which belies the extensive infiltrative nature of the process.

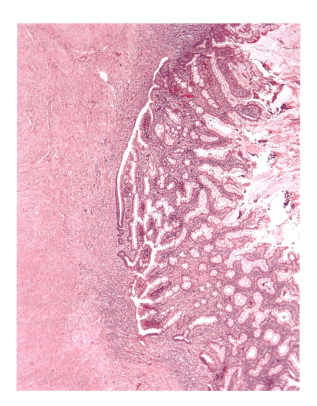 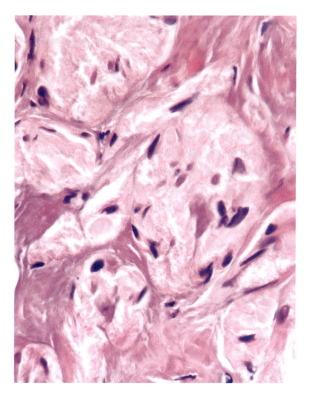

Figure 8-21

GRANULAR CELL TUMOR

Left: The tumor is subtle, merging with the smooth muscle of the muscularis propria, but centered in the submucosa.
Right: Colorectal examples often arise in the right colon, where they may display degenerative atypia that can cause concern for malignancy.

Histologically, they can be infiltrative or well-marginated, involving the mucosa, submucosa or both (fig. 8-21). Colorectal granular cell tumors may be associated with a lymphoid cuff and may display cytologic atypia and areas of calcification. Some cases show reactive surface epithelial changes, which may lead to misdiagnosis as adenoma. Mitoses and areas of necrosis are absent (82). There are rare reports of multicentric granular cell tumors of the colon (83).

Granular cell tumors may recur following incomplete excision but most are benign. There are two case reports of malignant granular cell colorectal tumors at the time of this writing, but neither has resulted in distant metastases or patient death (84,85).

Gangliocytic Paraganglioma

Gangliocytic paragangliomas are rare and fascinating tumors: most arise in the duodenum in adult patients of an average age of about 54 years (86–93). Rare examples are found in the jejunum or even the pylorus. We have seen rare lesions of the colon that fulfill the criteria for gangliocytic paraganglioma.

The typical presentation involves abdominal pain, gastric outlet obstruction, or bleeding. There are isolated reports of an association with neurofibromatosis (94), but the majority of cases are sporadic. These lesions are usually centered in the submucosa (fig. 8-22), with minor extensions into the mucosa, which are occasionally biopsied. Excised tumors are 3 to 4 cm, with a soft, yellowish cut surface. They have infiltrative borders.

These tumors display a histologic constellation of three cell types: spindle cells with the appearance of nerve sheath cells; ganglion-like cells; and epithelioid cells arranged in nests ("endocrine" pattern) and trabeculae or papillary structures (figs. 8-23, 8-24). The proportion of the cell types is variable; hence, these lesions are prone to causing diagnostic problems.

317

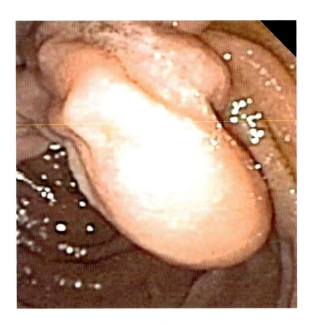

Figure 8-22

GANGLIOCYTIC PARAGANGLIOMA

This is a submucosal lesion. The overlying mucosa is intact, and the endoscopic appearance is similar to that of a well-differentiated neuroendocrine (carcinoid) tumor or a submucosal lipoma.

The tumors are reactive with S-100 protein in spindle/"supporting or sustentacular" cells, synaptophysin in ganglion-like cells, and NSE in all three cell types. About half of the cases display keratin in the epithelioid cells. A variety of hormones can be demonstrated including somatostatin, human pancreatic polypeptide, serotonin, gastrin, glucagon, insulin, and vasoactive intestinal peptide.

In spindle cell-predominant lesions, the differential diagnosis is with GIST and nerve sheath tumors. The sustentacular pattern of S-100 protein positivity excludes GIST and finding the admixture of other cell types excludes nerve sheath tumors. Epithelioid lesions are distinguished from WDNTs and carcinomas, again, by the admixture of other cell types.

Gangliocytic paragangliomas are benign in the majority of cases. There are rare reports of regional metastases (88,89) and a single report of a tumor-associated death (95).

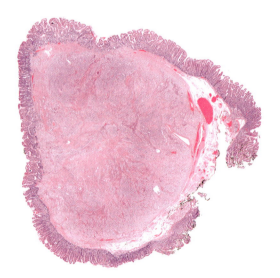

Figure 8-23

GANGLIOCYTIC PARAGANGLIOMA

Above: A perfect polypectomy sample with an uninvolved margin (inked black at the right side of the image). The neoplasm is lobulated and expands to fill the submucosa and muscularis mucosae.

Right: This image shows the three components with schwannian spindle cells at the left and epithelioid nests and gangliocytic cells at the right.

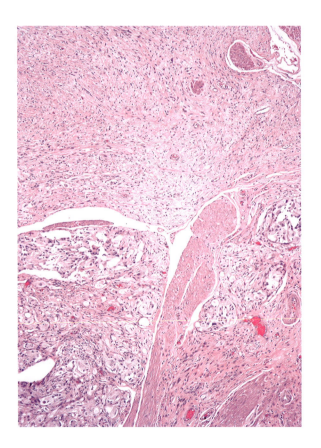

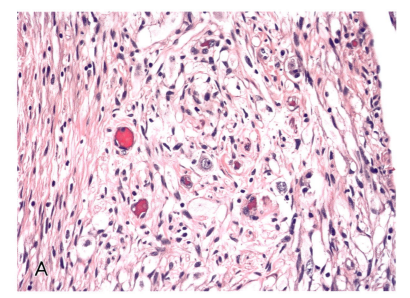

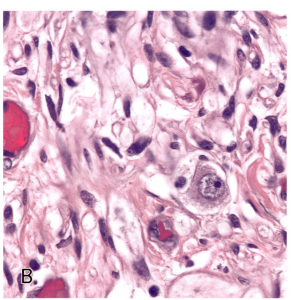

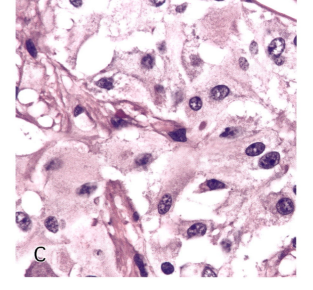

Figure 8-24

GANGLIOCYTIC PARAGANGLIOMA

A: The schwannian spindle cells predominate in this field, with a centrally placed ganglion cell.

B: At high power, the nuclear features of both the schwannian and gangliocytic components are seen.

C: The epithelioid component resembles well-differentiated neuroendocrine (carcinoid) tumor.

SMOOTH MUSCLE TUMORS

Colon

Most spindle cell tumors of the wall of the GI tract are stromal tumors (GISTs) except in the esophagus where leiomyomas predominate. However, if a brightly eosinophilic spindle cell lesion with bland cytologic features is encountered in the muscularis mucosae of the colon, it is, in all likelihood, an incidental *leiomyoma*, readily managed by simple polypectomy (96).

Miettinen et al. (96) studied 88 such tumors of the muscularis mucosae of the colon and rectum. All of the lesions, except one, were removed by snare polypectomy as incidental lesions at cancer or polyp surveillance; one small tumor was an incidental finding in a rectal resection specimen. The tumors had a significant male predominance (overall 2.4 to 1.0) and were found in adults (38 to 85 years; median age, 62 years). The lesions were typically small (range, 1 to 22 mm; median, 4 mm) and located predominantly in the rectum and sigmoid colon (72 percent). All were composed of well-differentiated, eosinophilic smooth muscle cells that were seen immediately beneath the mucosa,

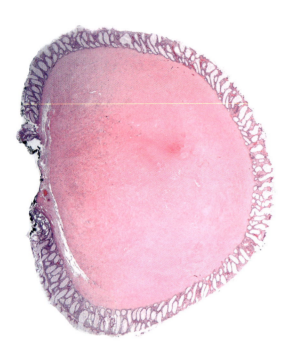
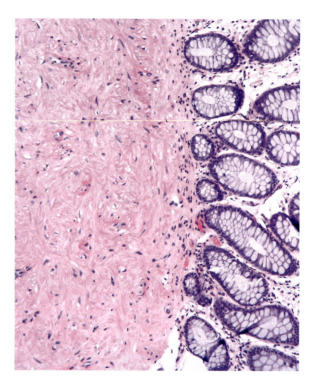

Figure 8-25

LEIOMYOMA

Left: Colonic leiomyomas arise in association with the muscularis mucosae and are detected at screening colonoscopy. This one was completely removed by polypectomy. The inked margin is seen at the bottom of the field.

Right: The tumor merges with the colonic muscularis mucosae.

obliterating the muscularis mucosae layer and merging with it (fig. 8-25). Two tumors had significant atypia ("symplastic leiomyoma"); mitotic activity was seen in one of these tumors, but not in the other. The lesional cells were uniformly positive for SMA and desmin, and negative for CD34, CD117, and S-100 protein, based on immunohistochemical studies on 20 to 24 cases with each marker. No GISTs were identified among the tumors of muscularis mucosae, and no CD117-positive cells, except mast cells, were seen in the muscularis mucosae layer. None of the patients had morbidity related to the tumor. Based on the authors' follow-up data on 29 patients, leiomyomas of muscularis mucosae are benign and do not transform to malignant neoplasms.

Leiomyosarcomas can also be encountered on colon biopsies (fig. 8-26), where they display the same features as leiomyosarcomas elsewhere in the body (fig. 8-27). Typically they involve the muscularis propria, as do GISTs. They tend to have perfectly perpendicular fascicles of spindle cells, with pleomorphic blunt-ended nuclei like leiomyosarcomas elsewhere in the body. The issue is distinguishing them from GISTs (below), which is usually readily accomplished since they are usually desmin-positive, CD117-negative. They are also more pleomorphic than GISTs. Most stromal tumors in the colorectum are GISTs rather than leiomyosarcomas. Leiomyosarcomas presenting as polypoid lesions may have a better outcome than GISTs but it is difficult to draw meaningful conclusions since leiomyosarcomas of the colorectum are so rare (27).

Small Intestine

Leiomyomas of the small bowel are rare and accounted for only 2.5 percent of smooth muscle and stromal tumors in one series of duodenal tumors (26); rare cases arise in association with muscularis mucosae (fig. 8-28) but most reported examples arise in the muscularis propria (fig. 8-29). The latter are differentiated

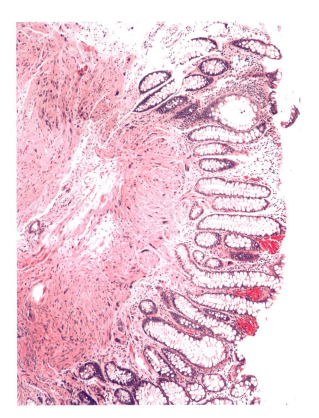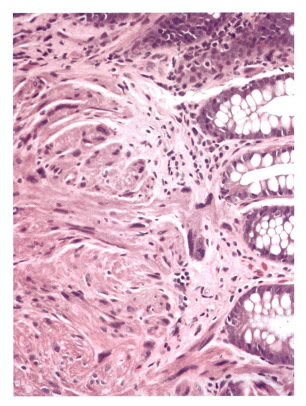

Figure 8-26

LEIOMYOSARCOMA

Left: This tumor extended into the colonic muscularis mucosae and could thereby be diagnosed on a mucosal biopsy. The cells are brightly eosinophilic, similar to the leiomyoma shown in figure 8-25, but their nuclei are large and hyperchromatic.
Right: Large hyperchromatic nuclei are present.

from GISTs because of their low cellularity, bright eosinophilia on routine stains, immuno-reactivity for desmin, and lack of CD117 and CD34 immunostaining (26).

Leiomyosarcomas in this location are similarly rare and show more nuclear pleomorphism when compared to GISTs. Their appearance is the same as that of leiomyosarcoma elsewhere in the body. In addition, they lack skeinoid fibers and are CD117 negative (26).

ADIPOSE TISSUE TUMORS

Submucosal Lipoma and Lipomatous Polyposis

Lipomas are common in the intestines (fig. 8-30). So-called lipomatous hypertrophy, or li-pohyperplasia, of the ileocecal valve is the most common adipose tissue lesion of the intestines but it is probably reflective of herniation of patulous submucosal fat at the site of the ileo-cecal valve rather that true neoplasia. Patients who are obese are more likely to have such a tumor (97). Most persons with this condition are asymptomatic, although intussusception has been documented (97).

Lipomas usually arise in the submucosa of the colon, where they are asymptomatic and detected at routine colonoscopy. They are not common: only one was detected in a study of 5,000 sigmoidoscopies (98). They are far rarer in the small bowel. Multiple lipomas can be a component of the PTEN hamartoma syndrome (99).

Submucosal lipomas are recognized at endos-copy by their yellow color and lack of firmness (whereas neuroendocrine tumors tend to be yellow and firm). They are usually covered by unremarkable mucosa but occasionally there is ulceration. Some can be removed endoscopi-cally although resection is sometimes required for large examples.

Figure 8-27

LEIOMYOSARCOMA

A: This small intestinal leiomyosarcoma has epithelioid features. The tumor is cellular and eosinophilic. It arose in the muscularis propria but has extended into the mucosa at the upper right, infiltrating between crypts.

B: Inclusion-like nucleoli and pink cytoplasm are seen in this epithelioid leiomyosarcoma. Inflammatory cells are rare in the lesion, in contrast to many epithelioid inflammatory myofibroblastic sarcomas (essentially a high-grade inflammatory myofibroblastic tumor), which can have overlapping features.

C: This colonic case contains an anaphase bridge, an indication of chromosome instability and not a feature of translocation-associated sarcomas.

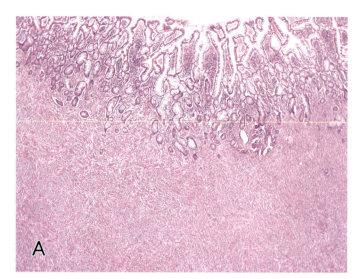

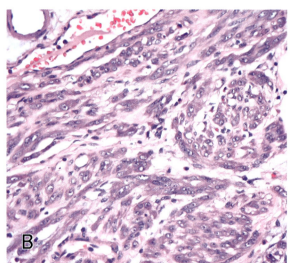

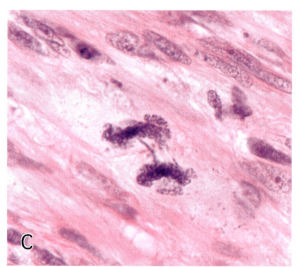

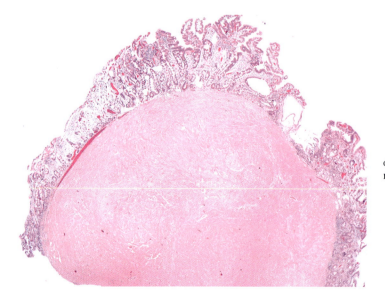

Figure 8-28

LEIOMYOMA

Small intestinal leiomyomas are rare. This one has arisen in association with the muscularis mucosae and extended into the submucosa.

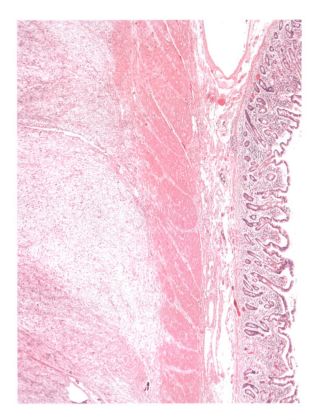
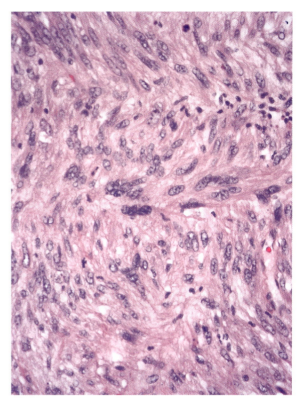

Figure 8-29

LEIOMYOSARCOMA: SMALL INTESTINE

Left: This neoplasm is centered in the muscularis propria.

Right: This degree of nuclear pleomorphism would be unusual for a GIST. The nuclei are blunt ended; in GISTs they are more tapered at their ends.

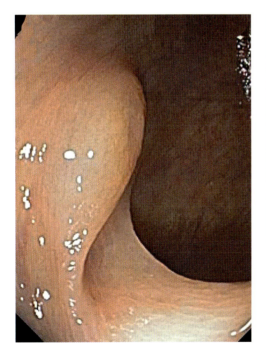
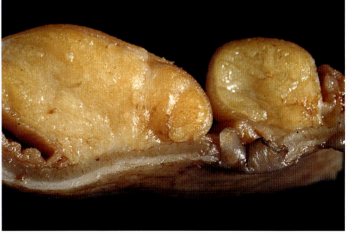

Figure 8-30

SUBMUCOSAL LIPOMA

Left: The overlying mucosa appears normal and glistening endoscopically.

Above: Colon lipomas maintain their oily adipose tissue appearance.

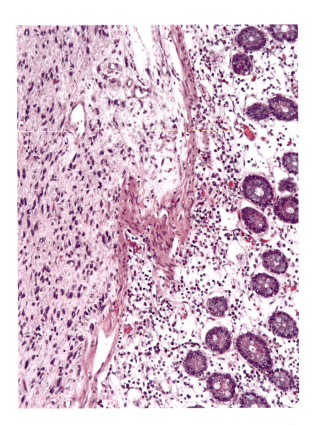 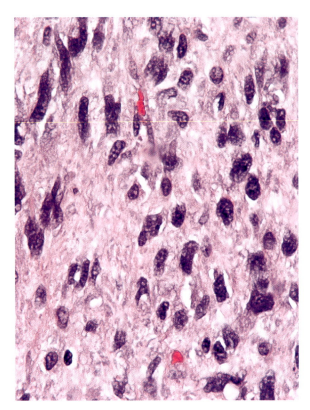

Figure 8-31

DEDIFFERENTIATED LIPOSARCOMA EXTENDING INTO SMALL BOWEL SUBMUCOSA

Left: This sarcoma is impossible to diagnose as such based on this image in isolation, which shows a pleomorphic spindle cell sarcoma proliferating in the submucosa. This component, however, arose in association with a well-differentiated liposarcoma.

Right: At higher magnification, the enlarged hyperchromatic nuclei are seen.

Microscopically, submucosal lipomas essentially consist of mature adipose tissue that cannot always be distinguished from normal submucosal fat on small biopsies. Ulcerated lipomas can display slightly enlarged cells but they lack the intense hyperchromasia associated with well-differentiated liposarcomas.

Liposarcomas

Liposarcomas found in the intestines reflect spread of retroperitoneal well-differentiated or de-differentiated liposarcomas (fig. 8-31) by direct extension or metastases from other types of liposarcomas (myxoid/round cell liposarcoma and pleomorphic liposarcoma). Apparent primary liposarcomas of the intestines are the subject of case reports based on their rarity and all types have been represented, as summarized by others (100). In daily practice, if such a tumor is encountered, it can be expected to be a secondary lesion.

RHABDOMYOSARCOMA

We are unaware of primary *rhabdomyosarcomas* of the colon, although they have been reported in the anal area (101–103) and small bowel (104).

VASCULAR TUMORS AND MIMICS

Angiomas

Lymphangiomas are uncommon benign tumors that occur more commonly in children and can involve any portion of small intestine including the ampulla of Vater (105). The tumor may exude milky fluid upon sectioning. The histologic appearance consists of numerous thin-walled lymphatic spaces filled with proteinaceous material. The vessel walls consist of fibrous tissue and may contain lymphoid aggregates. The term *lymphangiomatosis* has been applied to extensive, diffuse lesions, that

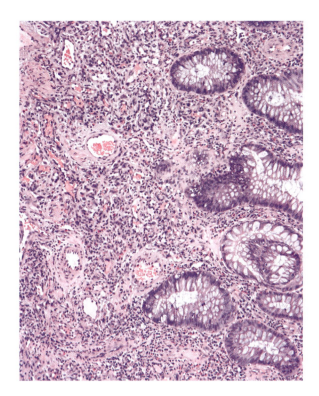 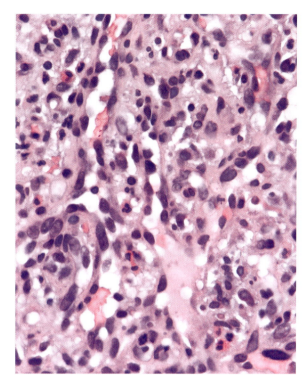

Figure 8-32

CAPILLARY HEMANGIOMA INVOLVING SMALL INTESTINE

Left: The lesion consists of congeries of tiny capillaries, emanating from larger ones. The endothelial cells lining the capillaries are supported by other cell types, a clue to the benign nature.

Right: High-power magnification.

are in a spectrum with vascular malformations (lymphatic malformations). Although lymphangiomas are predominantly located in the submucosa, dilated lymphatic channels may be seen in the lamina propria, allowing diagnosis via endoscopic biopsy.

Hemangiomas are also rarely encountered in biopsies of the small intestine, mainly because biopsies of these lesions may result in significant bleeding. These lesions may be seen in association with syndromic states such as Maffucci and blue rubber bleb nevus syndromes (BRBNS) or as solitary, sporadic lesions. Patients with BRBNS have multiple cutaneous and GI tract hemangiomas. The cutaneous lesions are present at birth and have the appearance of blue rubber blebs, hence the name. The extent of GI involvement may be dramatic and associated with severe GI bleeding and iron deficiency anemia. In some of these cases, the majority of the lesions may be localized in the small bowel and these may be diagnosed via capsule endoscopy (106).

Patients with Maffucci syndrome have multiple enchondromas and cutaneous hemangiomas, which may be quite deforming and asymmetrically involve the hands and feet preferentially. Involvement of the GI tract is much less frequent than in BRBNS, but is documented (107). Patients with Maffucci syndrome, unlike those with BRBNS, are at increased risk for malignancy (bone, vascular, and brain tumors among others).

If a hemangioma is biopsied or resected, histologic exam reveals cavernous vascular channels filled with blood. These are surrounded by an attenuated endothelial lining and a smooth muscle wall involving the submucosa and lamina propria, features that it shares with sporadic angiomas. Rare lesions that appear indistinguishable from capillary hemangiomas elsewhere can be found in the colon as well (fig. 8-32).

A rare variant of hemangioma is the *anastomosing hemangioma* (fig. 8-33) (108), which was first described in the male genital tract and later

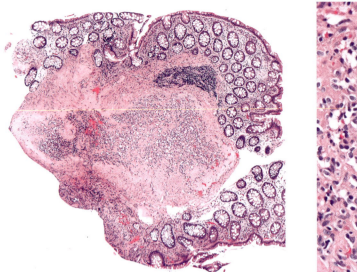 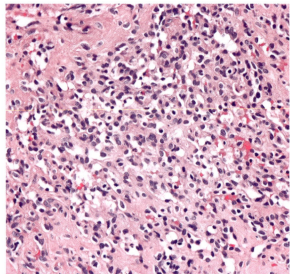

Figure 8-33

ANASTOMOSING HEMANGIOMA OF COLON

Left: The interanastomosing architecture raises the possibility of angiosarcoma, but the vaguely lobulated architecture is against this possibility.

Right: The endothelial cells have a hobnail appearance but they are devoid of mitotic activity and there is a backdrop of supporting cells.

in various other sites. These have been detected on screening colonoscopy in adults (109), presenting as colorectal polyps. They are composed of interanastomosing vessels lined by plump endothelial cells with a hobnail appearance. The vessels can be accompanied by extramedulary hematopoiesis and hyaline globules. The anastomosing appearance can suggest angiosarcoma, but the vessels are associated with supporting cells and the endothelial cells themselves lack mitotic activity, although there can be rare mitoses in the supporting cells that surround the unusual vessels.

Vascular Malformations

Vascular malformations are often best diagnosed on imaging studies and are not often encountered on endoscopic biopsies. When they are, a clue that a lesion is a vascular malformation rather than an hemolymphangioma is finding thick-walled small-caliber vessels in the lamina propria (110). Frequently, however, only an abnormal vascular proliferation on biopsies can be reported (figs. 8-34, 8-35).

Patients with GI tract vascular malformations present with obstruction or occult bleeding.

Vascular malformations of the GI tract tend to present in children and young adults as per their soft tissue counterparts.

Angiosarcoma

Angiosarcoma may involve the GI tract as a primary or metastatic malignancy. Because of its tendency to display epithelioid morphology when involving the GI tract, it may be easily confused with carcinoma. Allison et al. (111) studied a series of 8 GI angiosarcomas, 5 of which involved the small bowel. Of these, 3 were involved as the primary site, 1 represented direct extension from a retroperitoneal primary, and 1 was considered indeterminate because of widely metastatic disease at presentation. The last 3 cases involved the colon. The tumors were seen grossly as red, polypoid mucosal- or serosal-based, hemorrhagic, friable lesions. On histologic exam, the tumors predominantly involved the submucosa. Seven out of 8 cases displayed epithelioid morphology. The tumors were infiltrative and grew as diffuse sheets of epithelioid cells with areas of clefting, which suggested vascular differentiation. In cases where the tumor involved the mucosa, the malignant

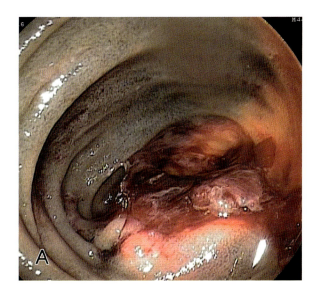

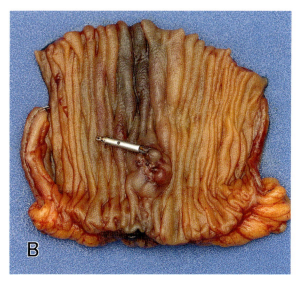

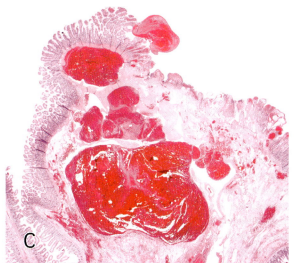

Figure 8-34

VASCULAR MALFORMATION

A: The patient presented with gastrointestinal hemorrhage.

B: Resection was performed to control the hemorrhage. Irregular blood coagulum is seen on the eroded surface.

C: Gaping vessels are seen in the resected small intestinal segment. An eroded area is present at the upper right.

D: This colon resection shows a large vascular malformation extending through all the layers of the bowel.

E: A lymphatic component (seen as delicate translucent blebs with milky fluid at the surface) as well as a venous component are present.

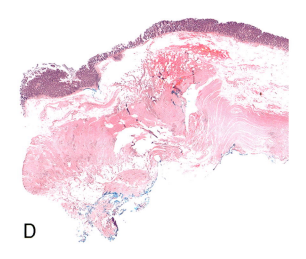

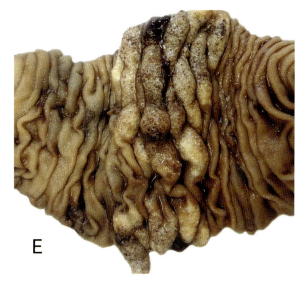

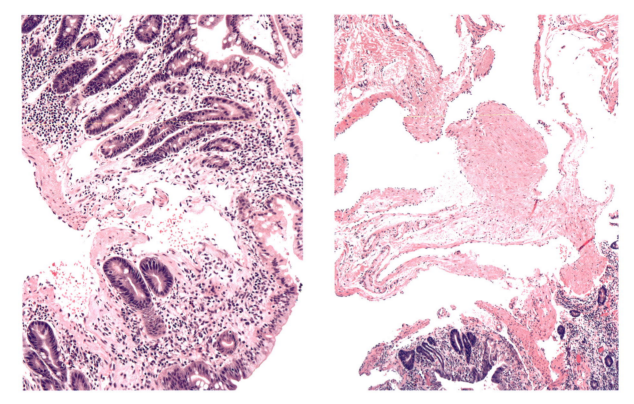

Figure 8-35

VASCULAR MALFORMATION DETECTED ON MUCOSAL BIOPSY

Left: In general, it is unsafe to biopsy such lesions because of the risk of hemorrhage but they sometimes masquerade as solid tumors and are sampled. A clue to the diagnosis is the presence of thick-walled, irregularly shaped lamina propria vessels.

Right: Irregular smooth muscle is present in the walls of the abnormal vascular channels.

cells were seen expanding the lamina propria in association with intact glands or areas of ulceration. Cytologically, the tumors showed uniform, epithelioid cells with eosinophilic cytoplasm and hyperchromatic nuclei with very prominent nucleoli (figs. 8-36, 8-37). Some cells had intracytoplasmic lumens containing red blood cells.

Immunohistochemical staining can lead the unsuspecting observer down the wrong path since the epithelioid variant of angiosarcoma is immunoreactive to AE1/AE3 and may also show immunoreactivity to other keratins such as CAM5.2, CK19, CK7, and EMA. These tumors, however, are consistently negative for CK20 and all are immunoreactive with the vascular markers CD31 (strongly and diffusely), CD34, and factor VIII. None of the examples in the series of Allison et al. (111) was associated with radiation exposure. This tumor displays aggressive behavior and, as a result, appropriate classification is important for prognostication.

A pitfall in diagnosis is the reactive vacular proliferations that are associated with intussusception (figs. 8-37, 8-38) (112). In such cases, the zone near the lead point can show a florid lobular proliferation of small vascular channels lined by plump endothelial cells, extending from the submucosa through the entire thickness of the bowel wall. The endothelial cells display minimal nuclear atypia, and mitotic figures are infrequent. The overlying mucosa is ulcerated, with ischemic-type changes and features of mucosal prolapse.

Kaposi Sarcoma

Similar to the rest of the GI tract, the small bowel and colon may be sites of involvement with *Kaposi sarcoma*, usually in the setting of severe immunosuppression as a result of human immunodeficiency virus (HIV) infection. In the current era of highly active antiretroviral therapy, GI tract Kaposi sarcoma is still detected,

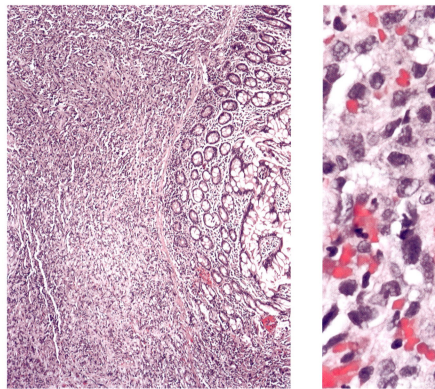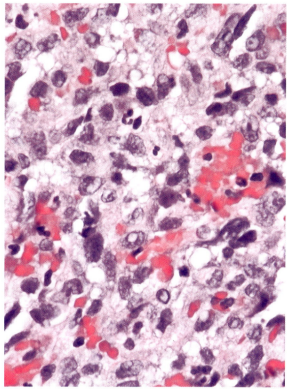

Figure 8-36

ANGIOSARCOMA

Left: Although there are some well-formed vessels, the neoplasm raggedly infiltrates the submucosa of the small bowel, with no lobulation.

Right: High magnification shows sheets of hyperchromatic malignant cells.

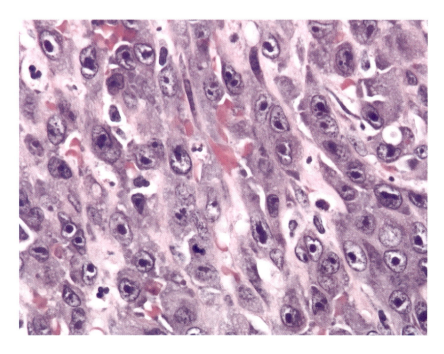

Figure 8-37

ANGIOSARCOMA

This example is epithelioid, a common phenotype for visceral angiosarcomas. These epithelioid angiosarcomas can express keratins, thereby mimicking carcinoma, so their diagnosis requires performance of a panel of immunostains.

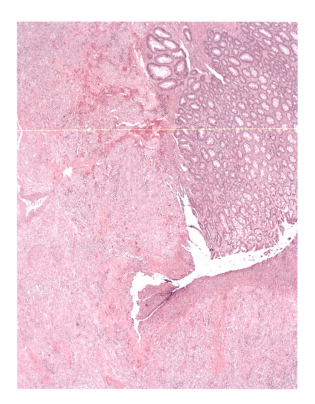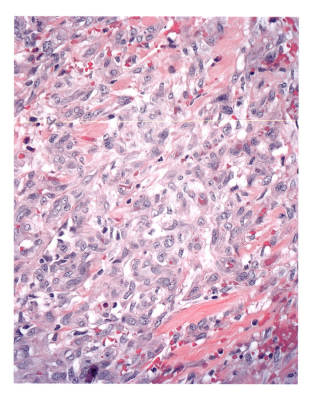

Figure 8-38

REACTIVE VASCULAR PROLIFERATION ASSOCIATED WITH INTUSSUSCEPTION

Left: This lesion is pale at low magnification compared to the angiosarcomas depicted in figures 8-36 and 8-37. It also appears sheet-like but individual vascular channels are seen at the upper right.

Right: Although this focus shows a sheet-like arrangement of the endothelial cells, the cytologic features are bland.

but it is most commonly encountered in the stomach rather than the intestines (113).

GI Kaposi sarcoma has the same appearance as it does in the rest of the body (fig. 8-39). Histologic exam shows a proliferation of human herpesvirus (HHV)8/LANA1- and CD34-reactive spindle cells, usually associated with extravasated red blood cells.

GI Kaposi sarcoma tends to resolve with restitution of immune function regardless of the initial cause of the dysfunction, although most examples are HIV/acquired immunodeficiency syndrome (AIDS)-associated and most gastrointestinal cases can be managed conservatively. Etoposide has been used with efficacy as well.

MESENTERIC TUMORS

Mesenteric Fibromatosis

Mesenteric fibromatosis is probably the most common entity in the intra-abdominal fibro-

matosis group. It usually is a slowly growing mass that involves small bowel mesentery or retroperitoneum, where clinical distinction may become extremely difficult from retroperitoneal fibrosis. There are cases associated with pregnancy and Crohn disease even though most are secondary to trauma in individuals with the appropriate predisposition.

In patients with Gardner syndrome, mesenteric fibromatosis appears to have a substantially higher recurrence rate than in patients without this syndrome. Gardner syndrome is an autosomal dominant familial disease with a female predilection. It consists of numerous colorectal adenomatous polyps, osteomas, cutaneous cysts, soft tissue masses, and other manifestations. Gardner syndrome is related to FAP, a disorder caused by germline adenomatous polyposis coli (*APC*) gene mutations. It is associated with an 8 to 12 percent incidence of developing fibromatosis.

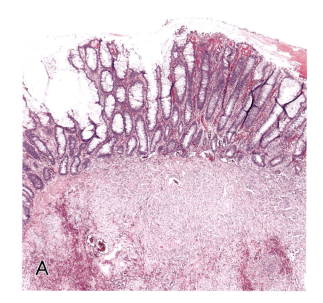

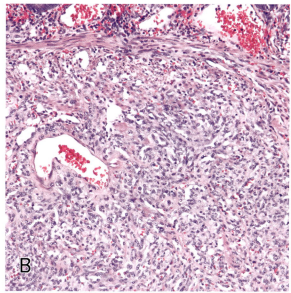

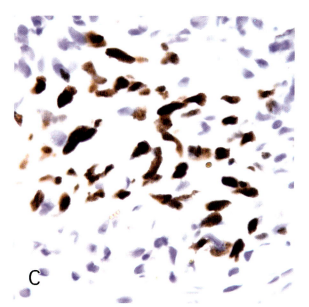

Figure 8-39

KAPOSI SARCOMA INVOLVING COLON

A: At low magnification, the tumor appears similar to the angiosarcoma seen in figure 8-38, but it is less hyperchromatic.

B: The tumor consists of well-formed spindle cells and areas of slit-like spaces.

C: An HHV8/LANA1 immunostain shows strong nuclear labeling.

Among patients with FAP, intestinal and extraintestinal neoplasms typically arise through bi-allelic (germline then somatic) inactivation of the *APC* gene, whereas the corresponding tumors in non-FAP patients occur either through somatic bi-allelic *APC* inactivation or somatic mutation of a single *CTNNB1* (the gene that encodes for β-catenin) allele.

Somatic alterations of the APC/β-catenin pathway were initially detected in the familial tumors and then subsequently demonstrated in the sporadic counterparts. The first tumors studied were GI adenomas, followed by des-

moid tumors, medulloblastomas, childhood hepatoblastomas, gastric fundic gland polyps, and nasopharyngeal angiofibromas, all of which occur more frequently in FAP patients than in controls. It has been estimated that FAP patients in general have an 852-fold increased risk of developing desmoid tumors, typically intra-abdominal lesions (114).

Mesenteric fibromatosis involves the mesentery and often infiltrates into the muscularis propria, but seldom into the submucosa or mucosa. Grossly, the tumor is firm with coarse white trabeculation resembling a scar and has

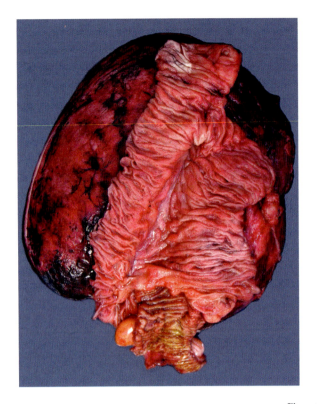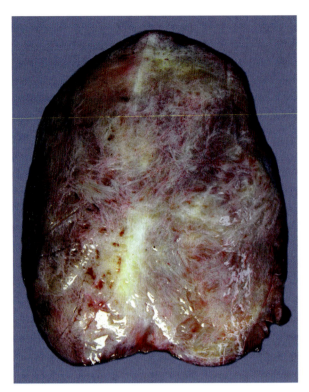

Figure 8-40

MESENTERIC FIBROMATOSIS EXTENDING INTO SMALL BOWEL

Left: The lesion forms a large well-circumscribed mass.
Right: The cut surface is densely fibrotic.

a gritty sensation when cut. Microscopically (figs. 8-40, 8-41), the lesion is poorly defined, with infiltrative margins consisting of spindled fibroblasts separated by abundant collagen. Cells and collagen are organized in parallel arrays. Keloid-like collagen and hyalinization may be so extensive as to obscure the original pattern of the tumor.

Scattered thin-walled, elongated, and compressed vessels are usually seen with focal areas of hemorrhage, lymphoid aggregates, and, rarely, calcification or chondro-osseous metaplasia. Typically the vessels, although thin-walled, appear conspicuous at scanning magnification. The nuclei of the proliferating lesion are typically tinctorially lighter than those of the endothelial cells and the smooth muscle cytoplasm in the vessel walls is pinker than the surrounding myo-fibroblastic cytoplasm of the tumor cells. Mitotic figures are infrequent. Mesenteric examples often have a storiform pattern similar to that of nodular fasciitis in the soft tissue of the extremities.

Since fibromatoses are myofibroblastic, they express actin but usually not desmin or CD34. These tumors frequently need to be distinguished from GISTs. Although their features are readily distinguishable on routine hematoxylin and eosin (H&E)-stained slides, pathologists should be aware that fibromatoses may react with some commercially available CD117 antibodies. Staining is typically weaker than that seen with true GISTs but in doubtful cases, β-catenin staining can be helpful, since nuclear staining is only seen in desmoid tumors (115).

Fibromatoses are treated surgically but frequently persist. Incomplete excision results in recurrences and intra-abdominal tumors can be challenging to fully resect. Treatment includes radiation therapy, high intensity focused ultrasound (116), hormone-directed therapy (since these tumors have estrogen receptors), nonsteroidal anti-inflammatory drugs, and chemotherapy, even including tyrosine kinase inhibitors (117).

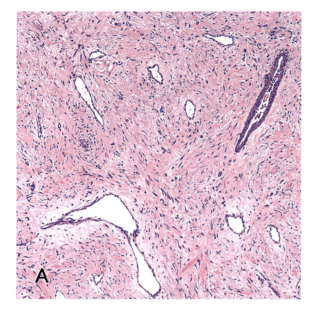

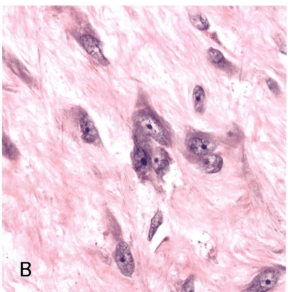

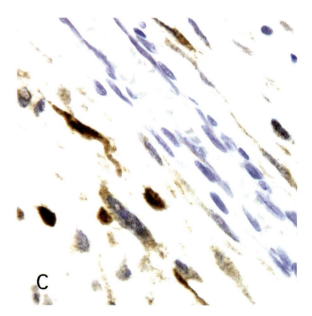

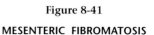

Figure 8-41

MESENTERIC FIBROMATOSIS

A: The tumor consists of stellate to spindle cells that are pale and uniformly spaced between collagen. The blood vessels are small but appear conspicuous because their slender walls are more brightly eosinophilic than the surrounding lesions. One at the lower left gapes open as though pulled open by the dense collagen.

B: Some of the cells have stellate cytoplasm. Delicate round nucleoli present in nearly every nucleus.

C: The capillary coursing diagonally from the upper left of the field to the lower right contains erythrocytes. The nuclei of the capillary cells are nonreactive (internal negative control) whereas some (but not all of the tumor nuclei are reactive. Seeing even focal nuclear labeling in the absence of nuclear labeling in endothelial cells may help confirm a diagnosis of fibromatosis (beta-catenin immunostain).

Inflammatory Myofibroblastic Tumor

Although *inflammatory myofibroblastic tumor* and so-called *inflammatory fibrosarcoma* were originally described as separate entities, they are now recognized as ends of a spectrum of tumors with a common molecular profile and grouped together by the World Health Organization (WHO) (118). Gene fusions involving the anaplastic lymphoma kinase (*ALK*) gene at chromosome 2p23 have been known for years (119,120). In their original description, these tumors were termed "inflamma-tory fibrosarcoma" (121). They are most common in childhood but with a wide age range.

Inflammatory myofibrotic tumor arises within the abdomen, involving mesentery, omentum, and retroperitoneum (over 80 percent of cases), with occasional cases in the mediastinum, abdominal wall, and liver. Sometimes there are associated systemic symptoms. The tumor can be solitary or multinodular (30 percent), and up to 20 cm in diameter.

The tumor is composed of myofibroblasts and fibroblasts in fascicles or whorls, with variable background inflammation (fig. 8-42).

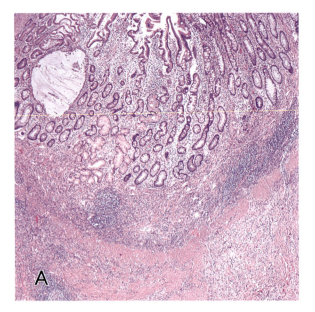

Figure 8-42

INFLAMMATORY MYOFIBROBLASTIC TUMOR

A: This inflammatory lesion extends from the mesentery into the small bowel. Overlying pyloric metaplasia is seen at the left center of the field.

B: The tumor consists of myofibroblastic cells, many with prominent nucleoli reminiscent of those seen in fibromatosis, in a background of prominent lymphoplasmacytic inflammation.

C: An ALK stain highlights the cytoplasm of the tumor cells.

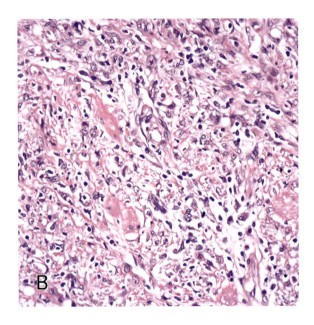

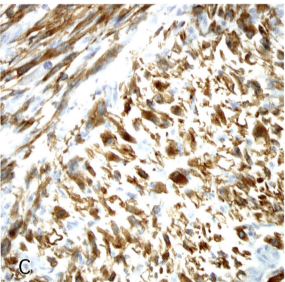

Pleomorphism is moderate, but mitoses are infrequently seen. There is a variable but often marked inflammatory infiltrate, predominantly plasmacytic, but with some lymphocytes and occasionally neutrophils or eosinophils. Fibrosis and calcification can be seen in the stroma.

Immunostaining is positive for SMA and many examples express cytokeratin, especially where there is submesothelial extension. ALK is detected immunohistochemically in 60 to 70 percent of cases, a finding that can be exploited for diagnosis and possibly prognosis (positive cases may have a better prognosis) (122). The tumors invade adjacent viscera; occasional examples metastasize and are aggressive but most are treated surgically and have indolent behavior.

A separate, more aggressive form of inflammatory myofibroblastic tumor (fig. 8-43) has been termed *epithelioid inflammatory myofibroblastic sarcoma*. It is characterized by an unusual nuclear membrane or perinuclear pattern of ALK expression and more aggressive clinical behavior than the classic form (123).

Inflammatory myofibroblastic tumors are generally managed surgically, but the presence of ALK and other tyrosine kinase rearrangements

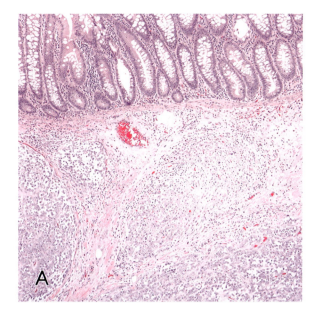

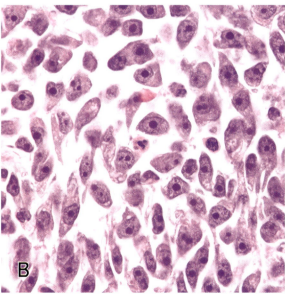

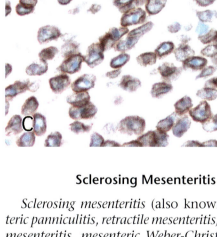

Figure 8-43

EPITHELIOID INFLAMMATORY MYOFIBROBLASTIC SARCOMA

A: This tumor is essentially a very aggressive form of inflammatory myofibroblastic tumor. Its appearance is similar to that of epithelioid leiomyosarcoma but the latter tends to be infiltrated with neutrophils and often labels with ALK.

B: Inclusion-like nucleoli are seen.

C: This example demonstrates a curious perinuclear labeling pattern on ALK immunostaining.

has allowed them to be treated with specific targeted therapy. About half of these tumors harbor *ALK* rearrangements with a host of fusion partners. Such tumors respond to treatment with crizotinib (124-128), including the more aggressive epithelioid inflammatory myofibroblastic sarcoma variant (which tends to be centered in the mesentery and omentum). About 10 percent of these tumors have *ROS1* rearrangements (129,130); these fusions tend to be found in tumors from children and are also amenable to crizotinib treatment.

Sclerosing Mesenteritis

Sclerosing mesenteritis (also known as *mesenteric panniculitis, retractile mesenteritis, liposclerotic mesenteritis, mesenteric Weber-Christian disease, xanthogranulomatous mesenteritis, mesenteric lipogranuloma, systemic nodular panniculitis, inflammatory pseudotumor,* and *mesenteric lipodystrophy*) most commonly affects the mesentery of the small bowel (131,132). It presents as an isolated large mass, although about 20 percent of patients have multiple lesions. The etiology remains unknown; it is assumed to reflect a reparative

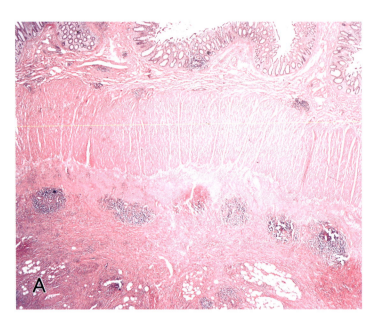

Figure 8-44

SCLEROSING MESENTERITIS

A: These lesions feature prominent fat necrosis and have also been called mesenteric panniculitis.

B: There is prominent fat necrosis.

C: Occasionally, these tumors display obliterative phlebitis, similar to the lesions found in IgG4-related fibrosclerosing disease, but they differ by lacking the storiform fibrosis. These tumors do not respond to steroid treatment.

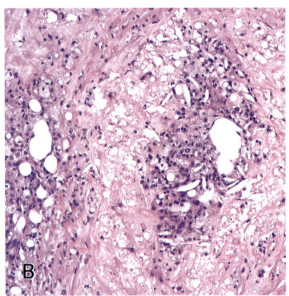

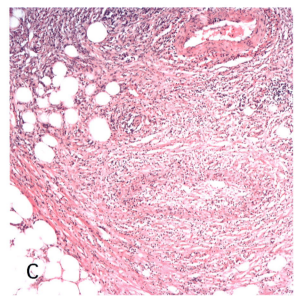

response although the stimulus is not clear. Prior trauma/surgery is usually not reported.

Lesions consist of fibrous bands infiltrating and encasing fat lobules, with an associated admixture of inflammatory cells, typically lymphocytes, plasma cells, and eosinophils (fig. 8-44). Sometimes these lesions have prominent IgG4-reactive plasma cells and they often display a lymphocytic phlebitis pattern similar to that in lymphoplasmacytic pancreatitis and retroperitoneal fibrosis (133). There seems to be some relationship between sclerosing mesenteritis and the family of "IgG4-related sclerosing disorders." In contrast to the latter, however, sclerosing mesenteritis usually does not respond to steroids and is less likely to display prominent IgG4 labeling.

This process is benign but a few affected patients die of complications, such as small bowel obstruction. The disease does not typically progress or recur, and the patients' symptoms are relieved by resection.

Calcifying Fibrous Pseudotumor

Calcifying fibrous pseudotumor was originally described as a childhood fibrous tumor with psammoma bodies (134). It is a rare, benign

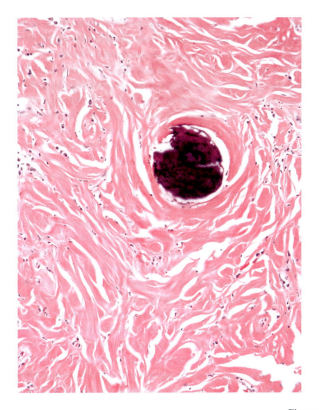 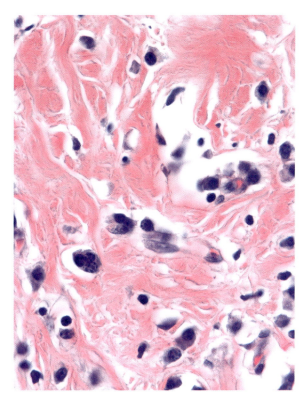

Figure 8-45

CALCIFYING FIBROUS PSEUDOTUMOR

Left: These tumors are paucicellular and contain psammomatous and dystrophic calcifications. They are densely collagenized and lightly sprinkled with plasma cells and occasional lymphocytes. They can arise in crops in the viscera but are benign.

Right: The tumoral fibroblasts appear benign.

fibrous lesion. Most soft tissue examples affect children and young adults without gender predilection, whereas visceral examples usually occur in adults. These tumors were originally described in the subcutaneous and deep soft tissues (extremities, trunk, neck, and scrotum) but have subsequently been reported all over the body, notably in the mesentery, peritoneum, and pleura (sometimes as multiple lesions) (118). Visceral examples may produce site-specific symptoms.

Radiographs show well-marginated, noncalcified tumors. Calcifications are apparent on CT and may be thick and band-like or punctuate. On MRI, the masses appear similar to fibromatoses, with a mottled appearance and a signal closer to that of muscle than fat. Although cases have followed trauma and occurred in association with Castleman disease and inflammatory myofibroblastic tumors, the pathogenesis remains unknown.

Grossly, these lesions are well-marginated but unencapsulated, ranging in size from less than 1 to 15 cm. Some show indistinct boundaries, with infiltration into the surrounding tissues. On occasion, a gritty texture is noted on sectioning, which reveals a firm white lesion.

Microscopically, calcifying fibrous tumor consists of well-circumscribed, unencapsulated, paucicellular, hyalinized fibrosclerotic tissue with a variable inflammatory infiltrate consisting of lymphocytes and plasma cells (fig. 8-45). Lymphoid aggregates may be present. Calcifications, both psammomatous and dystrophic, are scattered throughout.

Lesional cells express vimentin and factor XIIIa, but usually lack actins, desmin, factor VIII, S-100 protein, neurofilament protein, cytokeratins, CD34, and CD31. The immunophenotype differs from that of inflammatory myofibroblastic tumors in that most calcifying

337

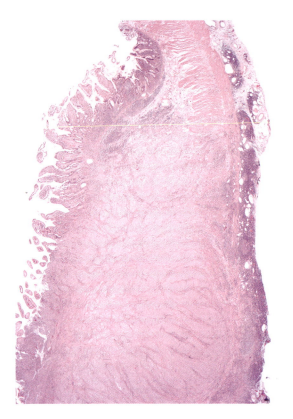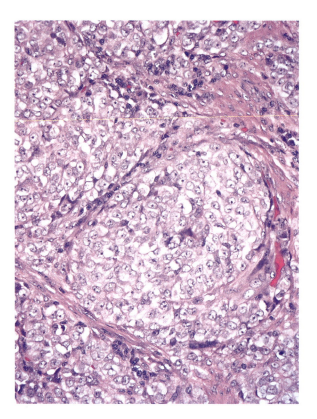

Figure 8-46

CLEAR CELL SARCOMA-LIKE TUMOR

Left: The ileum is the usual location, as in this case. The tumor has a nested appearance and is centered in the muscularis propria.
Right: The cells are uniform, an important feature of translocation-associated sarcomas.

fibrous pseudotumors lack actin and anaplastic lymphoma kinase (ALK). Occasional lesions express CD34. These tumors are benign; occasional recurrences are recorded.

TRANSLOCATION-ASSOCIATED SARCOMAS

There are several clues that can help in interpreting spindle cell tumors in the GI tract. The first is shown in Table 8-1, namely, that knowing which types of tumors are encountered in which layer (i.e., mucosa, submucosa, muscularis propria, serosa) can help suggest the type of tumor. The other is that sarcomas with characteristic translocations and gene fusions tend to have uniform cells, as do many neoplasms with characteristic mutations and fusions. For example, both inflammatory fibroid polyp and most GISTs have uniform cells without nuclear pleomorphism and without atypical mitoses. Inflammatory fibroid polyp is most commonly a submucosal gastric lesion, but it can be found in

the small bowel and colon; small bowel examples harbor *PDGFRA* mutations, a feature they share with gastric GISTs (which usually arise in the muscularis propria), but they are always benign.

The rare *translocation sarcomas* encountered in the small bowel (and rarely, the colon) follow this rule, but may require molecular techniques to confidently diagnose. For example, *Ewing sarcoma/ primitive neuroectodermal tumor* is rare in small intestinal samples (135,136), where it has the same characteristics as lesions elsewhere, namely labeling for CD99 and a small round cell phenotype, but in this location, it is usually only considered after an extensive immunolabeling panel is directed at small cell carcinoma and lymphomas.

GI-type clear cell sarcoma is fairly well described (figs. 8-46, 8-47). The classic location is the ileum and the patients tend to be young adults. The lesions consist of sheets of rounded to slightly spindled cells that are uniform. Sometimes there is a slightly nodular appearance and

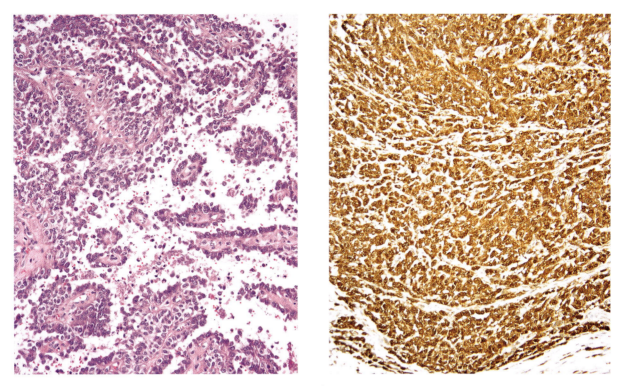

Figure 8-47

CLEAR CELL SARCOMA-LIKE TUMOR

Left: This example has a pseudopapillary appearance.
Right: These tumors strongly express S-100 protein.

some cases show cells with prominent uniform nucleoli. The lesional cells express S-100 protein but not invariably HMB45 or other so-called melanoma markers. This feature distinguishes them from clear cell sarcoma of the soft tissues, which usually express melanoma markers in addition to S-100 protein. While most soft tissue clear cell sarcomas have *EWSR1-ATF1* gene rearrangements, those in the GI tract often have *EWSR1-CREB1* rearrangements (137).

Clear cell sarcoma-like tumors tend to have overlapping features with neuroendocrine tumors, a concern that can be compounded by their synaptophysin labeling, but they lack keratins and show strong S-100 protein expression. They also overlap with metastatic melanoma and some cases require molecular confirmation. They are unlikely to express CD117. GI clear cell sarcomas are aggressive lesions. Some observers have suggesting renaming them malignant gastrointestinal neuroectodermal tumor (138). Regardless, they are worth separating from Ewing sarcoma (fig. 8-48) even if molecular testing

is required because the latter responds to treatment and clear cell sarcoma-like tumor of the GI tract does not. It is associated with a dismal outcome (138).

Rare cases of *low-grade fibromyxoid sarcoma* (which has a t(7;16) (q32-34;p11) or t(11;16) (p11;p11) translocation, resulting in *FUS-CREB3L2* or *FUS-CREB3L1*, have also been reported in the bowel (139), where they are centered in the mesentery and muscularis propria (figs. 8-49, 8-50). They appear similar to fibromatoses but differ by featuring more hyperchromatic nuclei.

Pseudosarcomatous Changes in Ulcers and Polyps

It is important to note that ulcers and polyps in the gastrointestinal tract can display striking pseudosarcomatous changes, which readily mimic carcinomas. These cells are arranged in a rind at the interface between the viable and nonviable tissue and can be ignored (fig. 8-51). If immunolabeling is performed, they lack expression of keratins and S-100 protein.

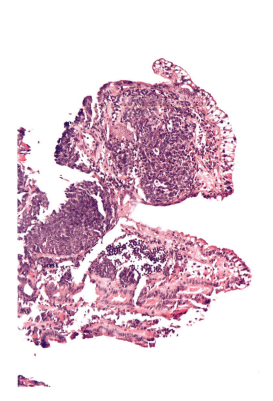

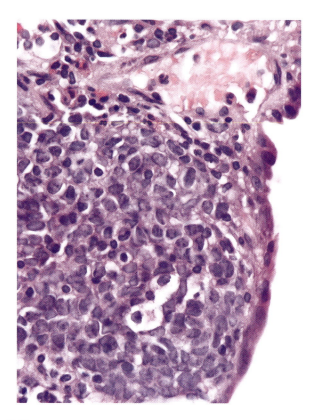

Figure 8-48

EWING SARCOMA PRIMARY IN DUODENUM

Left: These tumors are rare in the gastrointestinal tract but are important to identify as they are treated with specific protocols. The malignant cells are very uniform.

Right: The cells are primitive but extremely monotonous. A few lymphocytes and the endothelial cells at the top of the field serve as internal size controls. The tumor cell nuclei are small.

Figure 8-49

LOW-GRADE FIBROMYXOID SARCOMA INVOLVING COLONIC MESENTERY

These tumors are deceptively bland and known to mimic fibromatoses but the cellularity is variable throughout the lesion whereas fibromatoses have uniform cellularity.

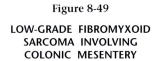

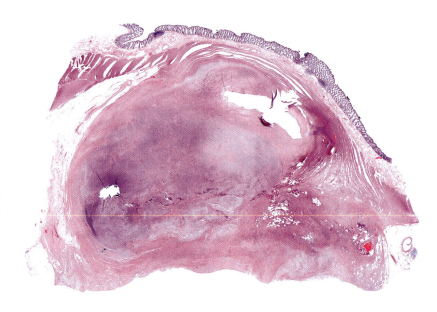

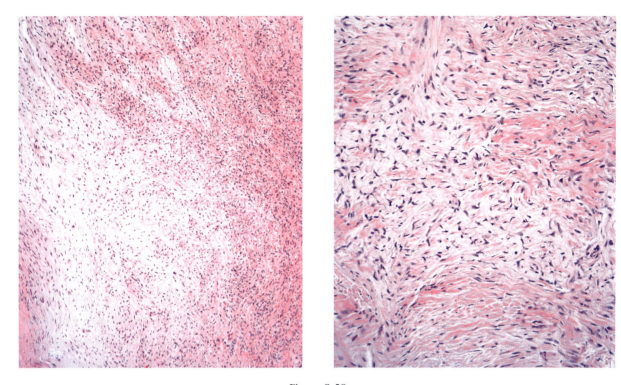

Figure 8-50

LOW-GRADE FIBROMYXOID SARCOMA INVOLVING COLONIC MESENTERY

Left: A fibrous area is at the upper right and a myxoid zone at the lower left.

Right: The architecture has a swirled appearance. Since this is a translocation-associated sarcoma, the nuclei are uniform.

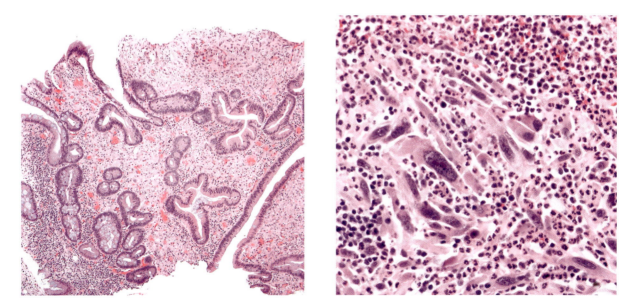

Figure 8-51

PSEUDOSARCOMATOUS STROMAL CHANGES

Left: This inflammatory polyp displays expansion of the lamina propria just under denuded surface by spindle cells restricted to a small area.

Right: The cytologic features are alarming, but there is a low nuclear cytoplasmic ratio.

REFERENCES

1. Miettinen M, Lasota J. Gastrointestinal stromal tumors. Gastroenterol Clin North Am 2013;42:399-415.
2. Kindblom LG, Remotti HE, Aldenborg F, Meis-Kindblom JM. Gastrointestinal pacemaker cell tumor (GIPACT): gastrointestinal stromal tumors show phenotypic characteristics of the interstitial cells of Cajal. Am J Pathol 1998;152:1259-1269.
3. Hameed M, Corless C, George S, et al. Template for reporting results of biomarker testing of specimens from patients with gastrointestinal stromal tumors. Arch Pathol Lab Med 2015;139:1271-1275.
4. Miettinen M, Lasota J. Gastrointestinal stromal tumors: review on morphology, molecular pathology, prognosis, and differential diagnosis. Arch Pathol Lab Med 2006;130:1466-1478.
5. Miettinen M, Lasota J. Gastrointestinal stromal tumors: pathology and prognosis at different sites. Semin Diagn Pathol 2006;23:70-83.
6. Miettinen M, Fetsch JF, Sobin LH, Lasota J. Gastrointestinal stromal tumors in patients with neurofibromatosis 1: a clinicopathologic and molecular genetic study of 45 cases. Am J Surg Pathol 2006;30:90-96.
7. Carney JA, Sheps SG, Go VL, Gordon H. The triad of gastric leiomyosarcoma, functioning extra-adrenal paraganglioma and pulmonary chondroma. N Engl J Med 1977;296:1517-1518.
8. Belinsky MG, Rink L, von Mehren M. Succinate dehydrogenase deficiency in pediatric and adult gastrointestinal stromal tumors. Front Oncol 2013;3:117.
9. Bolland M, Benn D, Croxson M, et al. Gastrointestinal stromal tumour in succinate dehydrogenase subunit B mutation-associated familial phaeochromocytoma/paraganglioma. ANZ J Surg 2006;76:763-764.
10. Celestino R, Lima J, Faustino A, et al. Molecular alterations and expression of succinate dehydrogenase complex in wild-type KIT/PDGFRA/BRAF gastrointestinal stromal tumors. Eur J Hum Genet 2013;21:503-510.
11. Doyle LA, Hornick JL. Gastrointestinal stromal tumours: from KIT to succinate dehydrogenase. Histopathology 2014;64(1):53-67.
12. Doyle LA, Nelson D, Heinrich MC, Corless CL, Hornick JL. Loss of succinate dehydrogenase subunit B (SDHB) expression is limited to a distinctive subset of gastric wild-type gastrointestinal stromal tumours: a comprehensive genotype-phenotype correlation study. Histopathology 2012;61:801-809.
13. Dwight T, Benn DE, Clarkson A, et al. Loss of SDHA expression identifies SDHA mutations in succinate dehydrogenase-deficient gastrointestinal stromal tumors. Am J Surg Pathol 2013;37:226-233.
14. Janeway KA, Kim SY, Lodish M, et al. Defects in succinate dehydrogenase in gastrointestinal stromal tumors lacking KIT and PDGFRA mutations. Proc Natl Acad Sci U S A 2011;108:314-318.
15. Jove M, Mora J, Sanjuan X, et al. Simultaneous KIT mutation and succinate dehydrogenase (SDH) deficiency in a patient with a gastrointestinal stromal tumour and Carney-Stratakis syndrome: a case report. Histopathology 2014;65:712-717.
16. Killian JK, Kim SY, Miettinen M, et al. Succinate dehydrogenase mutation underlies global epigenomic divergence in gastrointestinal stromal tumor. Cancer Discov 2013;3:648-657.
17. Mason EF, Hornick JL. Succinate dehydrogenase deficiency is associated with decreased 5-hydroxymethylcytosine production in gastrointestinal stromal tumors: implications for mechanisms of tumorigenesis. Mod Pathol 2013;26:1492-1497.
18. Miettinen M, Killian JK, Wang ZF, et al. Immunohistochemical loss of succinate dehydrogenase subunit A (SDHA) in gastrointestinal stromal tumors (GISTs) signals SDHA germline mutation. Am J Surg Pathol 2013;37:234-240.
19. Miettinen M, Lasota J. Succinate dehydrogenase deficient gastrointestinal stromal tumors (GISTs)—a review. Int J Biochem Cell Biol 2014;53:514-519.
20. Nannini M, Astolfi A, Paterini P, et al. Expression of IGF-1 receptor in KIT/PDGF receptor-alpha wild-type gastrointestinal stromal tumors with succinate dehydrogenase complex dysfunction. Future Oncol 2013;9:121-126.
21. Pantaleo MA, Nannini M, Astolfi A, Biasco G, Bologna GSG. A distinct pediatric-type gastrointestinal stromal tumor in adults: potential role of succinate dehydrogenase subunit A mutations. Am J Surg Pathol 2011;35:1750-1752.
22. Wang JH, Lasota J, Miettinen M. Succinate dehydrogenase subunit B (SDHB) Is expressed in neurofibromatosis 1-associated gastrointestinal stromal tumors (GISTs): Implications for the sdhb expression based classification of GISTs. J Cancer 2011;2:90-93.
23. Ricci R. Syndromic gastrointestinal stromal tumors. Hered Cancer Clin Pract 2016;14:15.
24. Xing GS, Wang S, Sun YM, Yuan Z, Zhao XM, Zhou CW. Small Bowel stromal tumors: different clinicopathologic and computed tomography features in various anatomic sites. PLoS One 2015;10:e0144277.

25. Miettinen M, Makhlouf H, Sobin LH, Lasota J. Gastrointestinal stromal tumors of the jejunum and ileum: a clinicopathologic, immunohistochemical, and molecular genetic study of 906 cases before imatinib with long-term follow-up. Am J Surg Pathol 2006;30:477-489.

26. Miettinen M, Kopczynski J, Makhlouf HR, et al. Gastrointestinal stromal tumors, intramural leiomyomas, and leiomyosarcomas in the duodenum: a clinicopathologic, immunohistochemical, and molecular genetic study of 167 cases. Am J Surg Pathol 2003;27:625-641.

27. Miettinen M, Furlong M, Sarlomo-Rikala M, Burke A, Sobin LH, Lasota J. Gastrointestinal stromal tumors, intramural leiomyomas, and leiomyosarcomas in the rectum and anus: a clinicopathologic, immunohistochemical, and molecular genetic study of 144 cases. Am J Surg Pathol 2001;25:1121-1133.

28. Tworek JA, Goldblum JR, Weiss SW, Greenson JK, Appelman HD. Stromal tumors of the abdominal colon: a clinicopathologic study of 20 cases. Am J Surg Pathol 1999;23:937-945.

29. Gold JS, Gonen M, Gutierrez A, et al. Development and validation of a prognostic nomogram for recurrence-free survival after complete surgical resection of localised primary gastrointestinal stromal tumour: a retrospective analysis. Lancet Oncol 2009;10:1045-1052.

30. Herawi M, Montgomery EA, Epstein JI. Gastrointestinal stromal tumors (GISTs) on prostate needle biopsy: A clinicopathologic study of 8 cases. Am J Surg Pathol 2006;30:1389-1395.

31. Miettinen M, Sarlomo-Rikala M, Sobin LH, Lasota J. Gastrointestinal stromal tumors and leiomyosarcomas in the colon: a clinicopathologic, immunohistochemical, and molecular genetic study of 44 cases. Am J Surg Pathol 2000;24:1339-1352.

32. Agaimy A, Pelz AF, Wieacker P, Roessner A, Wunsch PH, Schneider-Stock R. Gastrointestinal stromal tumors of the vermiform appendix: clinicopathologic, immunohistochemical, and molecular study of 2 cases with literature review. Hum Pathol 2008;39:1252-1257.

33. Chun JM, Lim KH. Gastrointestinal stromal tumor of the vermiform appendix mimicking Meckel's diverticulum: Case report with literature review. Int J Surg Case Rep 2016;21:20-22.

34. Miettinen M, Sobin LH. Gastrointestinal stromal tumors in the appendix: a clinicopathologic and immunohistochemical study of four cases. Am J Surg Pathol 2001;25:1433-1437.

35. Tran S, Dingeldein M, Mengshol SC, Kay S, Chin AC. Incidental GIST after appendectomy in a pediatric patient: a first instance and review of pediatric patients with CD117 confirmed GISTs. Pediatr Surg Int 2014;30:457-466.

36. Vassos N, Agaimy A, Gunther K, Hohenberger W, Schneider-Stock R, Croner RS. A novel complex KIT mutation in a gastrointestinal stromal tumor of the vermiform appendix. Hum Pathol 2013;44:651-655.

37. Herrera GA, Pinto de Moraes H, Grizzle WE, Han SG. Malignant small bowel neoplasm of enteric plexus derivation (plexosarcoma). Light and electron microscopic study confirming the origin of the neoplasm. Dig Dis Sci 1984;29:275-284.

38. Walker P, Dvorak AM. Gastrointestinal autonomic nerve (GAN) tumor. Ultrastructural evidence for a newly recognized entity. Arch Pathol Lab Med 1986;110:309-316.

39. Antonescu CR, Romeo S, Zhang L, et al. Dedifferentiation in gastrointestinal stromal tumor to an anaplastic KIT-negative phenotype: a diagnostic pitfall: morphologic and molecular characterization of 8 cases occurring either de novo or after imatinib therapy. Am J Surg Pathol 2013;37:385-392.

40. Espinosa I, Lee CH, Kim MK, et al. A novel monoclonal antibody against DOG1 is a sensitive and specific marker for gastrointestinal stromal tumors. Am J Surg Pathol 2008;32:210-218.

41. Gomez-Pinilla PJ, Gibbons SJ, Bardsley MR, et al. Ano1 is a selective marker of interstitial cells of Cajal in the human and mouse gastrointestinal tract. Am J Physiol Gastrointest Liver Physiol 2009;296:G1370-1381.

42. West RB, Corless CL, Chen X, et al. The novel marker, DOG1, is expressed ubiquitously in gastrointestinal stromal tumors irrespective of KIT or PDGFRA mutation status. Am J Pathol 2004;165:107-113.

43. Fletcher CD, Berman JJ, Corless C, et al. Diagnosis of gastrointestinal stromal tumors: A consensus approach. Hum Pathol 2002;33:459-465.

44. AJCC Cancer Staging Manual. Seventh ed. New York: Springer; 2010.

45. Bischof DA, Kim Y, Behman R, et al. A nomogram to predict disease-free survival after surgical resection of GIST. J Gastrointest Surg 2014;18:2123-2129.

46. Bischof DA, Kim Y, Dodson R, et al. Conditional disease-free survival after surgical resection of gastrointestinal stromal tumors: a multi-institutional analysis of 502 patients. JAMA Surg 2015;150:299-306.

47. Corless CL. Gastrointestinal stromal tumors: what do we know now? Mod Pathol 2014;27(Suppl 1):S1-16.

48. Falchook GS, Trent JC, Heinrich MC, et al. BRAF mutant gastrointestinal stromal tumor: first report of regression with BRAF inhibitor dabrafenib (GSK2118436) and whole exomic sequencing for analysis of acquired resistance. Oncotarget 2013;4:310-315.

49. DeMatteo RP, Ballman KV, Antonescu CR, et al. Long-term results of adjuvant imatinib mesylate in localized, high-risk, primary gastrointestinal stromal tumor: ACOSOG Z9000 (Alliance) intergroup phase 2 trial. Ann Surg 2013;258:422-429.

50. Vanek J. Gastric submucosal granuloma with eosinophilic infiltration. Am J Pathol 1949;25:397-411.

51. Helwig EB, Ranier A. Inflammatory fibroid polyps of the stomach. Surg Gynecol Obstet 1953;96:335-367.

52. Johnstone JM, Morson BC. Inflammatory fibroid polyp of the gastrointestinal tract. Histopathology 1978;2:349-361.

53. Liu TC, Lin MT, Montgomery EA, Singhi AD. Inflammatory fibroid polyps of the gastrointestinal tract: spectrum of clinical, morphologic, and immunohistochemistry features. Am J Surg Pathol 2013;37:586-592.

54. Allibone RO, Nanson JK, Anthony PP. Multiple and recurrent inflammatory fibroid polyps in a Devon family ('Devon polyposis syndrome'): an update. Gut 1992;33:1004-1005.

55. Righetti L, Parolini F, Cengia P, et al. Inflammatory fibroid polyps in children: a new case report and a systematic review of the pediatric literature. J Clin Pediatr 2015;4:160-166.

56. Lasota J, Wang ZF, Sobin LH, Miettinen M. Gain-of-function PDGFRA mutations, earlier reported in gastrointestinal stromal tumors, are common in small intestinal inflammatory fibroid polyps. A study of 60 cases. Mod Pathol 2009;22:1049-1056.

57. Pantanowitz L, Antonioli DA, Pinkus GS, Shahsafaei A, Odze RD. Inflammatory fibroid polyps of the gastrointestinal tract: evidence for a dendritic cell origin. Am J Surg Pathol 2004;28:107-114.

58. Schildhaus HU, Cavlar T, Binot E, Buttner R, Wardelmann E, Merkelbach-Bruse S. Inflammatory fibroid polyps harbour mutations in the platelet-derived growth factor receptor alpha (PDGFRA) gene. The J Pathol 2008;216:176-182.

59. Agaimy A, Markl B, Kitz J, et al. Peripheral nerve sheath tumors of the gastrointestinal tract: a multicenter study of 58 patients including NF1-associated gastric schwannoma and unusual morphologic variants. Virchows Arch 2010;456:411-422.

60. Voltaggio L, Murray R, Lasota J, Miettinen M. Gastric schwannoma: a clinicopathologic study of 51 cases and critical review of the literature. Hum Pathol 2012;43:650-659.

61. Miettinen M, Shekitka KM, Sobin LH. Schwannomas in the colon and rectum: a clinicopathologic and immunohistochemical study of 20 cases. Am J Surg Pathol 2001;25:846-855.

62. Kienemund J, Liegl B, Siebert F, Jagoditsch M, Spuller E, Langner C. Microcystic reticular schwannoma of the colon. Endoscopy 2010;42(Suppl 2):E247.

63. Lee SM, Goldblum J, Kim KM. Microcystic/reticular schwannoma in the colon. Pathology 2009;41:595-596.

64. Trivedi A, Ligato S. Microcystic/reticular schwannoma of the proximal sigmoid colon: case report with review of literature. Arch Pathol Lab Med 2013;137:284-288.

65. Emanuel P, Pertsemlidis DS, Gordon R, Xu R. Benign hybrid perineurioma-schwannoma in the colon. A case report. Ann Diagn Pathol 2006;10:367-370.

66. Hornick JL, Bundock EA, Fletcher CD. Hybrid schwannoma/perineurioma: clinicopathologic analysis of 42 distinctive benign nerve sheath tumors. Am J Surg Pathol 2009;33:1554-1561.

67. Lasota J, Wasag B, Dansonka-Mieszkowska A, et al. Evaluation of NF2 and NF1 tumor suppressor genes in distinctive gastrointestinal nerve sheath tumors traditionally diagnosed as benign schwannomas: s study of 20 cases. Lab Invest 2003;83:1361-1371.

68. Tashiro Y, Matsumoto F, Iwama K, et al. Laparoscopic resection of schwannoma of the ascending colon. Case Rep Gastroenterol 2015;9:15-19.

69. Lewin MR, Dilworth HP, Abu Alfa AK, Epstein JI, Montgomery E. Mucosal benign epithelioid nerve sheath tumors. Am J Surg Pathol 2005;29:1310-1315.

70. Gibson JA, Hornick JL. Mucosal Schwann cell "hamartoma": clinicopathologic study of 26 neural colorectal polyps distinct from neurofibromas and mucosal neuromas. Am J Surg Pathol 2009;33:781-787.

71. Chetty R, Vajpeyi R, Penwick JL. Psammomatous melanotic schwannoma presenting as colonic polyps. Virchows Arch 2007;451:717-720.

72. Agaimy A, Stoehr R, Vieth M, Hartmann A. Benign serrated colorectal fibroblastic polyps/intramucosal perineuriomas are true mixed epithelial-stromal polyps (hybrid hyperplastic polyp/mucosal perineurioma) with frequent BRAF mutations. Am J Surg Pathol 2010;34:1663-1671.

73. Eslami-Varzaneh F, Washington K, Robert ME, Kashgarian M, Goldblum JR, Jain D. Benign fibroblastic polyps of the colon: a histologic, immunohistochemical, and ultrastructural study. Am J Surg Pathol 2004;28:374-378.

74. Groisman GM, Polak-Charcon S. Fibroblastic polyp of the colon and colonic perineurioma: 2 names for a single entity? Am J Surg Pathol 2008;32:1088-1094.

75. Groisman GM, Polak-Charcon S, Appelman HD. Fibroblastic polyp of the colon: clinicopathological analysis of 10 cases with emphasis on its common association with serrated crypts. Histopathology 2006;48:431-437.

76. Hornick JL, Fletcher CD. Intestinal perineuriomas: clinicopathologic definition of a new anatomic subset in a series of 10 cases. Am J Surg Pathol 2005;29:859-865.

77. Shekitka KM, Sobin LH. Ganglioneuromas of the gastrointestinal-tract. Relation to Von-Recklinghausen disease and other multiple tumor syndromes. Am J Surg Pathol 1994;18:250-257.

78. Moon SB, Park KW, Jung SE, Lee SC. Vasoactive intestinal polypeptide-producing ganglioneuromatosis involving the entire colon and rectum. J Pediatr Surg 2009;44:e19-21.

79. Rescorla FJ, Vane DW, Fitzgerald JF, West KW, Grosfeld JL. Vasoactive intestinal polypeptide-secreting ganglioneuromatosis affecting the entire colon and rectum. J Pediatr Surg 1988;23:635-637.

80. Schaffer JV, Kamino H, Witkiewicz A, McNiff JM, Orlow SJ. Mucocutaneous neuromas: an underrecognized manifestation of PTEN hamartoma-tumor syndrome. Arch Dermatol 2006;142:625-632.

81. Johnston J, Helwig EB. Granular cell tumors of the gastrointestinal tract and perianal region: a study of 74 cases. Dig Dis Sci 1981;26:807-816.

82. Singhi AD, Montgomery EA. Colorectal granular cell tumor: a clinicopathologic study of 26 cases. The Am J Surg Pathol 2010;34:1186-1192.

83. Saleh H, El-Fakharany M, Frankle M. Multiple synchronous granular cell tumors involving the colon, appendix and mesentery: a case report and review of the literature. J Gastrointestin Liver Dis 2009;18:475-478.

84. Choi SM, Hong SG, Kang SM, et al. A case of malignant granular cell tumor in the sigmoid colon. Clin Endosc 2014;47:197-200.

85. Treglia G, Mormando M, Iacovazzo D, et al. A rare case of malignant granular cell tumor of the colon incidentally detected by (18) F-FDG positron emission tomography/computed tomography. Nucl Med Mol Imaging 2013;47:148-150.

86. Burke AP, Helwig EB. Gangliocytic paraganglioma. Am J Clin Pathol 1989;92:1-9.

87. Hamid QA, Bishop AE, Rode J, et al. Duodenal gangliocytic paragangliomas: a study of 10 cases with immunocytochemical neuroendocrine markers. Hum Pathol 1986;17:1151-1157.

88. Hashimoto S, Kawasaki S, Matsuzawa K, Harada H, Makuuchi M. Gangliocytic paraganglioma of the papilla of Vater with regional lymph node metastasis. Am J Gastroenterol 1992;87:1216-1218.

89. Inai K, Kobuke T, Yonehara S, Tokuoka S. Duodenal gangliocytic paraganglioma with lymph node metastasis in a 17-year-old boy. Cancer 1989;63:2540-2545.

90. Perrone T. Duodenal gangliocytic paraganglioma and carcinoid. Am J Surg Pathol 1986;10:147-149.

91. Perrone T, Sibley RK, Rosai J. Duodenal gangliocytic paraganglioma. An immunohistochemical and ultrastructural study and a hypothesis concerning its origin. Am J Surg Pathol 1985;9:31-41.

92. Reed RJ, Caroca PJ, Jr., Harkin JC. Gangliocytic paraganglioma. Am J Surg Pathol 1977;1:207-216.

93. Scheithauer BW, Nora FE, LeChago J, et al. Duodenal gangliocytic paraganglioma. Clinicopathologic and immunocytochemical study of 11 cases. Am J Clin Pathol 1986;86:559-565.

94. Castoldi L, De Rai P, Marini A, Ferrero S, De Luca V, Tiberio G. Neurofibromatosis-1 and Ampullary gangliocytic paraganglioma causing biliary and pancreatic obstruction. Int J Gastrointest Cancer 2001;29:93-98.

95. Li B, Li Y, Tian XY, Luo BN, Li Z. Malignant gangliocytic paraganglioma of the duodenum with distant metastases and a lethal course. World J Gastroenterol 2014;20:15454-15461.

96. Miettinen M, Sarlomo-Rikala M, Sobin LH. Mesenchymal tumors of muscularis mucosae of colon and rectum are benign leiomyomas that should be separated from gastrointestinal stromal tumors—a clinicopathologic and immunohistochemical study of eighty-eight cases. Mod Pathol 2001;14:950-956.

97. Tawfik OW, McGregor DH. Lipohyperplasia of the ileocecal valve. Am J Gastroenterol 1992;87:82-87.

98. Jain A, Falzarano J, Decker R, Okubo G, Fujiwara D. Outcome of 5,000 flexible sigmoidoscopies done by nurse endoscopists for colorectal screening in asymptomatic patients. Hawaii Med J 2002;61:118-120.

99. Mackay G, Spitz L, McHugh K. Lipomatosis of the colon complicating Proteus syndrome. Arch Dis Child 2002;86:265.

100. D'Annibale M, Cosimelli M, Covello R, Stasi E. Liposarcoma of the colon presenting as an endoluminal mass. World J Surg Oncol 2009;7:78.

101. Blakely ML, Andrassy RJ, Raney RB, et al. Prognostic factors and surgical treatment guidelines for children with rhabdomyosarcoma of the perineum or anus: a report of Intergroup Rhabdomyosarcoma Studies I through IV, 1972 through 1997. J Pediatr Surg 2003;38:347-353.

102. Jung SP, Lee Y, Han KM, et al. Breast metastasis from rhabdomyosarcoma of the anus in an adolescent female. J Breast Cancer 2013;16:345-348.

103. Sharp WC Jr., Helwig EB. Sarcoma botryoides (embryonal rhabdomyosarcoma) of the anus. AMA J Dis Child 1959;97:845-848.

104. Damiani S, Nappi O, Eusebi V. Primary rhabdomyosarcoma of the ileum in an adult. Arch Pathol Lab Med 1991;115:235-238.

105. Artaza T, Potenciano JM, Legaz M, Munoz C, Talavera A, Sanchez E. Lymphangioma of Vater's ampulla: a rare cause of obstructive jaundice. Endoscopic therapy. Scand J Gastroenterol 1995;30:804-806.

106. Badran AM, Vahedi K, Berrebi D, et al. Pediatric ampullar and small bowel blue rubber bleb nevus syndrome diagnosed by wireless capsule endoscopy. J Pediatr Gastroenterol Nutr 2007;44:283-286.

107. Shepherd V, Godbolt A, Casey T. Maffucci's syndrome with extensive gastrointestinal involvement. Australas J Dermatol 2005;46:33-37.

108. Montgomery E, Epstein JI. Anastomosing hemangioma of the genitourinary tract: a lesion mimicking angiosarcoma. Am J Surg Pathol 2009;33:1364-1369.

109. Lin J, Bigge J, Ulbright TM, Montgomery E. Anastomosing hemangioma of the liver and gastrointestinal tract: an unusual variant histologically mimicking angiosarcoma. Am J Surg Pathol 2013;37:1761-1765.

110. Handra-Luca A, Montgomery E. Vascular malformations and hemangiolymphangiomas of the gastrointestinal tract: morphological features and clinical impact. Int J Clin Exp Pathol 2011;4:430-443.

111. Allison KH, Yoder BJ, Bronner MP, Goldblum JR, Rubin BP. Angiosarcoma involving the gastrointestinal tract: a series of primary and metastatic cases. Am J Surg Pathol 2004;28:298-307.

112. Bavikatty NR, Goldblum JR, Abdul-Karim FW, Nielsen SL, Greenson JK. Florid vascular proliferation of the colon related to intussusception and mucosal prolapse: potential diagnostic confusion with angiosarcoma. Mod Pathol 2001;14:1114-1118.

113. Huppmann AR, Orenstein JM. Opportunistic disorders of the gastrointestinal tract in the age of highly active antiretroviral therapy. Hum Pathol 2010;41:1777-1787.

114. Gurbuz AK, Giardiello FM, Petersen GM, et al. Desmoid tumours in familial adenomatous polyposis. Gut 1994;35:377-381.

115. Montgomery E, Folpe AL. The diagnostic value of beta-catenin immunohistochemistry. Adv Anat Pathol 2005;12:350-356.

116. Zhao WP, Han ZY, Zhang J, et al. Early experience: high-intensity focused ultrasound treatment for intra-abdominal aggressive fibromatosis of failure in surgery. Br J Radiol 2016;89:20151026.

117. Eastley N, McCulloch T, Esler C, et al. Extra-abdominal desmoid fibromatosis: a review of management, current guidance and unanswered questions. Eur J Surg Oncol 2016;42:1071-1083.

118. Fletcher C, Bridge J, Hogendoorn P, Mertens F. World Health Organization Classification of Tumours. Pathology and Genetics of Tumours of Soft Tissue and Bone, Vol 4. Lyon: IARC Press; 2013.

119. Coffin CM, Patel A, Perkins S, Elenitoba-Johnson KS, Perlman E, Griffin CA. ALK1 and p80 expression and chromosomal rearrangements involving 2p23 in inflammatory myofibroblastic tumor. Mod Pathol 2001;14:569-576.

120. Griffin CA, Hawkins AL, Dvorak C, Henkle C, Ellingham T, Perlman EJ. Recurrent involvement of 2p23 in inflammatory myofibroblastic tumors. Cancer Res 1999;59:2776-2780.

121. Meis JM, Enzinger FM. Inflammatory fibrosarcoma of the mesentery and retroperitoneum. A tumor closely simulating inflammatory pseudotumor. Am J Surg Pathol 1991;15:1146-1156.

122. Coffin CM, Hornick JL, Fletcher CD. Inflammatory myofibroblastic tumor: comparison of clinicopathologic, histologic, and immunohistochemical features including ALK expression in atypical and aggressive cases. Am J Surg Pathol 2007;31:509-520.

123. Marino-Enriquez A, Wang WL, Roy A, et al. Epithelioid inflammatory myofibroblastic sarcoma: An aggressive intra-abdominal variant of inflammatory myofibroblastic tumor with nuclear membrane or perinuclear ALK. Am J Surg Pathol 2011;35:135-144.

124. Butrynski JE, D'Adamo DR, Hornick JL, et al. Crizotinib in ALK-rearranged inflammatory myofibroblastic tumor. N Engl J Med 2010;363:1727-1733.

125. Gaudichon J, Jeanne-Pasquier C, Deparis M, et al. Complete and repeated response of a metastatic ALK-rearranged inflammatory myofibroblastic tumor to crizotinib in a teenage girl. J Pediatr Hematol Oncol 2016;38:308-311.

126. Liu Q, Kan Y, Zhao Y, He H, Kong L. Epithelioid inflammatory myofibroblastic sarcoma treated with ALK inhibitor: a case report and review of literature. Int J Clin Exp Pathol 2015;8:15328-15332.

127. Murga-Zamalloa C, Lim MS. ALK-driven tumors and targeted therapy: focus on crizotinib. Pharmacogenomics Pers Med 2014;7:87-94.

128. Subbiah V, McMahon C, Patel S, et al. STUMP un"stumped": anti-tumor response to anaplastic lymphoma kinase (ALK) inhibitor based targeted therapy in uterine inflammatory myofibroblastic tumor with myxoid features harboring DCTN1-ALK fusion. J Hematol Oncol 2015;8:66.

129. Antonescu CR, Suurmeijer AJ, Zhang L, et al. Molecular characterization of inflammatory myofibroblastic tumors with frequent ALK and ROS1 gene fusions and rare novel RET rearrangement. Am J Surg Pathol 2015;39:957-967.

130. Hornick JL, Sholl LM, Dal Cin P, Childress MA, Lovly CM. Expression of ROS1 predicts ROS1 gene rearrangement in inflammatory myofibroblastic tumors. Mod Pathol 2015;28:732-739.

131. Akram S, Pardi DS, Schaffner JA, Smyrk TC. Sclerosing mesenteritis: clinical features, treatment, and outcome in ninety-two patients. Clin Gastroenterol Hepatol 2007;5:589-596; quiz 523-584.

132. Emory TS, Monihan JM, Carr NJ, Sobin LH. Sclerosing mesenteritis, mesenteric panniculitis and mesenteric lipodystrophy: a single entity? Am J Surg Pathol 1997;21:392-398.

133. Chen TS, Montgomery EA. Are tumefactive lesions classified as sclerosing mesenteritis a subset of IgG4-related sclerosing disorders? J Clin Pathol 2008;61:1093-1097.

134. Rosenthal NS, Abdul-Karim FW. Childhood fibrous tumor with psammoma bodies. Clinicopathologic features in two cases. Arch Pathol Lab Med 1988;112:798-800.

135. Prasertvit S, Stoikes N. A rare case of Ewing's sarcoma of the small intestine. Am Surg 2013;79:E78-79.

136. Vignali M, Zacche MM, Messori P, Natale A, Busacca M. Ewing's sarcoma of the small intestine misdiagnosed as a voluminous pedunculated uterine leiomyoma. Eur J Obstet Gynecol Reprod Biol 2012;162:234-235.

137. Antonescu CR, Nafa K, Segal NH, Dal Cin P, Ladanyi M. EWS-CREB1: a recurrent variant fusion in clear cell sarcoma—association with gastrointestinal location and absence of melanocytic differentiation. Clin Cancer Res 2006; 12:5356-5362.

138. Stockman DL, Miettinen M, Suster S, et al. Malignant gastrointestinal neuroectodermal tumor: clinicopathologic, immunohistochemical, ultrastructural, and molecular analysis of 16 cases with a reappraisal of clear cell sarcoma-like tumors of the gastrointestinal tract. Am J Surg Pathol 2012;36:857-868.

139. Laurini JA, Zhang L, Goldblum JR, Montgomery E, Folpe AL. Low-grade fibromyxoid sarcoma of the small intestine: report of 4 cases with molecular cytogenetic confirmation. Am J Surg Pathol 2011;35:1069-1073.

140. Shekitka KM, Helwig EB. Deceptive bizarre stromal cells in polyps and ulcers of the gastrointestinal tract. Cancer 1991;67:2111-2117.

141. Jessurun J, Paplanus SH, Nagle RB, Hamilton SR, Yardley JH, Tripp M. Pseudosarcomatous changes in inflammatory pseudopolyps of the colon. Arch Pathol Lab Med 1986;110:833-836.

9 HEMATOPOIETIC DISORDERS

The gastrointestinal tract hosts a large proportion of the extranodal lymphoid tissue and is the most common extranodal site of lymphoma involvement. Myeloid neoplasms, by comparison, are much less common. Although a comprehensive discussion of all hematopoietic neoplasms that can involve the gastrointestinal tract is beyond the scope of this chapter, the more common tumors and their mimics are discussed below.

BENIGN LYMPHOID HYPERPLASIA

Definition. *Lymphoid nodules* are normally present in the small bowel and colon, particularly among children. They tend to regress with increased age, and are mostly limited to the terminal ileum (i.e., Peyer patches), periappendiceal orifice, and rectum (i.e., rectal tonsil) in older adults. *Nodular lymphoid hyperplasia* describes a diffuse proliferation of benign lymphoid nodules in the small bowel and colon.

Clinical Features. Nodular lymphoid hyperplasia can be a normal finding in the distal ileum, or reflect an exuberant inflammatory response to a host of injuries ranging from infections to idiopathic inflammatory bowel disease (fig. 9-1). Large lesions can serve as a lead point for intussusception, resulting in intermittent obstructive symptoms (fig. 9-2).

Multiple duodenal lymphoid nodules can be a normal finding in pediatric patients, but are pathologic when present in older adult patients

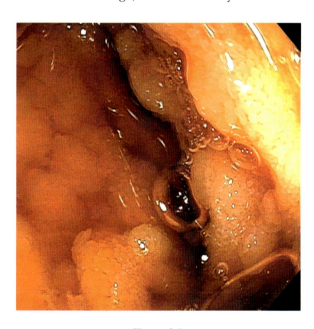

Figure 9-1

**PROMINENT LYMPHOID
AGGREGATES OF TERMINAL ILEUM**

This 21-year-old male with infectious diarrhea has a diffusely nodular ileum secondary to enlarged Peyer patches.

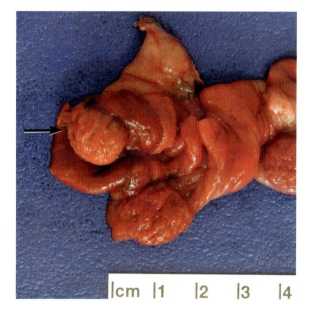

Figure 9-2

**INTUSSUSCEPTION DUE TO PROMINENT
LYMPHOID HYPERPLASIA IN TERMINAL ILEUM**

This 3-month-old baby presented with an acute abdomen secondary to intussusception of the terminal ileum into the cecum. The lead point (arrow), composed of large lymphoid follicles, formed a mass.

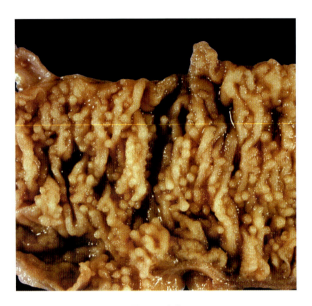

Figure 9-3

**NODULAR LYMPHOID HYPERPLASIA
IN TERMINAL ILEUM**

An ileal segment contains numerous sessile, yellow nodules corresponding to lymphoid follicles.

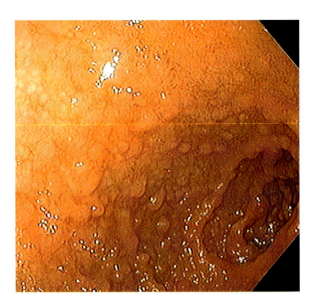

Figure 9-4

NODULAR LYMPHOID HYPERPLASIA IN DUODENUM

This patient had giardiasis. Endoscopic examination reveals innumerable sessile polyps carpeting the mucosa.

(1). They are commonly seen in patients with chronic giardiasis, in which case they presumably reflect a sustained immune response to chronic antigenic stimulation. The lymphoid hyperplasia may persist following successful eradication of the organism. Nodular lymphoid hyperplasia in the duodenum may also be a manifestation of an underlying immune disorder, such as selective IgA deficiency or common variable immunodeficiency (1–6).

Lymphoid nodules do not cause symptoms, but the underlying disorders associated with them have variable manifestations. Patients with giardiasis may complain of bloating, flatulence, or diarrhea. Those with primary immunodeficiencies have reduced serum IgA levels (IgA deficiency) or IgG, IgM, and IgA (common variable immunodeficiency). Individuals with common variable immunodeficiency have severe malabsorptive diarrhea, recurrent bacterial infections, or persistent giardiasis (1,4,7,8).

Lymphoid hyperplasia of the colon is usually most pronounced in the rectum. In this area it can produce a mass lesion.

Gross Findings. Large lymphoid nodules often show central umbilication with a yellow-white appearance, or rim of erythema that

simulates aphthous ulcers. In fact, clinicians often biopsy "aphthous ulcers" that prove to be prominent lymphoid aggregates at microscopy. Multiple nodules produce mucosa-based sessile polyps with smooth surfaces (figs. 9-3, 9- 4). The background mucosa is generally normal, but may show atrophy, scalloping, or inflammation in cases of common variable immunodeficiency.

Microscopic Findings. Lymphoid nodules stretch the overlying epithelium and distort adjacent crypts, but epithelial destruction is uncommon (figs. 9-5–9-7). The nodules are centered in the submucosa, and can focally transgress the muscularis mucosae (fig. 9-8). Adjacent crypts and the surface epithelium are commonly infiltrated by mononuclear cells, neutrophils, and eosinophils.

Immunohistochemical and Molecular Genetic Findings. Lymphoid nodules consist of B-cell–rich follicles surrounded by T cells. Primary (resting) follicles express BCL-2, but not BCL-6, whereas germinal centers express BCL-6 and are negative for BCL-2; BCL-2 expression is more pronounced in the mantle zone of reactive follicular hyperplasia (figs. 9-9–9-12).

The follicular cells are polyclonal without light chain restriction. The ratio of cells

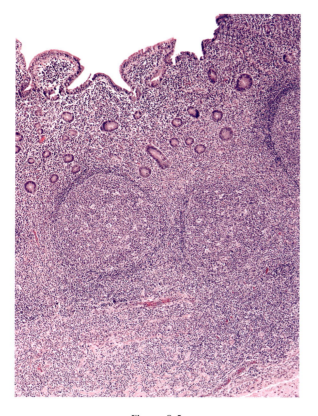

Figure 9-5

**NODULAR LYMPHOID HYPERPLASIA
OF TERMINAL ILEUM**

Polarized lymphoid follicles with germinal centers and
eccentric mantles diffusely expand the mucosa. Secondary
follicles push the crypts aside, but they are not destroyed.

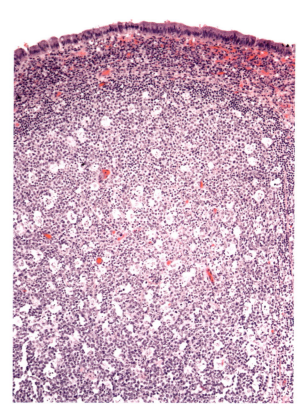

Figure 9-6

PROMINENT LYMPHOID AGGREGATE IN COLON

A large follicle contains tingible body macrophages.

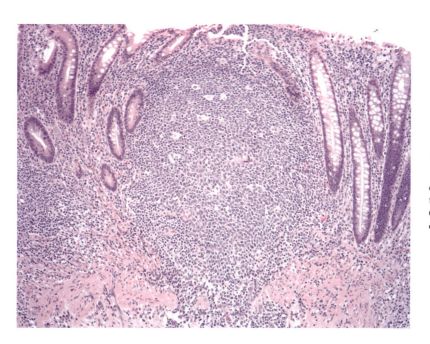

Figure 9-7

**DIVERSION COLITIS WITH
NODULAR LYMPHOID HYPERPLASIA**

A large follicle contains a germinal
center, expands the lamina propria, and
transgresses the muscularis mucosae.
Crypts are pushed aside, but destruction
of mucosal elements is lacking.

Figure 9-8

REACTIVE LYMPHOID HYPERPLASIA IN RECTUM

The submucosa is expanded by a lymphoid aggregate with node-like architecture. Large, irregularly shaped follicles show polarity and contain tingible body macrophages. Immunohistochemical stains demonstrate polytypic B-cell populations without aberrant expression of B- or T-cell markers.

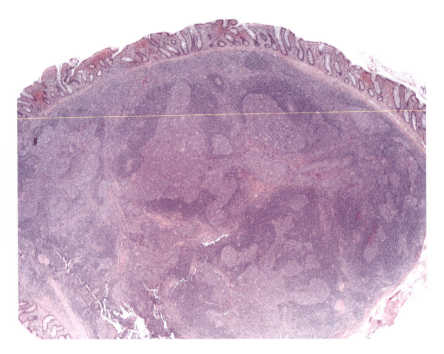

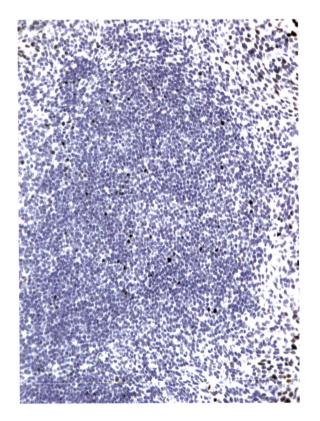

Figure 9-9

PRIMARY LYMPHOID FOLLICLE BCL-6 STAIN

Primary follicles contain small, mature B cells that are mostly negative for BCL-6.

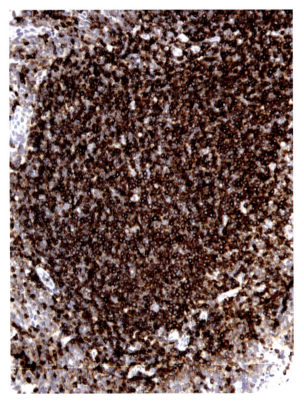

Figure 9-10

PRIMARY LYMPHOID FOLLICLE: BCL-2 STAIN

Primary follicles show strong uniform BCL-2 staining in small lymphocytes.

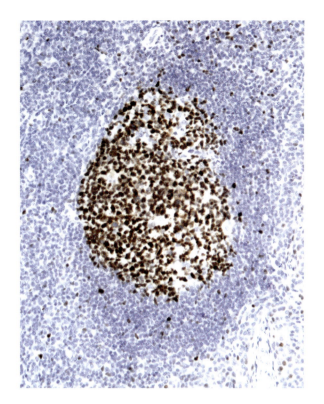

Figure 9-11

SECONDARY FOLLICLE: BCL-6 STAIN

Most mature B cells in the germinal center are positive for BLC-6. Scattered immunopositive cells are present in the mantle zone.

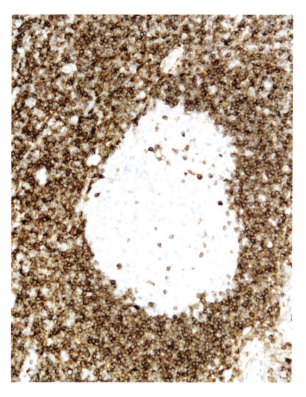

Figure 9-12

SECONDARY FOLLICLE: BCL-2 STAIN

Lymphocytes in the mantle zone show strong cytoplasmic staining for BCL-2, but only scattered positive cells are present in the germinal center.

expressing kappa compared to those expressing lambda is approximately 2 to 1.

Differential Diagnosis. Benign lymphoid proliferations can simulate low-grade B-cell neoplasms that display a nodular growth pattern. Primary lymphoid follicles contain mostly small lymphocytes, and tangential sections through the edge of a secondary follicle shows a monotonous cell population that mimics lymphoma in small or superficial samples. Exuberant lymphoid hyperplasia often distorts the crypt architecture and extends into the submucosa.

The primary follicles are recognizable because they tend to be small and do not distort normal mucosal elements. Other clues to a benign diagnosis include follicular polarization with an eccentric cuff of peripherally located small lymphocytes around germinal centers, tingible body macrophages within germinal centers, and heterogeneous cell populations nodules (fig. 9-13A).

The germinal centers contain a meshwork of CD23-positive follicular dendritic cells, as well as B cells that express BCL-6 (fig. 9-13B). Mantle zones that extend into the mucosa can simulate low-grade B-cell lymphoma because they appear to be monotonous and stain for BCL-2 (fig. 9-13C). Interfollicular areas contain CD3-positive T cells, but activated B cells may also be CD23 positive.

Treatment and Prognosis. Nodular lymphoid hyperplasia requires no specific treatment, although patients with obstructive symptoms may develop ischemic complications or intussusception that requires surgical intervention. Lymphoid hyperplasia resulting from infection may persist for some time following eradication of the infectious agent.

The relationship between nodular lymphoid hyperplasia and intestinal lymphoma is not clear; there is no statistically significant risk of lymphoma among patients with nodular

Figure 9-13

FOLLICULAR HYPERPLASIA IN COLON

A: Small, monotonous lymphocytes infiltrate the deep mucosa, simulating the appearance of a low-grade B-cell lymphoma. A large germinal center is also present. It contains a mixed population of small and large cells.

B: Germinal center B cells show strong BCL-6 staining.

C: Benign germinal center cells are essentially negative for BCL-2. However, cells in the mantle zone show strong positivity, which can represent a potential pitfall in limited, superficial samples. (All parts courtesy of Dr. S. Owens, Ann Arbor, MI.)

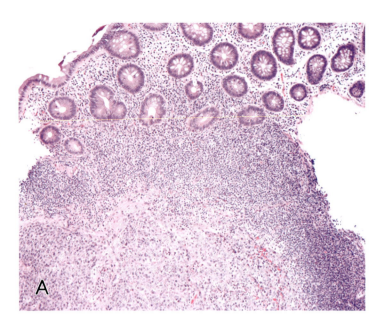

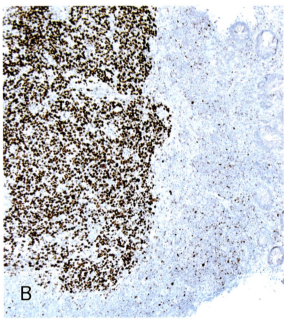

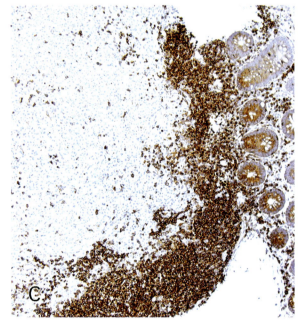

lymphoid hyperplasia, but lymphomas from both immunocompromised and immunocompetent patients often arise on a background of nodular lymphoid hyperplasia (8–11). Gradual transitions between nodular lymphoid hyperplasia and lymphoma may be apparent, and monoclonal lymphocytic populations can be detected in the former (fig. 9-14) (11,12). For this reason, older adult patients with nodular lymphoid hyperplasia in the proximal small bowel should be clinically monitored.

EXTRANODAL MARGINAL ZONE LYMPHOMA OF MUCOSA-ASSOCIATED LYMPHOID TISSUE

Definition. *Extranodal marginal zone lymphomas of mucosa-associated lymphoid tissue* (MALT) are the most common low-grade B-cell neoplasms affecting the small bowel and colon, and the second most common lymphoma type to affect the intestines overall. They may arise in patients with concomitant gastric extranodal marginal zone lymphoma, or as an isolated

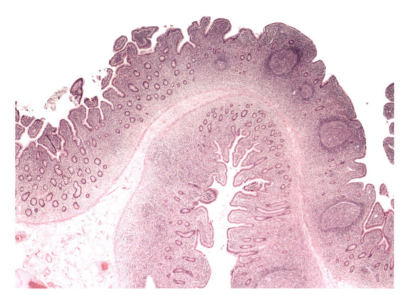

Figure 9-14

FLORID LYMPHOID HYPERPLASIA ASSOCIATED WITH DIFFUSE LARGE B-CELL LYMPHOMA

This 73-year-old woman with diffuse large B-cell lymphoma underwent resection of the small bowel due to obstructive symptoms. The background mucosa shows lymphoid hyperplasia with diffuse infiltration by a mixed lymphocyte-predominant infiltrate.

finding (13). *Immunoproliferative small intestinal disease* is a subtype of extranodal marginal zone lymphoma that results from chronic antigenic stimulation of IgA-secreting lymphoid tissue by *Campylobacter jejuni* (14,15).

Clinical Features. Extranodal marginal zone lymphoma of MALT type shows an equal predilection to affect men and women. With the exception of immunoproliferative small intestinal disease, which tends to occur in young adults (mean age, 25 years), tumors occur almost exclusively in middle-aged and older adults (16). Patients present with abdominal pain, weight loss, and features related to gastrointestinal bleeding.

Patients with immunoproliferative small intestinal disease are often of lower socioeconomic status and Middle Eastern descent (14). They are more likely to have malabsorptive diarrhea and digital clubbing, rather than obstructive symptoms or gastrointestinal bleeding. Approximately 50 percent of patients with immunoproliferative small intestinal disease have free alpha heavy chains in the serum (17).

Gross Findings. Most extranodal marginal zone lymphomas of the intestines develop in the rectum. They form polypoid masses or plaques, with surface erythema, erosions, or even ulcers (fig. 9-15). Superficial lesions lead to serpiginous expansion of mucosal folds, or a few clustered polyps. Extranodal marginal zone lymphoma is an infrequent cause of multiple lymphomatous polyposis (18).

Patients with immunoproliferative small intestinal disease tend to have bulky tumors that produce diffuse thickening of the bowel wall. Disease is more common in the proximal small intestine and is often accompanied by mesenteric lymphadenopathy.

Microscopic Findings. Extranodal marginal zone lymphomas consist of lymphoid nodules throughout the bowel wall (fig. 9-16). They often transgress the muscularis mucosae and obliterate the normal crypt architecture (fig. 9-17). Clusters of tumor cells can infiltrate the crypt epithelium and produce lymphoepithelial lesions. Lymphoepithelial lesions, however, are more common among gastric extranodal marginal zone lymphomas than intestinal tumors, and they may be seen in several other types of low-grade B-cell lymphoma (19). For these reasons, they are of limited diagnostic value in the morphologic classification of low-grade B-cell lymphomas of the intestine. Monocytoid tumor cells contain pale cytoplasm with round nuclei and are present on a background of plasma cell-rich inflammation (figs. 9-18, 9-19) (20).

Immunoproliferative small intestinal disease shows a continuous, band-like lymphoid infiltrate in the superficial submucosa and mucosa. The lamina propria is expanded, resulting in bulbous distortion of villi by lymphoid cells that consistently show plasmacytic differentiation (fig. 9-20). Intraepithelial lymphocytosis is more pronounced in the crypt region than the surface epithelium, but is not striking in most cases.

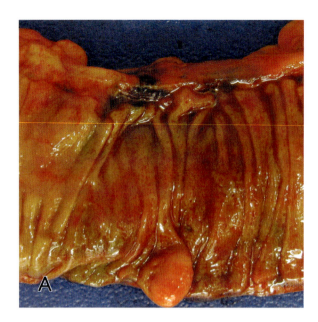

Figure 9-15

EXTRANODAL MARGINAL ZONE LYMPHOMA OF COLON

A: A 68-year-old man had a large sessile polyp in the descending colon that proved to be extranodal marginal zone lymphoma. Bleeding at the biopsy site ultimately led to a segmental colonic resection.

B: This tumor involves 50 percent of the luminal circumference, producing fusiform expansion of a mucosal fold.

C: A nodular irregular plaque is surfaced by otherwise normal-appearing mucosa.

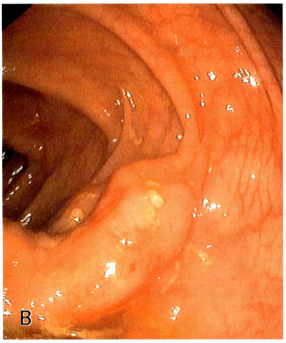

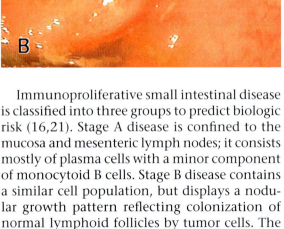

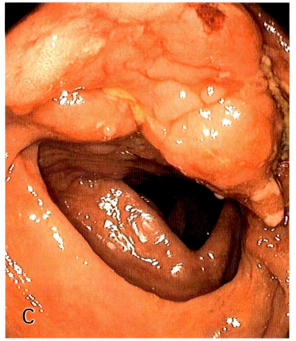

Immunoproliferative small intestinal disease is classified into three groups to predict biologic risk (16,21). Stage A disease is confined to the mucosa and mesenteric lymph nodes; it consists mostly of plasma cells with a minor component of monocytoid B cells. Stage B disease contains a similar cell population, but displays a nodular growth pattern reflecting colonization of normal lymphoid follicles by tumor cells. The infiltrate extends beyond the muscularis muco-sae and can show a minor population of large, atypical cells with high-grade cytologic features. Stage C tumors are high-grade, mass-forming lymphomas composed of tumor cells reminiscent of diffuse large B-cell lymphoma.

Immunohistochemical and Molecular Genetic Findings. Unfortunately, extranodal marginal zone lymphomas do not have a specific immunophenotype. The tumor cells uniformly express CD20, but expression of other markers is variable. Many stain for BCL-2, and staining for CD43 is present in approximately 30 percent of cases, whereas rare (fewer than 5 percent) tumors show CD5 positivity (fig. 9-21) (16). Tumor cells that show plasmacytic differentiation can be light chain restricted, or express PAX5 or CD79a (fig. 9-22).

Multiple molecular alterations have been described, including translocations that lead to *API2-MALT* fusions t(11;18)(q21;q21), dysregulation of *BLC10* [t(1;14)(p22;q32)], and altered expression of *MALT1* ([t(14;18)(q32;q21)] (22,23). Immunoproliferative small intestinal disease shows expression of alpha heavy chains without light chains, as well as clonal rearrangement of immunoglobulin heavy and light chains (14). Expression of α4β7 mucosal homing receptor is common among extranodal marginal zone lymphomas that involve the gastrointestinal tract (24).

Differential Diagnosis. Extranodal marginal zone lymphomas can be difficult to distinguish from benign inflammatory conditions and other types of B-cell lymphoma. Reactive lymphoid nodules in the rectum and terminal ileum can be large, with irregularly shaped germinal centers, infiltration of surface and crypt epithelium,

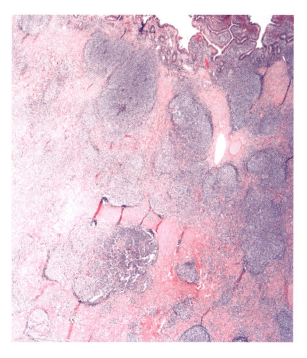

Figure 9-16

**EXTRANODAL MARGINAL ZONE
LYMPHOMA OF SMALL INTESTINE**

The entire bowel wall is infiltrated by a nodular proliferation of small lymphocytes.

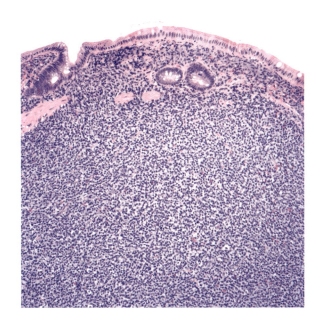 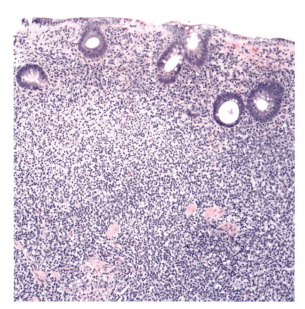

Figure 9-17

EXTRANODAL MARGINAL ZONE LYMPHOMA OF COLON

Left: A large lymphoid nodule expands the submucosa and disrupts the muscularis mucosae. The nodule contains a monotonous cell population without tingible-body macrophages.

Right: Tumor cells overrun normal mucosal elements; only a few residual crypts are present.

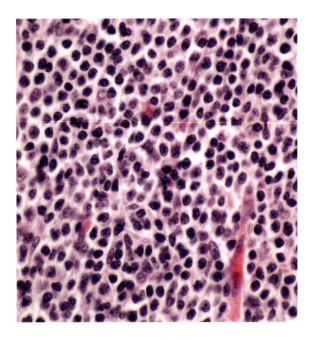

Figure 9-18

**EXTRANODAL MARGINAL ZONE
LYMPHOMA OF SMALL INTESTINE**

Monomorphic small lymphocytes contain round, slightly irregular nuclei and conspicuous nucleoli. Some tumor cells contain a moderate amount of faintly eosinophilic cytoplasm, whereas others have a plasmacytoid appearance.

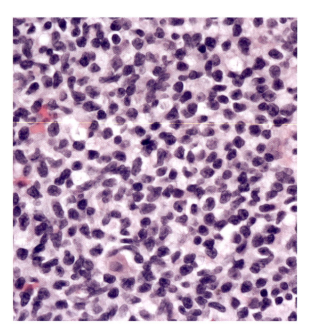

Figure 9-19

**EXTRANODAL MARGINAL ZONE
LYMPHOMA OF COLON**

The tumor cells are small, with pronounced nuclear grooves and irregularities that simulate follicular lymphoma.

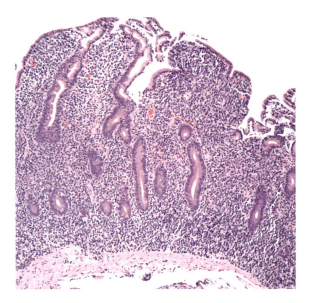
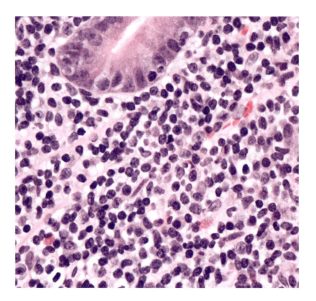

Figure 9-20

IMMUNOPROLIFERATIVE SMALL INTESTINAL DISEASE OF JEJUNUM

Left: This disorder is a variant of extranodal marginal zone lymphoma, a tumor that shows striking plasmacytic differentiation. Small bowel samples from this 45-year-old man show villous distention in combination with crypt hyperplasia and marked expansion of the lamina propria by a dense mononuclear cell-rich infiltrate.

Right: The lamina propria is infiltrated by plasma cells and clusters of monocytoid B cells.

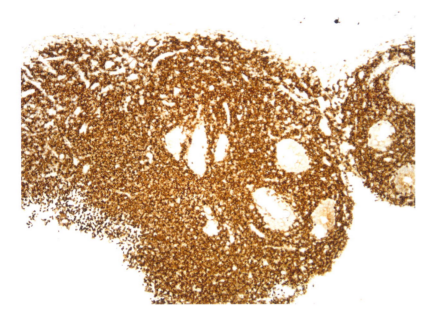

Figure 9-21

**EXTRANODAL MARGINAL
ZONE LYMPHOMA OF COLON**

The tumor cells show strong BCL-2 positivity. This marker is not specific for follicular lymphoma and may be seen in other low-grade B-cell neoplasms.

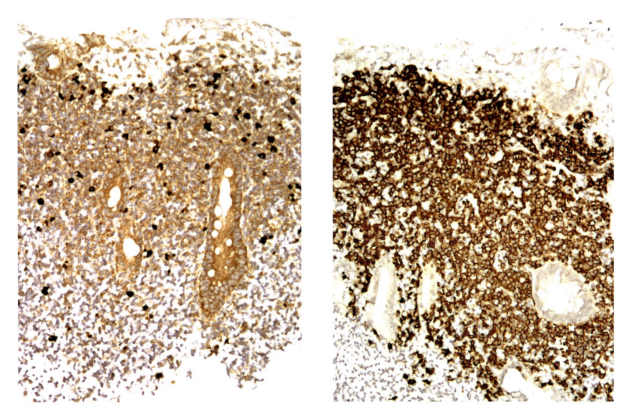

Figure 9-22

EXTRANODAL MARGINAL ZONE LYMPHOMA OF COLON

Left: In situ hybridization for light chains is a helpful diagnostic tool. This extranodal marginal zone lymphoma shows scattered kappa-positive cells.

Right: Virtually all of the lesional cells in the mucosa show lambda light chain restriction by in situ hybridization (same case as figs. 9-15C, 9-17, left).

and apparent crypt distortion. Unlike lymphomas, however, benign follicles are polarized and surrounded by a mixed population of B and T cells. Disruption of the muscularis mucosae is focal, if present.

The diffuse plasma cell-rich infiltrate of immunoproliferative small intestinal disease can mimic celiac disease and other forms of enteritis, particularly during its early stages. Failure to respond to gluten withdrawal is a helpful clue to pursue additional studies.

Distinguishing between subtypes of low-grade B-cell lymphoma is challenging, although follicular lymphoma, mantle cell lymphoma, and chronic lymphocytic leukemia all show characteristic immunophenotypic and molecular features that facilitate a diagnosis, as described in subsequent sections.

Treatment and Prognosis. The prognosis for patients with extranodal marginal zone lymphoma is generally better than that for patients with other intestinal B-cell lymphomas, with 5-year survival rates in excess of 90 percent and 10-year survival rates of approximately 80 percent, although they have higher relapse rates than comparable gastric tumors (25). Immunoproliferative small intestinal disease behaves in a stage-dependent fashion. Early-stage tumors may respond to broad-spectrum antibiotic therapy, whereas advanced, overtly malignant tumors have been historically associated with poor 5-year survival rates of up to 25 percent. Aggressive approaches in the modern era, however, combine antibiotic therapy with systemic chemotherapy and surgery. They induce complete remission in up to 60 percent of cases (26).

FOLLICULAR LYMPHOMA

Definition. *Follicular lymphomas* recapitulate the features of B cells in germinal centers. They can develop in the small bowel and colon, but show a predilection for the second part of the duodenum, particularly the ampulla, and are the most common lymphoma subtype to affect the duodenum (27). Most lymphomas of the proximal intestine are unassociated with generalized disease, whereas those of the distal small bowel and colon more commonly occur in patients with systemic disease and bone marrow involvement.

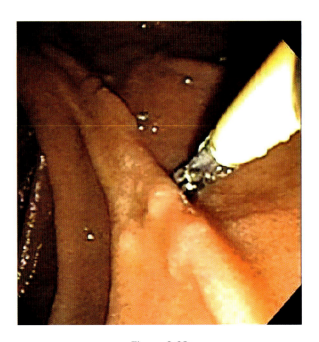

Figure 9-23

FOLLICULAR LYMPHOMA OF DUODENUM

Clustered polypoid nodules are present along a mucosal fold. The biopsy demonstrated the presence of low-grade follicular lymphoma.

Clinical Features. Follicular lymphomas occur in older adults and show a slight female predominance (27). Patients with small intestinal or colonic disease complain of abdominal pain, obstructive symptoms, weight loss, and chronic blood loss. Primary tumors of the ampulla can produce symptoms of obstructive jaundice, thereby mimicking the clinical features of pancreatic adenocarcinoma or biliary disease (28–30).

Gross Findings. Follicular lymphomas produce variable endoscopic abnormalities. Most commonly, superficial disease appears as an ill-defined mucosal nodularity or as multiple mucosa-based polyps, including multiple lymphomatous polyposis in some cases (fig. 9-23) (29,31,32). Large tumors infiltrate the entire bowel wall and mesentery (fig. 9-24). Secondary intestinal involvement among patients with systemic disease is generally associated with regional lymphadenopathy, whereas primary lesions partially involve regional lymph nodes or completely spare them (fig. 9-25). Rare patients have symptoms related to severe gastrointestinal hemorrhage.

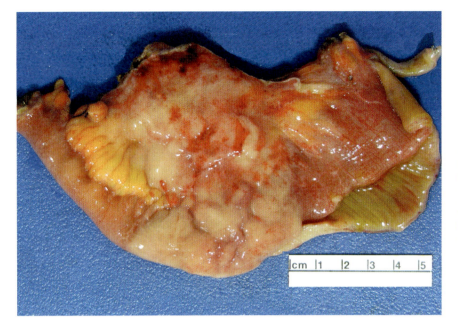

Figure 9-24

FOLLICULAR LYMPHOMA OF THE SMALL INTESTINE

This 49-year-old woman with a history of follicular lymphoma presented with acute abdominal pain and bowel obstruction. A segment of ileum contains a nodular, fleshy mass that transmurally involves the bowel wall and extends into the mesentery.

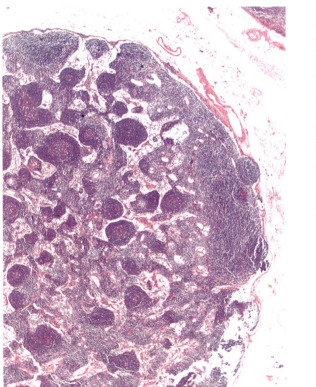

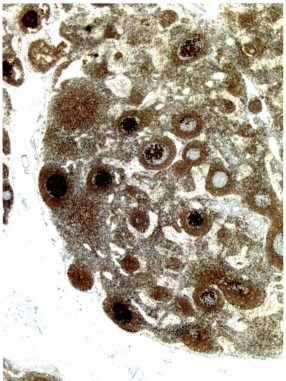

Figure 9-25

PARTIAL INVOLVEMENT OF A REGIONAL LYMPH NODE BY FOLLICULAR LYMPHOMA OF SMALL INTESTINE

Left: This lymph node has a normal architecture with prominent sinuses and numerous primary and secondary follicles.
Right: There is moderately intense BCL-2 staining of primary follicles and the mantle zones of germinal centers. Several germinal centers, however, are colonized by follicular lymphoma cells that show strong BCL-2 staining. (Both figures courtesy of Dr. S. Owens, Ann Arbor, MI.)

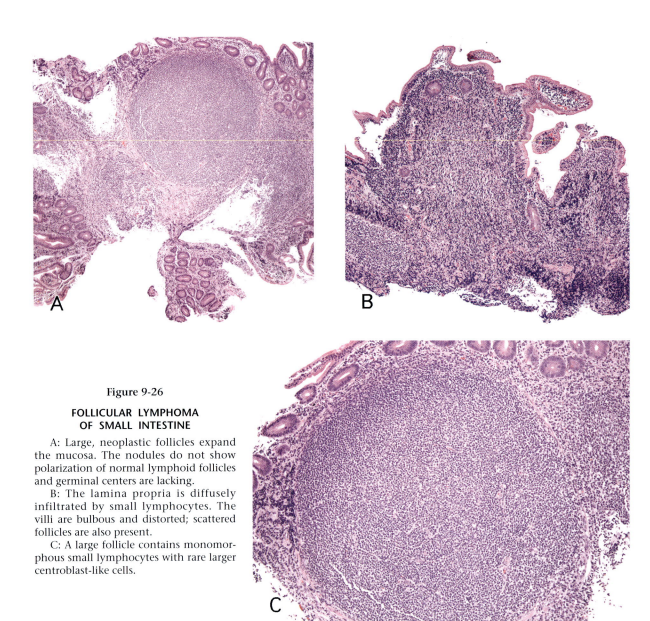

Figure 9-26

**FOLLICULAR LYMPHOMA
OF SMALL INTESTINE**

A: Large, neoplastic follicles expand the mucosa. The nodules do not show polarization of normal lymphoid follicles and germinal centers are lacking.

B: The lamina propria is diffusely infiltrated by small lymphocytes. The villi are bulbous and distorted; scattered follicles are also present.

C: A large follicle contains monomorphous small lymphocytes with rare larger centroblast-like cells.

Microscopic Findings. Intestinal follicular lymphomas are usually composed of nodular proliferations of neoplastic "follicles" (fig. 9-26). These nodules contain follicular dendritic cells and small, mature-appearing B cells, as well as occasional larger centroblast-like cells (fig. 9-27) (31). The former display a slight degree of nuclear irregularity, or appear to be grooved or cleaved, reminiscent of centrocytes that are normally present in germinal centers. Tumors are graded based on the proportion of small centrocyte-like cells to larger centroblast-like cells

(20). Most primary tumors are grade 1 lesions, with only scattered large cells (fig. 9-28) (33).

Immunohistochemical and Molecular Genetic Findings. The characteristic immunohistochemical features of follicular lymphoma include immunopositivity for CD20 and BCL-2 in combination with markers of follicular differentiation, namely, BCL-6 and CD10. Follicular lymphomas are negative for CD5, CD43, and cyclin-D1 (34). Molecular studies demonstrate clonal populations with respect to heavy and light chain genes, as well as *BCL-2* rearrangements (31).

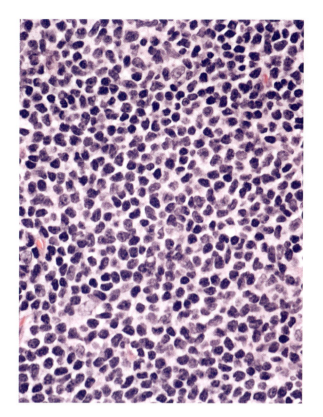

Figure 9-27

FOLLICULAR LYMPHOMA OF SMALL INTESTINE

The tumor cells are small, with dark, irregularly shaped nuclei and small, but conspicuous chromatin, reminiscent of centrocytes of a normal follicle.

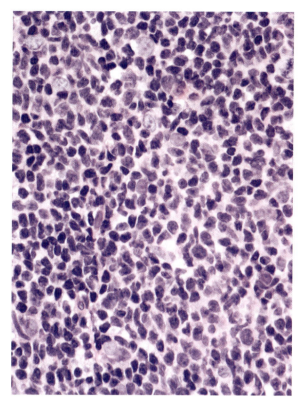

Figure 9-28

FOLLICULAR LYMPHOMA OF SMALL INTESTINE

Most of the tumor cells contain small cleaved nuclei, but scattered larger cells with one or more nucleoli are also present.

Differential Diagnosis. Follicular lymphomas should be distinguished from benign lymphoid nodules and other types of low-grade B-cell lymphoma. Benign follicles show polarization and distort the mucosa, but do not destroy epithelial elements. They generally contain mixed cell populations, including macrophages. Immunohistochemical staining patterns are extremely helpful in distinguishing between lymphoma subtypes. BCL-2 helps distinguish benign secondary follicles from follicular lymphoma, but it is not a specific stain for follicular lymphoma; several other types of low-grade B-cell lymphoma can also express this marker.

Treatment and Prognosis. Follicular lymphomas are indolent tumors that commonly involve the bone marrow and, thus, may be difficult to treat. Although nodal tumors often transform to high-grade lesions over time, primary intestinal

tumors seem to be particularly indolent and may persist as low-grade neoplasms for some time. Many patients with disease confined to the intestine do well without chemotherapy and are managed by observation (29).

SMALL LYMPHOCYTIC LYMPHOMA/ CHRONIC LYMPHOCYTIC LEUKEMIA

Definition. *B-cell chronic lymphocytic leukemia* is the most common B-cell neoplasm of adults. It is essentially the leukemic form of *small lymphocytic lymphoma*. Most patients with intestinal involvement have the leukemic form of the disease.

Clinical Features. Patients with gastrointestinal involvement are older adults (median age, 70 years) who have established chronic lymphocytic leukemia. They generally have elevated white blood cell counts with marked lymphocytosis. Men are affected more commonly than

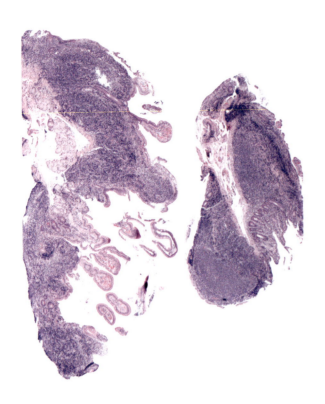

Figure 9-29

CHRONIC LYMPHOCYTIC LEUKEMIA IN ILEUM

Unlike Peyer patches, chronic lymphocytic leukemia is not confined to follicles; small lymphocytes permeate the mucosa and efface crypt architecture.

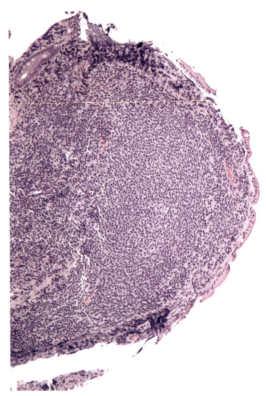

Figure 9-30

CHRONIC LYMPHOCYTIC LEUKEMIA IN ILEUM

A large pseudofollicle contains a uniform population of small, mature lymphocytes.

women. Patients may present with generalized lymphadenopathy, hepatosplenomegaly, fevers of unknown origin, or recurrent infections, although many cases are incidentally discovered as a result of routine blood work obtained for other reasons. Involvement of the gastrointestinal tract rarely dominates the clinical picture.

Gross Findings. Endoscopic findings are variable. In most cases, leukemic infiltrates are detected in endoscopically normal mucosa. Tumors may produce polyps, however, particularly in the terminal ileum.

Microscopic Findings. Tumors consist of a sheet-like, often vaguely nodular proliferation of monomorphic B cells that effaces the mucosal architecture (fig. 9-29). Nodular pseudofollicles lack germinal center architecture and mostly contain prolymphocytes and paraimmunoblasts (fig. 9-30). The tumor cells have scant cytoplasm, nuclei with dense chromatin, and small incon-

spicuous nucleoli. Their nuclei are mostly round, but can be somewhat irregular; they infrequently show clefts and grooves to the same extent seen in mantle cell lymphoma or follicular lymphoma (20). Occasional pseudofollicles contain pale-appearing areas composed of small lymphocytes with slightly more cytoplasm (proliferation centers). Large cell transformation to diffuse large B-cell lymphoma is common (35).

Immunohistochemical and Molecular Genetic Findings. Lesional cells show uniform staining for B-cell markers, including CD20, CD79a, and PAX5. They also show strong diffuse staining for CD5, as well as nearly universal positivity for CD43 (13).

Although no specific molecular alterations characterize chronic lymphocytic leukemia, many cases show numeric chromosomal abnormalities. Slightly more than 50 percent of tumors show deletions in 13q14 that lead to deregulation of apoptosis (36,37). Deletions in 17p that affect *TP53* are associated with a poor prognosis (38). Driver mutations affecting *SF3B1* and *NOTCH1* have been recently identified by next-generation sequencing (39).

Differential Diagnosis. The differential diagnosis of chronic lymphocytic leukemia includes non-neoplastic lymphoid infiltrates and other low-grade lymphomas. Chronic lymphocytic leukemia diffusely infiltrates the mucosa in biopsy samples, whereas non-neoplastic lymphoid proliferations are generally confined to lymphoid aggregates. Diffusely infiltrative monomorphic populations of small lymphocytes are not typically seen in most benign inflammatory conditions. Inflammatory conditions that are characterized by dense lymphoid infiltrates often contain secondary follicles and numerous plasma cells, both of which are lacking in chronic lymphocytic leukemia. Immunohistochemical stains reliably distinguish chronic lymphocytic leukemia from potential neoplastic mimics in most cases (see Table 9-1).

Treatment and Prognosis. Chronic lymphocytic leukemia is often an indolent disease and some patients may opt to receive no medical intervention. Others consider a combination of systemic chemotherapy, monoclonal antibodies, and/or targeted agents. Combination therapy with fludarabine, cyclophosphamide, and rituximab is the most effective regimen. Other agents include chlorambucil, bendamustine, obinutuzumab, ibrutinib, and, most recently, idelalisib (36,40,41). Stem cell transplantation is a consideration, particularly among individuals with large cell transformation. The prognosis is dependent upon the degree of cell maturation, as determined by expression of CD38 and Z-chain-associated protein kinase-70 (ZAP-70) (42).

MANTLE CELL LYMPHOMA

Definition. *Mantle cell lymphoma* is an aggressive form of B-cell lymphoma. The tumor cells share phenotypic and morphologic features of antigen-naïve pregerminal center B cells that normally reside in the mantle zone surrounding germinal centers in secondary follicles (43).

Clinical Features. Patients with gastrointestinal involvement by mantle cell lymphoma are older adults, and males are affected more frequently than females. They may complain of fevers, night sweats, or weight loss, and often have peripheral lymphadenopathy. Most patients have generalized disease, with bone marrow involvement and splenomegaly at the time of diagnosis. Gastrointestinal symptoms rarely dominate the clinical picture.

Gross Findings. Mantle cell lymphoma typically affects the small bowel and colon in the form of multiple lymphomatous polyposis. Lymphomatous involvement of the mucosa and submucosa produces smooth, round polyps that simulate the appearance of familial adenomatous polyposis (fig. 9-31A) (44). Tiny tumor nodules produce small, sessile plaques with central umbilication that simulate aphthous ulcers (fig. 9-31B).

The tumor nodules are fleshy and span up to 2 cm in diameter, particularly in the terminal ileum and right colon where nodules tend to be largest (fig. 9-31C). Solitary tumors can form polypoid or annular masses with associated regional lymphadenopathy or generalized disease (fig. 9-32) (45).

Microscopic Findings. Mantle cell lymphoma diffusely expands the mucosa in a band-like or nodular fashion, often extending into the superficial submucosa (fig. 9-33). The nodularity reflects colonization of preexisting benign follicles, some of which may be partially effaced by neoplastic cells (fig. 9-34) (44). Lesional cells are slightly larger than normal lymphocytes and contain irregular nuclei with prominent clefts or grooves (fig. 9-35). The cytoplasm is generally scant and nucleoli are inconspicuous. Occasional tumors are infiltrated by scattered macrophages (13).

Immunohistochemical and Molecular Genetic Findings. The tumor cells stain for CD20 and other B-cell markers; there is aberrant expression of the T-cell marker CD5 (fig. 9-36). They almost always stain for CD43 and cyclin-D1, and are negative for CD10 and CD23. They also show t(11;14) translocations involving *BCL-1* and *IgH* (44).

Differential Diagnosis. Mantle cell lymphomas that grow around reactive germinal centers closely simulate the mantle zone of a secondary follicle. Other low-grade lymphomas can usually be distinguished from mantle cell lymphoma following evaluation with a battery of B-cell markers (46). Cyclin D1 is a helpful marker of neoplasia; its expression is limited

Figure 9-31

MANTLE CELL LYMPHOMA OF COLON

A: Multiple lymphomatous polyposis appears as innumerable round, smooth nodules that fill the lumen.

B: Tumor nodules produce an indurated mucosa, with central depressions similar to aphthous ulcers.

C: Lymphoid infiltrates impart a nodular appearance to the mucosa with multiple plaques and aphthous ulcers; the latter reflect small lymphoid aggregates.

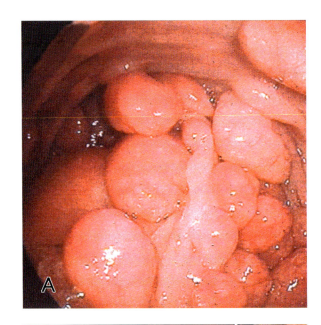

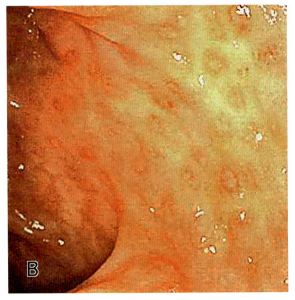

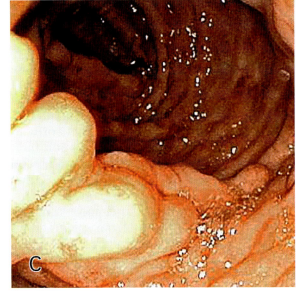

to mantle cell lymphoma, hairy cell leukemia, and plasma cell neoplasms.

Treatment and Prognosis. Intestinal involvement by mantle cell lymphoma is usually associated with systemic disease and the clinical course is aggressive. In the past, most patients died of disease within 3 to 5 years of diagnosis despite intensive chemotherapy and stem cell transplantation (43). However, increased use of high-dose therapy, autologous stem cell transplant, rituximab, and bendamustine, as well as targeted biologic agents, has improved prognosis among affected patients (47,48).

DIFFUSE LARGE B-CELL LYMPHOMA

Definition. *Diffuse large B-cell lymphoma* is the most common lymphoma of the small bowel and colon (49). It is a high-grade neoplasm composed of malignant B cells with nuclei that are at least twice the size of a normal lymphocyte nucleus. These tumors may develop de novo, or reflect transformation of low-grade lymphoma. Up to 50 percent of intestinal diffuse large B-cell lymphomas are associated with a preexisting low-grade lymphoma, usually an extranodal marginal zone lymphoma or follicular lymphoma (49).

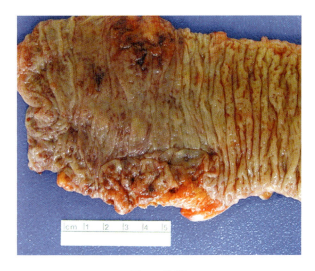

Figure 9-32

MANTLE CELL LYMPHOMA OF DESCENDING COLON

Marked lymphoid infiltration produced a large mass involving much of the colonic circumference. The background mucosa contains a few nodules and shows punctate erythema.

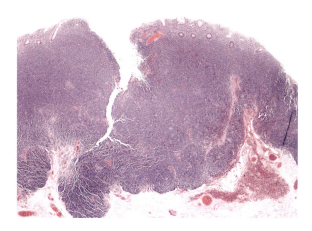

Figure 9-33

MANTLE CELL LYMPHOMA OF COLON

The tumor diffusely infiltrates the submucosa and mucosa. Mucosal architecture is largely effaced; only a few residual crypts are present.

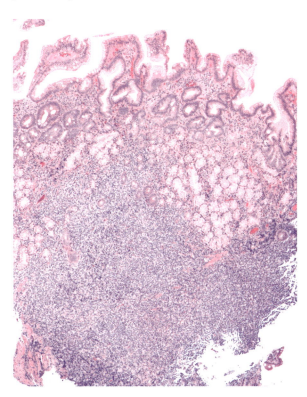

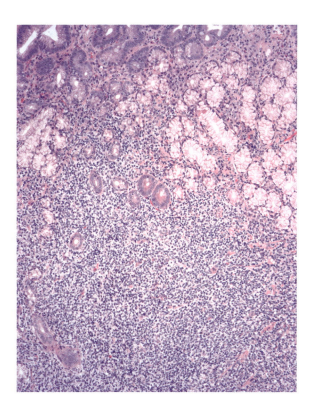

Figure 9-34

MANTLE CELL LYMPHOMA OF DUODENUM

Left: Large tumor nodules expand the submucosa and infiltrate the mucosa. They lack features of reactive germinal centers, and contain a monotonous population of small lymphocytes.

Right: The tumor cells infiltrate the mucosa and overrun Brunner glands as well as the deep crypts.

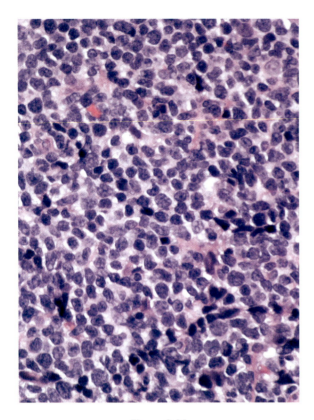

Figure 9-35

MANTLE CELL LYMPHOMA OF DUODENUM

The tumor cells are small to medium-sized, with irregular nuclear contours. No cells are completely round; they show variable degrees of irregularity and angulation. Nucleoli are conspicuous.

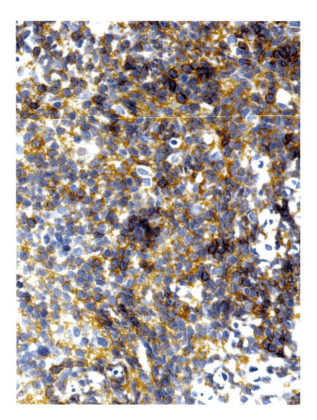

Figure 9-36

MANTLE CELL LYMPHOMA OF COLON

The cytoplasm of the tumor cells stains strongly for CD5.

Clinical Features. Diffuse large B-cell lymphoma develops in older patients, with a peak incidence in the seventh decade unless it occurs in the setting of immunosuppression. Males are affected slightly more commonly than females (49). Pediatric patients rarely develop diffuse large B-cell lymphomas of the intestines; virtually all cases occur in the ileocecal region, and almost exclusively develop in boys (50). The clinical symptoms include abdominal pain, weight loss, or anemia. Tumor perforation can occur following initiation of therapy.

Gross Findings. Intestinal tumors are usually large, ulcerated lesions that transmurally involve the bowel (fig. 9-37A). The overlying mucosa may be eroded or nodular (fig. 9-37B) (20). Occasional tumors form large annular or polypoid masses that cause obstructive symptoms (fig. 9-37C).

Endoscopic findings range from diffuse mucosal induration to a large luminal mass (fig. 9-38). Some cases associated with regional lymphadenopathy show bowel wall thickening and mucosal edema emanating from the mass. The latter may represent infiltrating tumor or secondary inflammatory changes resulting from intermittent obstruction.

Microscopic Findings. Tumors contain sheets of proliferating intermediate to large, dyscohesive cells that efface the normal architecture of the mucosa (fig. 9-39). Tumor cells overrun crypts and distort overlying villi. They contain large, vesicular nuclei with peripherally condensed chromatin and one or more nucleoli (fig. 9-40). Mitotic activity is generally brisk and necrosis is frequently present. Centroblast-like cells contain round nuclei with multiple small nucleoli and scant cytoplasm, whereas immunoblast-like cells contain prominent,

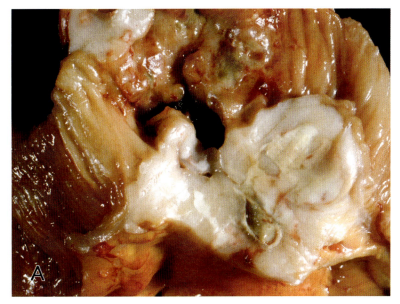

Figure 9-37

DIFFUSE LARGE B-CELL LYMPHOMA OF SMALL BOWEL

A: A fleshy, ulcerated tumor diffusely involves the bowel wall.

B: The tumor diffusely thickens the bowel wall, resulting in flattened mucosal folds, mucosal pallor, and nodularity.

C: This patient presented with acute obstructive symptoms and underwent small bowel resection. The polypoid mass forms the lead point for an intussusception.

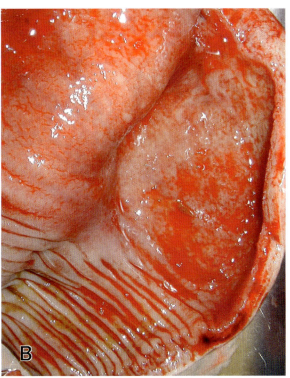

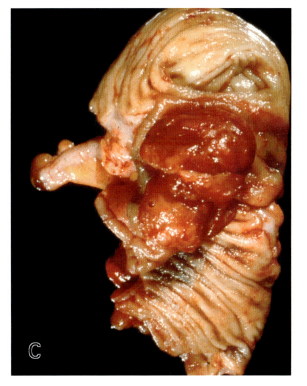

centrally located nucleoli and eosinophilic cytoplasm (fig. 9-41) (50,51). Other cells have more anaplastic features, with pleomorphic nuclei and abundant cytoplasm; some of these may simulate Reed-Sternberg cells (20,49).

Immunohistochemical and Molecular Genetic Findings. Diffuse large B-cell lymphomas show strong diffuse staining for B-cell markers such as CD20 and PAX5, as well as frequent staining for CD79a. This tumor type commonly stains for BCL-2 and approximately 50 percent of cases stain for CD43. Nearly 30 percent of tumors show a germinal center B-cell phenotype, with variable positivity for CD10 and BCL-6, and negativity for MUM1 52. The remaining cases are negative for CD10, positive for MUM1,

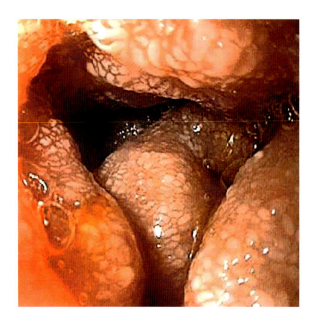 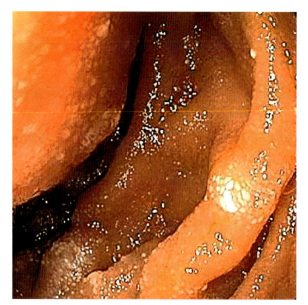

Figure 9-38

DIFFUSE LARGE B-CELL LYMPHOMA

Left: In this lymphoma of the duodenum, infiltration of the mucosa by tumor combined with obstructive regional lymphadenopathy to produce markedly thickened folds and lymphangiectasia.

Right: In the small bowel, a large, polypoid tumor occupies approximately 50 percent of the luminal circumference.

Figure 9-39

DIFFUSE LARGE B-CELL LYMPHOMA OF COLON

The tumor expands the submucosa and infiltrates the mucosa.

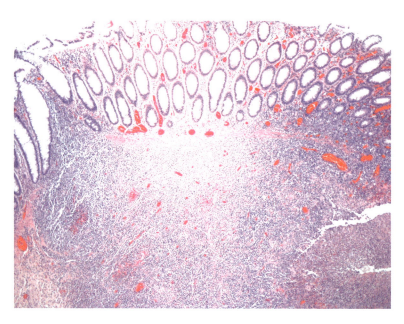

and show variable BCL-6 staining (20,49,53). The tumor cells are negative for T-cell markers, such as CD3, although up to 10 percent of cases are positive for CD5 (54).

A number of cytogenetic abnormalities have been described. Translocations at t(14;18) resulting in *BCL-2* alterations are seen in 20 to 30 percent of tumors; these cases may be derived from follicular lymphoma. Tumors derived from extranodal marginal zone lymphoma may express fusion proteins resulting from t(11;18) translocations affecting *API2* and *MALT1*. Approximately 30 percent of tumors have 3q27 abnormalities that affect *BCL-6* (55).

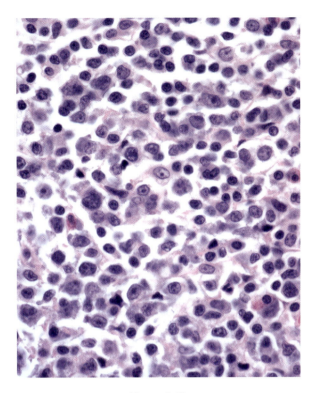

Figure 9-40

DIFFUSE LARGE B-CELL LYMPHOMA OF COLON

Tumor cells harbor large, round or slightly ovoid nuclei with prominent nucleoli. The chromatin is mostly clear with peripheral condensation. Many of the cells contain a moderate amount of eosinophilic cytoplasm.

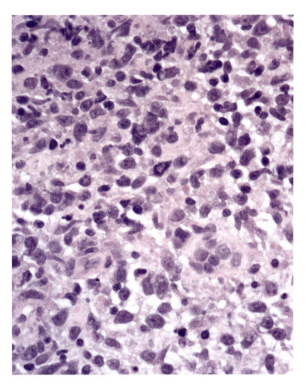

Figure 9-41

DIFFUSE LARGE B-CELL LYMPHOMA OF COLON

The tumor consists of neoplastic cells with large nuclei, irregular contours, and prominent nucleoli. Mitotic figures are easily identified, and scattered apoptotic debris is present.

Differential Diagnosis. Diffuse large B-cell lymphomas can simulate the gross appearance of invasive adenocarcinomas, as well as inflammatory conditions characterized by mucosal nodularity or ulcers. Anaplastic tumors may show cytologic changes that overlap with features of high-grade adenocarcinoma, metastatic malignant melanoma, or even sarcoma (56). Occasional carcinomas contain sheets of large, poorly cohesive cells, although they generally display a somewhat nested growth pattern. Melanomas contain plasmacytoid tumor cells with prominent nucleoli and open chromatin. Gastrointestinal stromal tumors can show plasmacytoid differentiation that resembles hematopoietic neoplasia with plasmacytic differentiation. A basic panel of immunohistochemical stains, including keratin, S-100 protein, DOG1, and CD45 can be useful in differentiation.

Other malignant hematopoietic neoplasms can also mimic diffuse large B-cell lymphoma, and, thus, a limited panel of B- and T-cell markers should be routinely used in suspected cases. Blastoid mantle cell lymphoma can contain cells that show morphologic overlap with diffuse large B-cell lymphoma; cyclin-D1 is useful in distinguishing these entities. Burkitt lymphoma should be a consideration whenever high-grade lymphomas are found in the distal small bowel or in children. In contrast to diffuse large B-cell lymphomas that show Ki-67 labeling of less than 70 percent of tumor cells, Burkitt lymphomas show staining in nearly 100 percent of the lesional cells (13). Involvement of the bowel by acute lymphoblastic leukemia typically shows expression of terminal deoxynucleotide transferase or other markers of immaturity.

Treatment and Prognosis. Most patients present with disease confined to the intestine; blood and bone marrow involvement are rare. Patients are offered chemotherapy, as well as radiation and/or surgery in some cases. Standard

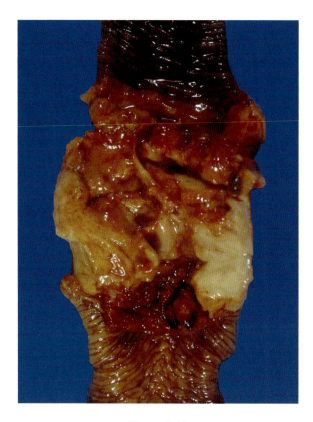

Figure 9-42

BURKITT LYMPHOMA OF DISTAL ILEUM

A circumferential fleshy mass involves the distal ileum. The overlying mucosa is ulcerated. (Courtesy of Dr. D. Beneck, New York, NY.)

agents include rituximab, cyclophosphamide, vincristine, doxorubicin, and dexamethasone (R-CHOP). Most tumors are chemosensitive, with a high rate of remission initially. Those that do not respond to chemotherapy, or recur, may be treated with ablative chemotherapy and stem cell transplantation. Poor prognostic factors include advanced age, high serum lactate dehydrogenase levels, and ascites (13).

BURKITT LYMPHOMA

Definition. *Burkitt lymphoma* is an aggressive B-cell lymphoma that occurs in three clinical situations: endemic, sporadic, and immunodeficiency associated. Most cases develop in association with Epstein-Barr virus (EBV) (57).

Clinical Features. Endemic Burkitt lymphoma especially is associated with EBV and specifically occurs in parts of Africa. Presumably, the virus is oncogenic in the setting of malaria-stimulated lymphoid hyperplasia (58,59). Sporadic tumors have a worldwide distribution and show a predilection for the gastrointestinal tract; they account for 1 to 2 percent of lymphomas in adults and 40 percent of pediatric lymphomas (59). Immunodeficiency-associated tumors usually occur in patients with acquired immunodeficiency due to human immunodeficiency virus (HIV) infection, although some patients have congenital immunodeficiency (60).

Gross Findings. Endemic Burkitt lymphoma generally presents with disease in the facial bones or the small intestine. Patients are usually young children, and males are affected more often than females. Sporadic tumors typically occur in the ileocecal region of young patients, particularly males. Burkitt lymphomas are usually large, bulky exophytic masses with mucosal ulceration (fig. 9-42). The cut surface is homogeneous, tan-white, and bulging (61).

Microscopic Findings. Burkitt lymphomas have very high proliferative and mitotic rates. They also have a high rate of cell turnover, with numerous tingible body macrophages that impart a "starry sky" appearance at low magnification (fig. 9-43).

Tumors are categorized as *classic Burkitt lymphoma*, *plasmacytoid Burkitt lymphoma*, and *atypical Burkitt/Burkitt-like variant*. The cells of classic Burkitt lymphoma are intermediate in size with a rim of basophilic cytoplasm (59). They contain round nuclei with granular chromatin and inconspicuous, often multiple nucleoli (fig. 9-44). Plasmacytoid differentiation is more common among patients with immunodeficiency (57). In this case, the cells contain more abundant, somewhat basophilic cytoplasm and eccentrically located nuclei with prominent nucleoli. Atypical Burkitt/Burkitt-like lymphoma cells also contain a moderate amount of cytoplasm and tend to show more nuclear pleomorphism with less numerous, more prominent nucleoli than are typically seen in classic cases.

Immunohistochemical and Molecular Genetic Findings. Burkitt lymphoma expresses monotypic surface IgM as well as several B-cell markers, including CD19, CD20, CD22, and CD79a. These tumors also stain for CD10, BCL-6, and CD43, but are negative for BCL-2 and CD138. Virtually 100 percent of tumor cells show Ki-67 labeling, and p53 staining is common (fig.

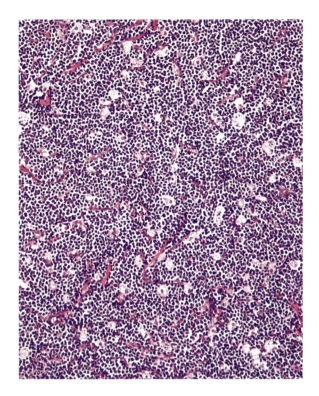

Figure 9-43

BURKITT LYMPHOMA OF TERMINAL ILEUM

The tumor consists of sheets of intermediate-size lymphocytes associated with numerous tingible body macrophages. Brisk mitotic activity is evident.

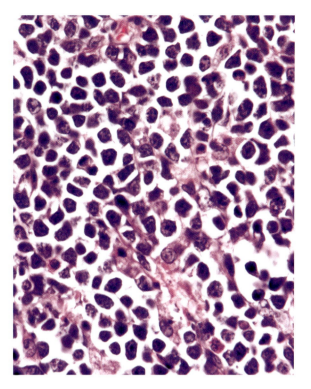

Figure 9-44

BURKITT LYMPHOMA OF TERMINAL ILEUM

The tumor cells contain nuclei with coarse chromatin, several nucleoli, and scant to moderate amounts of cytoplasm.

9-45) (50). The plasmacytoid variant expresses monotypic cytoplasmic immunoglobulin.

Translocations affecting *MYC* are universally present: 80 percent of cases show t(8;14) translocations between *MYC* and *IgH*, and 20 percent show translocations between *MYC* and genes encoding kappa [t(2;8)] or lambda [t(8;22)] (62).

Differential Diagnosis. The differential diagnosis of Burkitt lymphoma includes other high-grade lymphomas, most notably diffuse large B-cell lymphoma. In most cases, the problem can be resolved with a combination of immuno-histochemistry and molecular testing. Atypical Burkitt/Burkitt-like lymphomas are classified as Burkitt lymphomas, provided they harbor *MYC* rearrangements; lymphomas that show some morphologic features of Burkitt lymphoma, but lack *MYC* rearrangements, should not be classified as Burkitt lymphoma. These tumors represent a heterogeneous group of aggressive neoplasms with a poor prognosis. Some of them have biallelic alterations in *BCL-2* or *BCL-6* and

are termed "double-hit" lymphomas. Others show BCL-2 immunopositivity and comprise a subset of unclassifiable B-cell lymphomas.

Treatment and Prognosis. The highly proliferative nature of Burkitt lymphoma renders it potentially curable. Survival rates range from 80 to 90 percent among patients with endemic and sporadic disease who receive intensive chemotherapy (63). Decreased immunosuppression in the post-transplant setting, combined with chemotherapy and rituximab, may result in a good therapeutic response (64). Similarly, highly active antiretroviral therapy (HAART) can improve immunity among HIV-infected patients so that they can better tolerate chemotherapy.

HODGKIN LYMPHOMA OF THE GASTROINTESTINAL TRACT

Definition. *Primary Hodgkin lymphoma of the gastrointestinal tract* is extremely rare and accounts for less than 0.5 percent of all cases of Hodgkin lymphoma (65). Most cases of

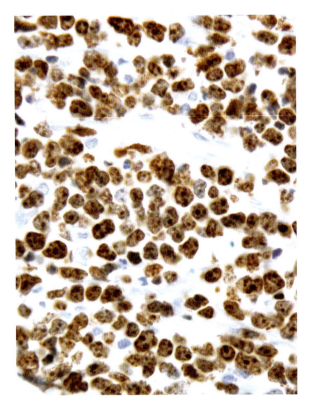

Figure 9-45

BURKITT LYMPHOMA OF TERMINAL ILEUM

The proliferative index is very high; virtually all the tumor cells display nuclear Ki-67 staining.

gastrointestinal Hodgkin lymphoma represent secondary involvement in patients with widespread disease.

Clinical Features. The clinical features of primary gastrointestinal Hodgkin disease are not well described owing to its rarity. Patients tend to be adults, and men are more commonly affected than women (66). Several cases have been described in patient with underlying Crohn disease and longstanding immunosuppressive therapy, as well as in patients with HIV infection (67). Symptoms include night sweats, fever, weight loss, abdominal pain, nausea, vomiting, diarrhea, and hematochezia.

Gross Findings. Regional lymph node involvement and distant spread are often evident even when the bulk of disease is located in the small bowel or colon. Tumors involve the full thickness of the bowel wall and form polypoid, ulcerated masses. Those that develop in patients with Crohn disease show a predilection for

areas of transmural injury, such as fistulae and strictures (68).

Microscopic Findings. Classic mixed cellularity and nodular sclerosing Hodgkin disease can occur as primary intestinal tumors, but lymphocyte-predominant disease has not been described (65). The morphologic features are similar to those of the extraintestinal lymphoma, showing characteristic Reed-Sternberg cells on a background of mixed inflammation rich in eosinophils, macrophages, and mononuclear cells (fig. 9-46). Reed-Sternberg cells and variants contain large nuclei with open chromatin and macronucleoli (fig. 9-47).

Immunohistochemical and Molecular Genetic Findings. Reed-Sternberg cells consistently label with CD15 and CD30, and are variably positive for CD20 (fig. 9-48) (67). They are negative for CD3, CD79a, and CD45, similar to nonintestinal Hodgkin lymphoma. Interestingly, in situ hybridization often demonstrates EBV-encoded RNA (EBER) in Reed-Sternberg cells, and immunostains can detect latent membrane protein in some cases (69).

Differential Diagnosis. The differential diagnosis includes other forms of non-Hodgkin lymphoma, which can usually be resolved using a targeted panel of immunostains. Hodgkin disease that features numerous Reed-Sternberg cells and large atypical variants may be confused with anaplastic carcinoma. In this situation, cytokeratin immunostains help establish a diagnosis, with the caveat that carcinomas can show CD15 positivity, similar to neoplastic cells of Hodgkin lymphoma.

Treatment and Prognosis. Treatment of intestinal Hodgkin lymphoma consists of systemic chemotherapy. Patients generally have a good prognosis, similar to that of patients without involvement of the gastrointestinal tract (65). Treatment may be complicated in patients who develop Hodgkin lymphoma in the setting of Crohn disease or longstanding immunosuppression.

POST-TRANSPLANT LYMPHOPROLIFERATIVE DISORDER

Definition and General Features. Patients who undergo solid organ or bone marrow transplantation are at risk for EBV-driven lymphoproliferative disorders. Post-transplant immunosuppression impairs T-cell–mediated immunity

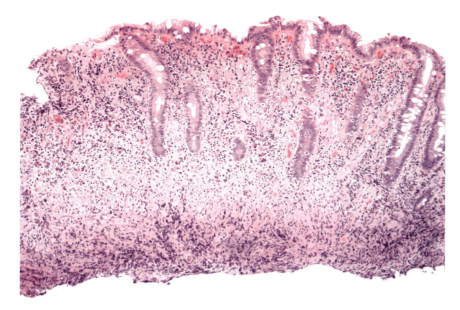

Figure 9-46

HODGKIN LYMPHOMA OF COLON

Tumor cells infiltrate the colonic mucosa in this superficial biopsy from a patient with Hodgkin disease. Large, atypical cells are associated with lymphocytes, macrophages, and eosinophils, many of which infiltrate the crypt epithelium.

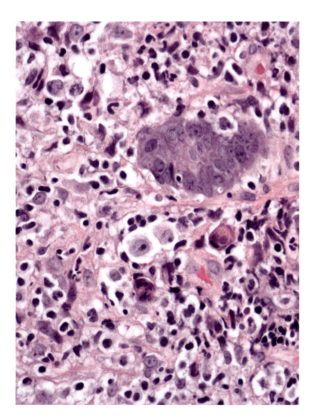

Figure 9-47

HODGKIN LYMPHOMA OF COLON

Reed-Sternberg-like cells contain large pale nuclei with folded membranes, bright red macronuclei, and abundant, faintly eosinophilic cytoplasm.

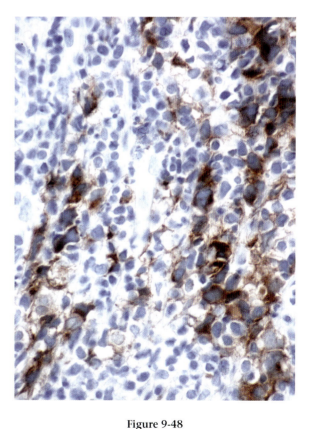

Figure 9-48

HODGKIN LYMPHOMA OF COLON

A CD30 immunostain decorates the Reed-Sternberg cells. The mixed inflammatory cells in the background are negative.

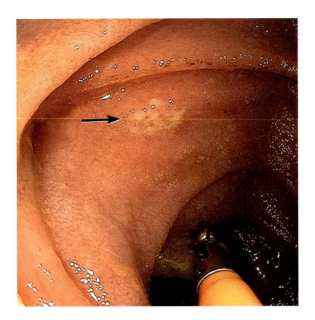

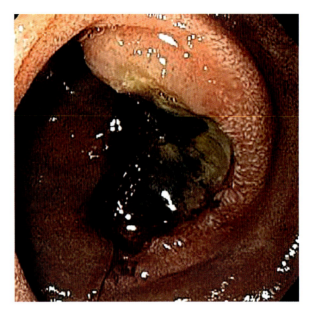

Figure 9-49

**POST-TRANSPLANT LYMPHOPROLIFERATIVE
DISORDER OF ILEUM**

A white fibrinous exudate overlies a small ulcer (arrow) in the terminal ileum. Biopsies revealed polymorphous post-transplant lymphoproliferative disease.

Figure 9-50

**POST-TRANSPLANT LYMPHOPROLIFERATIVE
DISORDER OF DUODENUM**

A large cratered ulcer developed in the proximal duodenum of this patient who underwent stem cell transplantation for acute myelogenous leukemia. Biopsies revealed monomorphic post-transplant lymphoproliferative disorder.

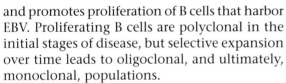

and promotes proliferation of B cells that harbor EBV. Proliferating B cells are polyclonal in the initial stages of disease, but selective expansion over time leads to oligoclonal, and ultimately, monoclonal, populations.

The oncogenic properties of EBV are probably related to expression of latent viral antigens in memory B cells. EBV nuclear antigen 2 upregulates latent membrane protein (LMP1). The latter induces CD23 expression in B cells and drives production of BCL-2, which has antiapoptotic properties.

Clinical Features. The risk of post-transplant lymphoproliferative disorder depends on several factors. Risk increases with higher levels of immunosuppression and among patients with nonrenal organ transplants, probably reflecting the higher doses of immunosuppression required for preservation of these grafts (70,71). It is also more common among pediatric patients, many of whom are seronegative for EBV prior to transplantation (72). These patients presumably acquire EBV infection either through the donor organ, or through primary infection following

transplantation. Gastrointestinal involvement by post-transplant lymphoproliferative disorder is directly linked to cyclosporine usage. It usually occurs within 12 months of transplantation, although it may develop after years of immunosuppression. Symptoms include fever, lymphadenopathy, gastrointestinal symptoms, mononucleosis-like syndrome, and declining graft function.

Gross Findings. The gross and endoscopic features of disease are variable. The small bowel is the most common site of involvement. Small lesions may appear as ulcers or erosions, whereas larger tumors may be bulky luminal masses or present as strictures (figs. 9-49, 9-50) (72,73).

Microscopic Findings. The World Health Organization (WHO) classifies post-transplant lymphoproliferative disorders according to morphologic and molecular features (74). Early lesions are polyclonal B-cell proliferations and do not efface tissue architecture. They consist of dense, slightly atypical lymphoid infiltrates associated with numerous plasma cells and scattered immunoblasts (75).

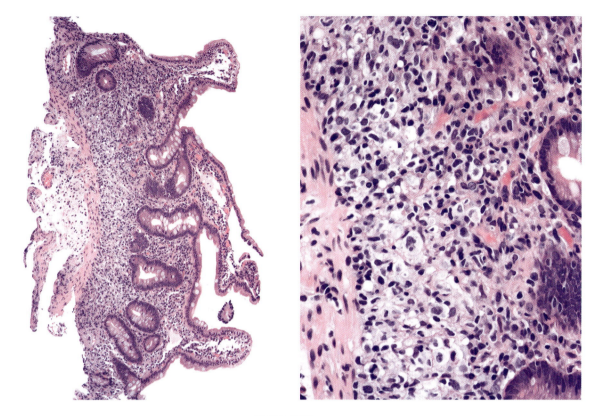

Figure 9-51

POLYMORPHOUS POST-TRANSPLANT LYMPHOPROLIFERATIVE DISORDER OF DUODENUM

Left: This 64-year-old male underwent allogeneic stem cell transplantation and subsequently developed diarrheal symptoms. Biopsies of the duodenum show a deep infiltrate of atypical cells that contain abundant eosinophilic cytoplasm.

Right: The lesional cells contain enlarged, convoluted nuclei with open chromatin and prominent nucleoli. Additional studies demonstrated a monoclonal B-cell population. The large cells showed strong labeling for EBV-encoded RNA (EBER).

The polymorphic variant is a destructive mass lesion consisting of lymphocytes, plasma cells, centrocytes, and immunoblasts (fig. 9-51). It may be polyclonal or monoclonal. The monomorphic variant is a high-grade neoplasm that can show B- or T-cell differentiation and resembles a variety of different tumor types (fig. 9-52) (76,77).

Approximately 85 percent of tumors are B-cell neoplasms that resemble diffuse large B-cell lymphoma, Burkitt and Burkitt-like lymphomas, plasmablastic lymphoma, plasma cell myeloma, or plasmacytoma (78,79). T-cell neoplasms account for 15 percent of cases and resemble peripheral T-cell lymphoma, not otherwise specified. Rare tumors simulate Hodgkin disease.

Immunohistochemical and Molecular Genetic Findings. Immunohistochemical features are variable and can be useful in subtyping disease (74). Early lesions show a mixed population of polyclonal B cells, plasma cells, and T cells. Oligoclonal populations may be detected by molecular methods. Polymorphic tumors contain B-cell populations, with or without light chain restriction, in a small proportion of lesional cells. If present, Reed-Sternberg-like cells are CD30 and CD20 positive, but CD15 negative. Genetic studies reveal clonal rearrangements of immunoglobulin genes in subpopulations of lesional cells (73).

Monomorphic variants show immunohistochemical features that vary with tumor morphology and extent of plasmacytic differentiation. Those of B-cell lineage show frequent monotypic immunoglobulin and many cases are CD30 positive, regardless of the degree of cytologic atypia.

Clonal immunoglobulin gene rearrangements are almost universally present. Alterations

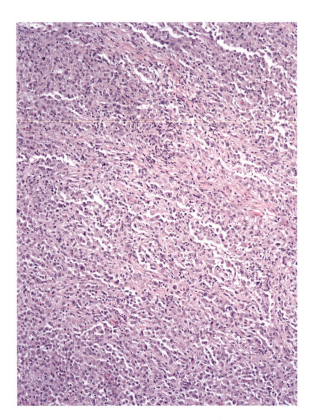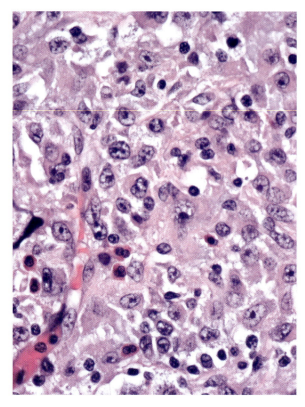

Figure 9-52

MONOMORPHIC POST-TRANSPLANT LYMPHOPROLIFERATIVE DISORDER

Left: This 51-year-old solid organ transplant patient developed a bowel obstruction secondary to a mass. The tumor is composed of sheets of large, atypical cells with abundant eosinophilic cytoplasm. Additional studies demonstrated a monoclonal B-cell population and the large cells showed strong labeling for EBER.

Right: The tumor cells contain large nuclei with open chromatin and prominent, centrally located nucleoli.

affecting *TP53*, *MYC*, and *BCL6* are often present in association with widespread chromosomal gains and losses (75).

In situ hybridization for EBER is a more sensitive method than immunohistochemistry for detecting EBV infection, and is often positive (fig. 9-52). Both methods may be negative in monomorphic T-cell neoplasms.

Differential Diagnosis. Post-transplant lymphoproliferative disorders can simulate the features of a variety of neoplastic and non-neoplastic intestinal disorders. Early lesions can simply be overlooked, or interpreted to represent an inflammatory response to infection, so a high index of suspicion is often necessary. It is worth remembering that mononuclear cell-rich infiltrates with immunoblasts are not common in the post-transplant setting; their detection

should always prompt consideration of an EBV-driven process.

A destructive growth pattern is typical of the polymorphic variant, but this finding is not a feature of non-neoplastic inflammatory conditions. Most polymorphic and monomorphic variants show enough cytologic atypia to warrant further investigation, which ultimately distinguishes them from other high-grade hematopoietic neoplasms.

Treatment and Prognosis. Treatment consists of decreased immunosuppression in combination with a number of approaches: chemotherapy, surgery, radiation to the site, and targeted therapies. Patients with early lesions and polymorphous variants usually respond well to reduced immunosuppression, whereas many patients with monomorphic disease succumb

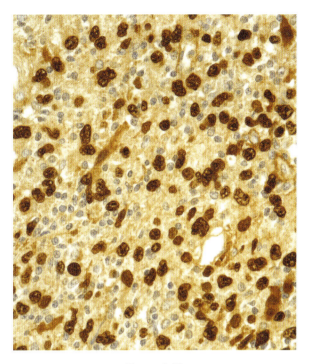

Figure 9-53

**MONOMORPHIC POST-TRANSPLANT
LYMPHOPROLIFERATIVE DISORDER**

In situ hybridization for EBER strongly labels the nuclei of the tumor (same case as figs. 9-48 and 9-49).

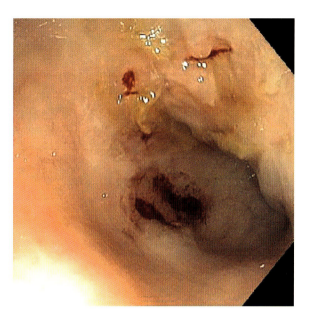

Figure 9-54

**DIFFUSE LARGE B-CELL LYMPHOMA OF
COLON ASSOCIATED WITH IMMUNOSUPPRESSION**

This 24-year-old male with human immunodeficiency virus (HIV) and acquired immunodeficiency syndrome (AIDS) presented with colonic obstruction and was found to have a nearly obstructing stricture in the sigmoid colon. The mucosa is indurated and nodular, with loss of the normal vascular pattern.

to their disease (77). Tumors that do not harbor EBV generally have a more aggressive course than those in which viral RNAs are detected.

LYMPHOPROLIFERATIVE DISORDERS ASSOCIATED WITH IMMUNOSUPPRESSION

Definition. Immunosuppression is a risk factor for lymphoma development in the gastrointestinal tract. In fact, lymphoma is the second most common malignancy among HIV-infected individuals. Up to one third of *HIV-related lymphomas* develop in the gastrointestinal tract (80). Unfortunately, lymphoma risk seems unaffected, or even increased, by HAART in HIV-positive patients (81). Intestinal lymphoma can also complicate longstanding immunosuppression due to other reasons, such as therapy for inflammatory bowel disease or other immune-mediated disorders, solid organ and stem cell transplantation, or a congenital immunodeficiency syndrome (82–84).

Clinical Features. Most patients with HIV-related lymphomas are young or middle-aged adult homosexual males. Tumors show a predilection for the colorectum and, thus, patients present with anal pain, small caliber stools, obstruction, and hematochezia. Small intestinal disease produces diarrheal symptoms. Patients with underlying inflammatory bowel disease may have symptoms that simulate worsening colitis, such as abdominal pain or rectal bleeding. Intestinal lymphomas are also increased among patients with X-linked lymphoproliferative disorder and common variable immunodeficiency. Infection with EBV is an important risk factor for lymphoma development in all of these groups (84).

Gross Findings. Most tumors that develop in immunosuppressed patients are high-grade lymphomas that form large, bulky masses associated with regional lymphadenopathy or fistulae (figs. 9-54, 9-55) (85). Tumors may cause intussusception, particularly when occurring in the ileocecal region. Diffuse infiltration of the wall is characteristic and ulcers are variably present (fig. 9-56).

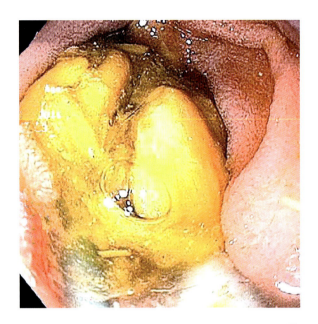
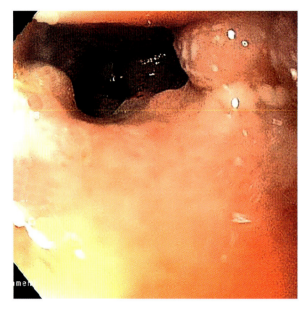

Figure 9-55

DIFFUSE LARGE B-CELL LYMPHOMA OF DUODENUM ASSOCIATED WITH IMMUNOSUPPRESSION

Left: Multiple polypoid projections fill the duodenal lumen of this 41-year-old woman.
Right: In another case, a large mural mass occupies nearly 50 percent of the duodenal circumference.

Figure 9-56

DIFFUSE LARGE B-CELL LYMPHOMA OF SMALL INTESTINE ASSOCIATED WITH IMMUNOSUPPRESSION

The tumor diffusely infiltrates the bowel wall, resulting in an ill-defined mural thickening.

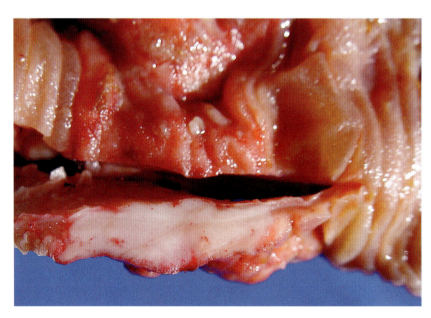

Microscopic Findings. Although low-grade B-cell lymphomas have been described in immunosuppressed patients, most of these are probably sporadic tumors that are unrelated to immunodeficiency. Immunosuppression-related lymphoproliferative lesions are typically high-grade tumors, most commonly diffuse large B-cell lymphomas (fig. 9-57). Diffuse large B-cell lymphomas that develop in HIV-infected patients often contain large immunoblasts or show prominent plasmacytoid differentiation, and are classified as plasmablastic lymphomas (fig. 9-58). Burkitt and Burkitt-like lymphomas also occur, as previously described (80). A number of lymphoma subtypes have been described in association with Crohn disease, including diffuse

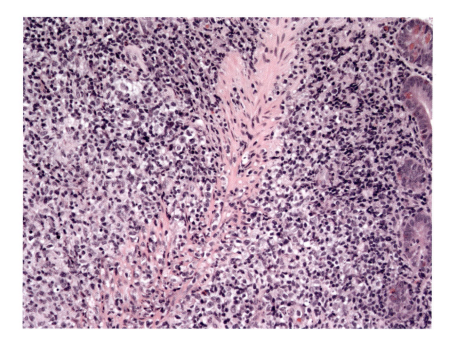

Figure 9-57

DIFFUSE LARGE B-CELL LYMPHOMA OF DUODENUM

Large, atypical cells infiltrate and expand the mucosa. They contain abundant, faintly eosinophilic cytoplasm and large, multilobated nuclei. Numerous mature T cells are present in the background.

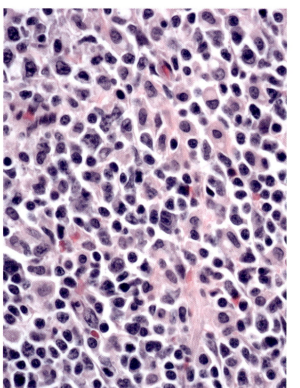

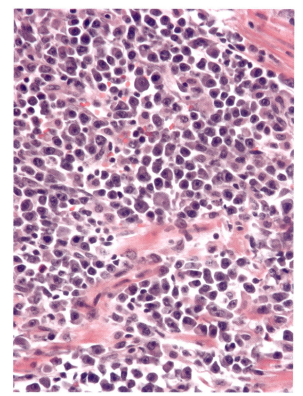

Figure 9-58

DIFFUSE LARGE B-CELL LYMPHOMA OF COLON ASSOCIATED WITH HIV INFECTION

Left: The tumor contains large immunoblast-like cells and others that show plasmacytic differentiation (same case as fig. 9-53).

Right: This tumor also shows plasmablastic differentiation. Lesional cells contain abundant eccentric cytoplasm with a perinuclear hoff and large round nuclei with macronucleoli.

large B-cell lymphoma, Hodgkin disease, T-cell lymphomas, and Burkitt lymphoma (85).

Immunohistochemical and Molecular Genetic Findings. The immunohistochemical features of lymphoproliferative disorders associated with immunodeficiency are indistinguishable from those of morphologically similar tumors that develop in immunocompetent individuals (86). A high number of the former harbor EBV, supporting the concept that the virus is oncogenic in the setting of altered immunity (87).

Treatment and Prognosis. Patients with immunodeficiency-related lymphoproliferative disease have a slightly worse prognosis than those with sporadic intestinal lymphomas of similar subtype. Rituximab and newer chemotherapeutic agents have improved 2-year survival rates to at least 75 percent. Approximately 50 percent of tumors are cured with a combination of chemotherapy and surgery (88). Prognosis is strongly associated with the achievement of complete remission (89).

T-CELL LYMPHOMA, NOT OTHERWISE SPECIFIED

Primary gastrointestinal T-cell lymphoma is extremely uncommon outside the setting of immunosuppression or an immunodeficiency syndrome, as described above. Most examples represent secondary involvement of the gastrointestinal tract in patients with an established T-cell lymphoma affecting other organs. Two entities that show a predilection for the small bowel and colon, extranodal NK/T-cell lymphoma and enteropathy associated T-cell lymphoma, are described below.

Extranodal NK/T-cell Lymphoma

Definition. *Extranodal NK/T-cell lymphomas of nasal type* are extremely rare tumors that can affect the gastrointestinal tract. They are generally regarded as high-grade neoplasms, similar to other T-cell lymphomas, and are highly associated with EBV. Angiocentric T-cell lymphoma, lethal midline granuloma, and angiocentric immunoproliferative lesion are older terms now classified in the extranodal NK/T-cell lymphoma category (90).

Clinical Features. Extranodal NK/T-cell lymphoma is a disease of adults and has a predilection to affect Asian patients as well as indigenous persons from Mexico, Central America, and South America (91). Most patients are adults, and males are affected more commonly than females.

Systemic manifestations include fever, malaise, weight loss, and lymphadenopathy. Some patients present with hematophagocytic syndrome (92). Patients may present with symptoms related to bowel obstruction or chronic blood loss, although intestinal perforation may be the first manifestation of disease.

Gross Findings. Tumors are large, bulky masses that have a polypoid luminal component. Lesions are often extensively ulcerated and friable, with recent signs of bleeding.

Microscopic Findings. NK/T-cell lymphoma displays a sheet-like proliferation of variably sized, markedly atypical tumor cells that diffusely permeate all layers of the bowel wall. An angiocentric growth pattern with destructive invasion of blood vessels (fig. 9-59) is characteristic. Some tumor cells contain small hyperchromatic nuclei with irregular, angulated contours and coarse chromatin; others contain larger nuclei with open chromatin and prominent nucleoli, or anaplastic features (93). Most tumor cells contain abundant clear or eosinophilic cytoplasm. Mitotic activity is usually brisk, and most tumors show extensive tumor necrosis, often with abundant apoptotic cellular debris in viable areas (90).

Immunohistochemical and Molecular Genetic Findings. Extranodal NK/T-cell lymphomas express CD2 and CD56, but are negative for most other T-cell markers, including CD3 (94). However, they do show cytoplasmic staining for CD3ε (95). Virtually all cases are positive for EBV by in situ hybridization, and approximately 40 percent overexpress p53 (96). Tumors that show cytotoxic T-cell differentiation may express granzyme B and TIA-1 (97).

Mutations are generally lacking in both T-cell receptor and immunoglobulin genes, although tumors that show cytotoxic T-cell differentiation may have T-cell receptor-gamma (*TCRX*) gene rearrangements (96). Extranodal NK/T-cell lymphomas show a wide variety of chromosomal abnormalities, but characteristic molecular alterations have not yet been identified.

Differential Diagnosis. The differential diagnosis includes hematopoietic and non-hematopoietic malignancies. High-grade B-cell

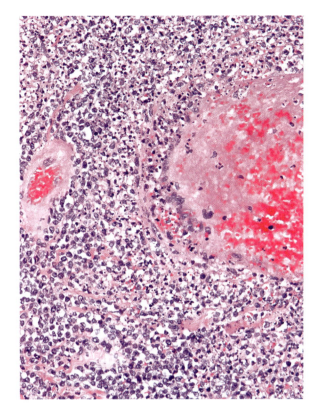

Figure 9-59

EXTRANODAL NK/T-CELL LYMPHOMA, NASAL TYPE

Sheets of pleomorphic, highly atypical tumor cells diffusely infiltrate the tissue and destructively invade a large caliber vessel. Numerous mitotic figures are present and readily identified. (Courtesy of Dr. S. Owens, Ann Arbor, MI.)

and T-cell neoplasms can contain tumor cells that have features that overlap with those of extranodal NK/T-cell lymphoma. An angiocentric, destructive growth pattern and extensive necrosis are characteristic features of extranodal NK/T-cell lymphoma, and less commonly seen in high-grade B- or T-cell lymphomas. Extranodal NK/T-cell lymphomas can also simulate malignant melanoma, anaplastic carcinoma, and epithelioid sarcoma. Immunohistochemical stains help facilitate the differential diagnosis.

Treatment and Prognosis. The prognosis of patients with extranodal NK/T-cell lymphoma is variable. The tumor is aggressive and generally presents at an advanced stage of disease, although several recent advances have improved overall survival. Extranodal NK/T-cell lymphoma cells express P-glycoprotein, which effectively exports chemotherapeutic agents

out of the cell. Combination therapy with l-asparaginase, corticosteroids, methotrexate, ifosfamide, and etoposide has improved remission rates and overall survival (98). Response to therapy can be monitored through the detection of free EBV DNA fragments in peripheral blood; higher levels reflect a greater tumor burden and predict poorer survival (99).

ENTEROPATHY-ASSOCIATED T-CELL LYMPHOMA

Definition. *Enteropathy-associated T-cell lymphomas* (EATLs) are rare and account for less than 5 percent of all gastrointestinal lymphomas. The WHO subclassified them as type I and type II in the past but has changed the classification as of 2016.

The WHO 2016 classification divides intestinal T-cell lymphomas into two types. The first is *enteropathy-associated T-cell lymphoma*. This is associated with celiac disease and tends to be found in persons of European origin. It generally displays pleomorphic cytologic features. Immunophenotypes are CD3+, CD5-, CD7+, CD8+/-, CD4-, and CD56-.

The second type, *monomorphic epitheliotropic intestinal T-cell lymphoma* (termed EATL, type 2 in the past), is unassociated with celiac disease and found in Asians and Hispanics. It often has *STAT5B* mutations, is derived from gamma delta T cells, and has monomorphic cytologic features. Immunophenotypes are CD3+, CD4-, CD8+, and CD56+.

Classic EATL has been regarded as a lesion that arises in association with so-called refractory sprue, which has been subclassified based on the nature of intraepithelial T cells. Type 1 refractory sprue is characterized by the presence of polyclonal populations, whereas monoclonal T cells are present in type 2 disease (101).

Clinical Features. EATL typically affects older patients, with onset 15 to 20 years after the diagnosis of celiac disease. Most patients have a diagnosis of celiac disease and present with recurrent sprue-like symptoms despite gluten withdrawal, abdominal pain, gastrointestinal bleeding, or symptoms related to small intestinal perforation (101). Some patients, however, have no prior malabsorptive symptoms. A subset of patients in the latter group have histologic evidence of celiac disease, with villous shortening,

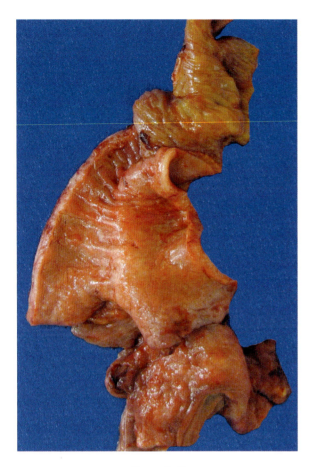

Figure 9-60

ENTEROPATHY-ASSOCIATED T-CELL LYMPHOMA

The proximal jejunum is diffusely infiltrated by lymphoma. The bowel wall is thickened with loss of the normal fold pattern.

crypt hyperplasia, and intraepithelial lymphocytosis in the background mucosa at the time of lymphoma resection; these patients are best classified as having type I EATL. Patients without a history of malabsorption or sprue-like changes in the duodenal mucosa are considered to have type II disease.

Gross Findings. Refractory sprue may be accompanied by benign-appearing ulcers in the proximal small bowel, which have been termed "ulcerative jejunitis." These ulcers contain monoclonal T-cell populations and are generally considered to represent incipient lymphomas at risk for progression to EATL (102). Overt lymphomas appear as solitary or multiple raised, often ulcerated, plaques or masses, or diffuse

mural thickening (fig. 9-58). Imaging studies may reveal features of intestinal perforation, mesenteric lymphadenopathy, or cavitary lesions in the spleen and regional lymph nodes.

Microscopic Findings. EATL may display high-grade or intermediate- to low-grade cytologic features. EATL tumors are more commonly high grade and contain neoplastic lymphocytes with sheet-like growth punctuated by tingible body macrophages. Tumor cells tend to be medium to large in size, with vesicular nuclei, coarse chromatin, and inconspicuous nucleoli (fig. 9-60) (101). Nuclei are ovoid or round with irregular contours and, in some cases, a cerebriform appearance (fig. 9-61). Mitotic activity, cellular necrosis, and a mixed inflammatory infiltrate composed of eosinophils and macrophages are common. The background mucosa may show features of celiac disease, with villous architectural abnormalities, crypt hyperplasia, mononuclear cell-rich inflammation in the lamina propria, and intraepithelial lymphocytes, which often contain monoclonal populations as well.

Monomorphic epitheliotropic intestinal T-cell lymphomas are more likely to have a monomorphic appearance owing to the presence of monotonous, small to medium-sized lymphocytes. They have slightly irregular nuclei and a rim of pale or clear cytoplasm (103).

Immunohistochemical and Molecular Genetic Findings. EATLs typically express CD2, CD3, and CD7, and decreased CD5 (104). Genetic abnormalities, including amplifications of chromosome 9q31.3 or deletions in 16q12.1, are common (105,106). In addition to these features, EATLs are usually negative for CD8 (80 percent) and CD56 (90 percent). They show frequent gains of genetic material on chromosomes 1q and 5q, and tend to have the HLA-DQ2/DQ8 genotype (107). Monomorphic epitheliotropic intestinal T-cell lymphoma tumor cells are CD8 positive and may coexpress both CD56 and cytotoxic granule-associated protein, TIA-1 (108). They also show more frequent amplifications of 8q24 affecting *MYC* (106).

Patients with refractory celiac disease symptoms who lack overt lymphoma may also harbor abnormal T-cell populations in their mucosae (109). Some have intraepithelial lymphocyte populations that show loss of CD3 and CD8, as

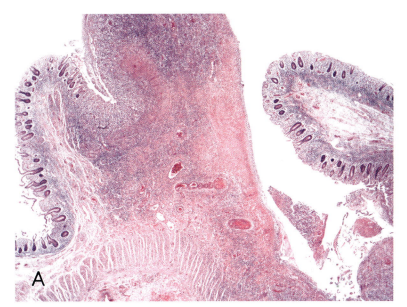

Figure 9-61

ENTEROPATHY-ASSOCIATED T-CELL LYMPHOMA

A: The proximal jejunum is infiltrated by lymphoma that diffusely expands the mucosa and submucosa. Surface ulceration is present.

B: Atypical cells infiltrate the mucosa; they contain convoluted cerebriform nuclei. The surface epithelium is infiltrated by mature-appearing T cells typical of gluten sensitivity.

C: The tumor cells are large and contain convoluted nuclei with coarse chromatin. Scattered mitotic figures are present.

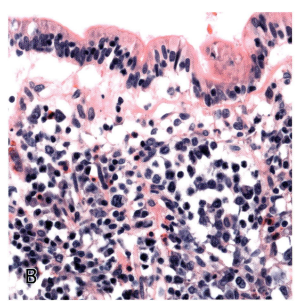

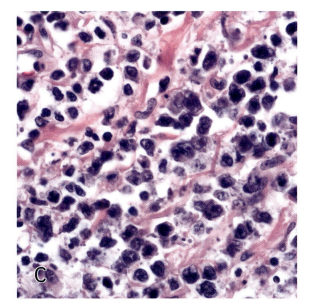

well as 1q trisomy. A subset later develops EATLs that display identical molecular alterations. For this reason, patients who have abnormal T-cell populations in their intestinal mucosae are considered to have cryptic (in situ) EATL and require surveillance for potential evolution of disease.

Differential Diagnosis. The differential diagnosis includes other types of T-cell lymphoma, as well as large B-cell lymphoma. Anatomic location can be helpful, as most diffuse large B-cell lymphomas of the small bowel affect the ileum, whereas EATLs show a predilection for the duodenum and jejunum. T- and B-cell lym-phomas can show a broad spectrum of cytologic abnormalities, but are readily distinguished based on a combination of morphologic features and immunohistochemical staining patterns. For example, extranodal NK/T-cell lymphomas frequently contain angiocentric intermediate-sized to large cells with angioinvasion and necrosis. They express CD56 and TIA-1, similar to monomorphic epitheliotropic intestinal T-cell lymphoma, but are negative for CD8 and βF1, and show cytoplasmic CD3 staining, rather than surface staining. Unlike EATLs, extranodal NK/T-cell lymphomas are EBV positive.

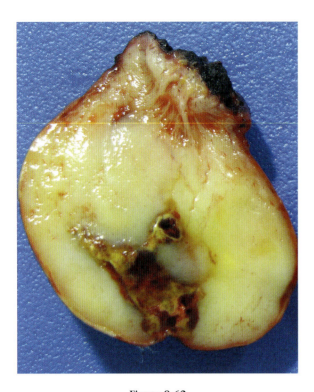

Figure 9-62

FOLLICULAR DENDRITIC CELL SARCOMA

A 19-year-old man had a 3-cm perirectal mass that proved to be a follicular dendritic cell sarcoma. The tumor has a fleshy, lobulated cut surface with an area of cystic degeneration and necrosis.

EATL should also be distinguished from NK-cell enteropathy, which has also been termed "lymphomatoid gastropathy." Patients with NK-cell enteropathy are generally asymptomatic or have vague abdominal complaints, but lack a history of celiac disease (110,111). Infiltrates may affect one or more sites and appear as discrete plaques, ulcers, or nodules that usually span less than 1 cm. The lesions contain diffuse infiltrates composed of intermediate-sized to large atypical lymphocytes. They express cytoplasmic CD3, as well as CD56 and TIA-1, similar to extranodal NK/T-cell lymphoma. Unlike the latter, however, NK-cell enteropathy does not contain EBV and is associated with an indolent clinical course with an excellent prognosis (112).

Treatment and Prognosis. Patients with obstructive symptoms, uncontrolled bleeding, or perforation are treated with surgical resection. Intensive adjuvant chemotherapy is generally recommended. This includes cyclophosphamide, doxorubicin, vincristine, and prednisone (CHOP) or cyclophosphamide, vincristine, doxorubicin, and dexamethasone (hyper-CVAD). Some patients may benefit from aggressive chemotherapy followed by bone marrow transplantation. Nevertheless, the prognosis is generally poor, even with aggressive treatment (113).

FOLLICULAR DENDRITIC CELL SARCOMA

Definition. *Follicular dendritic cell sarcomas* are rare neoplasms that simulate the features of antigen-presenting cells found in the follicles of lymph nodes and extranodal lymphoid tissue.

Clinical Features. Follicular dendritic cell sarcomas show no age or gender predilection (114). They rarely cause systemic symptoms; patients present with complaints related to a mass lesion, including abdominal pain, diarrhea, or gastrointestinal bleeding (115).

Gross Findings. The tumors are multinodular, well-circumscribed, bulging masses (fig. 9-62). They can be quite large, in which case they can show cystic degeneration or frank necrosis (115).

Microscopic Findings. The histologic features are variable. Most tumors contain plump spindle or ovoid cells, with ill-defined cell borders and faintly eosinophilic cytoplasm. Tumor cells are arranged in sweeping fascicles, storiform patterns, or whorls (fig. 9-63, left). Nuclei are elongated, with vesicular or granular chromatin and conspicuous nucleoli.

Follicular dendritic cell sarcomas are often highly cellular, although mitotic figures are generally few in number, ranging up to 10 per 10 high-power fields (116). Some tumors contain cells with large pleomorphic nuclei, prominent nucleoli, and abundant cytoplasm; mitotic activity is more brisk in these cases. Regardless of the degree of cytologic atypia, mature small B and T lymphocytes are frequently present throughout the tumor, particularly in a perivascular distribution (fig. 9-63, right) (115). Cases that simulate the features of inflammatory pseudotumor may be associated with hyaline-vascular Castleman disease and EBV positivity, but they have not been described in the tubular gut.

Immunohistochemical and Molecular Genetic Findings. Follicular dendritic cell sarcomas generally show strong immunopositivity for follicular dendritic cell markers, including

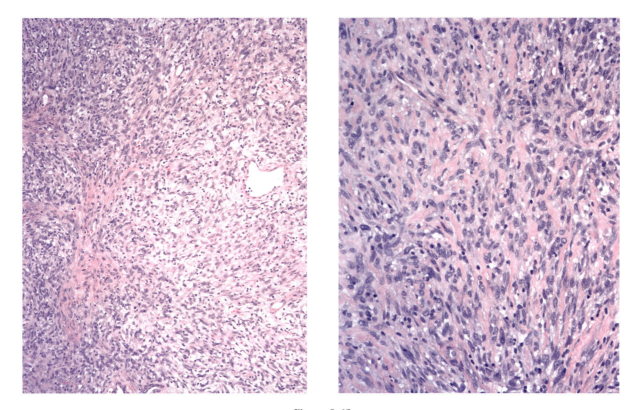

Figure 9-63

FOLLICULAR DENDRITIC CELL SARCOMA

Left: The tumor contains sheets and fascicles of plump, spindled cells with fibrillar cytoplasm and indistinct cell borders. Despite the highly cellular nature of the tumor, mitotic figures are infrequent. The tumor also contains a sprinkling of small lymphocytes (same case as fig. 9-61).

Right: The tumor cells contain ovoid, elongated nuclei with vesicular chromatin and small nucleoli.

CD21, CD23, and CD35 (117). They are positive for vimentin, fascin, epithelial membrane antigen (EMA), and epidermal growth factor receptor. Variable positivity for S-100 protein and CD68 may be seen. Aberrant staining for CD45RO and CD4 has been reported, although staining for other pan-T-cell markers is generally lacking (118). Mutations affecting *BRAF* have been described in nearly 20 percent of follicular dendritic cell sarcomas (119).

Differential Diagnosis. More than 50 percent of cases are initially misdiagnosed. Follicular dendritic cell sarcomas arising in extranodal sites can simulate interdigitating dendritic cell sarcoma, spindle cell carcinoma, malignant melanoma, and gastrointestinal stromal tumor. Interdigitating dendritic cell sarcomas generally lack the whorled appearance of follicular dendritic cell sarcomas and show diffuse S-100 protein positivity. Carcinomas and melanomas

tend to show a greater degree of nuclear and cellular pleomorphism, and can be distinguished with immunohistochemistry. Gastrointestinal stromal tumors often contain monotonous cell populations, but lack dense lymphocytic infiltrates and show strong immunostaining for CD117 and DOG1.

Treatment and Prognosis. Surgical resection is the most effective treatment modality for patients with follicular dendritic cell sarcomas, although those with advanced disease may be offered a combination of surgery and chemotherapy (114). A role for adjuvant radiotherapy has not been established. Poor prognostic features include young age at diagnosis, advanced tumor stage, intra-abdominal disease, necrosis, increased mitotic activity, and an absence of lymphoplasmacytic infiltration. Patients may show an initial response to therapy, although 40 to 50 percent of tumors recur and metastases occur in 25 percent (116). Up to one fifth of patients ultimately die of their disease.

MYELOID SARCOMA

Definition. *Myeloid sarcomas* are solid, extramedullary tumors composed of neoplastic myeloid cells. They also have been termed *granulocytic sarcoma*, *extramedullary myeloid tumor*, and *chloroma*. By definition, they form mass lesions that efface the underlying tissue architecture.

Clinical Features. Myeloid sarcoma occurs across a wide age distribution, similar to that of acute myelogenous leukemia (AML), although it is more common among older adults and more common in men than women (120). Myeloid sarcoma can result from leukemic involvement of the intestine by a known malignancy, relapse of previously treated leukemia, or transformation of a low-grade lesion, such as myelodysplastic syndrome (MDS) (121). Although most tumors develop in patients without a prior history of leukemia, they may represent harbingers of AML: at least 50 percent of myeloid sarcomas progress to AML within 3 years (122,123).

Lesions of the gastrointestinal tract show a predilection for the small intestine and, thus, produce symptoms related to intermittent bowel obstruction (124). Patients with ulcerated tumors may present with iron deficiency anemia or rectal bleeding. Other symptoms include nausea, vomiting, fever, and weight loss.

Gross Findings. Myeloid sarcoma can appear as a polypoid, exophytic mass, or as a bulky, transmurally invasive tumor involving the intestinal wall in a circumferential fashion. Tumors may be solitary or multiple in the gastrointestinal tract, or occur in combination with extraintestinal tumors. They often have a pink or fleshy cut surface; green discoloration typical of "chloroma" is uncommon among intestinal tumors. Regional lymph nodes are often enlarged.

Microscopic Findings. Tumors are composed of a sheet-like proliferation of infiltrating, medium to large dyscohesive cells. They contain large nuclei that may be round, ovoid, or multilobated, often with a prominent nucleolus (fig. 9-64). The tumor cells typically contain a moderate amount of granular eosinophilic cytoplasm, which can be a helpful diagnostic clue (123). A variable number of mature-appearing granulocytes may

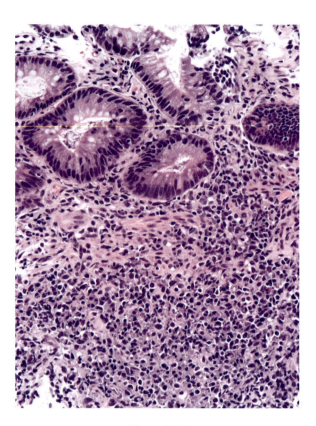

Figure 9-64

MYELOID SARCOMA OF COLON

The deep mucosa contains a monotonous population of plasmacytoid cells with enlarged, hyperchromatic nuclei.

be present, particularly in differentiated lesions. Blasts contain irregularly shaped or folded nuclei (fig. 9-64). Tumors are often mitotically active, with scattered tingible body macrophages, but necrosis is generally lacking (125).

Most myeloid sarcomas consist of myeloblasts, with or without promyelocytes or neutrophilic differentiation. Some tumors show mostly myelomonocytic or monoblastic differentiation; most of these occur in combination with acute monoblastic leukemia (126,127).

Immunohistochemical and Molecular Genetic Findings. Myeloid sarcoma most commonly shows strong staining with CD68, followed by myeloperoxidase, lysozyme, and chloroacetate esterase. Antigenic profiles are similar to those of lesional cells of AML, with expression of CD13, CD33, and CD117 (124). Monoblasts express CD14, CD116, and CD11c, as well as lysozyme in many cases. Most myeloid

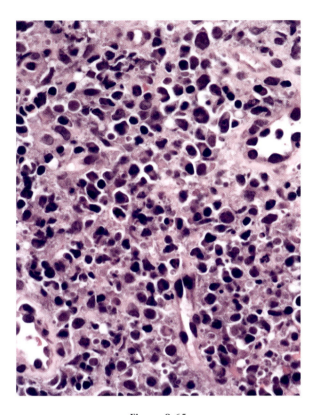

Figure 9-65

MYELOID SARCOMA OF COLON

Sheets of large, atypical cells are associated with apoptotic cellular debris. Many of the tumor cells contain abundant eosinophilic cytoplasm.

sarcomas also stain for CD43, but are negative for other T-cell markers.

Molecular alterations are detected in slightly more than 50 percent of cases and include monosomy 7, trisomy 8, t(8;21)(q22;q22), inv(16)(p13q22), and t(16;15)(p13;q22), similar to leukemic infiltrates (120,127,128). Monoblastic sarcomas may show 11q23 translocations (129,130).

Differential Diagnosis. The differential diagnosis of myeloid sarcoma includes lymphoma, undifferentiated carcinoma, melanoma, sarcoma, and small round blue cell tumors. At least 50 percent of myeloid sarcomas are initially misdiagnosed as other entities. A battery of immunostains for keratins, S-100 protein, and a limited panel of mesenchymal markers excludes nonhematopoietic tumors. Distinction between myeloid sarcoma and lymphoma requires a high index of suspicion, particularly when unusual immunohistochemical staining patterns are present.

Treatment and Prognosis. Myeloid sarcomas that develop in association with MDS or myeloproliferative disorder are essentially equivalent to blast transformation. Patients with tumors that occur in combination with AML have a prognosis comparable to that of the underlying leukemia. Systemic chemotherapy with possible peripheral stem cell/bone marrow transplantation is more effective than surgery and radiation.

Approximately 80 percent of myeloid sarcomas that occur in isolation transform to leukemia within 1 year following surgery and/or radiotherapy (124). The addition of systemic chemotherapy improves outcome: nearly 60 percent of patients are disease free at 1 year, and nearly 20 percent are disease free at 2 years (123).

SYSTEMIC MASTOCYTOSIS

Definition and General Features. *Systemic mastocytosis* is a neoplastic proliferation of mast cells that involves the bone marrow and extracutaneous organs, including the spleen, liver, and gastrointestinal tract (131). The diagnosis can be rendered when multifocal aggregates of 15 or more mast cells are detected in the intestine in combination with three or more of the following features: 1) over 25 percent of mast cells are atypical or spindled, 2) activating *KIT* mutations at codon 816 are detected, 3) mast cells express CD2 and/or CD25 as well as other mast cell markers, and 4) serum tryptase levels persistently exceed 20 ng/mL in the absence of another myeloid disorder (132).

Systemic mastocytosis is classified based on the presence of B findings (more than 30 percent bone marrow mast cells on biopsy and/or serum tryptase levels over 200 ng/mL, increased marrow cellularity without meeting the criteria for another myeloid neoplasm, or enlargement of liver, spleen, or lymph nodes without evidence of organ damage) and C findings (evidence of organ damage due to a mast cell infiltrate, hypersplenism, cytopenias, osteolytic lesions or fractures, and malabsorption with weight loss due gastrointestinal involvement) (133). Indolent systemic mastocytosis is defined by the absence of C findings, whereas advanced systemic mastocytosis includes aggressive

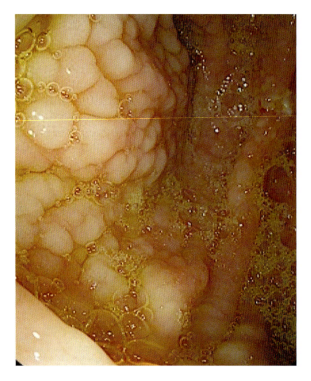

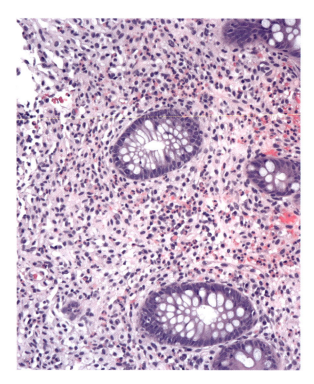

Figure 9-66

SYSTEMIC MASTOCYTOSIS

The mucosa is diffusely nodular secondary to massive infiltration by lesional cells. A few normal folds are present in the background mucosa.

Figure 9-67

SYSTEMIC MASTOCYTOSIS OF COLON

The lamina propria is expanded by a infiltrate of ovoid to spindled neoplastic mast cells. Numerous eosinophils are present in the background.

systemic mastocytosis, mast cell leukemia, mast cell sarcoma, and extracutaneous mastocytoma.

Clinical Features. The systemic manifestations of mastocytosis include anorexia, fever, and weight loss, as well as histamine-induced flushing and hypotension. The gastrointestinal tract is involved in 70 to 80 percent of patients. They may complain of abdominal pain and diarrhea, often with increased urgency or even incontinence. Histamine stimulates gastric acid secretion, so patients may develop one or more duodenal ulcers that simulate the clinical features of Zollinger-Ellison syndrome. Portal hypertension can be a late manifestation of histamine-induced hepatic fibrosis.

Gross Findings. Any site within the gastrointestinal tract may be affected, although involvement of the stomach and duodenum are most common. Mucosal abnormalities include loss of normal folds, nodularity, erosions, and ulcers (fig. 9-66). Abdominal imaging may reveal splenomegaly and retroperitoneal lymphadenopathy.

Microscopic Findings. Mucosal biopsy samples show expansion of the lamina propria and superficial submucosa by an atypical infiltrate that effaces the crypt architecture or overruns mucosal glands (fig. 9-66). Neoplastic mast cells may form a compact cellular cuff around epithelial elements, or be dispersed in the mucosa (134). The cells have an epithelioid or spindle appearance, with abundant, pale eosinophilic cytoplasm and ovoid or reniform nuclei. The nuclei contain dense chromatin with inconspicuous nucleoli and perinuclear cytoplasmic clearing (fig. 9-68). Eosinophils are usually present and may be numerous. The Giemsa stain decorates the cytoplasmic granules of mast cells and improves their detection.

Immunohistochemical and Molecular Genetic Findings. Immunohistochemical stains facilitate the diagnosis. Systemic mastocytosis shows strong diffuse staining for CD117 and mast cell tryptase. Stains for CD25 are particularly helpful in identifying systemic

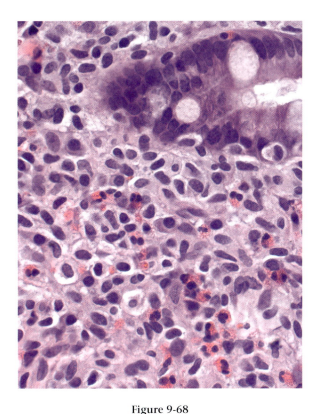

Figure 9-68

SYSTEMIC MASTOCYTOSIS OF COLON

Atypical mast cells contain ovoid nuclei with dense chromatin and inconspicuous nucleoli. Most contain abundant, faintly eosinophilic cytoplasm.

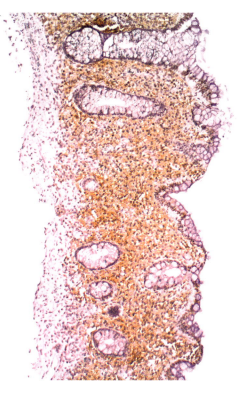

Figure 9-69

SYSTEMIC MASTOCYTOSIS OF COLON

Abnormal mast cells stain for CD25.

mastocytosis, as it labels abnormal mast cells (fig. 9-69) (135). Neoplastic mast cells can also stain for CD68, CD43, and CD30.

Most patients have *KIT* mutations that affect D816V in exon 17. The resultant mutant isoform is resistant to tyrosine kinase inhibitor therapy (136). Mutations in *TET2* are less common, occurring in approximately 30 percent of patients.

Differential Diagnosis. Systemic mastocytosis can be easily overlooked in mucosal biopsy samples, particularly when other cell types are prominent. Eosinophil-rich infiltrates can mask the presence of mast cells, simulating the appearance of eosinophilic enterocolitis or even inflammatory bowel disease. However, neutrophils, plasma cells, and lymphocytes are not prominent in systemic mastocytosis, and crypt architectural distortion is generally lacking.

The spindled appearance of mast cells can mimic Langerhans cells, raising the possibility of Langerhans cell histiocytosis. Most patients with Langerhans cell histiocytosis, however, are young children, whereas systemic mastocytosis tends to be a disease of adults. Langerhans cells also have more eosinophilic cytoplasm, with folded, grooved, or multilobated nuclei and delicate chromatin. They express langerin and CD1a.

Treatment and Prognosis. Patients with systemic mastocytosis are generally resistant to imatinib because they have a mutant isoform resulting from a D816V *KIT* mutation that is resistant to targeted therapies. Cytoreductive chemotherapy is of limited value and rarely induces complete remission. Prognosis depends on disease category: most patients with aggressive systemic mastocytosis succumb to their disease within a few months, whereas those with indolent disease may have a normal life expectancy (137,138).

REFERENCES

1. Case records of the Massachusetts General Hospital. Weekly clinicopathological exercises. Case 8-1997. A 65-year-old man with recurrent abdominal pain for five years. N Engl J Med 1997; 336:786-793.

2. Albuquerque A. Nodular lymphoid hyperplasia in the gastrointestinal tract in adult patients: a review. World J Gastrointest Endosc 2014;6:534-540.

3. de Weerth A, Gocht A, Seewald S, et al. Duodenal nodular lymphoid hyperplasia caused by giardiasis infection in a patient who is immunodeficient. Gastrointest Endosc 2002;55:605-607.

4. Luzi G, Zullo A, Iebba F, et al. Duodenal pathology and clinical-immunological implications in common variable immunodeficiency patients. Am J Gastroenterol 2003;98:118-121.

5. Spodaryk M, Mrukowicz J, Stopyrowa J, et al. Severe intestinal nodular lymphoid hyperplasia in an infant. J Pediatr Gastroenterol Nutr 1995;21:468-473.

6. Daniels JA, Lederman HM, Maitra A, Montgomery EA. Gastrointestinal tract pathology in patients with common variable immunodeficiency (CVID): a clinicopathologic study and review. Am J Surg Pathol 2007;31:1800-1812.

7. Onbasi K, Gunsar F, Sin AZ, Ardeniz O, Kokuludag A, Sebik F. Common variable immunodeficiency (CVID) presenting with malabsorption due to giardiasis. Turk J Gastroenterol 2005;16:111-113.

8. Washington K, Stenzel TT, Buckley RH, Gottfried MR. Gastrointestinal pathology in patients with common variable immunodeficiency and X-linked agammaglobulinemia. Am J Surg Pathol 1996;20:1240-1252.

9. Jonsson OT, Birgisson S, Reykdal S. Resolution of nodular lymphoid hyperplasia of the gastrointestinal tract following chemotherapy for extraintestinal lymphoma. Dig Dis Sci 2002;47:2463-2465.

10. Rubio-Tapia A, Hernandez-Calleros J, Trinidad-Hernandez S, Uscanga L. Clinical characteristics of a group of adults with nodular lymphoid hyperplasia: a single center experience. World J Gastroenterol 2006;12:1945-1948.

11. Matuchansky C, Touchard G, Lemaire M, et al. Malignant lymphoma of the small bowel associated with diffuse nodular lymphoid hyperplasia. N Engl J Med 1985;313:166-171.

12. Matuchansky C, Morichau-Beauchant M, Touchard G, et al. Nodular lymphoid hyperplasia of the small bowel associated with primary jejunal malignant lymphoma. Evidence favoring a cytogenetic relationship. Gastroenterology 1980;78:1587-1592.

13. Burke JS. Lymphoproliferative disorders of the gastrointestinal tract: a review and pragmatic guide to diagnosis. Arch Pathol Lab Med 2011; 135:1283-1297.

14. Al-Saleem T, Al-Mondhiry H. Immunoproliferative small intestinal disease (IPSID): a model for mature B-cell neoplasms. Blood 2005;105:2274-2280.

15. Lecuit M, Abachin E, Martin A, et al. Immunoproliferative small intestinal disease associated with Campylobacter jejuni. N Engl J Med 2004; 350:239-248.

16. Isaacson PG, Chott A, Nakamura S, Muller-Hermelink HK, Harris NL, Swerdlow SH. Extranodal marginal zone lymphoma of mucosa-associated lymphoid tissue (MALT lymphoma). In: Swerdlow SH, Campo E, Harris NL, et al., eds. WHO Classification of Tumours of Haematopoietic and Lymphoid Tissues. Lyon, France: IARC Press; 2008:214-217.

17. Price SK. Immunoproliferative small intestinal disease: a study of 13 cases with alpha heavy-chain disease. Histopathology 1990;17:7-17.

18. Kyung Shin B, Lee H, Choi J, et al. Primary marginal zone B-cell lymphoma of gastrointestinal tract presenting as multiple lymphomatoid polyposis. Int J Colorectal Dis 2007;22(8):991-992.

19. Isaacson PG, Du MQ. MALT lymphoma: from morphology to molecules. Nat Rev Cancer 2004; 4:644-653.

20. O'Malley DP, Goldstein NS, Banks PM. The recognition and classification of lymphoproliferative disorders of the gut. Hum Pathol 2014;45:899-916.

21. Isaacson PG, Dogan A, Price SK, Spencer J. Immunoproliferative small-intestinal disease. An immunohistochemical study. Am J Surg Pathol 1989;13:1023-1033.

22. Murga Penas EM, Hinz K, Roser K, et al. Translocations t(11;18)(q21;q21) and t(14;18)(q32;q21) are the main chromosomal abnormalities involving MLT/MALT1 in MALT lymphomas. Leukemia 2003;17:2225-2229.

23. Remstein ED, James CD, Kurtin PJ. Incidence and subtype specificity of API2-MALT1 fusion translocations in extranodal, nodal, and splenic marginal zone lymphomas. Am J Pathol 2000;156:1183-1188.

24. Geissmann F, Ruskone-Fourmestraux A, Hermine O, et al. Homing receptor alpha4beta7 integrin expression predicts digestive tract involvement in mantle cell lymphoma. Am J Pathol 1998; 153:1701-1705.

25. Raderer M, Streubel B, Woehrer S, et al. High relapse rate in patients with MALT lymphoma warrants lifelong follow-up. Clin Cancer Res 2005;11:3349-3352.

26. Ben-Ayed F, Halphen M, Najjar T, et al. Treatment of alpha chain disease. Results of a prospective study in 21 Tunisian patients by the Tunisian-French Intestinal Lymphoma Study Group. Cancer 1989;63:1251-1256.

27. Misdraji J, Harris NL, Hasserjian RP, Lauwers GY, Ferry JA. Primary follicular lymphoma of the gastrointestinal tract. Am J Surgical Pathol 2011;35:1255-1263.

28. Nadal E, Martinez A, Jimenez M, et al. Primary follicular lymphoma arising in the ampulla of Vater. Ann Hematol 2002;81:228-231.

29. Shia J, Teruya-Feldstein J, Pan D, et al. Primary follicular lymphoma of the gastrointestinal tract: a clinical and pathologic study of 26 cases. Am J Surg Pathol 2002;26:216-224.

30. Tang Z, Jing W, Lindeman N, Harris NL, Ferry JA. One patient, two lymphomas. Simultaneous primary gastric marginal zone lymphoma and primary duodenal follicular lymphoma. Arch Pathol Lab Med 2004;128:1035-1038.

31. Harris NL, Swerdlow SH, Jaffe ES, et al. Follicular lymphoma. In: Swerdlow SH, Campo E, Harris NL, et al., eds. WHO classification of tumours of haematopoietic and lymphoid tissues. Lyon, France: IARC Press; 2008:220-226.

32. Damaj G, Verkarre V, Delmer A, et al. Primary follicular lymphoma of the gastrointestinal tract: a study of 25 cases and a literature review. Ann Oncol 2003;14:623-629.

33. Yoshino T, Miyake K, Ichimura K, et al. Increased incidence of follicular lymphoma in the duodenum. Am J Surg Pathol 2000;24:688-693.

34. Sato Y, Ichimura K, Tanaka T, et al. Duodenal follicular lymphomas share common characteristics with mucosa-associated lymphoid tissue lymphomas. J Clin Pathol 2008;61:377-381.

35. Muller-Hermelink HK, Montserrat E, Catovsky D, Campo E, Harris NL, Stein H. Chronic lymphocytic leukemia/small lymphocytic lymphoma. In: Swerdlow SH, Campo E, Harris NL, et al., eds. World Health Organization classification of tumours, pathology and genetics of tumours of haematopoietic and lymphoid tissues. Lyon, France: IARC Press; 2008:180-182.

36. Rossi D, Gaidano G. The clinical implications of gene mutations in chronic lymphocytic leukaemia. Br J Cancer 2016;114:849-854.

37. Jiang Y, Chen HC, Su X, et al. ATM function and its relationship with ATM gene mutations in chronic lymphocytic leukemia with the recurrent deletion (11q22.3-23.2). Blood Cancer J 2016;6:e465.

38. Pospisilova S, Gonzalez D, Malcikova J, et al. ERIC recommendations on TP53 mutation analysis in chronic lymphocytic leukemia. Leukemia 2012;26:1458-1461.

39. Bogusz AM, Bagg A. Genetic aberrations in small B-cell lymphomas and leukemias: molecular pathology, clinical relevance and therapeutic targets. Leuk Lymphoma 2016;57:1991-2013.

40. Weidner AS, Panarelli NC, Geyer JT, et al. Idelalisib-associated colitis: histologic findings in 14 patients. Am J Surg Pathol 2015;39:1661-1667.

41. Louie CY, DiMaio MA, Matsukuma KE, Coutre SE, Berry GJ, Longacre TA. Idelalisib-associated enterocolitis: clinicopathologic features and distinction from other enterocolitides. Am J Surg Pathol 2015;39:1653-1660.

42. Shanafelt TD, Byrd JC, Call TG, Zent CS, Kay NE. Narrative review: initial management of newly diagnosed, early-stage chronic lymphocytic leukemia. Ann Intern Med 2006;145:435-447.

43. Swerdlow SH, Campo E, Seto M, Muller-Hermelink HK. Mantle cell lymphoma. In: Swerdlow SH, Campo E, Harris NL, et al., eds. WHO classification of tumours of haematopoietic and lymphoid tissues. Lyon: France; 2008:229-232.

44. Salar A, Juanpere N, Bellosillo B, et al. Gastrointestinal involvement in mantle cell lymphoma: a prospective clinic, endoscopic, and pathologic study. Am J Surg Pathol 2006;30:1274-1280.

45. Kohno S, Ohshima K, Yoneda S, Kodama T, Shirakusa T, Kikuchi M. Clinicopathological analysis of 143 primary malignant lymphomas in the small and large intestines based on the new WHO classification. Histopathology 2003;43:135-143.

46. Tomita S, Kojima M, Imura J, et al. Extranodal diffuse follicular center lymphoma mimicking mantle cell lymphoma of the intestine. Am J Hematol 2003;74:287-289.

47. Chen R, Sanchez J, Rosen ST. Clinical management updates in mantle cell lymphoma. Oncology (Williston Park) 2016;30:353-360.

48. Cheah CY, Seymour JF, Wang ML. Mantle cell lymphoma. J Clin Oncol 2016;34:1256-1269.

49. Stein H, Warnke RA, Chan WC, et al. Diffuse large B-cell lymphoma, not otherwise specified. In: Swerdlow SH, Campo E, Harris NL, et al., eds. WHO classification of tumours of haematopoietic and lymphoid tissues. Lyon: IARC Press; 2008:233-237.

50. Harris NL, Jaffe ES, Stein H, et al. A revised European-American classification of lymphoid neoplasms: a proposal from the International Lymphoma Study Group. Blood 1994;84:1361-1392.

51. Engelhard M, Brittinger G, Huhn D, et al. Subclassification of diffuse large B-cell lymphomas according to the Kiel classification: distinction of centroblastic and immunoblastic lymphomas is a significant prognostic risk factor. Blood 1997;89:2291-2297.

52. Nagakita K, Takata K, Taniguchi K, et al. Clinico-pathological features of 49 primary gastrointestinal diffuse large B-cell lymphoma cases; comparison with location, cell-of-origin, and frequency of MYD88 L265P. Pathol Int 2016;66:444-452.

53. Tagawa H, Suguro M, Tsuzuki S, et al. Comparison of genome profiles for identification of distinct subgroups of diffuse large B-cell lymphoma. Blood 2005;106:1770-1777.

54. Matolcsy A, Chadburn A, Knowles DM. De novo CD5-positive and Richter's syndrome-associated diffuse large B cell lymphomas are genotypically distinct. Am J Pathol 1995;147:207-216.

55. Ohno H, Fukuhara S. Significance of rearrangement of the BCL6 gene in B-cell lymphoid neoplasms. Leuk Lymphoma 1997;27:53-63.

56. Smith LB, Owens SR. Gastrointestinal lymphomas: entities and mimics. Arch Pathol Lab Med 2012;136:865-870.

57. Leoncini L, Raphael M, Stein H, Harris NL, Jaffe ES, Kluin PM. Burkitt lymphoma. In: Swerdlow SH, Campo E, Harris NL, et al., eds. WHO classification of tumours of haematopoietic and lymphoid tissues. Lyon, France: IARC Press; 2008:262-264.

58. Burkitt D. A sarcoma involving the jaws in African children. Br J Surg 1958;46:218-223.

59. Wright DH. Burkitt's lymphoma: a review of the pathology, immunology, and possible etiologic factors. Pathol Annu 1971;6:337-363.

60. Raphael M, Gentilhomme O, Tulliez M, Byron PA, Diebold J. Histopathologic features of high-grade non-Hodgkin's lymphomas in acquired immunodeficiency syndrome. The French Study Group of Pathology for Human Immunodeficiency Virus-Associated Tumors. Arch Pathol Lab Med 1991;115:15-20.

61. Magrath IT, Sariban E. Clinical features of Burkitt's lymphoma in the USA. IARC Sci Publ 1985:119-127.

62. Haralambieva E, Boerma EJ, van Imhoff GW, et al. Clinical, immunophenotypic, and genetic analysis of adult lymphomas with morphologic features of Burkitt lymphoma. Am J Surg Pathol 2005;29:1086-1094.

63. Soussain C, Patte C, Ostronoff M, et al. Small non-cleaved cell lymphoma and leukemia in adults. A retrospective study of 65 adults treated with the LMB pediatric protocols. Blood 1995;85:664-674.

64. Thomas DA, Faderl S, O'Brien S, et al. Chemoimmunotherapy with hyper-CVAD plus rituximab for the treatment of adult Burkitt and Burkitt-type lymphoma or acute lymphoblastic leukemia. Cancer 2006;106:1569-1580.

65. Ma J, Wang Y, Zhao H, et al. Clinical characteristics of 26 patients with primary extranodal Hodgkin lymphoma. Int J Clin Exp Pathol 2014;7:5045-5050.

66. Gobbi PG, Ferreri AJ, Ponzoni M, Levis A. Hodgkin lymphoma. Crit Rev Oncol Hematol 2013;85:216-237.

67. Kumar S, Fend F, Quintanilla-Martinez L, et al. Epstein-Barr virus-positive primary gastrointestinal Hodgkin's disease: association with inflammatory bowel disease and immunosuppression. Am J Surg Pathol 2000;24:66-73.

68. Moran NR, Webster B, Lee KM, et al. Epstein Barr virus-positive mucocutaneous ulcer of the colon associated Hodgkin lymphoma in Crohn's disease. World J Gastroenterol 2015;21:6072-6076.

69. Anagnostopoulos I, Hummel M, Stein H. Frequent presence of latent Epstein-Barr virus infection in peripheral T cell lymphomas. A review. Leuk Lymphoma 1995;19:1-12.

70. Caillard S, Dharnidharka V, Agodoa L, Bohen E, Abbott K. Posttransplant lymphoproliferative disorders after renal transplantation in the United States in era of modern immunosuppression. Transplantation 2005;80:1233-1243.

71. Caillard S, Lelong C, Pessione F, Moulin B, French PTLD Working Group. Post-transplant lymphoproliferative disorders occurring after renal transplantation in adults: report of 230 cases from the French Registry. Am J Transplant 2006;6:2735-2742.

72. Webber SA, Naftel DC, Fricker FJ, et al. Lymphoproliferative disorders after paediatric heart transplantation: a multi-institutional study. Lancet 2006;367:233-239.

73. Nalesnik MA, Jaffe R, Starzl TE, et al. The pathology of posttransplant lymphoproliferative disorders occurring in the setting of cyclosporine A-prednisone immunosuppression. Am J Pathol 1988;133:173-192.

74. Knowles DM, Cesarman E, Chadburn A, et al. Correlative morphologic and molecular genetic analysis demonstrates three distinct categories of posttransplantation lymphoproliferative disorders. Blood 1995;85:552-565.

75. Vakiani E, Nandula SV, Subramaniyam S, et al. Cytogenetic analysis of B-cell posttransplant lymphoproliferations validates the World Health Organization classification and suggests inclusion of florid follicular hyperplasia as a precursor lesion. Hum Pathol 2007;38:315-325.

76. Swerdlow SH. T-cell and NK-cell posttransplantation lymphoproliferative disorders. Am J Clin Pathol 2007;127:887-895.

77. Swerdlow SH, Webber SA, Chadburn A, Ferry JA. Post-transplant lymphoproliferative disorders. In: Swerdlow SH, Campo E, Harris NL, et al., eds. WHO classification of tumours of haematopoietic and lymphoid tissues. Lyon, France: IARC Press; 2008:343-349.

78. Borenstein J, Pezzella F, Gatter KC. Plasmablastic lymphomas may occur as post-transplant lymphoproliferative disorders. Histopathology 2007;51:774-777.

79. Colomo L, Loong F, Rives S, et al. Diffuse large B-cell lymphomas with plasmablastic differentiation represent a heterogeneous group of disease entities. Am J Surg Pathol 2004;28:736-747.

80. Raphael M, Said J, Borisch B, Cesarman E, Harris NL. Lymphomas associated with HIV infection. In: Swerdlow SH, Campo E, Harris NL, et al., eds. WHO classification of tumours of haematopoietic and lymphoid tissues. Lyon, France: IARC Press; 2008:340-342.

81. Clifford GM, Polesel J, Rickenbach M, et al. Cancer risk in the Swiss HIV Cohort Study: associations with immunodeficiency, smoking, and highly active antiretroviral therapy. J Natl Cancer Inst 2005;97:425-432.

82. Kamel OW. Iatrogenic lymphoproliferative disorders in non-transplantation settings. Recent Results Cancer Res 2002;159:19-26.

83. Haramura T, Haraguchi M, Irie J, et al. Case of plasmablastic lymphoma of the sigmoid colon and literature review. World J Gastroenterol 2015;21:7598-7603.

84. Hoshida Y, Xu JX, Fujita S, et al. Lymphoproliferative disorders in rheumatoid arthritis: clinicopathological analysis of 76 cases in relation to methotrexate medication. J Rheumatol 2007; 34:322-331.

85. Gaulard P, Swerdlow SH, Harris NL, Jaffe ES, Sundstrom C. Other iatrogenic immunodeficiency-associated lymphoproliferative disorders. In: Swerdlow SH, Campo E, Harris NL, et al., eds. WHO classification of tumours of haematopoietic and lymphoid tissues. Lyon, France: IARC Press; 2008:350-351.

86. Vega F, Chang CC, Medeiros LJ, et al. Plasmablastic lymphomas and plasmablastic plasma cell myelomas have nearly identical immunophenotypic profiles. Mod Pathol 2005;18:806-815.

87. Dong HY, Scadden DT, de Leval L, Tang Z, Isaacson PG, Harris NL. Plasmablastic lymphoma in HIV-positive patients: an aggressive Epstein-Barr virus-associated extramedullary plasmacytic neoplasm. Am J Surg Pathol 2005;29:1633-1641.

88. Teruya-Feldstein J, Chiao E, Filippa DA, et al. CD20-negative large-cell lymphoma with plasmablastic features: a clinically heterogenous spectrum in both HIV-positive and -negative patients. Ann Oncol 2004;15:1673-1679.

89. Wolf T, Brodt HR, Fichtlscherer S, et al. Changing incidence and prognostic factors of survival in AIDS-related non-Hodgkin's lymphoma in the era of highly active antiretroviral therapy (HAART). Leuk Lymphoma 2005;46:207-215.

90. Chan JK, Quintanilla-Martinez L, Ferry JA, Peh S-C. Extranodal NK/T-cell lymphoma, nasal type. In: Swerdlow SH, Campo E, Harris NL, et al., eds. WHO Classification of Tumours of Haematopoietic and Lymphoid Tissues. Lyon, France: IARC Press; 2008:285-288.

91. Quintanilla-Martinez L, Franklin JL, Guerrero I, et al. Histological and immunophenotypic profile of nasal NK/T cell lymphomas from Peru: high prevalence of p53 overexpression. Hum Pathol 1999;30:849-855.

92. Kwong YL, Chan AC, Liang R, et al. CD56+ NK lymphomas: clinicopathological features and prognosis. Br J Haematol 1997;97:821-829.

93. Ding W, Wang J, Zhao S, et al. Clinicopathological study of pulmonary extranodal nature killer/T-cell lymphoma, nasal type and literature review. Pathol Res Pract 2015;211:544-549.

94. Tsang WY, Chan JK, Ng CS, Pau MY. Utility of a paraffin section-reactive CD56 antibody (123C3) for characterization and diagnosis of lymphomas. Am J Surg Pathol 1996;20:202-210.

95. Jaffe ES. Nasal and nasal-type T/NK cell lymphoma: a unique form of lymphoma associated with the Epstein-Barr virus. Histopathology 1995;27:581-583.

96. Ng SB, Lai KW, Murugaya S, et al. Nasal-type extranodal natural killer/T-cell lymphomas: a clinicopathologic and genotypic study of 42 cases in Singapore. Mod Pathol 2004;17:1097-1107.

97. Elenitoba-Johnson KS, Zarate-Osorno A, Meneses A, et al. Cytotoxic granular protein expression, Epstein-Barr virus strain type, and latent membrane protein-1 oncogene deletions in nasal T-lymphocyte/natural killer cell lymphomas from Mexico. Mod Pathol 1998;11:754-761.

98. Suzuki R. Pathogenesis and treatment of extranodal natural killer/T-cell lymphoma. Semin Hematol 2014;51:42-51.

99. Ito Y, Kimura H, Maeda Y, et al. Pretreatment EBV-DNA copy number is predictive of response and toxicities to SMILE chemotherapy for extranodal NK/T-cell lymphoma, nasal type. Clin Cancer Res 2012;18:4183-4190.

100. Swerdlow SH, Campo E, Pileri SA, et al. The 2016 revision of the World Health Organization classification of lymphoid neoplasms. Blood 2016;127:2375-2390.

101. Isaacson PG, Chott A, Ott G, Stein H. Enteropathy-associated T-cell lymphoma. In: Swerdlow SH, Campo E, Harris NL, et al., eds. WHO classification of tumours of haematopoietic and lymphoid tissues. Lyon, France: IARC Press; 2008:289-291.

102. Ashton-Key M, Diss TC, Pan L, Du MQ, Isaacson PG. Molecular analysis of T-cell clonality in ulcerative jejunitis and enteropathy-associated T-cell lymphoma. Am J Pathol 1997;151:493-498.

103. Zettl A, deLeeuw R, Haralambieva E, Mueller-Hermelink HK. Enteropathy-type T-cell lymphoma. Am J Clin Pathol 2007;127:701-706.

104. Kikuma K, Yamada K, Nakamura S, et al. Detailed clinicopathological characteristics and possible lymphomagenesis of type II intestinal enteropathy-associated T-cell lymphoma in Japan. Hum Pathol 2014;45:1276-1284.

105. Du MQ, Isaacson PG. First steps in unraveling the genotype of enteropathy-type T-cell lymphoma. Am J Pathol 2002;161:1527-1529.

106. Zettl A, Ott G, Makulik A, et al. Chromosomal gains at 9q characterize enteropathy-type T-cell lymphoma. Am J Pathol 2002;161:1635-1645.

107. Verkarre V, Romana SP, Cellier C, et al. Recurrent partial trisomy 1q22-q44 in clonal intraepithelial lymphocytes in refractory celiac sprue. Gastroenterology 2003;125:40-46.

108. Krenacs L, Smyth MJ, Bagdi E, et al. The serine protease granzyme M is preferentially expressed in NK-cell, gamma delta T-cell, and intestinal T-cell lymphomas: evidence of origin from lymphocytes involved in innate immunity. Blood 2003;101:3590-3593.

109. Carbonnel F, Grollet-Bioul L, Brouet JC, et al. Are complicated forms of celiac disease cryptic T-cell lymphomas? Blood 1998;92:3879-3886.

110. Leventaki V, Manning JT Jr, Luthra R, et al. Indolent peripheral T-cell lymphoma involving the gastrointestinal tract. Hum Pathol 2014;45:421-426.

111. Vega F, Chang CC, Schwartz MR, et al. Atypical NK-cell proliferation of the gastrointestinal tract in a patient with antigliadin antibodies but not celiac disease. Am J Surg Pathol 2006;30:539-544.

112. Takeuchi K, Yokoyama M, Ishizawa S, et al. Lymphomatoid gastropathy: a distinct clinicopathologic entity of self-limited pseudomalignant NK-cell proliferation. Blood 2010;116:5631-5637.

113. Belhadj K, Reyes F, Farcet JP, et al. Hepatosplenic gammadelta T-cell lymphoma is a rare clinicopathologic entity with poor outcome: report on a series of 21 patients. Blood 2003;102:4261-4269.

114. Saygin C, Uzunaslan D, Ozguroglu M, Senocak M, Tuzuner N. Dendritic cell sarcoma: a pooled analysis including 462 cases with presentation of our case series. Crit Rev Oncol Hematol 2013;88:253-271.

115. Wu A, Pullarkat S. Follicular Dendritic cell sarcoma. Arch Pathol Lab Med 2016;140:186-190.

116. Chan JK, Fletcher CD, Nayler SJ, Cooper K. Follicular dendritic cell sarcoma. Clinicopathologic analysis of 17 cases suggesting a malignant potential higher than currently recognized. Cancer 1997;79:294-313.

117. Soriano AO, Thompson MA, Admirand JH, et al. Follicular dendritic cell sarcoma: a report of 14 cases and a review of the literature. Am J Hematol 2007;82:725-728.

118. Yamada Y, Haga H, Hernandez M, et al. Follicular dendritic cell sarcoma of small intestine with aberrant T-cell marker expression. Pathol Int 2009;59:809-812.

119. Go H, Jeon YK, Huh J, et al. Frequent detection of BRAF(V600E) mutations in histiocytic and dendritic cell neoplasms. Histopathology 2014;65:261-272.

120. Kohl SK, Aoun P. Granulocytic sarcoma of the small intestine. Arch Pathol Lab Med 2006;130:1570-1574.

121. Bekassy AN, Hermans J, Gorin NC, Gratwohl A. Granulocytic sarcoma after allogeneic bone marrow transplantation: a retrospective European multicenter survey. Acute and Chronic Leukemia Working Parties of the European Group for Blood and Marrow Transplantation. Bone Marrow Transplant 1996;17:801-808.

122. Yamauchi K, Yasuda M. Comparison in treatments of nonleukemic granulocytic sarcoma: report of two cases and a review of 72 cases in the literature. Cancer 2002;94:1739-1746.

123. Neiman RS, Barcos M, Berard C, et al. Granulocytic sarcoma: a clinicopathologic study of 61 biopsied cases. Cancer 1981;48:1426-1437.

124. Byrd JC, Edenfield WJ, Shields DJ, Dawson NA. Extramedullary myeloid cell tumors in acute nonlymphocytic leukemia: a clinical review. J Clin Oncol 1995;13:1800-1816.

125. Meis JM, Butler JJ, Osborne BM, Manning JT. Granulocytic sarcoma in nonleukemic patients. Cancer 1986;58:2697-2709.

126. Pileri SA, Orazi A, Falini B. Myeloid sarcoma. In: Swerdlow SH, Campo E, Harris NL, et al., eds. WHO Classification of Tumours of Haematopoietic and Lymphoid Tissues. Lyon, France: IARC Press; 2008:140-141.

127. Pileri SA, Ascani S, Cox MC, et al. Myeloid sarcoma: clinico-pathologic, phenotypic and cytogenetic analysis of 92 adult patients. Leukemia 2007;21:340-350.

128. Muss HB, Moloney WC. Chloroma and other myeloblastic tumors. Blood 1973;42:721-728.

129. Julia A, Nomdedeu JF. Eosinophilic gastroenteritis or eosinophilic chloroma? Acta Haematol 2004;112:164-166.

130. Russell SJ, Giles FJ, Thompson DS, Scanlon DJ, Walker H, Richards JD. Granulocytic sarcoma of the small intestine preceding acute myelomonocytic leukemia with abnormal eosinophils and inv(16). Cancer Genet Cytogenet 1988;35:231-235.

131. Valent P, Horny HP, Escribano L, et al. Diagnostic criteria and classification of mastocytosis: a consensus proposal. Leuk Res 2001;25:603-625.

132. Horny HP, Metcalfe DD, Bennett JM, Bain BJ, Akin, C., Escribano L, Valent P. Mastocytosis. In: Swerdlow SH, Campo E, Harris NL, et al., eds. WHO Classification of Tumours of Haematopoietic and Lymphoid Tissues. Lyon, France: IARC Press; 2008:54-63.

133. Gotlib J, Pardanani A, Akin C, et al. International Working Group-Myeloproliferative Neoplasms Research and Treatment (IWG-MRT) & European Competence Network on Mastocytosis (ECNM) consensus response criteria in advanced systemic mastocytosis. Blood 2013;121:2393-2401.

134. Bedeir A, Jukic DM, Wang L, Mullady DK, Regueiro M, Krasinskas AM. Systemic mastocytosis mimicking inflammatory bowel disease: A case report and discussion of gastrointestinal pathology in systemic mastocytosis. Am J Surg Pathol 2006;30:1478-1482.

135. Hahn HP, Hornick JL. Immunoreactivity for CD25 in gastrointestinal mucosal mast cells is specific for systemic mastocytosis. Am J Surg Pathol 2007;31:1669-1676.

136. Garcia-Montero AC, Jara-Acevedo M, Teodosio C, et al. KIT mutation in mast cells and other bone marrow hematopoietic cell lineages in systemic mast cell disorders: a prospective study of the Spanish Network on Mastocytosis (REMA) in a series of 113 patients. Blood 2006;108:2366-2372.

137. Valent P, Akin C, Escribano L, et al. Standards and standardization in mastocytosis: consensus statements on diagnostics, treatment recommendations and response criteria. Eur J Clin Invest 2007;37:435-453.

138. Valent P, Akin C, Sperr WR, et al. Diagnosis and treatment of systemic mastocytosis: state of the art. Br J Haematol 2003;122:695-717.

10 METASTASES TO THE INTESTINES

Essentially any neoplasm can spread to the intestines, either as a metastasis or by direct extension. Also, several benign processes can result in findings that mimic such neoplasms. Although a comprehensive discussion of every tumor that can secondarily involve the gastrointestinal tract is beyond the scope of this section, a few of the more common entities, as well as those that can cause diagnostic challenges, are discussed in the following paragraphs.

SMALL INTESTINE

The primary differential diagnostic consideration of adenocarcinoma in the small bowel is metastatic disease or direct spread of neoplasm from organs that lie within the peritoneal cavity. Data from autopsy-based studies demonstrate that metastases outnumber primary carcinomas by over two-fold (1) and the small bowel is the favored gastrointestinal tract site for metastases (2). Features that favor secondary involvement

of the small bowel by tumor originating in another site include the presence of multiple lesions, lack of a precursor adenoma or inflammation-associated dysplasia, "bottom heavy" histologic growth pattern, and lack of mucosal ulceration. These features are summarized in Table 10-1.

The presence of an apparent in situ lesion does not necessarily imply a primary carcinoma; neoplasms that spread from other sites readily "colonize" the basement membrane of the enteric epithelium and are induced to apparent maturation, imparting an appearance of an in situ component (figs. 10-1–10-4) (3). Moreover, carcinoma in the lamina propria seldom elicits a desmoplastic stromal reaction and, thus, a metastasis may show mucosal features that simulate a primary malignancy. Immunolabeling can be of value in separating primary from secondary neoplasms in many instances, although metastases from elsewhere in

Table 10-1

FEATURES THAT DISTINGUISH PRIMARY AND SECONDARY INTESTINAL NEOPLASMS

Feature	Primary Neoplasm	Secondary Neoplasm
Gross Findings		
Single mucosa-based lesions	Common	Common
Multifocal tumor	Uncommon	May be present
Adenomatous polyps	May be present	Uncommon
Background of ileocolitis	May be present	Uncommon
Microscopic Findings		
Extensive serosal tumor deposits	Uncommon	Common
Extensive lymphovascular invasion	Uncommon	May be present
Associated adenoma	Common	Uncommon
Malignant glands with cribriform architecture	Common	Uncommon
Mixed architecture (papillary, acinar, solid)	Uncommon	May be present
Cords of cytologically bland cells	Uncommon	May be present
Dirty necrosis	Common	Uncommon
Solid growth pattern without lymphocytosis	Uncommon	May be present
Small glands with bland cytology	Uncommon	May be present
Nested, trabecular growth	Uncommon	Common
Clear cells	Uncommon	May be present
Psammomatous calcifications	Absent	May be present

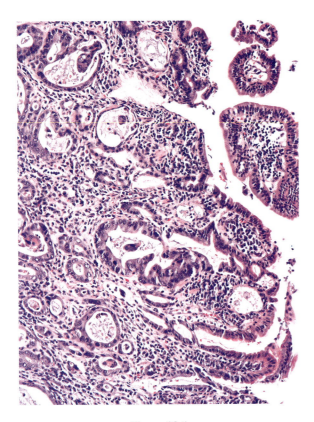

Figure 10-1

**PANCREATOBILIARY ADENOCARCINOMA
EXTENDING ONTO DUODENAL SURFACE**

The adenocarcinoma at the bottom of the image merges with the benign surface epithelium.

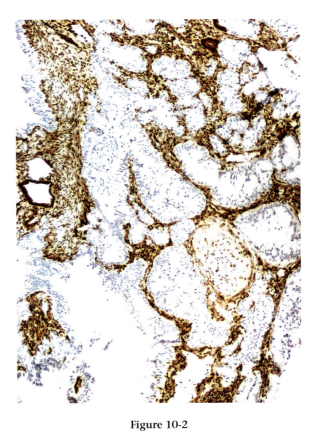

Figure 10-2

**PANCREATOBILIARY ADENOCARCINOMA
EXTENDING ONTO DUODENAL SURFACE**

Using a SMAD4/DPC4 immunostain, there is loss of staining in the nuclei of the carcinoma cells but not in the nuclei of benign glands and stroma.

Figure 10-3

**PANCREATOBILIARY
ADENOCARCINOMA
EXTENDING ONTO
DUODENAL SURFACE**

A subtle adenocarcinoma (one gland is indicated by a white arrow) is seen. Once this gland is spotted, it is easy to see similar malignant glands near it. Pancreatic adenocarcinomas can display a deceptively bland appearance but, in this example, their appearance does not match that of the reactive small bowel crypts.

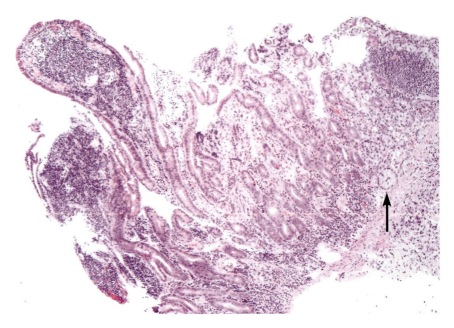

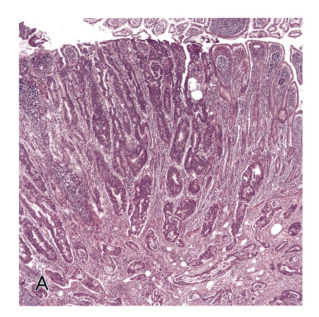

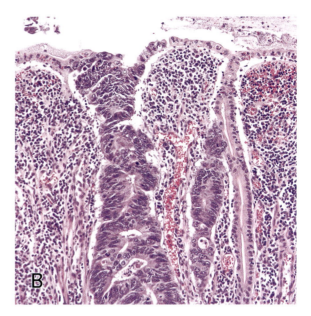

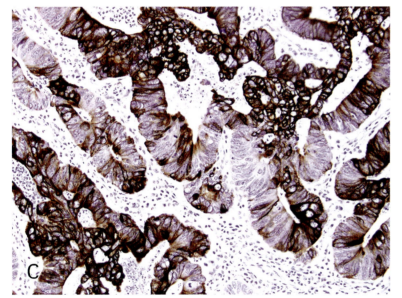

Figure 10-4

COLORECTAL ADENOCARCINOMA COLONIZING SMALL BOWEL MUCOSA

A: The non-neoplastic mucosa is at the right and malignant glands are present in the submucosa at the bottom. On the upper left, the colorectal carcinoma has extended onto the luminal surface.

B: High-magnification view.

C: Strong CK20 expression favors metastatic colorectal adenocarcinoma over primary small intestinal adenocarcinoma.

the tubular gut show enough morphologic and immunohistochemical overlap that they cannot always be distinguished. In such instances, it is best to report "adenocarcinoma involving the small intestine" with a note suggesting imaging studies to address alternate primary sources.

The most common metastatic lesions that spread to the small bowel are melanoma (figs. 10-5, 10-6), colonic adenocarcinoma (fig. 10-4), renal cell carcinoma, and malignancies of the breast and gynecologic tract (fig. 10-7). Colorectal carcinomas spread to the small intestine with some frequency, where they are especially likely to mimic an in situ component. Occasionally, immunolabeling is of value because small intestinal primary carcinomas display alterations of their CK7/CK20 immunoprofiles: some are CK7/CK20 "double positive" or CK7 reactive and CK20 negative (4).

Pancreatobiliary adenocarcinomas are especially prone to involve the small intestine, especially the duodenum, which they involve by direct extension. Pancreaticobiliary carcinomas can "colonize" the small bowel mucosa and simulate a duodenal adenoma (fig. 10-3, see also chapter 4, figs. 4-42 and 4-52).

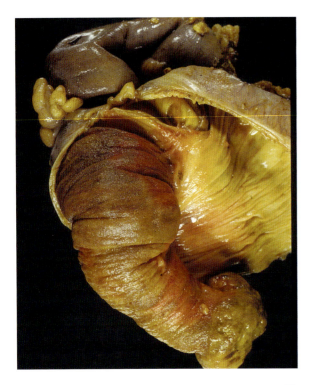
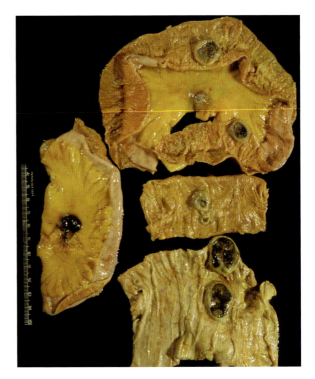

Figure 10-5

MELANOMA METASTATIC TO SMALL INTESTINE

Left: This lesion has caused intussusception.
Right: There are multiple pigmented deposits.

Figure 10-6

MELANOMA METASTATIC TO SMALL INTESTINE

The melanoma cells have replaced the lamina propria between the intact crypts. This pattern can also occur with metastatic lobular breast carcinoma. Small intestinal biopsies sometimes provide the first diagnosis of metastatic melanoma and breast carcinoma.

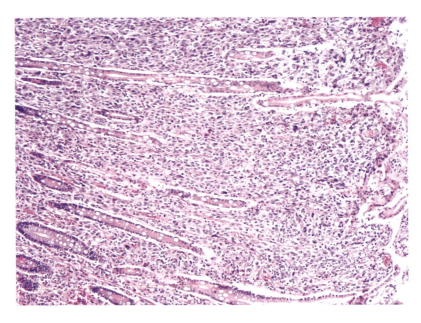

Immunohistochemical stains for SMAD4/DPC4 help identify a pancreatobiliary primary since 60 percent of these carcinomas show loss of nuclear staining for this marker (fig. 10-2) (5).

Intraductal papillary mucinous neoplasms of the pancreas can also extend along the common bile duct onto the surface of the duodenum (fig. 10-8). It is almost impossible to determine

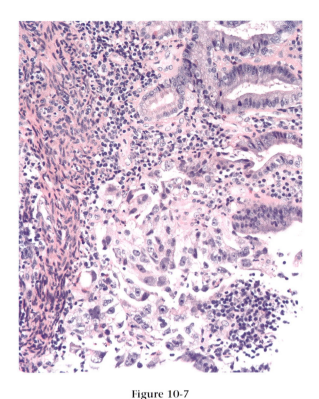

Figure 10-7

**OVARIAN SEROUS CARCINOMA
METASTATIC TO SMALL INTESTINE**

A "bottom up" appearance and marked cytologic alterations.

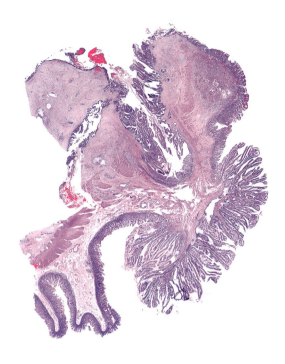

Figure 10-8

PANCREATIC INTRADUCTAL PAPILLARY MUCINOUS NEOPLASM EXTENDING ONTO DUODENAL SURFACE

The normal duodenal mucosa is at the right side of the image.

whether a mucinous neoplasm is a mucinous carcinoma or an intraductal papillary mucinous neoplasm when evaluation is limited to superficial mucosal sampling, although both are similarly treated so distinguishing them on biopsy samples is not critical for management. Imaging studies are useful for identifying the primary site of origin as well as the nature of the neoplasia. Other types of pancreatic neoplasia can directly invade the duodenum and be detected in mucosal biopsies (fig. 10-9).

Although any type of neoplasm, including sarcomas, can spread to the small bowel, most metastases are carcinomas. Thus, sarcomatoid carcinoma should be excluded when an overtly malignant spindle cell tumor is encountered (fig. 10-10). Most gastrointestinal stromal tumors are morphologically homogeneous and show low-grade cytologic abnormalities; striking nuclear pleomorphism is unusual and should suggest alternative diagnoses (figs. 10-11, 10-12). The occasional extension of mesothelioma into

submucosa or mucosa of the small intestine can mimic carcinoma (fig. 10-13).

Probably the most important entity to exclude when confronted with a small bowel malignancy is a metastatic germ cell tumor; virtually any type of germ cell tumor can metastasize to the small intestine. These lesions can be cured with appropriate treatment and confer a much better prognosis than primary intestinal carcinomas. Approximately 5 percent of testicular germ cell tumors metastasize to the gastrointestinal tract, usually to the proximal small intestine (6). Embryonal carcinomas show abortive glandular differentiation and, thus, may colonize the mucosa and simulate in situ neoplasia (fig. 10-14). This possibility should always be considered when evaluating a malignant neoplasm in a young male, particularly when the tumor shows unusual morphologic features, such as a sheet-like growth pattern or an absence of glandular differentiation (figs. 10-15, 10-16).

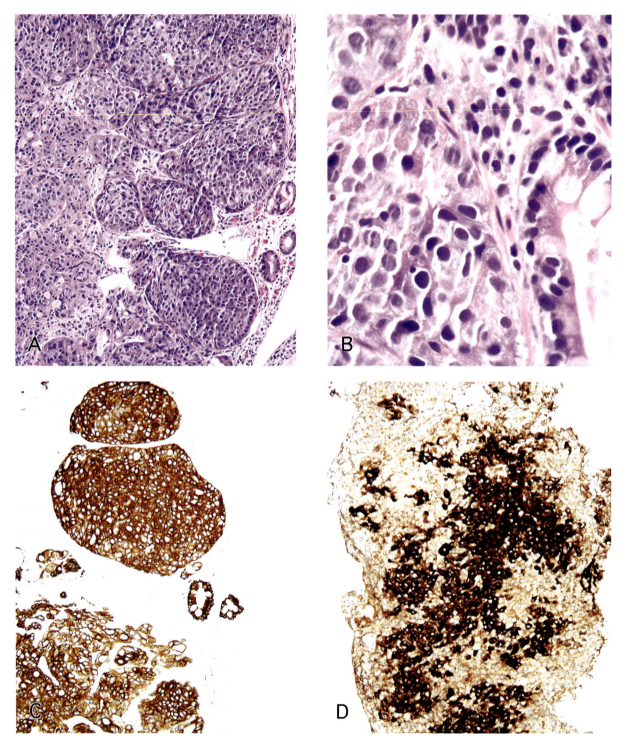

Figure 10-9

PANCREATIC ACINAR CELL CARCINOMA WITH SPREAD TO DUODENUM

A: A duodenal biopsy shows cells with finely granular cytoplasm. The lesion mimics a carcinoid tumor.
B: The duodenal biopsy shows macronucleoli, which would be unusual for a neuroendocrine (carcinoid) tumor.
C: This is a keratin CAM5.2 immunostain.
D: This is a BCL-10 immunostain.

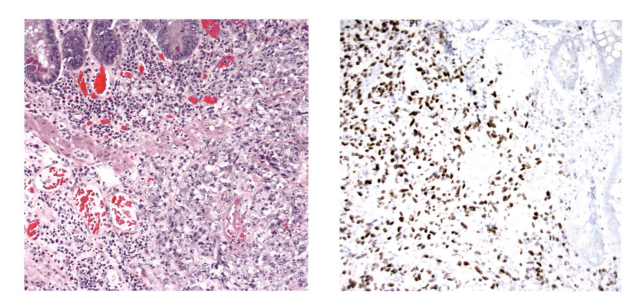

Figure 10-10

SARCOMATOID UROTHELIAL CARCINOMA METASTATIC TO SMALL BOWEL

Left: The malignant cells are epithelioid to spindled.

Right: This GATA3 immunostain labels the malignant nuclei. GATA3 is also expressed in lymphoid cells, which can be a diagnostic pitfall.

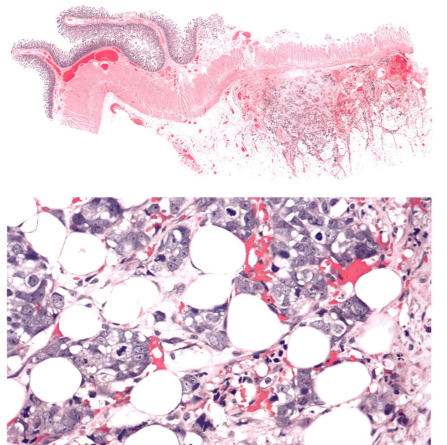

Figure 10-11

PROSTATIC ADENOCARCINOMA METASTATIC TO SMALL BOWEL SEROSA AND MUSCULARIS PROPRIA

Top: This lesion was believed to be a gastrointestinal stromal tumor (GIST) on clinical grounds. It is centered in the serosa, a clue that it is not likely a GIST.

Bottom: High-power magnification shows a high-grade neoplasm.

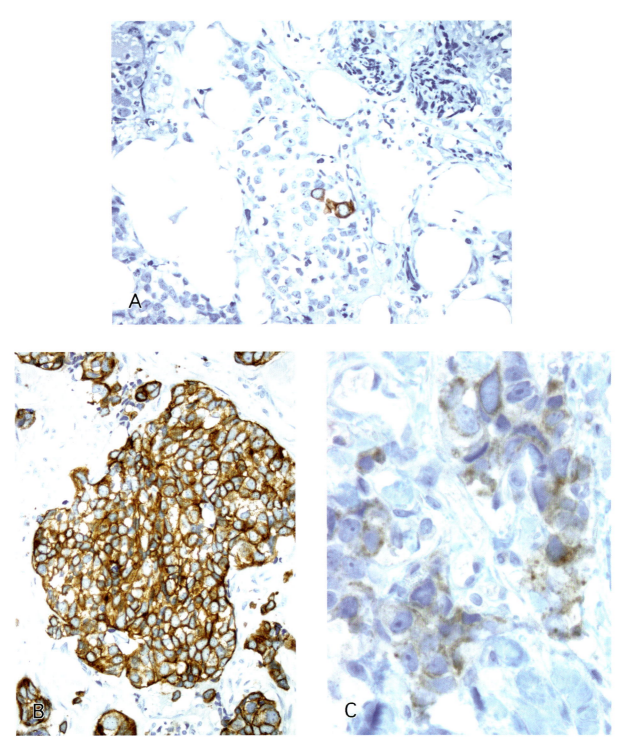

Figure 10-12

PROSTATIC ADENOCARCINOMA METASTATIC TO SMALL BOWEL SEROSA AND MUSCULARIS PROPRIA

A: With a keratin AE1/3 immunostain, only rare cells label. High-grade prostate adenocarcinomas are frequently negative using AE1/3, an occasional diagnostic pitfall.

B: CAM5.2 immunostain is usually reactive in even high-grade prostate adenocarcinomas.

C: A reactive prostate specific membrane antigen (PSMA) preparation.

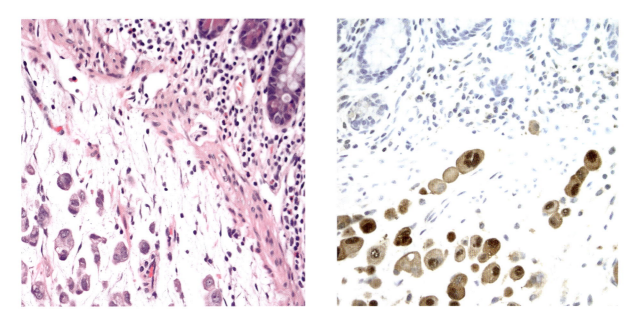

Figure 10-13

MESOTHELIOMA EXTENDING INTO SMALL INTESTINE

Left: Mesotheliomas occasionally present as either small bowel or colorectal nodules that are diagnosed on mucosal biopsies.
Right: A calretinin immunostain shows both cytoplasmic and nuclear labeling.

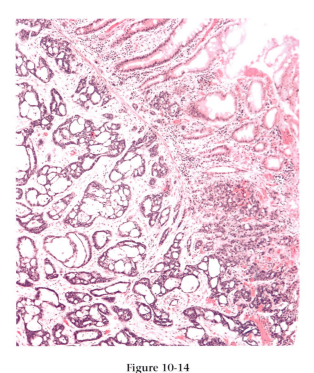

Figure 10-14

**EMBRYONAL CARCINOMA
METASTATIC TO SMALL BOWEL**

Such tumors are readily mistaken for adenocarcinomas out of context. This lesion was detected in a young man in his twenties.

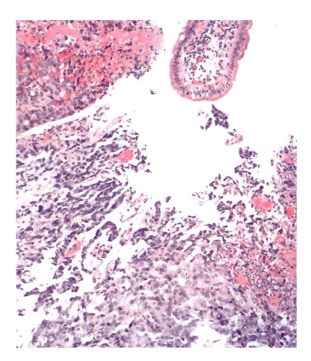

Figure 10-15

YOLK TUMOR METASTATIC TO SMALL BOWEL

The diagnostic clue was simply the age of the patient.

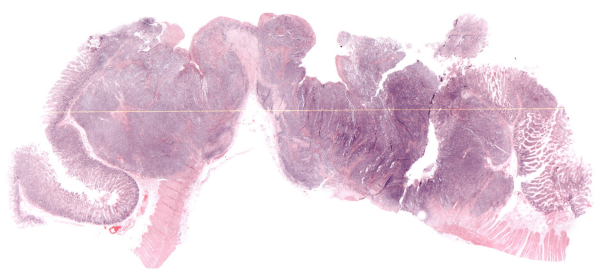

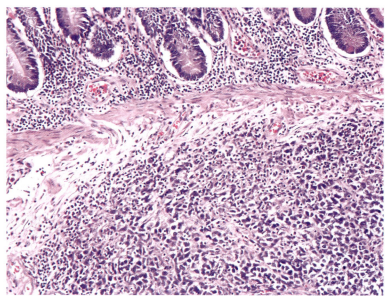

Figure 10-16

SEMINOMA METASTATIC TO SMALL BOWEL

Above: This impressive bulky metastasis was from a very small testicular primary that was only detected on imaging. There was no palpable scrotal mass.

Right: The backdrop of lymphocytes and young age of the patient were the diagnostic clues in this case.

Endometriosis is a common benign mimic of either primary or metastatic carcinoma, particularly in the ileum (7). Most endometriotic foci have a lobular appearance and show a combination of glandular elements and compact, cellular stroma. Inspissated secretions, ciliated epithelial cells, and an absence of prominent apoptotic debris and mitotic activity are characteristic features.

COLON

Extracolonic malignant neoplasms involve the colon via direct extension, peritoneal seeding, or hematogenous spread, thereby simulating the appearance of a primary carcinoma. In women, the main sources of metastases to the colon are neoplasms of the gynecologic tract, breast, and lung (figs. 10-17–10-19). Women may also develop mullerian malignancies within colonic endometriotic foci. More frequently, colonic endometriosis simulates the appearance of colorectal adenocarcinoma or even a sarcoma, if only stroma is present in the sample. Metastases from the extracolonic gastrointestinal tract and lung are most common in men. The colon is also often a site of metastasis from, or direct extension of, carcinomas of the bladder, kidney, pancreas, prostate gland, and cervix, as well as anal or cutaneous melanoma (figs. 10-20–10-24).

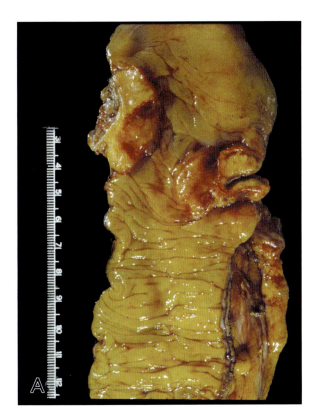

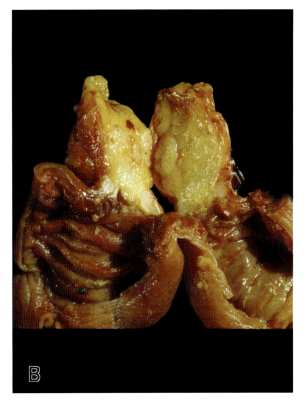

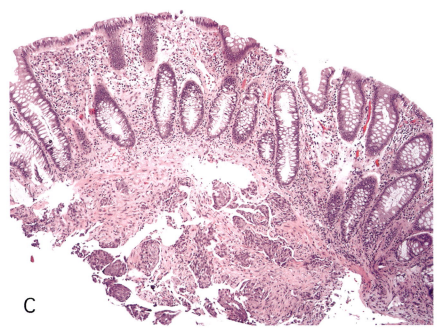

Figure 10-17

OVARIAN SEROUS CARCINOMA METASTATIC TO COLON

A: This bulky metastasis resulted in obstruction.
B: On careful examination of the cut surface, the mucosa is not involved.
C: The "bottom heavy" appearance and the lack of a precursor lesion led to the diagnosis by biopsy.

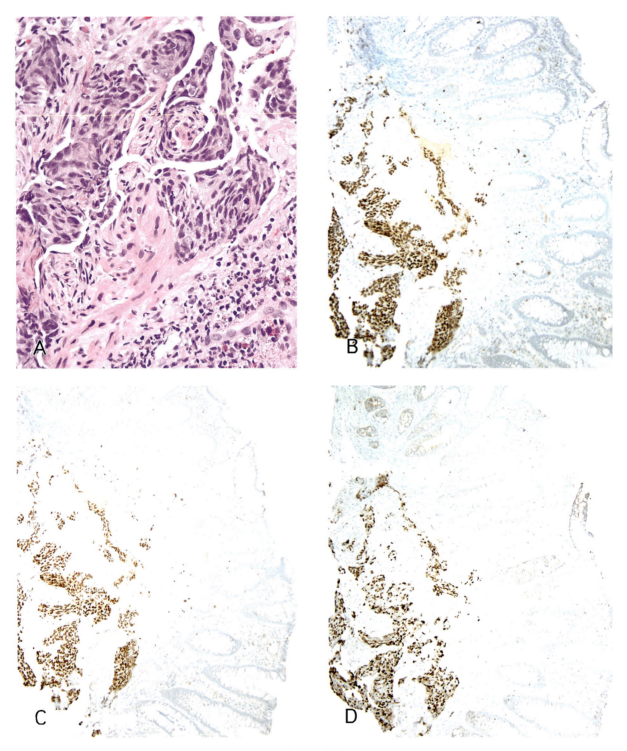

Figure 10-18

OVARIAN SEROUS CARCINOMA METASTATIC TO COLON

A: The appearance is nonspecific but the hyperchromatic nuclei are a clue.
B: A PAX8 immunostain.
C: An estrogen receptor immunostain.
D: A p53 immunostain.

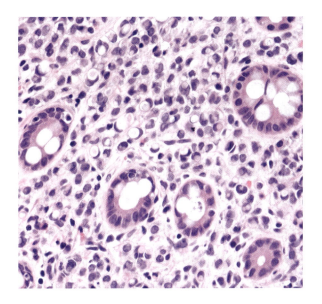

Figure 10-19

**LOBULAR BREAST CARCINOMA
METASTATIC TO COLON**

The malignant cells proliferate in the lamina propria between the crypts. In this case, they contain mucin vacuoles.

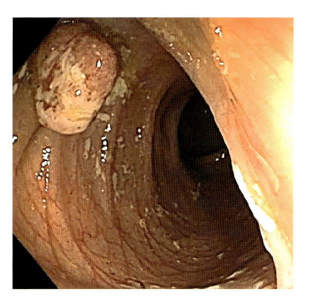

Figure 10-20

METASTATIC RENAL CELL CARCINOMA

This tumor masquerades as a colorectal polyp.

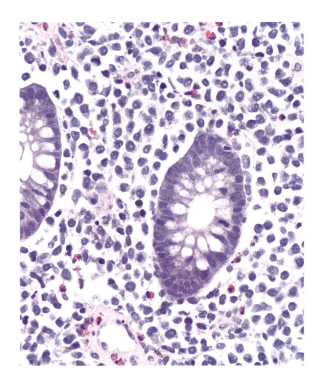

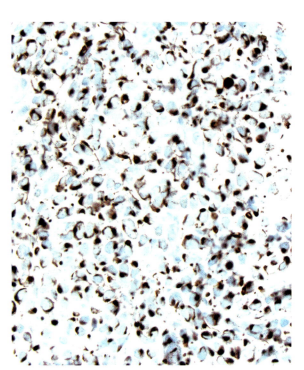

Figure 10-21

MERKEL CELL CARCINOMA OF SKIN METASTATIC TO COLON

Left: The cells are monotonous and infiltrate the lamina propria without damaging the crypts.
Right: CD20 labels in a dot-like pattern.

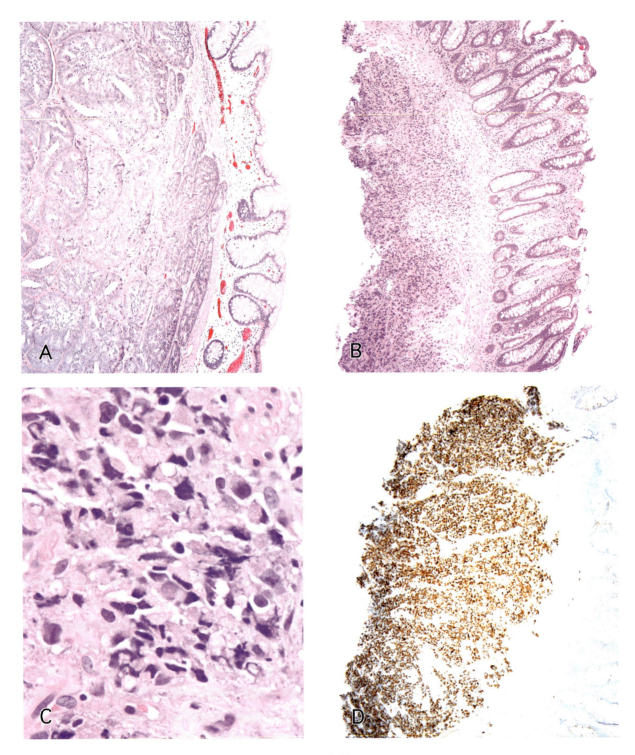

Figure 10-22

PROSTATE ADENOCARCINOMA DIRECTLY INVADING RECTUM

A: This lesion is easy to recognize as prostatic; the mucosa is wholly spared.

B: This high-grade example is more difficult to diagnose than the gland-forming carcinoma.

C: At high-power magnification of "B" the nucleoli are prominent. This, along with the location, are clues to the diagnosis.

D: A P501S immunostain of "B".

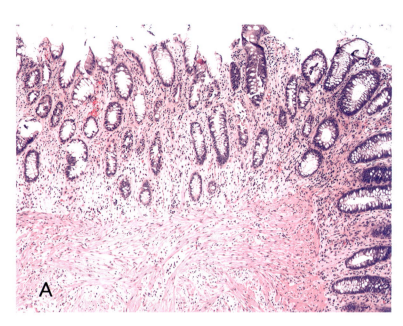

Figure 10-23

**UROTHELIAL CARCINOMA
DIRECTLY INVADING RECTUM**

A: The scarred appearance of the lamina propria and muscularis mucosae should prompt close scrutiny.

B: A malignant cell is in the center of the field.

C: A GATA3 immunostain.

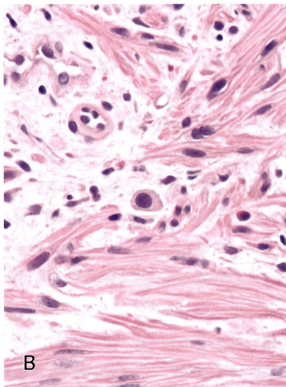

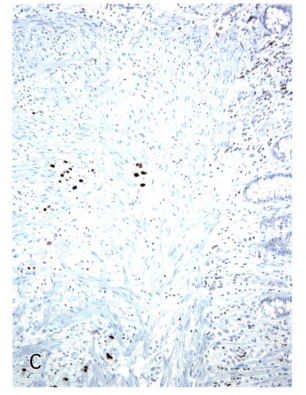

Most patients with secondary involvement of the colon by another malignancy undergo preoperative imaging and endoscopic mucosal sampling and, thus, the diagnosis is infrequently unexpected. However, colonic involvement by an extraintestinal malignancy may not be suspected, especially when patients present acutely with obstructive symptoms or colonic perforation. Some tumors, namely, breast carcinoma and melanoma, present with metastatic disease years or decades after the original diagnosis; others initially manifest as metastatic disease. Hematopoietic malignancies also simulate the gross and endoscopic appearance of colonic carcinomas.

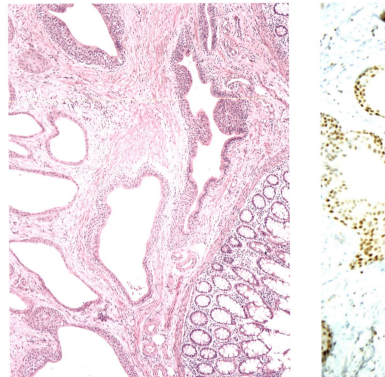 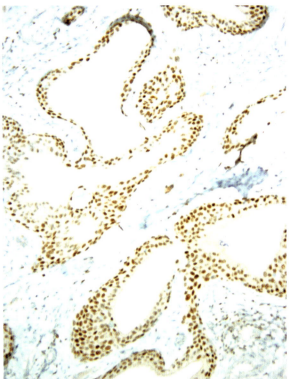

Figure 10-24

UROTHELIAL CARCINOMA DIRECTLY INVADING RECTUM

Left: This is a nested urothelial carcinoma.
Right: A GATA3 immunostain.

PRIMARY COLORECTAL CANCER VERSUS SECONDARY MALIGNANCIES OF THE COLON

Gross Features of Colorectal Carcinoma versus Secondary Neoplasms

Most colorectal adenocarcinomas are solitary, exophytic, polypoid tumors or endophytic, mucosa-based ulcerative lesions (see chapter 4). Some colorectal carcinomas are multiple, particularly in patients with underlying polyposis disorders or inflammatory bowel disease, but the presence of several lesions should always suggest metastatic disease.

Tumors that directly invade the colon or spread hematogenously generally involve the outer layers of the bowel wall and generally spare the mucosa. A secondary neoplasm should be suspected whenever the epicenter of the tumor lies in the outer aspect of the muscularis propria or in the mesenteric fat (figs. 10-17C, 10-22B, 10-23A, 10-25). Metastases that extend to the mucosa can ulcerate and simulate a primary carcinoma, but they are often ill-defined and undermine the mucosa with prominent lymphovascular invasion. Malignant melanoma typically expands the mucosa and submucosa, producing a polypoid mass. Both mammary carcinoma and melanoma may metastasize in the form of multiple nodules. Carcinomas of the gynecologic and extracolonic gastrointestinal tract are often associated with peritoneal disease.

Microscopic Features of Colorectal Carcinoma versus Secondary Neoplasms

Invasive carcinomas of the colorectum are usually associated with precursor lesions (dysplasia or adenoma) overlying the tumor, and consist of infiltrating single or cribriform glands with luminal necrosis. They lack architectural heterogeneity and show inconspicuous lymphovascular invasion.

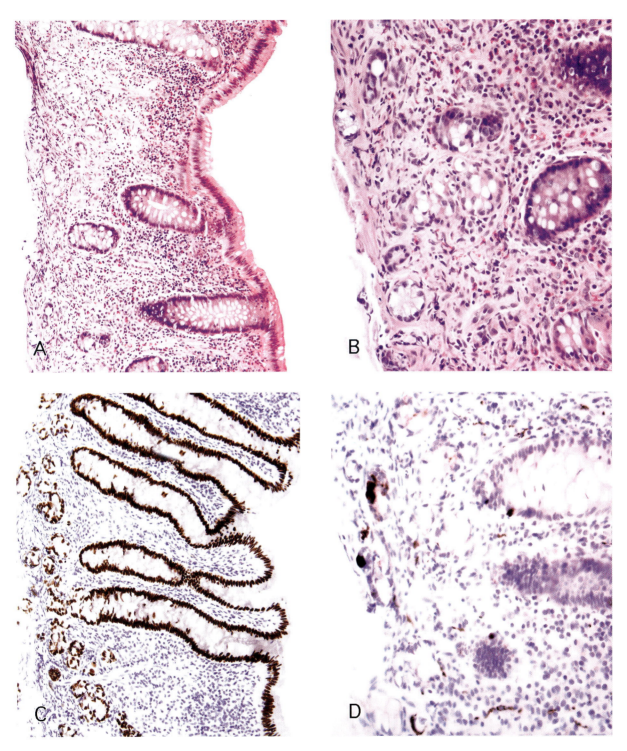

Figure 10-25

APPENDICEAL GOBLET CELL CARCINOID PRESENTING AS A FLAT LESION NEAR THE APPENDICEAL ORIFICE

A: The tumor is subtle, seen in the deep lamina propria in this mucosal biopsy.
B: High-power magnification.
C: A CDX2 immunostain.
D: A chromogranin immunostain.

Secondary malignancies of the colon commonly involve the serosal surface and outer muscularis propria more than the inner layers, and may show striking lymphovascular invasion. In fact, pronounced lymphovascular invasion should always suggest a metastasis. Gland-forming tumors that colonize the basement membrane appear to mature, simulating the appearance of an adenoma. However, they generally show more diffuse high-grade nuclear features than are typically observed in colorectal adenomas. Mixed architectural growth patterns, including papillae, acini, and solid nests are not typical of colorectal carcinoma, so a combination of these features should raise concern for an extraintestinal neoplasm. Diffuse-type gastric cancers and lobular breast cancers lack gland formation, but show low-grade nuclear features. In contrast, metastatic melanomas display prominent nucleoli, often with abundant eosinophilic cytoplasm and striking lymphovascular invasion.

Some features are unusual for colorectal carcinoma and their presence, especially in frozen section slides, should alert the pathologist to the possibility of a metastasis. Glands with slit-like spaces lined by cells with high-grade nuclei and prominent nucleoli should raise suspicion for serous carcinoma, especially if these glands are accompanied by psammomatous calcifications. Small glands with bland cytology and prominent nucleoli suggest a prostatic origin. Solid tumors composed of nests of tumor cells with a prominent vascular pattern suggest metastatic renal cell carcinoma or hepatocellular carcinoma. Metastatic endometrioid carcinomas may be histologically indistinguishable from colonic carcinomas, but those examples arising from endometriosis generally display low-grade cytologic atypia and a background of endometriosis and atypical endometrial hyperplasia (8). Primary colonic squamous cell and adenosquamous carcinomas are rare, so that squamous differentiation in an adenocarcinoma should suggest an endometrioid carcinoma in female patients.

There are some pitfalls associated with the interpretation of immunohistochemical stains. Well-differentiated neuroendocrine (carcinoid) tumors express prostatic acid phosphatase (PSAP) (fig. 10-26) (9); such expression can also be encountered in high-grade neuroendocrine carcinomas (fig. 10-27). High-grade prostatic carcinomas can show a lack cytokeratin expression when investigation is limited to cytokeratin AE1/3 and CK7, whereas CAM5.2 is almost always reactive.

NON-NEOPLASTIC PROCESSES THAT MIMIC COLORECTAL MALIGNANCY

Several non-neoplastic processes induce a variety of mucosal and mural changes that clinically simulate cancers. Preoperative imaging studies may demonstrate findings suggesting a malignancy, yet mucosal biopsy samples obtained at colonoscopy often fail to yield a diagnosis. Such processes include diverticular disease-associated colitis, proctitis associated with sexually transmitted infections (illustrated in chapter 6) (10), tuberculosis, and cytomegalovirus, among others: biopsies show clearly non-neoplastic features in these instances. Endometriosis and related processes merit special mention.

Endometriosis

Intestinal endometriosis induces hypertrophy of the muscularis propria in combination with serosal adhesions, thereby readily simulating a primary neoplasm. Endometriotic foci are most commonly observed in the outer muscularis propria and pericolic soft tissue of the rectosigmoid colon. Endometriosis occasionally involves the submucosa and mucosa, where it may induce a striking inflammatory response with inflammatory pseudopolyps, ulcers, induration, and regenerative cytologic atypia in the surface epithelium that can simulate a neoplasm (7,8).

Endometriosis consists of well-circumscribed aggregates of endometrial glands intimately associated with variable amounts of endometriotic stroma (figs. 10-28, 10-29), sometimes with accompanying hemorrhage and hemosiderin deposition. Endometriotic deposits form well-circumscribed lobules, predominantly in the pericolic tissues and muscularis propria, where they induce inflammation and fibrosis. The endometriotic glands are lined by bland columnar epithelium, and are often cystically dilated. They may show mild cytologic abnormalities, with nuclear enlargement and pseudostratification, but features typical of colonic epithelial neoplasia are lacking: mitotic figures, apoptotic debris, and luminal necrosis (fig. 10-30) (7). Examples that consist mostly of endometriotic stroma

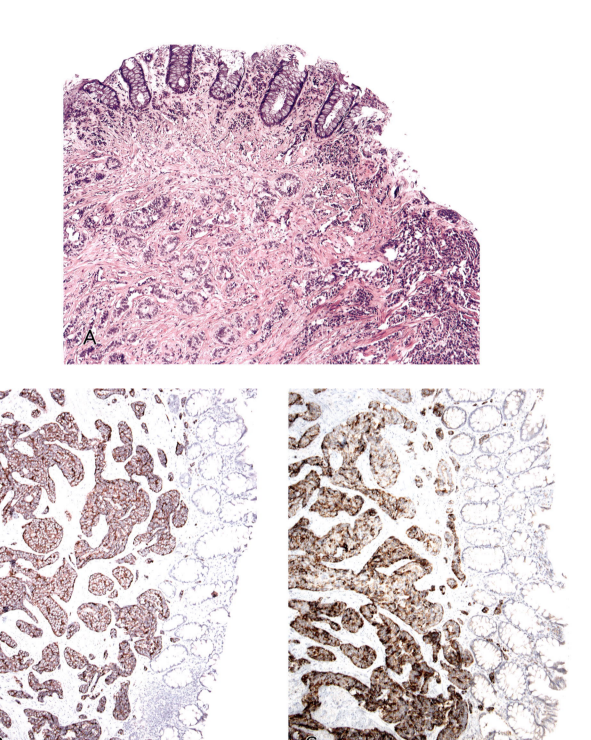

Figure 10-26

RECTAL WELL-DIFFERENTIATED NEUROENDOCRINE (CARCINOID) TUMOR

A: The tumor is centered in the lamina propria and submucosa.

B: A synaptophysin stain.

C: Prostate-specific acid phosphatase (PSAP) stain is positive. This pitfall has been known for years.

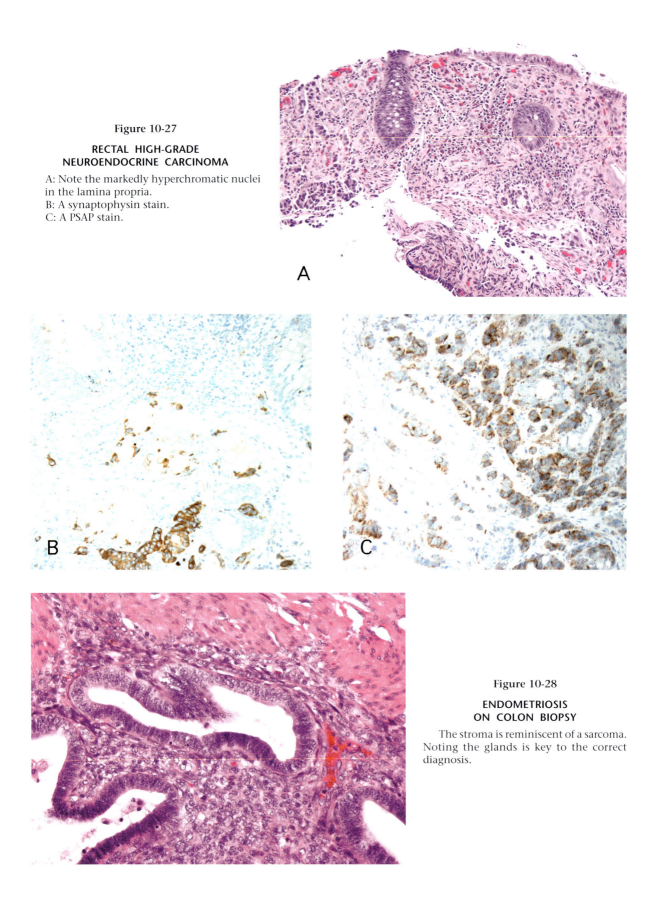

Figure 10-27

RECTAL HIGH-GRADE NEUROENDOCRINE CARCINOMA

A: Note the markedly hyperchromatic nuclei in the lamina propria.
B: A synaptophysin stain.
C: A PSAP stain.

Figure 10-28

ENDOMETRIOSIS ON COLON BIOPSY

The stroma is reminiscent of a sarcoma. Noting the glands is key to the correct diagnosis.

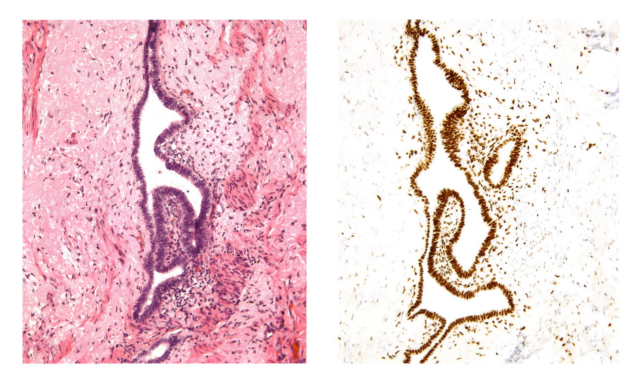

Figure 10-29

ENDOMETRIOSIS ON COLON BIOPSY

Left: This example is sclerotic, which mimics desmoplasia.
Right: An estrogen receptor immunostain shows strong nuclear labeling in both glands and stroma.

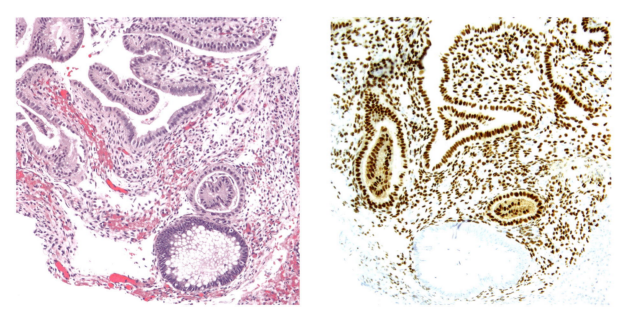

Figure 10-30

ENDOMETRIOSIS ON COLON BIOPSY

Left: The process has colonized the surface, a feature that can mimic dysplasia. A rim of stroma is beneath the surface endometrial-type epithelium.
Right: An estrogen receptor immunostain shows strong nuclear labeling in both surface and stromal cells.

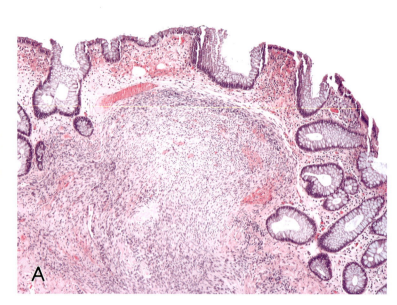

Figure 10-31

ENDOMETRIAL STROMAL SARCOMA, LOW GRADE, DIAGNOSED ON COLON BIOPSY

A: This example presented as a colon polyp. Even at low magnification, the tumor cells appear monotonous.

B: This pattern of collagen, termed "starburst collagen" by some, is a characteristic feature and a diagnostic pearl.

C: This is an estrogen receptor immunostain.

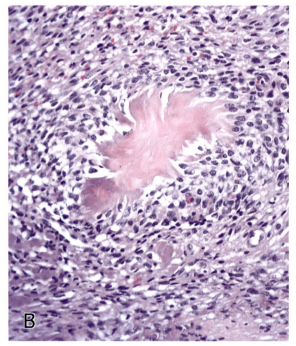

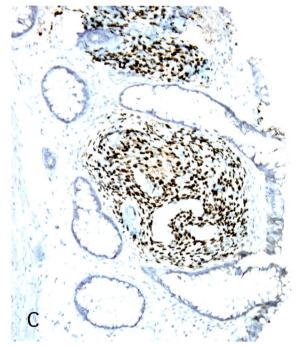

closely simulate sarcoma, although deeper tissue sections to detect glands or appropriate immuno-labeling stains point to the correct diagnosis.

Endometrial stromal sarcomas occasionally masquerade as gastrointestinal stromal tumors (fig. 10-31). Like other translocation sarcomas, they have monomorphic nuclei with characteristic "starburst collagen" (fig. 10-31B), a clue that separates them from synovial sarcoma and gastrointestinal stromal tumor (11).

Some patients with colonic endometriosis develop neoplasms similar to those in the gynecologic tract. Endometrioid-type adenocarcinomas and atypical hyperplasia are the usual types, although clear cell carcinomas (fig. 10-32), low-grade endometrial stromal sarcomas, and adenosarcomas, although less common, occur as well. In some cases, the ovary may be adherent to the external surface of the colon and can mimic a mesenchymal neoplasm (figs. 10-33, 10-34).

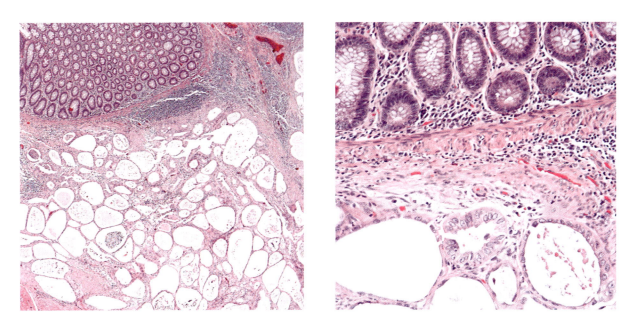

Figure 10-32

ENDOMETRIAL CLEAR CELL CARCINOMA ARISING IN ENDOMETRIOSIS IN COLON

Left: Low-power magnification shows a submucosal lesion.
Right: There are marked nuclear alterations.

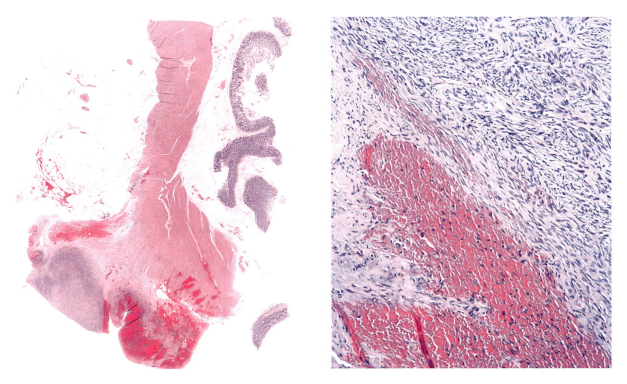

Figure 10-33

OVARIAN TISSUE ADHERENT TO COLON MIMICKING A GASTROINTESTINAL STROMAL TUMOR

Left: The serosal-based location is a clue that GIST is not the most likely interpretation.
Right: High-power magnification.

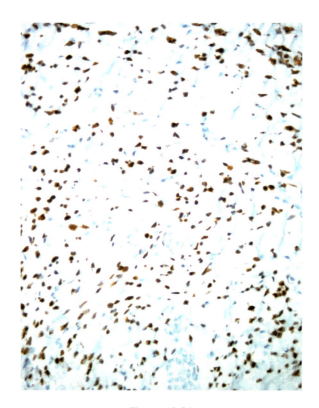

Figure 10-34

OVARIAN TISSUE ADHERENT TO COLON MIMICKING A GASTROINTESTINAL STROMAL TUMOR

An estrogen receptor immunostain.

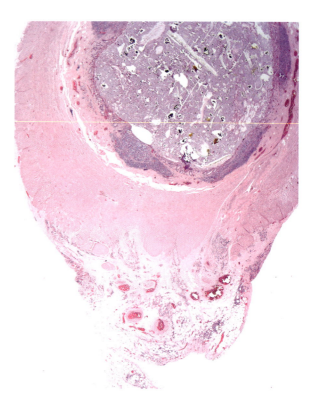

Figure 10-35

PROSTATE CARCINOMA METASTATIC TO APPENDIX

The tumor involves the subserosa and outer muscularis propria.

APPENDIX

Almost any type of neoplasm can spread to the appendix (figs. 10-35–10-37), and an immunolabeling panel can facilitate identification of the most likely primary source. Some tubular carcinoids express CK7, although the bland cytomorphology usually allows ready separation from metastatic disease (12).

The most common issue in interpreting appendiceal lesions is distinction between appendiceal mucinous neoplasia and its mimics. The process mostly likely to result in confusion with a mucinous neoplasm of the appendix is appendiceal diverticular disease, which is common (fig. 10-38) (13). When appendiceal diverticula rupture, they spill mucinous contents into the connective tissue, and exhibit mucosal hyperplasia that can simulate the low-grade appearance of mucinous neoplasia. The extruded mucin elicits an exuberant fibroinflammatory response that includes the presence of keratin-positive submesothelial spindle cells. The mucin may even mineralize over time. Features that aid in the recognition of appendiceal diverticula include the lack of mucinous neoplasia in the surface epithelium, the presence of retained lamina propria supporting the epithelium of a diverticulum, and detection of normal crypts with Paneth cells within the diverticulum.

Endometriosis commonly occurs in the appendix, although it rarely colonizes the mucosal surface. Most cases are easily identified and they only rarely cause confusion with adenocarcinomas. However, some cases of endometriosis undergo intestinal metaplasia (14) that simulates a low-grade appendiceal mucinous neoplasm. When this occurs, the intestinal-type epithelium attains an intestinal immunophenotype, with co-expression of CDX2 and CK20. Fortunately, endometriotic glands with mucinous metaplasia are accompanied by a cuff of cellular stroma and are usually seen in association with more conventional endometrioid glands (figs. 10-39, 10-40).

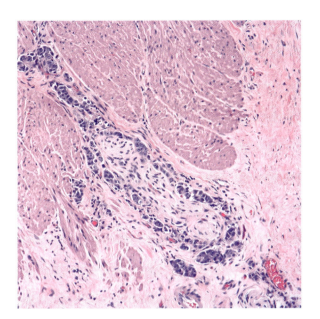 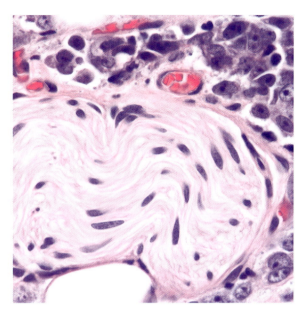

Figure 10-36

PROSTATE CARCINOMA METASTATIC TO APPENDIX

Left: The tumor cuffs the perineurium.
Right: Macronucleoli are present.

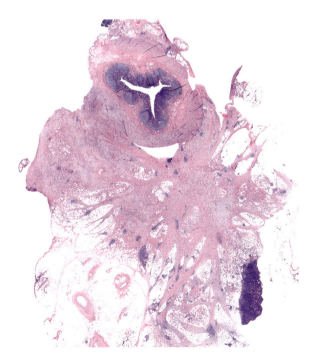 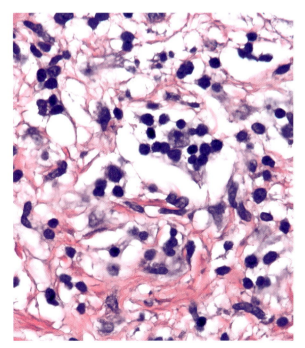

Figure 10-37

ROSAI-DORFMAN DISEASE IN PERIAPPENDICEAL TISSUE

Left: The overall appearance of the lesion is pale (since it is composed of histiocytic cells), punctuated by dark lymphoid aggregates.

Right: There is striking emperipolesis by the histiocytic cell at the center left. The engulfed lymphocytes are not damaged as they nestle in the cytoplasm.

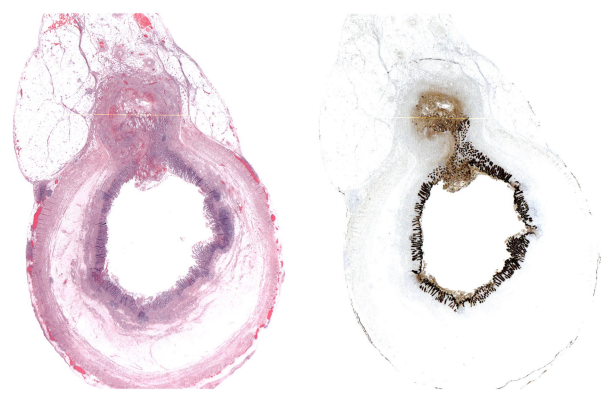

Figure 10-38

RUPTURED APPENDICEAL DIVERTICULUM

Left: Damaged residual mucosa can be seen in the diverticulum at the left.
Right: This pankeratin stain highlights the process to advantage.

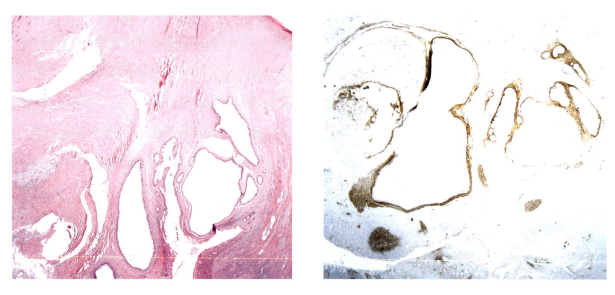

Figure 10-39

APPENDICEAL ENDOMETRIOSIS WITH INTESTINAL METAPLASIA MIMICKING MUCINOUS NEOPLASM

Left: Typical endometriosis with stroma is seen at left whereas the glands at the right appear intestinalized.
Right: A CD10 highlights the endometrial stroma that surrounds the intestinalized glands.

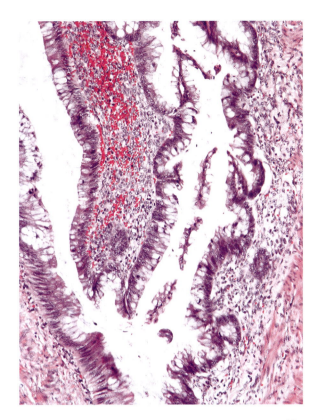 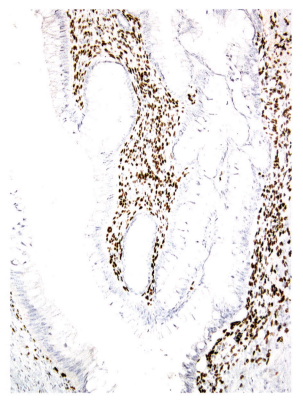

Figure 10-40

APPENDICEAL ENDOMETRIOSIS WITH INTESTINAL METAPLASIA MIMICKING MUCINOUS NEOPLASM

Left: The stroma around intestinalized glands is readily apparent at high magnification. Goblet cells are seen.
Right: Estrogen receptor immunolabeling highlights the stromal but not the intestinalized glands.

REFERENCES

1. Disibio G, French SW. Metastatic patterns of cancers: results from a large autopsy study. Arch Pathol Lab Med 2008;132:931-939.

2. Bosman FT, World Health Organization., International Agency for Research on Cancer. WHO classification of tumours of the digestive system. 4th ed. Lyon: International Agency for Research on Cancer; 2010.

3. Estrella JS, Wu TT, Rashid A, Abraham SC. Mucosal colonization by metastatic carcinoma in the gastrointestinal tract: a potential mimic of primary neoplasia. Am J Surg Pathol 2011;35:563-572.

4. Chen ZM, Wang HL. Alteration of cytokeratin 7 and cytokeratin 20 expression profile is uniquely associated with tumorigenesis of primary adenocarcinoma of the small intestine. Am J Surg Pathol 2004;28:1352-1359.

5. Wilentz RE, Su GH, Dai JL, et al. Immunohistochemical labeling for dpc4 mirrors genetic status in pancreatic adenocarcinomas: a new marker of DPC4 inactivation. Am J Pathol 2000;156:37-43.

6. Chait MM, Kurtz RC, Hajdu SI. Gastrointestinal tract metastasis in patients with germ-cell tumor of the testis. Am J Dig Dis 1978;23(10):925-928.

7. Yantiss RK, Clement PB, Young RH. Endometriosis of the intestinal tract: a study of 44 cases of a disease that may cause diverse challenges in clinical and pathologic evaluation. Am J Surg Pathol 2001;25:445-454.

8. Yantiss RK, Clement PB, Young RH. Neoplastic and pre-neoplastic changes in gastrointestinal endometriosis: a study of 17 cases. Am J Surg Pathol 2000;24:513-524.

9. Kimura N, Sasano N. Prostate-specific acid phosphatase in carcinoid tumors. Virchows Arch A Pathol Anat Histopathol 1986;410:247-251.

10. Arnold CA, Limketkai BN, Illei PB, Montgomery E, Voltaggio L. Syphilitic and lymphogranuloma venereum (LGV) proctocolitis: clues to a frequently missed diagnosis. Am J Surg Pathol 2013;37:38-46.

11. Oliva E, Clement PB, Young RH. Endometrial stromal tumors: an update on a group of tumors with a protean phenotype. Adv Anat Pathol 2000;7:257-281.

12. Matsukuma KE, Montgomery EA. Tubular carcinoids of the appendix: the CK7/CK20 immunophenotype can be a diagnostic pitfall. J Clin Pathol 2012;65:666-668.

13. Hsu M, Young RH, Misdraji J. Ruptured appendiceal diverticula mimicking low-grade appendiceal mucinous neoplasms. Am J Surg Pathol 2009;33:1515-1521.

14. Misdraji J, Lauwers GY, Irving JA, Batts KP, Young RH. Appendiceal or cecal endometriosis with intestinal metaplasia: a potential mimic of appendiceal mucinous neoplasms. Am J Surg Pathol 2014;38:698-705.

Index*

*In a series of numbers, those in boldface indicate the main discussion of the entity.

I

K

L

M

N